VASCULAR DISEASE IN THE ELDERLY

Edited by

WILBERT S. ARONOW, MD

Adjunct Professor of Geriatrics and Adult Development
Mount Sinai School of Medicine
New York, New York
Medical Director, Hebrew Hospital Home
Bronx, New York

EDWARD A. STEMMER, MD

Professor of Surgery, University of California at Irvine
Irvine, California
Chief of Surgical Service, Veterans Affairs Medical Center
Long Beach, California

SAMUEL ERIC WILSON, MD

Professor of Surgery
Chairman of Department of Surgery
University of California at Irvine
Irvine, California

Futura Publishing
Company, Inc.
Armonk, NY

Vascular disease in the elderly / edited by Wilbert S. Aronow, Edward
A. Stemmer, Samuel Eric Wilson.
    p.   cm.
Includes bibliographical references and index.
ISBN 0–87993–646–0 (alk. paper)
1. Cardiovascular diseases in old age. I. Aronow, Wilbert S. II. Stem-
mer, Edward A. III. Wilson, Samuel E., 1941– .
[DNLM: 1. Vascular Diseases—in old age. 2. Vascular Diseases—ther-
apy. 3. Vascular Diseases—diagnosis. WG 500 V33127 1997]
RC669.7.V37   1997
618.97′613—dc21
DNLM/DLC
for Library of Congress   96–50375
                                                             CIP

Copyright © 1997
Futura Publishing Company, Inc.

Published by
Futura Publishing Company, Inc.
135 Bedford Road
Armonk, New York 10504

LC#: 96-50375
ISBN#: 0-87993-646-0

Every effort has been made to ensure that the information in this book
is up to date and accurate at the time of publication. However, due to
the constant developments in medicine, neither the authors, nor the
editor, nor the publisher can accept any legal or any other responsibility
for any errors or omissions that may occur.

Printed in the United States of America.

Printed on acid-free paper.

Contributors

Paul Anain, MD [5]
Chief Surgical Resident,
Cleveland Clinic Foundation
Hospital Pepper Pike, Ohio

Wilbert S. Aronow, MD
[6,13,15,16,17,26]
Adjunct Professor, Geriatrics and
Adult Development, Mount Sinai
School of Medicine; Medical
Director, Hebrew Hospital Home
Bronx, New York

Allen W. Averbook, MD [5]
Assistant Professor, Department of
Surgery, Case Western Reserve
University; Chief, Vascular
Surgery Section, Veterans Affairs
Medical Center, Cleveland, Ohio

Jeffrey L. Ballard, MD [7]
Associate Professor, Division of
Vascular Surgery, Loma Linda
University; Consultant, Veterans
Affairs Medical Center, Loma
Linda, California

Steven J. Barker, PhD, MD [9]
Professor and Head, Department
of Anesthesiology, The University
of Arizona College of Medicine
Tucson, Arizona

Percy Bracamonte, MD [3]
Fellow, Geriatric Medicine
University of South Florida
College of Medicine; James A.
Haley Veterans Hospital, Tampa
Florida

T. J. Bunt, MD [/]
Professor of Surgery, Division of
Vascular Surgery, Loma Linda
University; Staff, Veterans Affairs
Medical Center, Loma Linda
California

Jennifer Daley, MD [24]
Staff, Beth-Israel Hospital
Director, Health Services Research
and Development, Brockton/West
Roxbury VA Medical Center, West
Roxbury, Massachusetts; Assistant
Professor, Harvard Medical
School, Boston, Massachusetts

Robert Forman, MD [17]
Montefiore Medical Center
Professor of Medicine, Albert
Einstein College of Medicine
Bronx, New York

Ian L. Gordon, MD, PhD [21]
Assistant Professor of Surgery
University of California at Irvine
Irvine, California; Chief, Vascular
Surgery, Veterans Affairs Medical
Center, Long Beach, California

James M. Guernsey, MD [8]
Professor of Surgery, University of
California, San Francisco; Chief
Surgical Service, VA Medical
Center, Fresno, California

Waleed Hassanein, MD [24]
Research Fellow, Cardiac Surgery
Harvard Medical School
Brockton/West Roxbury VA
Medical Center, West Roxbury
Massachusetts

William Henderson, PhD [24]
Associate Professor, Department
of Pharmacology, Stritch School
of Medicine, Loyola University
Maywood, Illinois; Veterans
Affairs Medical Center, Hines
Illinois; Adjunct Associate
Professor, Biometry Program
School of Public Health
University of Chicago, Chicago
Illinois

Numbers in brackets indicate chapters written or cowritten by the contributor.

Larry H. Hollier, MD [22]
Franz W. Sichel Professor of
Surgery, Chairman, Department of
Surgery, Mount Sinai Medical
Center, New York, New York

Kwan Hur, MS [24]
Biostatistician, Veterans Affairs
Medical Center, Hines, Illinois

Fernando E. Kafie, MD [25]
Surgical Fellow, University of
California at Irvine, Irvine
California

William B. Kannel, MD, MPH, FACC
[11]
Professor of Medicine and Public
Health, Section of Preventive
Medicine and Epidemiology,
Evans Memorial Department of
Research and Department of
Medicine University Hospital
Boston University, School of
Medicine Boston, Massachusetts

Shukri F. Khuri, MD [24]
Professor of Surgery, Harvard
Medical School; Vice Chairman
Department of Surgery, Brigham
and Women's Hospital, Boston
Massachusetts; Chief, Surgical
Service, Brockton/West Roxbury
VA Medical Center, West
Roxbury, Massachusetts

Adrienne Knight, MD [9]
Clinical Instructor, Department of
Anesthesiology, University of
California at Irvine, Irvine
California; Director, Recovery
Room Services, Veterans
Administration Medical Center
Long Beach, California

John Menezes, MD [23]
Resident in Surgery, University of
California at Irvine, Irvine
California

Debra E. Morrison, MD [9]
Assistant Clinical Professor
Department of Anesthesiology
University of California at Irvine
Director, Preoperative Services
Veterans Administration Medical
Center, Long Beach, California

Harold G. Olson, MD [16]
Associate Professor, Department
of Medicine, University of
California at Irvine, Irvine
California; Chief, Coronary Care
Unit, Veterans Affairs Medical
Center, Long Beach, California

Jean M. Panneton, MD [22]
St. Boniface General Hospital and
Health Sciences Centre; Assistant
Professor, Division of Vascular
Surgery, University of Manitoba
Winnipeg, Manitoba, Canada

Bruce E. Robinson, MD, MPH [3]
Professor and Chairman, Geriatric
Medicine, University of South
Florida, College of Medicine
James A. Haley VA Medical
Center, Tampa, Florida

Luis A. Sanchez, MD [20]
Montefiore Medical Center
Assistance Professor, Division of
Vascular Surgery, Albert Einstein
College of Medicine, Bronx, New
York

Stewart M. Scott, MD ‡ [19]
Clinical Professor, Department of
Surgery, Duke University
Durham, North Carolina; Chief
Surgical Service, Veterans Affairs
Medical Center, Asheville, North
Carolina

Edward A. Stemmer, MD
[1,2,12,19,26]
Professor of Surgery, University of
California at Irvine, Irvine
California; Chief, Surgical Service
Veterans Affairs Medical Center
Long Beach, California

‡ deceased

William D. Suggs, MD [20]
Montefiore Medical Center
Assistant Professor, Division of
Vascular Surgery, Albert Einstein
College of Medicine, Bronx, New
York

Randall C. Thompson, MD [18]
Consultant in Cardiology, Mid-
America Heart Institute, Kansas
City, Missouri

Donald D. Tresch, MD [15,26]
Professor of Medicine
Departments of Cardiology and
Geriatrics, Medical College of
Wisconsin, Milwaukee, Wisconsin

Frank J. Veith, MD [20]
Montefiore Medical Center
Professor and Chief, Division of
Vascular Surgery, Albert Einstein
College of Medicine, Bronx, New
York

John P. Walsh, PhD [4]
Andrus Gerontology Center
Associate Professor USC Program
in Neuroscience, University of
Southern California, Los Angeles
California

Russell A. Williams, MD [25]
Professor and Vice-Chairperson
Department of Surgery, University
of California at Irvine, Irvine
California

Samuel Eric Wilson, MD
[14,23,26]
Professor and Chairperson
Department of Surgery, University
of California at Irvine, Irvine
California

David H. Wong, PharmD, MD
[10]
Associate Clinical Professor
Department of Anesthesiology
University of California at Irvine
Irvine, California; Chief
Anesthesiology, Veterans Affairs
Medical Center, Long Beach
California

Patrick Yoon, MD [14]
Research Associate
Department of Surgery, University
of California at Irvine, Irvine
California

Foreword

The American population is an aging population. Every decade since the turn of the century has experienced a growth in the numbers of Americans who have passed the age of 65 years. Thus, 12.5% of the United States' population has reached this age at this time. Similarly, this century has seen a progressive increase in the percentage of the population that has exceeded 85 years of life. The unprecedented expansion of the older age groups has brought with it an enhanced awareness of the problems of senior citizens.

This awareness has brought a heightened appreciation of the social issues, personal care, and health care problems of senior citizens. We, as physicians, have had to become increasingly familiar with osteoporosis, dementia, delirium, and degenerative arthritis. In addition, physicians have had to better understand other unique problems related to aging, such as incontinence, hearing and visual impairment, behavioral problems, pressure sores, falls, and other issues more common to the older patient population.

Among the most important questions surrounding the many dilemmas related to aging are those concerning vascular disease. All of us are aware that diseases of the heart and vessels are often seen in older patients. We commonly associate cardiac disease and stroke with aging, but there are many other major vascular problems facing the elderly. Hypertension of a chronic nature may be seen in nearly half of individuals over the age of 65, and peripheral vascular problems may occur in 2% of males and 1% of females over this same age. Aneurysms of the aorta are another common vascular problem seen in older citizens. Superimposed upon the difficulties caused by atherosclerosis are those associated with venous insufficiency and those occurring as complications of vascular disease, such as ulcers of the extremities.

Many very important questions arise regarding these vascular problems. They often center on issues related to the genetics, pathogenesis, and prevention of these disorders. However, critical questions also exist regarding the therapy of these problems; these questions include the cost-effectiveness of these therapies, the effect of these treatments on the quality of life, and the implications of these therapies and interventions particularly on longevity. The answers to these questions are critical to a better approach to the aging patient, and will have a dramatic impact on the diagnosis and treatment of disease by physicians in the era of managed care and cost consciousness.

It is the purpose of this text to explore these issues and to arrive at reasonable conclusions regarding them based on the available evidence. This volume, therefore, addresses the important controversies facing the practitioner of primary care internal medicine, family practice, surgery, and geriatrics. It is with these thoughts in mind that the authors confront the problems of vascular disease in the elderly.

Thomas C. Cesario, MD
Professor of Medicine and Dean
UCI College of Medicine
University of California
Irvine, California

Preface

The stimulus for the development of this book arose from a request from an editor of a geriatric journal to submit an article dealing with vascular disease in the elderly.

In the process of writing that manuscript, it became apparent that the scope of the subject far exceeded our ability to cover it adequately in the limited space of a journal article. While we were developing the background information for the article, it also became apparent that use of the terms *elderly* or *geriatric* evoked, at least in the minds of the public, the picture of a group of individuals who are housed in nursing homes and have severe physical and mental impairments, as well as limited quality and duration of life. Even in medical schools, courses dealing with geriatric diseases are often centered about nursing homes and the care of their indigenous population. While some 5% to 10% of the older population might indeed be long-term nursing home residents, the majority of senior citizens in the United States live independently with surprisingly few serious disabilities. Appropriate medical and surgical management can not only extend the lives of these individuals, but can preserve and increase their quality.

Thus, what might have been a relatively uncomplicated problem 50 to 75 years ago has now become a major social, economic, and political issue as the elderly population, however it is defined, continues to grow both in absolute and in relative numbers. As physicians, we are faced with the need to learn how and when to provide sophisticated treatment for this group of individuals.

The authors who were asked to write the chapters in this text were selected because of their knowledge and experience in dealing with older individuals. They had access to large databases from which factual information could be drawn to provide an accurate picture of the medical status of our older population and their potential to benefit from both preventive and therapeutic measures, particularly as these relate to the prevention and treatment of vascular disease.

While some of the information in this volume is technical and detailed, the book is intended for a wider audience to include physicians, nurses, students, and other health care providers, as well as nonmedical individuals with an interest in vascular disease in the geriatric population.

Wilbert S. Aronow, MD
Edward A. Stemmer, MD
Samuel Eric Wilson, MD

Editors

Dedication

We dedicate this text to our wives, since without their support and patience we could not have pursued our careers; to our children and grandchildren who make it all worthwhile; to our secretaries without whom this text would not be; to the senior citizens who are the subjects and (hopefully) the beneficiaries of our efforts; and last, but not least, to the memory of our longtime friend and colleague, Stew Scott.

In addition, we wish to acknowledge the efforts of our coauthors who have given so freely of their knowledge and experience.

The Editors

Contents

Chapter 1

Introduction

Edward A. Stemmer, MD

Marcus Tullius Cicero, in the first century B.C., commented that, "As I give thought to the matter, I find four causes for the apparent misery of old age: first, it withdraws us from active accomplishments; second, it renders the body less powerful; third, it deprives us of almost all forms of enjoyment; and fourth, it stands not far from death." An excellent orator, a good philosopher, an able trial attorney, and a fair politician, Cicero was wise enough not to try to define old age. Even today, despite the growing numbers of men and women living well into their seventies and eighties, there is little doubt that society emphasizes youth and negatively values old age. In part, this is due to the reality that with increasing age comes loss of physical function, limitation of activity, assorted disabilities, increased prevalence of chronic diseases, and a greater likelihood of death. Also, it is due to the prevalence of several misconceptions about the elderly.

Physicians typically discuss sick or institutionalized individuals rather than the well, giving the public the impression that the majority of elderly are sick, physically impaired, or mentally compromised. Because the elderly, as a group, consume a greater share of the national health care expenditures, social planners question whether funds expended on the elderly are a proper "investment of scarce resources." They point out that the ratio of government expenditures on the elderly compared to children is 4 to 1.[1] The alarm is raised that, by some date in the future, all resources will go to support the elderly.[2] Nevertheless, in most discussions of medical care of the elderly, not only are the terms *old age* and *elderly* poorly defined, but the characteristics of the elderly population as a whole are left unstated. What are the chronic illnesses that affect the elderly? Are they treatable or preventable? How often are the common illnesses of themselves fatal? How often do the chronic conditions produce limitations of activities? How severe are those limitations? How real is the concern that medical resources will be diverted from the young, productive citizenry to the old, dependent

From: Aronow WS, Stemmer EA, Wilson SE (eds). *Vascular Disease in the Elderly.* Armonk, NY: Futura Publishing Company, Inc., © 1997.

population? How did it develop that society, through various levels of government, has become responsible for the care of the elderly?

The purpose of this text is, of course, to describe the management of vascular disease in the elderly. To place the information contained in this book in proper perspective, however, it is important to first provide a more detailed overview of the characteristics of the elderly population from whom we have drawn our subjects, and to provide a historical background for the government programs responsible for funding a large share of their medical treatment. In the process, an attempt is made in this and subsequent chapters to answer the questions posed above.

Overview

The number of individuals over the age of 65 has been growing in both absolute and relative measurements since 1900. The growth is expected to continue well into the twenty-first century. Since 1950, the number of individuals over the age of 65 in the United States has grown 260%; the number of those between 65 and 74 years has grown by 219%; the number of those between 75 and 84 years has grown by 318%; and the number of individuals over 85 years has grown from 577,000 in 1950 to 3,160,000 in 1991, an astounding 548%. Octagenarians are, in fact, the fastest growing segment of the population in the United States. In 1991, the total population of the United States was 252,177,000. Those over 65 years of age accounted for 12.6% of the population. In the over 65 years group, 57.5% were between the ages of 65 and 74; 32.5% were between the ages of 75 and 84; and 10% were over the age of 85.[3] Life expectancy over the age of 80 in the United States (9 years for women and 7.1 years for men) is greater than that in Sweden, France, England, or Japan.[4]

In 1991, 51.1% of the resident population in the United States were women. Men outnumber women until middle age, but thereafter women increasingly make up a larger percentage of the population. Women constitute 59.7% of all individuals over the age of 65; 56.1% of those aged 65 to 74; 62.3% of those 75 to 84; and 71.9% of those over 85 years. Thus, the individuals who are the subjects of this text are predominantly women.[3]

Survival, however, is not the only criterion by which an elderly population can be characterized. Functional or active life expectancy is another and equally important consideration. Of the population over 65 years of age, 80% have one or more chronic conditions, but only 1 in 5 is disabled by illness in even a minor way. It is only in the mid-eighties that the elderly run a high risk of marked disability from chronic disease.[5,6] It is important to make the distinction between the existence of chronic disease and the existence of disability from chronic disease.

Table 1 lists the top 15 chronic diseases that afflict the over 65 population. Only 5 of the 15 diseases are likely to be lethal. All five

Table 1
Prevalence of Chronic Diseases and Conditions
in the Population Age 65 or Older

	Prevalence (%)	
Disease/Condition	*Men*	*Women*
Arthritis	36	50
Hearing impairment	33	25
Hypertension	32	43
Heart condition	27	28
Chronic sinusitis	14	17
Arteriosclerosis	12	12
Visual impairment	12	12
Ortho (back, spine)	8	11
Diabetes mellitus	7	8
Hernia	7	XX
Emphysema	7	XX
Prostatic disease	6	XX
Hemorrhoids	5	8
Ortho (leg, hip)	5	6
Hay fever	4	XX
Varicose veins	XX	13
Frequent constipation	XX	8
Corns, calluses	XX	7
Urologic diseases	XX	7

XX Not in top 15 chronic conditions

(Reproduced with permission from Reference 7.)

are treatable by current medical and surgical techniques. Four of these five are subjects of this text. Table 2 lists the top 15 diseases that produce disability in people over 65. With some exceptions, the same diseases that are listed in Table 1 appear in Table 2 as well. However, the frequency with which they produce major limitations of activity is much less than the frequency with which they occur in the same population. Again, 5 of the 15 diseases are subjects of this book. Table 3 describes the degree of limitation that exists in noninstitutionalized individuals as they enter their sixties, seventies, and eighties. Two thirds of the individuals between the ages of 65 and 74 have no limitations of their activities, even with their chronic diseases. Over half of the noninstitutionalized individuals over the age of 75 have no limitation of their activities.[7,8]

Mental impairment of the elderly receives a great deal of attention, particularly when it afflicts public figures. While the concern is certainly appropriate, it needs to be put into the same perspective as the

Table 2
Percentage of Population Aged 65 or Older With Major Limitations
of Activities Because of Specific Chronic Conditions

Disease/Condition	Major Limitations (%)	
	Men	Women
Heart disease	12	10
Arthritis	8	13
Visual impairment	4	5
Emphysema	4	XX
Hypertension	3	5
Cerebrovasc disease	3	2
Diabetes mellitus	3	3
Other circulatory	3	3
Lower extremity/hips	2	3
Paralysis	2	1
Other respiratory	2	XX
Hernia	2	1
Back/spine	2	1
Other musculoskeletal	2	2
Mental/nervous	2	2
Other digestive	XX	2
Hearing impairment	XX	1

XX Not in top 15 chronic conditions
(Reproduced with permission from Reference 7.)

Table 3
Percentage of Noninstitutionalized Population Whose Activities are
Limited by One or More Chronic Conditions (1992).

Age-Group	Degree of Limitation			
	None	Minor	Major	Severe
65 years or older	61.2	15.6	12.5	10.6
65 to 74 years of age	65.6	13.6	10.4	10.4
75 years or older	54.7	18.6	15.7	11.1

(Reproduced with permission from Reference 8.)

physical impairments described above. In the community, about 5% of those older than 65 have some clinically detectable impairment of cognitive function. However, only 2% of the community-based population over 65 have major limitations of their activity because of mental or nervous conditions. The incidence of clinically detectable mental impairment rises with age, reaching 20% in those older than 75 years and almost 50% in those over 85 years.[7,9] The two chapters covering carotid arterial disease will deal with some aspects of the prevention and treatment of mental and neurologic impairment in the elderly population.

From the standpoint of the elderly themselves, 40% rate their health as very good or excellent. An additional 30% rate their health as good.[2] Those who have their own households account for 77%; 51% live with a spouse, while 26% live alone.[5] More than half of those 85 years old or older still live alone or with their spouse.[10] Among men and women aged 85 years or older living in the community, only 35% need help with one or more of the activities of daily living.[2]

While the comments above emphasize the characteristics of those living in the community (the group of elderly who are noninstitutionalized), do they represent the majority of the elderly or are they the exception? In fact, only 5% of the elderly reside in institutions. Many of these are temporary residents. Over half of the persons admitted to a nursing home are discharged within 3 months.

About three fourths of nursing home admissions come from hospitals. Even then, only 6% of men and 11% of women 65 or older are discharged from a hospital to a nursing home. Often, this has more to do with the economics of hospital care than it does with the need for prolonged care. The need to admit an older person to a nursing home or long-term care facility is age dependent. Less than 2% of those aged 65 to 74 reside in nursing homes. The percentage rises to about 7% for those aged 75 to 84, and to 20% for those 85 years old or older. Of those who do enter a nursing home, 55% spend at least 1 year there and 21% will spend 5 years or more.[2]

Table 4 lists the major causes of death in the elderly along with their relative ranks and rates per 100,000 individuals in the age-group 65 to 74 years. It is noteworthy that except for vascular disease and chronic obstructive pulmonary disease, the causes of death are not the same as the causes of disability (Table 2). Nonfatal diseases such as arthritis, orthopedic problems, and musculoskeletal conditions are at least as likely to produce major disabilities as are the fatal diseases.[11]

In summary, the generally held impression that old age is synonymous with sickness, disability, mental incapacitation, institutionalization, and death is incorrect. Of the top four chronic diseases that exist in the over 65 population—arthritis, hearing impairment, hypertension, and heart disease—only the last two pose any direct threat to life. Six of the top 15 chronic diseases that exist in this population and 5 of the 15 diseases that produce major limitations of activity in the elderly are due directly or indirectly to vascular disease. Three fourths of the el-

Table 4
Major Causes of Death in Population Ages 65 Years through 74 Years.
Rank and Rate per 100,000 (1989).

Causes of Death	Men		Women	
	Rank	Rate	Rank	Rate
Heart disease	1	1255.3	2	636.1
Malignancies	2	1079.1	1	670.9
Chronic obstr pulm dis	3	194.7	4	112.1
Cerebrovasc dis	4	164.3	3	128.9
Influenza, pneumonia	5	78.6	6	40.2
Diabetes mellitus	6	73.1	5	71.8
Accidents	7	65.7	7	34.6
Other arterial disease	8	57.1	10	9.9
Chronic liver disease	9	48.6	9	25.3
Suicide	10	33.1	12	5.9
Nephritis/nephrosis	11	25.5	11	9.1
Atherosclerosis	12	20.4	8	30.4

(Reproduced with permission from Reference 11.)

derly have no or only minor limitations of their activities. Over half of the elderly are vigorous and completely independent, often fiercely so. We can help improve not only their length of life, but its quality.

Historical Background of Government Programs

Traditionally, care for the invalid, the widowed, the orphaned, and the aged was the responsibility of the family, the religious, and the donors to private charities. The basic principles are clearly enunciated in the Old Testament. Even today in the United States, family and friends provide over a third of the informal care that allows the elderly to live in the community. Wives, daughters, and other women constitute the bulk of these caregivers.[2] How, then, did it become the responsibility of the state to fund medical and nursing home care?

It was the passage of the Poor Laws during the reign of Elizabeth I in the sixteenth century that fixed responsibility on the local community for the care of the disabled, poor, and elderly. When emigration (or deportation) to the New World took place, this pattern was adopted in the American colonies. As the industrial revolution of the eighteenth and nineteenth centuries progressed and urbanization of the population took place, individuals became more dependent on wages and their ability to work for their livelihood. Provision for the care of those too old or too disabled to work became an increasing problem. As a result, the belief was fostered that society as a whole should bear at least some responsibility for the economic protection of its members. Social insurance for various purposes began during the nineteenth century, when trade unions and working men's societies established funds to provide for their disabled workers, a practice that continues even today.[12]

Compulsory, nationwide programs of social insurance were instituted in Germany in 1883 by Chancellor Otto von Bismarck, largely as a result of pressure from labor unions. Initially, these programs provided for sickness insurance and workman's compensation, but in 1889, an old age insurance program was added. Workers, employers, and the government shared in the funding of the programs. It was in Germany, in 1870, that 65 was first established as the formal age of retirement. Anecdotally, von Bismarck picked this age not on the basis of any biological data, but as a way of eliminating his rivals in the federal government.[13] By 1930, all western European countries had programs combining social insurance, pensions, and public assistance. In light of future events to take place in the United States, it is interesting to note that von Bismarck has been described as "militantly conservative" and even as a "violent conservative."[14]

In the United States, the Social Security Act of 1935 was passed as part of President Franklin D. Roosevelt's New Deal legislative program. Initially intended to provide for unemployment insurance and retirement pensions, it grew in scope. In 1957, the National Disability Insurance program was introduced to provide for totally and permanently disabled workers over the age of 50. In 1965, Medicare was introduced. In 1974, the federal Supplemental Security Income Program began providing aid to the blind, disabled, and indigent aged.

When age 65 was established as a retirement age, life expectancy at birth was less than 49 years. At the turn of the century, men spent an average of 1.2 years in retirement before dying.[15] In 1900, life expectancy at birth was 49.6 years and at age 65 it was 11.5 years. There were 3 million individuals over the age of 65 and 125,000 over the age of 85 years in the United States. By 1980, life expectancy at birth had increased to 69.9 years and at age 65, to 14.0 years. There were 25 million people over the age of 65 and 2 million over the age of 85 years in the United States. By the year 2000, these numbers are projected to grow to 77.0 years, 15.7 years, 35 million people, and 4.6 million people, respectively. Those over age 65 will account for 13% of the entire population in the year 2000.[11] The number of people years over the age of 65 has grown from 35 million in 1900 to 550 million at present.

Society, or more accurately the federal government, now finds itself in a dilemma; that is, how to fund health care for a population that is not only growing in number, but growing in longevity. To add to the dilemma, patients now have available to them sophisticated medical and surgical treatments, some of which were only dimly envisioned in 1935. The percentage of the Gross National Product (GNP) spent on health care grew from 5.3% in 1960 to 13.2% in 1991.[16] Those 65 years of age or over constituted 12% of the population in 1991, but accounted for over one third of the national health expenditures.[2] Dire predictions about the future solvency of Medicare and Social Security abound. The opinion is expressed that expending resources to maintain the elderly would be better spent on the younger, more productive population.[1] A recent ex-governor of Colorado is alleged to have said that the elderly have an obligation to die.

The total cost of health care is indeed steadily increasing. The average annual percentage of change in national health expenditures in the United States has varied from a low of -3.6% during the years 1929 through 1935, to a high of 16.0% during the interval 1980 to 1981. The average annual percentage change for the time period 1929 through 1965 was 7.0%. From 1965 through 1991, it was 11.8%.[17] Are the escalating costs of medical care in the United States really due to the cost of providing care for the growing number of elderly? Or, are the elderly easily identified scapegoats being used to explain more serious problems of management?

Kane, Ouslander, and Abrass[9] countered what they referred to as "this ageist misimpression" with data provided by several agencies of the federal goverment. They made three points. First, that medical costs due to aging of the population alone would increase the proportion of the GNP spent on health care from 12% in 1990 to only 13.4% in 2020. Second, and in contrast to the first statement, continuation of the current rate of annual increase attributed to intensity of care and technology would increase the proportion of GNP devoted to health care to 36%. Third, the dependency ratio, which compares the proportion of the population under 18 and over 65 to that between 18 and 64, was highest in 1900 and, at least until the year 2050, will not exceed what it was in the mid-1960s.[2] Thus, individuals between ages 18 and 64, often represented as the group working to support the "dependent" population, will not be supporting an ever increasing proportion of the residents in the United States, although it is true that a larger share of the "dependent" population will be the elderly.[2] As pointed out earlier in this chapter, over half of the elderly are vigorous and completely independent.

The composition of the elderly population, as well as the costs of providing medical care to the older patient are, of necessity, the background against which the information provided in this text must be evaluated. From the foregoing, it is certainly clear that the great majority of the elderly is not sickly, incapacitated, confused, useless, or about to die. It is equally clear that vascular disease in one or more of its forms is the responsible cause for the majority of the chronic diseases, disabilities, and mortality of the elderly population. It will be apparent from other chapters in this book that currently available techniques of medical and surgical management can, if applied, prolong life, increase its quality, make it more active, and even prevent the diseases that would otherwise result in disability and death. Is the effort worth the cost? The authors will leave that decision to the elderly and to the 76 million "baby boomers" who will be joining that group shortly.

Organization of the Text

The motivation to write this text came from the publication of two earlier journal articles written by the editors on the subject of vascular disease in the elderly.[18,19] In the process of preparing those manuscripts, it became apparent that while a great deal of information about the management of vascular disease in the elderly was available, it was widely scattered, particularly when both the medical and surgical aspects were to be considered. In addition, it was clearly evident that there was a biased approach to the treatment of the elderly even as the techniques or treatments were being presented. This was notably the case when scientific information was presented in the lay press. Often, authors present a distorted picture of the elderly population as a whole not by intent, but because disease and disabilty of a specific patient population are the subject of the scientific presentation.

All of the authors selected by the editors have both special expertise in the areas of their subjects, as well as access to large databases from which to develop their presentation, conclusions, and recommendations. When it was possible, we were particularly interested in acquiring hard data from which valid conclusions could be drawn. Not surprisingly, in some of the areas of the text, hard data is difficult and sometimes impossible to find. Aside from assigning a specific subject to each of the authors, no effort was made to limit or direct their remarks or opinions. The development of each of the chapters was solely the prerogative of the author(s) responsible for that chapter. Thus, there might be some overlapping of coverage and, perhaps, some contrary opinions about the same subject. If there are, hopefully, it will assist the reader in arriving at the truth.

The organization of the text is intended to cover the general subject of aging as it might affect the vasculature, medical, and surgical risks that are unique to the elderly, and the medical and surgical management of specific vascular diseases.

References

1. Schlosberg S: Age. *Los Angeles Times.* E1-E4, May 15, 1995.
2. Kane RL, Ouslander JG, Abrass, IB: The elderly patient: demography and epidemiology. In: Kane RL, Ouslander JG, Abrass IB (eds). *Essentials of Geriatrics.* 3rd Ed. New York: McGraw-Hill, Inc.; 19-43, 1994.
3. Table one: resident population, according to age, detailed race, and hispanic origin. United States: selected years 1950-1991. In: *Health United States 1993.* Hyattsville, MD: US Printing Office; 61, 1994.
4. Manton KG, Vaupel JW: Survival after the age of 80 in the United States, Sweden, France, England, and Japan. *N Engl J Med* 333:1232-1235, 1995.

5. Healthy older adults. In: *Healthy People: The Surgeon General's Report on Health Promotion and Disease Prevention.* Washington, D.C.: US Goverment Printing Office; 71-80, 1979.
6. Belsky JK: Disability and health care. In: Belsky JK (ed). *Here Tomorrow: Making the Most of Life After Fifty.* New York: Ballantine Books; 244-280, 1988.
7. Verbrugge LM: Longer life but worsening health? Trends in health and mortality of middle-aged and older persons. *Milbank Q* 62:475-519, 1984.
8. Table 69: limitation of activity caused by chronic conditions, according to selected characteristics: United States, 1987 and 1992. In: *Health United States 1993.* Hyattsville, MD: US Printing Office; 153, 1994.
9. Kane RL, Ouslander JG, Abrass IB: Confusion. In: Kane RL, Ouslander JG, Abrass IB (eds). *Essentials of Geriatrics.* 3rd Ed. New York: McGraw-Hill, Inc.; 83-115, 1994.
10. Gartner M: Two faces of the elderly. *USA Today* 13A, November 15, 1994.
11. Table 117: Death rates, by selected causes and selected characteristics: 1970-1989. In: *Statistical Abstract of the United States: the National Data Book.* Washington, D.C.: US Government Printing Office; 85, 1992.
12. Bingham J: Social security. In: Fontaine EO, Couch WT (eds). *Collier's Encyclopedia.* Vol. 17. New York: PF Collier and Son Corp.; 674D-681D, 1955.
13. Hayflick L: A long and healthy life. In: Hayflick L (ed). *How and Why We Age.* New York: Ballantine Books; 89-108, 1994.
14. Lutz RH: von Bismarck or Bismarck-Schoenhausen, Prince Otto Eduard Leopold. In: Fontaine EO, Couch WT (eds). *Collier's Encyclopedia.* Vol. 17. New York: PF Collier and Son Corp.; 473-475, 1955.
15. Belsky JK: Retirement. In: Belsky JK (ed). *Here Tomorrow: Making the Most of Life After Fifty.* New York: Ballantine Books; 143-163, 1988.
16. Table 124: gross domestic product, national health expenditures, and federal and state and local government expenditures. United States, selected years 1960-1991. In: *Health United States 1993.* Hyattsville, MD: US Printing Office; 219, 1994.
17. Table 128: national health expenditures and average annual percent change, according to source of funds. United States, selected years 1929-1991. In: *Health United States 1993.* Hyattsville, MD: US Printing Office; 223, 1994.
18. Stemmer EA, Aronow WS, Wilson SE: Peripheral vascular disease in the elderly: part I. *Clin Geriatr* 3(2):17-29, 1995.
19. Stemmer EA, Aronow WS, Wilson SE: Peripheral vascular disease in the elderly: part II. *Clin Geriatr* 3(3):16-33, 1995.

Chapter 2

Definitions

Edward A. Stemmer, MD

In Chapter 1, a major goal of this text was identified as the provision of specific, objective information about vascular disease in the elderly. The editors expended great effort to give the reader access to large, well-analyzed databases. Conclusions drawn from those databases form the core of the chapters to follow. It seemed appropriate, therefore, that one of the first chapters should provide definitions of some of the terms that will appear in subsequent chapters. Many of these terms are in common use, but are often confused with one another or lack specific meanings. What follows is intended to help the reader interpret and make use of the data being presented.

Elderly

The first term that obviously needs definition is the word *elderly*, since that group of individuals is the subject of this text. According to the Little and Ives version of Webster's Dictionary, the word *elder* comes from the Old English *eldre* meaning older. The definition of elderly is given as "oldish, fairly old, rather old, past middle age, or approaching old age."[1,2] Clearly these definitions lack precision and, indeed, reflect the changing meaning of the term old during the past 100 years.

Jaffe cites the 1848 to 1852 autopsy/death log of Charity Hospital in New Orleans. In that log, men and women in their forties were said to have died of old age.[3] In the early years of this century, elderly patients were defined as those over the age of 50.[4] Today, studies of surgical outcomes in patients over 70 years of age are common and, as described in Chapter 18 dealing with the surgical treatment of coronary artery disease, studies of outcomes in octagenarians are easily found. In current commercial transactions, the benefits of senior citizenship regularly begin at age 55. In *Healthy People 2000*, a federal publication concerned with the nation's health into the future, the term *older adults* is used to designate those over the age of 65.[5]

From: Aronow WS, Stemmer EA, Wilson SE (eds). *Vascular Disease in the Elderly.* Armonk, NY: Futura Publishing Company, Inc., © 1997.

For the purposes of this text, we include individuals over the age of 60 in the elderly category, although we certainly do not use the term in a pejorative sense.

Age

Chronological age is usually determined by establishing the date of birth of the individual. As obvious as this appears, establishing someone's age is sometimes open to question, either because accurate records do not exist or because the individuals concerned have a motive to conceal their true age. Lady Astor is said to have commented, "I refuse to admit I'm more than 52, even if that does make my sons illegitimate." The belief that individuals in certain areas of the world have lived far into their hundreds is difficult to substantiate. The stories of superlongevity of residents in the Caucasus region of Georgia in the former Soviet Union had more to do with avoiding conscription into the Czar's army than it did with good health.[6]

The term *physiological age* is sometimes used to describe age in terms of functional status. The classic description of the functional changes that occur with increasing age appears in Shakespeare's *As You Like It* when Jaques presents the seven ages of man. Written in the last decade of the sixteenth century, the portrayal summarizes with surprising accuracy the functional changes that were to be documented in the second half of the twentieth century. In the seventeenth century, Thomas Sydenham supposedly made the comment that, "a man is as old as his arteries," a comment relevant to this text. Certainly the incidence and prevalence of chronic and degenerative diseases increases with age. The functional changes in specific organ systems with age have been described often. One of the best summaries of these changes has been reported from the Baltimore Longitudinal Study of Aging.[7] Even so, the great variability of the relationship between functional and chronological age of specific organ systems renders the physiological age of an indidual even more difficult to define than is the term elderly.

Aging

Victor Hugo commented that 40 is the old age of youth, 50 is the youth of old age. Irvine Page noted that after a certain age, one is elderly, aged, venerable, patriarchal, or just plain old.[8] *Aging* is, however, a process by which both animate and inanimate objects change. In contrast to advancing chronological age, the progress of aging consists of events that occur in time rather than because of time. *Gerontology* is the science that studies the process of aging in living organisms. While aging often implies the accumulation of chronic diseases or the development of disability and may make the individual more vulnerable to disease, it is, of itself, not a disease, even if it is inevitable from the time of birth onward. The nature of the process of aging will be discussed extensively in other chapters. Suffice it to say, at this point, that the process that leads to maturity of the infant and child is the same process that is involved later in life, although other factors, such as toxicity of the environment, may be involved as well. *Geriatrics* is concerned with the medical problems of the elderly.

Life Span

Life span is defined as the biological limit of life. Obviously, there is great variation in life span among both plant and animal species. In general, life span or the maximum years of life that can be achieved by a species is determined by documenting the age of the longest surviving member of that species. Thus, it is not an average number as is the situation when life expectancy is determined. Because of the difficulty encountered in establishing definite birth dates for the oldest members of our society, the real life span for human beings is a matter for speculation. Psalm 90 in the Book of Psalms (Moses) contains the verse, "the years of our life are three score and ten or even by reason of strength fourscore." In view of the fact that the most rapidly growing segment of the population is the octagenarians, the true life span certainly exceeds 80 years. Most gerontologists believe that the maximum life span of the human being is 115 to 120 years.

Hayflick, in his text *How and Why We Age,*[7] notes that the life span of many mammals in whom life span can be documented correlates with the average weight of the adult brain in comparison to the average weight of the adult body: the greater the brain/body ratio, the greater the longevity of the species.[9] As stated in Hayflick's text, life span or longevity of mammals can be stated as a formula with weights expressed in grams:

Maximum life span in years = $23(\text{brain weight})^{0.6} \times (\text{body weight})^{-0.267}$. Other variables such as metabolic rate also correlate with life span among mammals.

In terms of the goals of this text, attaining the maximum human life span, whatever its length, can only be considered a theoretical goal and one that might not be desirable of itself. Life expectancy and active life expectancy as described below are more pertinent to the discussions contained in this text.

Life Expectancy

Life expectancy is the average number of years that individuals may expect to live beyond any given age. Until early Roman times, the average life expectancy was about 18 years. By 1991, the average life expectancy had grown to 76 years.[10] Approximately half of this increase in life expectancy has occurred since 1900, largely as a result of control or elimination of deaths from infectious diseases.[11] The elimination or control of chronic diseases has been much less successful. Therefore, the absolute and relative gains in life expectancy have been greatest in the young and progressively decrease with increasing age. For example, in 1850 the average life expectancy was approximately 38 years. By 1989, the average life expectancy at birth was approximately 75 years.[12] In contrast, in 1841 in England and Wales the average life expectancy of a 65-year-old man was 11 years. By 1981, his life expectancy had increased by only 2 years to 13 years.[13] Vandenbroucke, in a study of the Knighthood Order of the Golden Fleece, reported that in the mid-1300s the average number of years for a man to live after age 85 was 1.75. By the mid-1800s, this had risen to only 3.6 years.[14] An 85 year old man in the United States in 1989 could expect to live another 5.3 years. Thus, the gains in life expectancy at the upper ranges of life are modest. Nevertheless, both the absolute and relative numbers of individuals over the age of 80 has grown steadily and are projected to continue to grow into the next century. There appear to be limits, however, to our ability to extend life expectancy. There has been little or no detectable change in the maximum age attained by individuals.[15] What has been achieved is the deferral of death or the rectangularization of the human survival curve.

Active Life Expectancy

Increased life expectancy is only one of the goals of modern medicine and surgery. Preservation of function and useful life is clearly an important consideration, regardless of the length of life. The term *active life expectancy* is used to distinguish the years of life spent free of disability from the years spent with restricted activity or in dependent status requiring aid in the activities of daily living or even total care. In a 1974 study of elderly, noninstitutionalized individuals in Massachusetts, the years spent in dependent status increased from 25% at ages 65 to 69 to 50% in men over the age of 85. In women, the percentage increased from 50% to 65% in the same age-groups. As expected, there was a larger number of women in each group.[16] Nevertheless, it is crucial to realize that in 1994 more than half of the individuals over the age of 85 still lived alone or with their spouse.[17] Another of the goals of this text is to describe medical and surgical treatment that is or should be available to elderly citizens in their quest for an active life.

Population

Since the presentation of data dealing with vascular disease in the elderly is a major consideration of this book, providing definitions for selected statistical terms seems appropriate. The basic units in statistical analyses are the populations from which the data are drawn and to which the conclusions apply. In common speech, the term *population* refers to the total number of inhabitants in a country, town, district, or other geographical area. In statistics, however, the term *population* refers to any collection of individuals or things that are to be studied or analyzed. The population may be finite or infinite. Since most statistical populations are very large (such as all the people over 60) or are, in fact, infinite (such as blood pressure measurements), it is a common practice to use *samples* of the population for analysis. *Parameters* are the measurements by which the sample is evaluated. Statistical analyses of these parameters then allow conclusions to be drawn about the whole population from which the sample was drawn. It is important to realize that the conclusions are only valid if the sample was representative of the population being studied. Even when the conclusions are valid, they apply only to the population as it was originally defined and only in terms of the parameters used. For example, studies in animals may not apply to humans; conclusions drawn from a study of coronary artery disease in men may not apply to women.

Multiple samples may be taken from the same population to study several specific aspects of the larger population. The results of treatment of carotid arterial disease in patients over the age of 60, outcome of the management of hypertension in elderly patients, or management of peripheral vascular disease in diabetics are examples of *subsets* of the original population of elderly patients with vascular disease. Each of these subpopulations will have its own parameters, with conclusions applying to that subset. Statistical analysis of the data from each subset may justify conclusions that apply to the original larger population. Samples may also be divided into *cohorts* so that the same individuals or objects can be followed prospectively over time.

Incidence

The *incidence rate* is defined as the number of new events that occur during a specific time period divided by the number of individuals in the appropriate population at risk. The time period is usually 1 year. The statistic is usually expressed as the number of new events per 1000 or 100,000 population per year. The number of individuals in the population at risk must be known or accurately estimated (as by a census). It needs to be emphasized that incidence refers only to new events or cases that arise within the time period selected. The term *incidence* is often confused with the term *prevalence*, an error which can grossly distort conclusions drawn from data.

Prevalence

Prevalence is defined as the number of events or cases that exist at any point in time divided by the number of individuals in the population at risk at that time. The term includes: those individuals in whom the characteristic existed prior to the point of measurement and continued into the interval of measurement; those in whom the characteristic being measured existed only during the interval of measurement; those in whom the characteristic persisted past the time interval selected; and those in whom the characteristic developed prior to the time interval, persisted through the time interval, and continued beyond the time interval. Prevalence may be expressed as a rate or as a percentage of the population at risk. For either incidence or prevalence, the population at risk may be limited by definition in several ways such as by age, nationality, or year. For example, in 1982 the prevalence of diabetes mellitus was 57.6 per 1000 people 45- to 64-years-old and 88.9 per 1000 people age 65 or older.

Variance

In any population, it is unlikely that the characteristic being measured, such as blood pressure, will be the same for each individual in the population. In an effort to describe a population, the *mean* or average is usally determined. However, by itself, the mean does not provide an adequate description of the population, since the spread of measurement or the degree of variation in the characteristic (in this case, the blood pressure) is also an important piece of information. When data are coming from a sample of the population rather than from the entire population, there is the additional problem of deciding whether or not the variation seen in the sample is representative of the variation that would have been observed in the entire population had it been possible to measure it.

When dealing with a sample, it is possible to evaluate the variation by plotting each data point relative to the mean. Since some of the individual measurements will have the same value, the location of identical measurements or a *frequency distribution* can be plotted about the mean with the result that a curve will be generated. If the curve is fairly symmetrical, it is referred to as a normal distribution, a concept fundamental to statistical analysis. The degree of dispersion of data under the curve is estimated by the variance and the standard deviation, two related measurements.

If the variations of each measurement from the mean were to be added to each other, their sum would necessarily be zero since the values would have both positive and negative signs. Because of the difficulties inherent with using zero in mathematical equations, it is more useful to square the individual variations from the mean, thus eliminating zero as a problem. To obtain an estimate of the average variation from the mean, the individual squared variations are first added. This number is referred to as the sum of the squares about the mean or simply the *sum of squares*. This number is then divided by the number of observations in the sample to produce an estimate of the average variation. This quotient is referred to as the *variance*. In actuality, when dealing with samples (that are a relatively small part of the whole population from which the sample was drawn), the sum of squares is divided by the number of observations less one (n-1), because this maneuver gives a better estimate of the scatter within the whole population. Because the variance is calculated from the square of the observations, it is not in the same units as the observations. To return the variance to the same units as the observations, the obvious solution is to take the square root of the variance. This number is referred to as the *standard deviation*.[18]

Standard Deviation

A large standard deviation indicates that the data are widely spread from the mean, while a small standard deviation shows that the data points are more closely concentrated about the mean. If the frequency distribution of the data in the population being studied is fairly symmetrical, the standard deviation can be used to determine the percentage of all the observations that will fall within a given range of standard deviations. For example:

1. 1 standard deviation on either side of the mean will encompass 68.27% of all observations;
2. 1.64 standard deviations on either side of the mean will encompass 90% of all observations;
3. 1.96 will encompass 95% of all observations;
4. 2 standard deviations on either side of the mean will encompass 95.45% of all observations;
5. 2.50 will encompass 98.75%;
6. 2.58 will encompass 99% of all observations;
7. 3 standard deviations on either side of the mean will encompass 99.73% of all observations.

The use of ±1.96 standard deviations is often used to establish confidence limits as described below.[19]

Coefficient of Variation

The *coefficient of variation* is defined as the standard deviation of a sample, divided by the mean of the sample multiplied by 100 to give a percentage. It is useful as a method for comparing the variabilities of frequency distributions expressed in different units. For example, if a study sought to compare the variability in weight with the variability of blood pressure, comparison of the respective standard deviations would not help since each of the standard deviations is in different units. The comparison could be made, however, using the coefficient of variation since that calculation is independent of units.

Standard Error of the Mean

The *standard error of the mean* (SEM), or as it is more commonly called the *standard error* (SE), estimates the amount by which the sam-

ple mean differs from the population mean. That is, the SE estimates
the degree to which the sample mean reflects the true mean of the
population being studied. It is calculated by dividing the standard deviation of the sample mean by the square root of the number of observations in the sample. The SE derives its usefulness from the obvious fact
that, as the size of the sample approaches the size of the population
from which the sample was drawn, the sample mean will approach the
true mean of the population. Clearly, the SE will decrease as the size
of the sample increases and, thus, will more accurately estimate the
true mean of the population. The terms *standard error* and *standard
deviation* are sometimes confused or used interchangeably. Standard
deviation measures the variability of samples, populations, or distributions. The SE measures the precision of estimates.

Confidence Intervals and Limits

Confidence intervals define a range of values within which the true
population mean is likely to lie. *Confidence limits* are those values
which set upper and lower limits to the confidence interval. When
confidence intervals are given, they are expressed as percentages; that
is, a 90% confidence interval or more commonly a 95% confidence
interval. Confidence intervals are based on the normal distribution
curve and the standard deviation.

The upper and lower limits of a 90% confidence interval would
be the mean of the sample ±1.64 standard deviations of the mean. The
upper and lower limits of a 95% confidence interval would be the mean
of the sample ± or −1.96 standard deviations of the mean. The term
95% confidence interval should be interpreted to mean that the true
value of the characteristic or parameter being studied will lie between
the limits of the confidence interval 95% of the time. A confidence
interval of 90% (or 95%) does not mean that there is a 90% or 95%
probability that the observed value of the characteristic or parameter
is the true value, even if it falls between the limits of the confidence
interval.[20,21]

The Null Hypothesis

The hypothesis that there is no real difference between two or more
statistical populations, or that there is no real difference in the effect
of different courses of action on the same population, is called the *null
hypothesis*. If the null hypothesis can be shown to be false, then an
alternative hypothesis (that there is a real difference between populations or courses of action) must be true. Since differences in outcome
can occur by chance, statistical tests are used to determine the probability that this was or was not the case.

Probability

In mathematics, *probability* is the chance of occurrence of any one of a number of possible events, some one of which is bound to occur. It is also a means of evaluating the likelihood that a conclusion drawn from a set (or sets) of data is correct. Probability can be expressed in terms of odds as in the likelihood ratio (LR) of the Bayes Theorem, or it can be expressed as a percentage as in the design of a confidence interval. More commonly in medicine, however, probability is expressed as a p-value which can range in value from zero to one. As used in medical statistics, the p-value measures the probability that the null hypothesis is correct. Therefore, the lower the p-value, the more likely it is that the alternative hypothesis is correct and that the differences being observed between population samples are real. Demanding too low a p-value to reject the null hypothesis risks the possibility of not detecting a true difference in populations (a type II error). Accepting to high a p-value makes it more likely that concluding that two or more populations are different is incorrect (a type I error). A p-value of 0.05 is typically chosen as a compromise between too stringent and too lax requirements for proof. A p-value of less than 0.05 is interpreted to mean that the probability of the observed differences in data being significant (real or true) is at least 95%. However, it is important to realize that statistically significant differences can occur with very large samples, without there being a clinically significant difference in outcome. Because of this possibility, the data themselves must be presented along with the evaluation of significance.

References

1. Wyld HC, Partridge EH: *The Little and Ives Webster Dictionary.* New York: JJ Little and Ives Company, Inc.; 409-410, 1957.
2. Ochsner JL, Douglas JR Jr: Surgery in the aged. In: Messerli FH (ed). *Cardiovascular Disease in the Elderly.* Boston: Martinus Nijhoff; 311-329, 1984.
3. Jaffe BM: Death be not proud. *Surg Rounds* 17:571-572, 1994.
4. Zenilman ME: Considerations in surgery in the elderly. In: Zenilman ME, Rosenthal RA, Roslyn JR, et al (eds). *Advances in Surgery in the Elderly.* New York: NY World Medical Press; 1-21, 1993.
5. Chapter 2. The nations health: age groups. In: *Healthy People 2000: National Health Promotion and Disease Prevention Objectives.* Washington, DC: US Printing Office; 9-28, 1991.
6. Hayflick L: *How and Why We Age.* New York: Ballantine Books; 200, 1994.
7. Hayflick L: *How and Why We Age.* New York: Ballantine Books; 137-149, 1994.
8. Page IH: Foreword. In: Messerli FH (ed). *Cardiovascular Disease in the Elderly.* Boston: Martinus Nijhoff; xiii-xiv, 1984.
9. Sacher GA: Relation of life span to brain weight and body weight in mammals. In: Wolstenholme GEW, O'Conner M (eds). *The Life Spans of Animals.* Boston: Little, Brown and Co.; 115-133, 1959.
10. Dublin LI, Lotka AJ, Spiegelman M: *Length of Life: A Study of the Life-Table.* New York: The Ronald Press, Co.; 26-43, 1949.

11. Cotran RS, Kumar V, Robbins SL: Diseases of aging. In: Cotran RS, Kumar V, Robbins SL (eds). *Pathologic Basis of Disease*. 4th Ed. Philadelphia: WB Saunders, Co.; 543-551, 1989.
12. National Center for Health Statistics: *Vital Statistics of the United States*. Vol. 2. Washington, DC: Public Health Service; 229, 1992.
13. Bland M: Mortality statistics and population structure. In: Bland M (ed). *An Introduction to Medical Statistics*. 2nd Ed. New York: Oxford University Press; 291-305, 1995.
14. Vandenbroucke JP: Survival and expectation of life from the 1400s to the present: a study of the Knighthood Order of the Golden Fleece. *Am J Epidemiol* 122: 1007-1016, 1985.
15. Ochsner JL, Douglas JR Jr: Surgery in the aged. In: Messerli FH (ed). *Cardiovascular Disease in the Elderly*. Boston: Martinus Nijhoff; 314, 1984.
16. Katz S, Branch LG, Branson MH, et al: Active life expectancy. *N Engl J Med* 309:1218-1224, 1983.
17. Gartner M: Two faces of the elderly. In: *USA Today*. Vol. 13, No. 44. Arlington, VA: Gannett Company, Inc.; 13A, 1994.
18. Bland M: Summarizing data. In: Bland M (ed). *An Introduction to Medical Statistics*. New York: Oxford University Press; 59-60, 1995.
19. Hill AB: The variability of observations. In: Hill AB (ed). *A Short Textbook of Medical Statistics*. 10th Ed. Philadelphia: JB Lippincott; 84, 1977.
20. Bland M: Estimation. In: Bland M (ed). *An Introduction to Medical Statistics*. New York: Oxford University Press; 124, 1995.
21. Hill AB: Problems of sampling. In: Hill AB (ed). *A Short Textbook of Medical Statistics*. 10th Ed. Philadelphia: JB Lippincott; 117, 1977.

Chapter 3

Health Care for the Aged

Percy Bracamonte, MD
Bruce E. Robinson, MD, MPH

Older People as Patients

The primary goal of health care for the elderly is to reduce the chance of dying from specific diseases and, therefore, maximize their survival. However, older people arrive at health care settings with broader and more complex expectations. They seldom identify survival as the primary focus for their health care; instead, the preservation and restoration of function are most often chosen as principal objectives. The focus on function is a major defining characteristic of good health care for the aged.[1]

A different health care target requires different methods. In younger patients, treatment decisions can generally be made by considering only the relevant medical facts, assuming that all other factors are relatively constant. However, as we age we become more different in every way and, therefore, less predictable. Older people may present with no relevant difficulties, or have multiple problems, extending through physical, mental, social, and functional areas. These problems may be observable, but at times are best understood as reductions in the body's reserve capacity in a given function. They can be identified only by careful assessment and with difficulty. Any decision to perform a medical act needs to consider the impact of, and the consequences anticipated toward, all dimensions of health. Therefore, some understanding of health in every dimension should be attempted before a decision on treatment is reached. In the elderly, physical, mental, social, and functional problems combine to produce the disability, as well as the opportunity for improvement of health.

Another critical requirement for good health care of the elderly is the ability to make the right decision, when so often one is faced with multiple imperfect options. The complexities of the usual clinical decisions in the context of aged and disabled older people often reach levels

From: Aronow WS, Stemmer EA, Wilson SE (eds). *Vascular Disease in the Elderly.* Armonk, NY: Futura Publishing Company, Inc., © 1997.

associated with ethical dilemmas. The medical outcomes of interventions become less certain and more complex, and must be estimated in terms of survival and quality. The variability characteristic of older people in physiological functions, psychology, and anatomy also applies to the philosophy held by the patients toward their own survival, and their personal tolerance for suffering and dysfunction which might occur in the course of intervention. Understanding the approach to the difficult decisions regarding medical and surgical intervention in later life, which requires true advocacy on the part of the provider and careful attention to communications skills, is the topic of this chapter.

Aging and Function

The World Health Organization (WHO) stated over three decades ago that, "Health in the elderly is best measured in terms of function . . . the degree of fitness rather than extent of pathology may be used as the measure of the amount of services the aged will require from the community."[2] The ability to function is both a target of health care services and a predictor of health care needs. A separate dimension of the value of functional information is the contribution it makes to clinical diagnosis. Older people often fail to develop the characteristic signs and symptoms associated with various medical and surgical conditions: heart attacks occur without chest discomfort, infections without fever, and appendicitis without reported pain. Functional disturbances may target correctable medical and surgical problems, as well as provide important information about the severity of disease. For example, new cognitive impairment may suggest adverse drug reactions, and incontinence may lead to diagnosis of obstructing prostatic carcinoma.

The figure illustrates the frequency of common functional disabilities in persons of increasing age. In general, a 65-year-old person differs little from his or her middle-aged counterpart in prevalence of disability. However, both disability and many serious chronic diseases exhibit logarithmic patterns of growth in later life: a 70-something is much more likely to be impaired than a 60-year-old, and a 90-something is many times more likely to be disabled. Despite the rising disability rate with age, Table 1 shows that people of any age can be expected to not only survive but, if independent, remain so for much of their remaining years. There is no age at which most people are unable to function reasonably well.

The importance of functional loss to older people and society is felt in areas of resource requirements and quality of life. Functional status is a powerful indicator of health services needs.[3] In particular, functional loss often requires expensive, continuous supportive care, such as home nursing and nursing home care, which is beyond the means of most older people for anything more than a few months, and requires substantial public funding. There is also a positive correlation between functional status and a patient's sense of well-being.[4] As a

Prevalence of Functional Disability
by age and sex

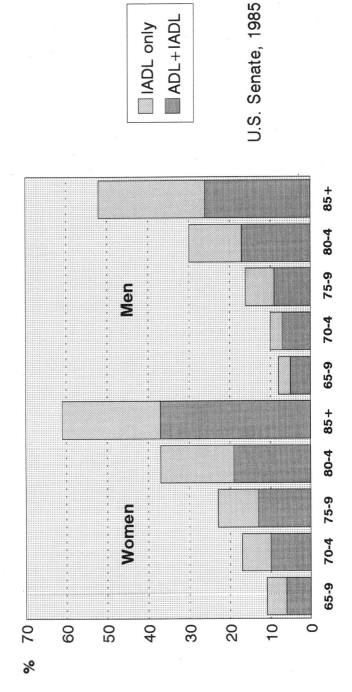

U.S. Senate, 1985

Table 1
Life Expectancy and Number of Remaining Years Free of Dependency in ADL

Age	Life Expectancy*		Disability-Free Years Remaining	
	Men	Women	Men	Women
65–68	13	20	9	11
70–74	12	16	8	8
75–79	10	13	7	7
80–84	7	10	5	5
>85	7	8	3	3

*Independent noninstitutionalized elderly men and women in Massachusetts.
ADL = activities of daily living
(Adapted with permission from Reference 19.)

group, older people are much more concerned about issues of disability (blindness, paralysis, having to live in a nursing home), and worry very little about dying.[5] Therefore, physicians caring for the elderly must shift their focus from dealing with organ-specific disease toward identifying and restoring a patient's corresponding loss of function.

The concept of function goes beyond the physical aspects of the typical medical evaluation. Social and psychological dimensions play crucial roles in how we feel about our health, and the ability of an elderly person to live independently in the community. Mental health problems are more common among the aged than any other group. Cognitive impairment is another age-associated problem, exhibiting logarithmic growth patterns among the older population. One recent study found the prevalence of dementia in those over 85 to be 47%.[6] Undetected cognitive impairment can lead to embarrassingly inaccurate histories and unexpected hospital events. Depression rates also increase in older persons. About 5% of all community elders have diagnosable major depression.[7] In a hospital setting, 23% of men over 70 exhibited a depressive disorder.[8] Depression is the most common confounder of medical illness in older persons—it clouds differential diagnosis, and often accompanies serious medical illness. Physical losses, reduced sensory capacities, losses of job, income, and death of relatives or friends are predisposing factors to depression in the elderly. On the other hand, depression both mimics and accompanies physical illness, leading to decreased mobility, malnutrition, delayed recovery from medical events, and an overall failure to improve.

Understanding "social function" is critical in medical management. For every impaired individual living in a nursing home, there are several equally impaired persons living at home. The difference is the availability and motivation of caregivers. The need for expensive and scarce, publicly funded home and institutional long-term care greatly depends on the availability of such caregivers, and the ability of the medical system to empower and protect them. Another relevant aspect of social function is the availability of money to meet personal needs. Many problems of personal care and function can be solved with enough money. The medical system also has the ability to quickly exhaust economic resources of retired older persons, through copayments, deductibles, and uncovered costs.

The impact of the environment on the health and well-being of older people must also be considered. Some individuals will clearly prefer death to disability that would require them to live in a nursing home. Others do not mind being cared for, and some seem to prefer it. Only by knowing how patients view a change in environment can you determine what target a medical or surgical intervention should choose.

The Multidimensional History and Physical Evaluation

Applying this broader understanding of the multiple dimensions of health to the clinical decisions we make for our patients requires that we have reasonable information about each dimension before we act. A cardinal skill in caring for elderly patients is to know how to evaluate health in multiple dimensions. As individuals age, the combination of disease, disability, side effects of drugs, and decreased physiological reserves makes older patients more vulnerable to functional loss when challenged with injuries, surgery, infections, or new drugs. The question of how to do this quickly and accurately has been studied extensively in geriatrics, and a practical approach can be suggested.

Table 1 is a modified version of a multidimensional screening assessment. The critical dimensions of health are listed in the first column. The suggested screening method is listed in the second column, and the abnormal result listed in the third. The listed items represent concepts and issues critical to good decisions in older persons that are often poorly evaluated in the traditional evaluations performed by physicians. Accurate diagnosis and treatment is always critical to good health care at any age, and is assumed.

The eventual goal of the evaluation is to develop accurate clinical expectations about the effectiveness of health services in achieving the specific goals, and to anticipate the consequences of intervention on the multiple dimensions of health. This process is related to the concept of prognosis, but is more general with respect to goals other than survival: goals such as regaining independence, going home, avoiding nursing home placement, etc.

Several items of physical health require additional attention. The concept of endurance is critical to tolerance of restorative activities and should be considered. The need for medical treatments and therapies can require specific settings to be successfully performed; tracheostomy care, tube feedings, wound care, and similar issues should be noted and considered. Medical stability is another powerful issue in the type of care required for patients. Discharge settings vary in their tolerance for acute changes in health, and vary in the availability of evaluation when changes occur. Nutritional state is important, but is often ignored in medical plans for care. Older persons are at risk for developing nutritional deficiencies because of reduced nutrients reserves associated with aging and an inability to respond adequately to periods of stress. Malnutrition frequently reflects concurrent medical illness, depression, inability to shop or cook, inability to feed oneself, or financial hardship.

Screening for abnormalities in mental health can be briefly performed. As older patients with dementia can be quite skilled in covering their disability, it is often missed unless specifically assessed. One should be alert for vague answers and reliance on family during the clinical interview. As memory is the earliest and most common deficit in dementia, the three-word memory screen is quite sensitive to cognitive impairment. However, temporal orientation is somewhat less threatening and also sensitive, if any error is considered a sign of potential dysfunction. Patients who fail either screen should be more thoroughly evaluated for cognitive disorders. As these screens are designed to be sensitive, an abnormal response is not diagnostic of impairment.

Our culture does not encourage the open expression of abnormal thoughts and feelings. Doctors on rounds often encourage patients to be upbeat and positive: it may be hard for patients to expose sadness, thoughts of dying, and hopelessness. The identification of depression in clinical practice often only requires that patients be given permission to talk about their bad feelings. A single question giving permission to patients to speak of how they feel inside is a good start. Patients who volunteer feelings of hopelessness and sadness should be asked about thoughts of suicide: it is disturbingly common in older persons, particularly men.[9] Further clinical evaluation is required for serious depressive thoughts and feelings. Therapy for depression is generally very successful and gratifying.

Screening for social support begins with the identification of caregivers. The most restrictive situation is when no one is available to help older persons who are ill. When caregivers are identified, it may be useful to determine whether they are fit and available to help with care. Problems thus identified can be referred to other providers (social workers, community nursing agencies) for further evaluation and action.

Determining patients' philosophy toward their medical care is an important component of evaluation. Older patients differ greatly in their perspective on the value of additional years of life, and their willingness to accept intervention toward that goal. Some openly wish for death, in the absence of depression: it's simply the last thing they feel they have to do. Others are as vigorous in their pursuit of additional life as any 20-year-old. There is simply no strategy toward health care decisions that does not require understanding of the patients' goals.

Identifying the discharge environment is critical to planning. The tolerance of the location of care for illness must be matched with the circumstances of the patient. Home, nursing home, and boarding home differ in tolerance for disability and sickness, and facilities differ within categories. Hospital staff and families may provide the necessary information about the capability and willingness of facilities to deal with specific problems in health and function.

Physical functioning has been grouped into two classes of measures. Instrumental activities of daily living (IADLs) refer to tasks to maintain an independent household. IADLs include using the telephone, managing money, shopping, preparing meals, doing light housework, and getting around the community. The ability to carry out basic self-care activities is described as activities of daily living (ADLs) and include eating, using the toilet, dressing, transferring, walking, and bathing. This way of categorizing function has become very common in reporting public health issues as well as clinical status. For example, it has been stated that persons 85 years of age or older have extraordinarily great demands for health care since 46% of the community in this age group need some assistance in ADLs or home management, 18% require assistance with at least three of the six ADLs, and 10% are essentially totally dependent.[10]

The evaluation of function can be approached in two ways. One way of doing it is to evaluate the physical and mental components of the ability to perform functional activities. The second is to ask patients or families about the ability to perform specific tasks. Practical and systematic tools to screen functional status have been developed to help clinicians.[11]

In performance-based appraisal, the clinicians assess the components of functional performance (leg function, arm function, vision, hearing, gait) (Table 1). In other words, limbs are evaluated for the capability to perform important tasks such as feeding or grooming, in the case of the arms, and mobility and transferring in the case of the legs. Physical exams on aged persons may uncover multiple abnormalities that may produce dysfunction in the legs: degenerative joint disease, decreased range of motion, deformities, podiatric problems, peripheral neuropathy, and many more. However, the most useful method to assess the significance of a finding is to observe patients getting out of a chair and walking around the room.

The second approach to determining functional competence is to ask patients or families about the abilities to perform functional tasks. This is less useful when acute change is expected, as when evaluating during an acute hospital stay. The evaluation of functional ability can take advantage of the hierarchical nature of personal functions: most persons with no limitation in dressing will also be independent in lesser functions, such as feeding. Persons competent in IADLs (shopping, housework) are unlikely to experience difficulty with basic functions. Thus, one or two well-chosen questions can often lead to good information about the level of function in an individual. Sensory impairment is screened because visual and hearing problems are highly prevalent, and significantly affect function and independence. They are linked to isolation, confusion, or depression. If a problem is found in this area, it may be evaluated and corrected.

Urinary incontinence is a common, disruptive, and potentially disabling condition in older persons. Physical health, psychological well-being, and the willingness of others to provide care can be adversely affected by incontinence. Even when not curable, incontinence can always be managed in a manner that will keep patients comfortable and make life easier for caregivers. Since many elderly patients are embarrassed and frustrated by their incontinence, it is rarely volunteered and, therefore, an essential part of this screening.

Home environment and social support are dimensions that are far from what many physicians consider their domain. However, these dimensions indicate who the patients are, and who can help them, and provide safety at home after intervention; they also help physicians to write an appropriate environmental prescription. Such an environmental prescription may include alterations in the physical environment (e.g., ramps, ground floor apartment, grab bars, and elevated toilet seats), special services (e.g., meals on wheels, homemaking, home nursing), increased social contact (e.g., friendly visiting, telephone reassurance, participation in recreational activities), or provision of critical elements to success at home (e.g., food, money).

The complexity of the problem requires teamwork for many patients. A multidisciplinary team is typically compounded by a physician, a nurse, a social worker, a physical therapist, an occupational therapist, a psychologist, and others. Multidisciplinary evaluations in which the multiple problems of older persons are uncovered, described, and explained are the basis of the so-called *Comprehensive Geriatric Assessment*. Its purpose is to deal with the exceedingly difficult health care issues posed by frail, old people. By using this method, the resources and the strengths of older persons are catalogued, the need for service assessed, and coordinated care plans developed to focus interventions on their problems.[12] Although a growing body of data suggest that frail, elderly people benefit from these assessment programs, the value of this approach has not been established in all the clinical settings,[13] and the cost is high. The brief screening proposed here may allow targeting of services to areas of identified need, and improve the efficiency of the use of other providers.

Developing Clinical Expectations

E.G. is a 74-year-old man with moderate vascular dementia. He is brought in from a nursing home for evaluation of bilateral heel ulcers, which developed 4 weeks earlier while he was hospitalized for a urinary infection. He has a history of moderate aortic stenosis, and angina pectoris which has been treated conservatively. Examination reveals a coarse, IV/VI systolic heart murmur, markedly diminished femoral pulses, and no detectable pulse below the groin. The feet are cool, the skin dusky in the sitting position, and both heels are covered with black eschar. Noninvasive arterial studies provide an ankle/brachial index of 0.24 on the right, and 0.20 on the left. The clinical impression is severe arterial insufficiency due to intra-abdominal arterial stenosis. Perfusion is considered inadequate for wound healing.

Typically, when physicians decide the best therapy for their patients, they intuitively break down that action into three steps[14]:

1. Establish the ultimate objective of treatment, i.e., to prolong survival, to prevent amputation of a limb with severe vascular disease, to heal a necrotic ulcer.
2. Choose the specific treatment, i.e., bypass surgery, amputation, antibiotics.
3. Decide the treatment target, i.e., improvement of vascular flow, vitality of tissue.

While this approach is frequently used to treat illness in younger people and those highly functional elders, going through the three steps is particularly challenging when applied to persons with accumulated chronic diseases and disabilities. When providing medical care to persons in the tail of the survival distribution for the human species, one often finds traditional medical decisions challenged. Families and patients often reject interventions on the basis of advanced age, with insufficient consideration of the consequences of the decision.

Good decisions require both a philosophy (the patient's) and specific information on the anticipated consequences of the choices available, often best understood by the doctor. Bringing these together is the challenge of good clinical decision making. Arriving at a decision for even a straightforward medical problem takes on the characteristics of an ethical dilemma when advanced age and disability are added. Stated briefly, good solutions to difficult medical decisions require merging medical information on choices and consequences with the values held by the patient, while attending to the context.

E.G. lives with his only relative, a niece. She is a capable caregiver, but has no other help, and must leave him alone when she shops. E.G. requires some help with dressing and encouragement to bathe, but otherwise is independent. He cannot remember for more than a moment, and sometimes mistakes the niece for his dead wife. The niece enjoys his company, but cannot handle the wound care currently being provided. She is also aware that he has expressed little pleasure at remaining alive in the years since the death of his wife. He has been very unhappy at the nursing home.

The quality of extended years is an important part of a reasonable judgment on therapeutic options. It is always treacherous for anyone to attempt to determine the quality of life of another. Many family members of patients with dementia feel strongly that their loved one would prefer death to life with severe dementia, and reject even simple therapy which would prolong life.[15] However, the clinical facts (coexisting conditions, stage of disease, and risks) are likely to be different in every patient.

Making decisions for cognitively impaired older persons requires that both the doctors and the families ponder the issue of what the patients would want, could they now decide. As this is the point of view required, it is always appropriate to provide patients with information and try to interpret any responses obtained—even when dementia limits the value of the response. Clinical assessments of decision capacity are dependent on the patients' abilities to comprehend options and reflect on personal preferences, more than on memory test results. It should be pointed out that many patients with different degrees of dementia can still make an informed decision about their health care. Physicians should avoid any kind of bias that could take away the cognitively impaired patients' rights to participate in their health care.

In a conference with both E.G. and the niece in attendance, the options of major arterial surgery, bilateral amputation, and conservative care are laid out, along with the attendant risks. The niece is distraught. She cannot bear the thought of putting E.G. through major surgery or bilateral amputation. However, she also feels that E.G. would not wish to remain alive in the nursing home. E.G. himself offers no opinions on the choices described, and defers to his niece for a decision.

In this case, a broad range of acceptable options is evident, and are displayed in Table 2. If the perspective of the family is that the patient's preferred choice is a quick and comfortable death, then no effort to interfere with natural processes need be made. However, if the dominant view is that the patient's only worthwhile existence is with both legs, at home, then surgery to restore flow to the legs might be considered. This could be attempted, despite the high risk of death in the process, and the real possibility of continuing difficulty in healing the wounds. The choice of wound care and antibiotics, with further hospital care for acute changes in health, is likely to result if no effort is made to reach a decision. This choice may be the most dangerous. Nutritional decline and progression of the wounds make acute infection likely. Hospitalizations to treat acute infection will only prolong the dying process without allowing a reasonable chance at regaining function and a life worth living. Additional morbid events are likely if the patient survives with rapidly declining nutrition and overall health. Specific counsel to the niece should help her overcome the paralysis that often occurs when faced with bad choices. No achievable goals may lead to the worst outcomes of all.

A decision is reached to provide E.G. with a comfortable death. The daily whirlpool treatments which had been producing substantial pain are discontinued. Therapy is also stopped. Morphine is given liberally for any sign of pain. Food and fluids are offered, but mostly refused. The local hospice spends time with the niece, helping her accept the choice she has made. Death occurs about 10 days later, and is peaceful.

Table 2
The Multidimensional History and Physical

Target Area	Assessment Procedure	Abnormal Result
Physical Health		
Endurance	Can you walk half a mile without stopping? Can you participate in daily activities without losing your breath or becoming exhausted?	No
Treatment needs	Record review, examination	Need for dressing changes, tube feedings, trach care, etc.
Stability	Record review, Hx., and P.E.	Frequent acute medical events requiring medical attention
Nutrition	Weigh the patient: measure height	Weight is below acceptable range for height
Prognosis and clinical trajectory	Record review, Hx., and P.E.	Short survival, disease state predicts continued deterioration
Mental Health		
Cognition	Instruct: "I am going to name three objects (pencil, truck, book). I will ask you to repeat their names now and then again a few minutes from now," or Orientation to month, day, year, and time of day	Inability to recall all three objects after 1 minute or Any incorrect
Depression	Ask: "Do you often feel sad or depressed?"	Yes
Social Support		
Social support	Ask: "Who would be able to help you in case of illness or emergency."	No support
Preferences	Ask: "Are there any medical treatments which you would reject, even it required to save your life?"	Yes
Environment	Consider: Is discharge environment tolerant of current identified disability and does it support improvement?	Intolerance of discharge site to level of physical or mental disability

Table 2 *(continued)*
The Multidimensional History and Physical

Target Area	Assessment Procedure	Abnormal Result
Function		
ADL-IADL	Ask: "Can you get out of bed by yourself?"; "Can you dress yourself?"; "Can you do your own shopping?"	No to any question
Vision	Test each eye with Jaeger card while patient wears corrective lenses (if applicable)	Inability to read greater than 20/40
Hearing	Whisper a short, easily answered question such as, "What is your name?"	Inability to answer question
Arm	Proximal: "Touch the back of your head with both hands." Distal: "Pick up the spoon."	Inability to do task
Leg	Observe the patient after asking: "Rise from your chair, walk ten feet, return, sit down."	Inability to walk or to transfer out of chair
Urinary incontinence	Ask: "Do you ever lose your urine and get wet?"	Yes

(Reproduced with permission from Reference 11.)

Medical care of the last 40 years has nearly forgotten how to comfort and allow death to proceed. Good health care for older people cannot ignore this traditional and still important goal. Medical care and advances in public health have successfully pushed life expectancy closer to life span: that theoretical, species-specific limit to survival. Medicine has not, however, altered life span, nor has it changed the fact that all living organisms are born, and all die. Refusing to accept death as a reasonable choice can produce suffering in patients, and loss of value within the system: half of Medicare expenditures are directed toward those in their last year of life. Providing a comfortable death against the challenges of painful diseases with unpredictable courses requires diligence and commitment.

The final principle of a good decision of this type is the principle of trepidation—whatever decision is made, the very real possibility of a bad outcome must be accepted. A decision to intervene recognizes a substantial chance that this man will die in surgery or fail to improve. Foregoing treatment may allow him to suffer substantial consequences from a disease which we at present could possibly cure. Our best service to the patient is to live with our concern, use it to keep us alert and flexible, but not allow it to drive us toward decisions which do not fairly represent the patient.

Table 3
Bilateral Heel Ulcers With Arterial Insufficiency

Action	Consequences
Amputation	Moderate surgery, poor functional outcome
Vascular surgery	Major surgery, morbidity,? chance of success
Abx., nutrition, wnd care	Increasing local wound related suffering
Narcotics only	Short survival, death by infection

Making good decisions in the "tail" of human survival is a skill requiring attention to process, flexibility, and the willingness to consider information from a variety of sources. For older patients with multiple medical problems, there are many decisions with no single option that is strongly favored by available data. The clinical judgment required is indeed a dilemma with strong ethical dimensions. The only wrong decision would be one made in isolation from the broader context of the philosophy of the patient and family.

Physicians have the ability to drive decisions toward their own preferences, often for intervention, with overly dramatic descriptions of the frequency and severity of complications without intervention, and optimistic presentations of the burdens and benefits of therapy. However, the proper outlook with which to weigh the facts should be that of the patients having their families as valuable sources of information as to what the outlook might be. The decision process involves the basic principle of true advocacy: acting on the best interest of each person by weighing the benefits and the burdens of treatments.

It has been suggested that age is a risk factor for inadequate treatment.[16,17] This can occur when decisions are driven by the concept that a person is *"too old"* to benefit from a therapeutic intervention.[18] There is no age at which a healthly older person cannot expect significant additional independent existence. Current evidence shows that the average life expectancy is 17 years at the age 65, 11 years at the age 75, 6 years at the age 85, 4 years at the age 90, and 2 years at the 100 (Table 3). In addition, many people remain functional throughout the last part of their lives.[19] Even the most disabled older human being deserves to be considered a candidate for any therapeutic option consistent with the medical facts and the patient's philosophy. The care of older persons requires one to develop the art of decisions in the face of uncertainty. Making intelligent choices when none are clearly "right" is the skill to be developed. The data required for good choices is the detailed understanding of the medical benefits of care, a broader set of information on health which considers the elements of the multidimensional assessment, and the philosophy of patients and families toward the outcomes anticipated. The mental attitude required is that of an advocate for the older persons, free from the bias of our personal philosophy and training. We must strive for good decisions in the face of ambivalence and confusion, ever mindful of the last of the Hippocratic charges: to comfort always.

References

1. Kennie DC: Good health care for the aged. *JAMA* 249:770-773, 1983.
2. *The Public Health Aspects of the Aging of the Population.* Copenhagen: World Health Organization; 1959.
3. Shanas E: Health status of older people: cross-national implications. *Am J Public Health* 64:261-264, 1974.
4. Shanas E, Towsend B, Wedderburn D, et al: The psychology in health. In: Newgarten BL (ed). *Middle Age and Aging.* Chicago: University of Chicago Press; 1968.
5. Stein S, Linn MW, Stater E, et al: Future concerns and recent life events of elderly community residents. *J Am Geriatr Soc* 32:431-434, 1984.
6. Evans DA, Funkenstein HH, Alberts MS, et al: Prevalence of Alzheimer's disease in a community population of older persons: higher than previously reported. *JAMA* 262:2551-2556, 1989.
7. NIH Concensus Conference: *Diagnosis and Treatment of Depression in Late Life.* NIH, November, 1991.
8. Koenig HG, Meador KG, Cohen HJ, Blazer DG: Depression in elderly hospitalized patients with medical illness. *Arch Intern Med* 148:1929-1936, 1988.
9. Osgood NJ: *Suicide in the Elderly.* Rockville, MD: Aspen; 1985.
10. Special Commmittee on Aging, United States Senate: *Aging America Trend and Projections.* 1985-1986 Ed. Washington, DC: US Government Printing Office; Publication No. 1986-498-116-814/42395, 1986-1987.
11. Lachs MS, et al: A simple procedure for general screening for functional disability in elderly patients. *Ann Intern Med* 112:699-706, 1990.
12. National Institutes of Health Consensus Development Conference Statement: Geriatric assessment methods for clinical decision making. *J Am Geriatr Soc* 36:342-347, 1988.
13. Solomon DH, Judd HL, Sier HC, Rubenstein LZ, morley JE: New issues in geriatric care (UCLA Conference). *Ann Intern Med* 108:718-732, 1988.
14. Sackett DL, et al: *Clinical Epidemiology: A Basic Science for Clinical Medicine.* 2nd Ed. New York: Little, Brown and Company; 1991.
15. Balducci L: Perspective of quality of life in older patients with cancer. *Drugs Aging* 4:313-324, 1994.
16. Avorn J: Benefits and cost analysis in geriatric care: turning age discrimination into health policy. *N Engl J Med* 310:1294-1301, 1984.
17. Wetle T: Age as a risk factor for inadequate treatment. *JAMA* 258:516, 1987.
18. Thibault GE: Too old for what? *N Engl J Med* 328(13):946-950, 1993.
19. Katz S, et al: *N Engl J Med* 309:1218-1224, 1983.

Chapter 4

Vascular Aging

John P. Walsh, PhD

Senescence can be viewed as an adaptation to ensure the survival of the species. In the face of finite resources and the advantages inherent to genetic variation, species have evolved to limit survival beyond the reproductive period. Nonetheless, the elderly have always been viewed as an invaluable source of wisdom in human societies and, consequently, we make every effort to increase their life span. In pursuit of this goal, clinicians use knowledge obtained from gerontological investigations to guide patients and to develop appropriate methods of intervention. A major problem faced by researchers, however, is that aging is a deteriorative process upon which pathology and disease are superimposed. Aging is often the soil from which diseases arise and it is, therefore, a difficult task for gerontologists to isolate the effects of "normative" aging. Consequently, we can only tentatively draw demarcations between aging, degenerative processes, and disease. For example, is an atheroma representative of a degenerative process or a disease? Is it a consequence of several age-related molecular changes in the arterial wall, or a response to mechanical injury, viral infections, or dietary flaws? Categorization of "normal" aging is further clouded by the similarities that exist between changes associated with aging and those associated with disuse (i.e., bed rest and space travel).

The purpose of this chapter is to describe age-related structural, physiological, and molecular alterations underlying the increased vulnerability and decreased viability associated with aging. While arbitrary, the cutoff between the mature phase of the life span and old age or senescence is usually 65 years of age for humans. Most human studies on aging compare the physiology of individuals greater than 65 years with a control, younger group. Similarly, in the most heavily studied animal model, the rat, a young adult is considered 3 to 6 months of age and an aged rat is considered older than 24 months of age. Each type of study has its own set of advantages and problems. Animal studies have the advantage of controlling environmental influences, as well as

From: Aronow WS, Stemmer EA, Wilson SE (eds). *Vascular Disease in the Elderly.* Armonk, NY: Futura Publishing Company, Inc., © 1997.

being permissive for performing invasive investigations. Comparative generalizations about the aging process must be guarded, however, since species-specific and tissue-specific responses to aging occur. Human studies are limited by the prevalence of occult coronary stenosis, with 60% of men over the age of 60 having a 75% to 100% block in at least one coronary artery.[1]

Through rigorous screening of coronary disease, it has been demonstrated that cardiovascular reserve capacity decreases with aging.[2] Much of the cardiovascular alterations can be explained by changes in cardiac muscle and connective tissue, and decreases in cardiac β-adrenoreceptors. A series of excellent reviews by E.G. Lakatta have described cardiac aging and it will, therefore, not be covered in this chapter.[1-3] An additional area not covered by this chapter is the age-related change in renal function, which alters fluid homeostasis and contributes to age-dependent reactions to therapies for vascular tension.[4]

In this chapter, the discussion is restricted to vascular aging, independent from age-related changes in the heart. Attempts at establishing a cutoff for disease versus aging in the vascular system are artificial, however, since many aspects of atherosclerosis stem from "basic age-related changes" in vascular remodeling, vascular modulation, and dietary handling of circulating lipids.

Functional Changes in Vascular Performance

Age-related decreases occur in vascular compliance and cardiac output.[5] The aorta functions as an elastic buffering chamber that dissipates the pressure wave resulting from ventricular contraction. During diastole, the large arteries supply the volume of blood to the periphery as a continuous peripheral blood flow. This elastic property of the aorta decreases left ventricular afterload and improves coronary blood flow. Age-related decreases in vascular compliance cause increases in systolic blood pressure, a decrease in diastolic blood pressure, an increase in systolic blood velocity, and a decrease in diastolic coronary blood flow.[6] In addition, cardiac perfusion is further compromised by age-related decreases in capillary and arteriole density.[7] There are also age-related decreases in blood volume and baroreceptor responses that contribute to alterations in cardiovascular reflex regulation.[8-10] Our scale of "normative" aging must be a sliding scale, however, since interventions to improve aerobic capacity reduce the stiffening of the arterial tree that accompanies aging.[11]

Morphological Changes

Decreases in vascular compliance are associated with thickening of the subendothelial layer, due to increased connective tissue, and thickening of the intimal layer due to migration of smooth muscle cells (SMCs).[12] In hypertension, these normal age-related increases in the cross-sectional thickness of the heart and large capacitance arteries are exacerbated.[13] Thickening of the vascular wall not only decreases compliance, but it also alters the permeability of the tunica media. This latter change may facilitate the accumulation of subendothelial lipids and proteins originating from plasma, and thus may constitute a link between aging and increased risk for atherosclerosis.[14] There is also evidence for a decrease in the permeation of oxygen to the outer vascular layers. For example, a 35% decrease in the oxygen tension was seen in the outer wall of arteries from aged rats.[15] Aging also results in an increase in the caliber of the arterial lumen. The increased luminal diameter partially compensates for the effects of arterial wall rigidity, but it limits functional changes in hemodynamics.[12] Similar changes also occur in the venous return system, although to a lesser extent.[5]

Molecular Modifications

Age-related increases in the content of lipids, collagen, and minerals contribute to a reduction in arterial distensibility.[16] These changes occur mainly around the internal elastic membrane.[17] Progressive fibrosis of the matrix occurs with age and there are prominent elastin modifications, such as elastin fragmentation.[18,19] Age-related changes in the geometric arrangement of the vessel wall are also caused by alterations in smooth muscle layering and changes in elastin and collagen content in the tunica media.[20] The collagen fraction and, specifically, the collagen-bound calcium increases. The elastin/collagen ratio also undergoes a dramatic decline with age.[14,21] These molecular changes underlie medial and intimal fibrosis, and may be a result of an age-related dedifferentiation of smooth muscles into a synthetic phenotype.[18] There is also evidence for age-related changes in the behavior of smooth muscle myosin that may increase the stiffness of vascular smooth muscles.[14] It is also proposed that age-related molecular alterations in elastin and collagen can be partially attributed to age-related increases in lysyl oxidase activity.[19]

Molecular Remodeling of the Matrix

Remodeling of the vessel wall occurs in response to differing hemodynamic conditions and disease. Release of nitric oxide (NO) (relaxant) and endothelin (contractile) from the endothelium have acute vasoactive effects, as well as chronic trophic effects on SMC remodeling of the matrix. SMCs control vascular tone and compliance, and synthesize and excrete structural proteins that form the vessel wall matrix (i.e., collagens I, III, IV, and V, elastin, proteoglycans, and glycoproteins). The matrix formed by this network of proteins provide blood vessels with their elastic physical characteristics. The matrix also participates in vascular remodeling through a release of stored growth factors and growth factor activation of matrix Zn^{2+} and Ca^{2+} metalloproteinases (i.e., collagenases, gelatinases, and stromelysins).[21,22] These proteinases can degrade all of the extracellular matrix (ECM).

Cytokines and growth factors (interleukin-1 [IL-1], platelet-derived growth factor (PDGF), and tumor necrosis factor-α [TNF-α], potent inflammatory and immunoregulatory cytokine) stimulate the synthesis of these matrix proteinases while TGF-β, heparin, and corticosteroids inhibit their synthesis.[23] Proenzymes, already synthesized and found in the matrix, are activated by plasmin. For example, prostromelysin is cleaved by plasmin activation to produce stromelysin, which in turn cleaves procollagenase which produces a huge increase in proteolytic enzyme activity.[24] There are also tissue inhibitors of metalloproteinases and circulating inhibitors (i.e., heparin and corticosteroids).

Metalloproteinases may also contribute to the development of atherosclerosis.[22] Initial vascular lesions begin with adherence of circulating monocytes to the vascular endothelium, through which they gain entry to the subintimal tissue. The monocytes secrete TNF-α, IL-1, and PDGF to stimulate metalloproteinase synthesis in SMCs and some endothelial cells.[25,26] One of these metalloproteinases, gelatinase A, degrades collagen IV of the basement membrane allowing for migration of SMCs to the intima. Eventually, there is a migration and proliferation of SMCs and a new deposition of ECM. In the formation of atheromas, the matrix forms a fibrous cap over a lipid core. The cellular content of these plaques is predominantly macrophages, SMCs, and foam cells. Gelatinase A secreted by SMCs and foam cells acts to weaken the fibrous matrix cap.[21]

Iatrogenic angioplasty restenosis may trigger smooth muscle migration and subsequent neointima formation. Beta-fibroblast growth factor (bFGF), released by injured or dying SMCs, induces SMC replication, and PDGF regulates their migration.[27] Initially, however, injury of SMCs induces collagenase and stromelysin induction that is postulated to lead to the degradation of both the basement membrane and the ECM.[28]

Nonenzymatic Glycosylation of Vascular Proteins (Maillard Reaction)

Nonenzymatic glycosylation is proposed to form protein and DNA adducts, and cross-links in aging and diabetes. Advanced glycation end-products are formed by the interaction of aldoses with proteins. These covalently linked sugars eventually produce a group of compounds that emit a fluorescent brown-yellow color. Aged vasculature and penile erectile tissue have been shown to express a sixfold increase in the level of pentosidine, which causes cross-linking of collagen and may impair collagen turnover.[29] Glycated proteins accumulated with aging make collagen fibers rigid and resistant to proteolysis.[18] Similar nonenzymatic glycosylations may also contribute to glomerular sclerosis in aging.[29,30] An additional problem associated with glycosylated proteins is that they may scavenge NO, which contributes to age-related decreases in endothelium-derived vascular relaxations.[29]

It is proposed that glycation end-products occur in SMCs, endothelial cells, and mononuclear monocytes by binding to a novel receptor.[31,32] The advanced glycation end-products also bind oxygen intermediates, possibly focussing oxidant stress on cellular targets and quenching released NO.[10,32] Glycation and oxidation of vascular proteins are also hypothesized to precipitate amyloid formation, which may contribute to the deterioration of the vasculature and heart with age.[33]

Responses to Neurotransmitters and Modulators

Some controversy exists with respect to the direction and extent of age-related changes in vascular responses to neurotransmitter and hormonal modulation. The disagreement in the literature is due in part to the varied tissue and species examined. Noradrenaline acts on vascular tissue through β- and α_1- and α_2-receptors. Evidence exists for β-adrenergic relaxations mediated by the direct action of β-receptors located on SMCs as well as by NO released by endothelial cells consequent to β-receptor activation. The overwhelming evidence, however, is in support of an endothelium-dependent mechanism.[10] Aging seems to cause a consistent decline in the response to vascular β-adrenergic receptor activation.[34] The age-related decrease in β-adrenergic responses appears to be due to a decrease in receptor number and affinity,[35] although, there is also evidence for age-related decreases in G-protein and cyclase activation.[36-38]

α_1-Adrenergic receptors are located on SMCs, and they mediate contractions that produce a decrease in vascular compliance.[10,34] α_1-Receptors increase smooth muscle Ca^{2+} through phosphoinositide hydrolysis and subsequent mobilization of stored Ca^{2+}. There is also evidence for α_1-mediated increases in smooth muscle calcium through a secondary activation of nifedipine sensitive voltage- dependent Ca^{2+} channels located in the plasma membrane.[39] No consistent age difference has been observed in the α_1-response, although it has been reported that α_1-mediated contractions decrease with age in coronary arteries.[40] Conversely, α_1-responses were shown to be unaffected by age in rat carotid arteries and there is evidence for both an increased vasoconstricting effect by α-agonists and a decreased vasodilatative action by α-receptor blockade in aging.[41]

α_2-Adrenergic receptors are located on both presynaptic terminals of sympathetic neurons and postsynaptically, predominantly on vascular SMCs.[5,42] Negative feedback activation of presynaptic α_2-receptors reduces release of noradrenaline and activation of postsynaptic α_2-receptors induces vascular relaxation. In aging, there appears to be a reduction in both pre- and postsynaptic α_2-receptors. The reduction in presynaptic α_2-receptors contributes to age-related increases in circulating noradrenaline levels, and the decrease in postsynaptic α_2-receptors further reduces compliance in aged vasculature. The change in presynaptic receptor function is considered to be an adaptive compensation for general age-related reductions occurring in the number of nerve fibers innervating the vascular system.[43] Decreases in nerve terminals, increases in the gap formed at the synaptic cleft, and reductions in presynaptic α_2-receptors all reduce noradrenaline uptake. The end effect is to increase circulating levels of noradrenaline. Since α_2-receptors and β-receptors decline with age, while α_1-receptors are unaffected, the predominant tonic effect of circulating noradrenaline in the elderly is to increase blood pressure.[44] Age-related increases in heart rate are not observed, despite the increased circulating levels of noradrenaline, because of the decline cardiac β-receptors.[1-3]

No age differences have been observed in α_2-adrenoreceptor-mediated phosphoinositide (PI) turnover, but with age, the α_2-receptor-mediated Ca^{2+} influx relies more and more on voltage-dependent Ca^{2+} channels.[39] This age-related shift in calcium source may also explain the age-dependent increase in sensitivity to dihydropyridine antagonists (i.e., veratridine).[39] The postsynaptic α_2-adrenergic response utilizing PI turnover is mediated through G-protein activation. Inositol triphosphate (IP3), formed by PI hydrolysis, causes a release of calcium from intracellular stores and calcium triggers the synthesis of NO.[45]

Other endothelial-dependent vasodilators that lose their efficacy with aging include acetylcholine, through muscarinic receptor activation, histamine, and adenosine.[46] Acetylcholine is linked to noradrenaline in the activation of guanine nucleotide regulatory proteins (G-proteins) to elevate intracellular Ca^{2+} and cause NO release from the endothelium.[45] It is of interest that other relaxing factors that elevate intracellular Ca^{2+} without the participation of G-proteins show less of an effect of aging in NO release (i.e., substance P, bradykinin, ATP, and Ca^{2+} ionophores). In addition, it has been shown that endothelium-dependent responses to acetylcholine (ACh) are decreased with aging, but that NO release and vascular muscle responses to nitroprusside are unaffected.[47] Together, these data indicate an age-related alteration in the coupling between ACh receptor activation and NO synthesis. Another vasodilator, atrial natriuretic peptide (ANP), shows an age-related reduction in vasodilation due to a decreased ability to increase cellular cyclic guanosine monophosphate (cGMP).[46] There is also some evidence for G-protein function being altered in aging and hypertension.[37,38] Alternatively, in the aged heart, G-protein number has been shown to be unaltered by aging, but β-adrenergic activation is decreased due to a decrease in the activation of adenylate cyclase.[48]

Nitric Oxide Metabolism

NO (formally known as endothelium-derived relaxing factor [EDRF]) is synthesized from its precursor molecule arginine by NO synthetase (NOS), which is inhibited by nitroarginine and L–N mono-methylarginine (L-NMMA).[49,50] NOS is activated by calcium increases occurring in vascular smooth muscle and the vascular endothelium. ACh, noradrenaline, and bradykinin induce hydrolysis of phosphoino-sitide to produce IP3, which causes calcium release from internal stores. In addition, shear stress and vascular deformation (i.e., pulsatile flow) cause release of NO through undefined mechanisms.[49] NO released from endothelial cells migrates across the plasma membrane of receptive SMCs to activate guanyl cyclase, which in turn reduces intracellular calcium. The decreased calcium reduces the level of contraction within the SMC, causing a general relaxation of the vasculature.

NO also decreases blood pressure through mechanisms other than its direct effect on SMCs. For example, NO decreases sympathetic out-flow and decreases blood pressure by acting at the central nervous system (CNS) to increase baroreceptor responses.[51,52] NO also inhibits the adhesion and activation of platelets and leukocytes to the endothe-lium,[53,54] and thus blocks the vasoconstriction produced by products of activated platelets (i.e., 5HT, adenine nucleotides, PDGF, thrombox-ane). NO also inhibits vascular smooth muscle proliferation.[55] Separate from NO, there is evidence for endothelium-derived hyperpolarizing factor that relaxes SMCs through an activation of SMC K^+ channels. Prostacyclin is also released by endothelial cells to produce vasodilator activity.[53] NO can be buffered, however, by hemoglobin which binds NO, and thus prevents its access to target tissue. This hemoglobin effect acts most often in resistance vessels to maintain flow hemodynamics.[56]

Aging and Nitric Oxide

The normal life span of an adult human endothelial cell is approxi-mately 30 years, after which it undergoes age-related death and replace-ment.[53] The replaced endothelial cells lose some of their ability to re-lease NO and, consequently, endothelial-dependent relaxations have decreased efficacy.[57] Age-related decreases in responses to acetylcho-line, histamine, adenosine, and activation of β-adrenoreceptors can all be tied to decreased production or release of NO.[58] There is also evidence that hypertension and atherosclerosis compound the age-related de-crease in NO release.[53,59] Aging is also associated with increases in the level of free radicals and end-product lipid peroxidation compounds (i.e., malondialdehyde), which further decrease the vascular relaxations mediated by ACh activation of endothelial cells.[10] This age-related de-crease in NO release is compounded by an age-related increase in the release of the contracting factor endothelin-1 (ET-1), which further re-duces vascular compliance.[58]

Calcium Physiology

There is evidence for a generalized impairment of Ca^{2+} homeostasis with aging in almost every tissue examined.[60] Ca^{2+} serves as part of the intracellular cascade mediating NO release from endothelial cells, and is integral to the sequence of events leading to actin-myosin interactions during smooth muscle contraction. For example, noradrenaline causes contraction of SMCs by α_1-receptor-mediated increases in intracellular Ca^{2+}. The source of calcium is both through a mobilization of intracellular stores and direct activation of plasmalemma voltage-dependent Ca^{2+} channels. SMC voltage-dependent Ca^{2+} channels are blocked by dihydropyridine antagonists (i.e., nifedipine, diltiazem, or felodipine).[61] It has been suggested that age produces an enhancement of binding sites for dihydropyridines and that this change underlies their greater effect on aged, vascular SMCs.[62] This finding is in contrast to the age-related decrease in cardiac myocyte sarcolemma dihydropyridine sensitive Ca^{2+} channels.[63] There is also evidence for an age-related decrease in the expression of sarcolemma Ca^{2+} pump proteins, which has the net effect of increasing basal cytosolic Ca^{2+}.[3] This latter change serves as an adaptive change to increase the duration of myocyte contraction and, thus, the ventricular ejection volume. Changes in cardiac Ca^{2+} physiology are also associated with increased Ca^{2+} oscillations and resulting functional abnormalities.[64] Some of these changes in cardiac Ca^{2+} physiology may also underlie the dihydropyridine-induced reduction in cardiac hypertrophy and ventricular filling rate when they are used to treat hypertension in the elderly.[3,64]

Cellular Changes in the Intima

Significant variation exists in the presence and extent of vascular intima. The intima develops spontaneously in humans after birth and continues to grow through the first 6 to 9 months of age.[65] The most heavily studied animal model for intimal growth is the rat. The rat differs in the relative paucity of vascular intima, although it does appear to increase in incidence with aging.[66] The rat does, however, express intimal proliferation as a response to vascular injury and has, thus, served as a model for intima in stenosis and the restenosis following angioplasty. The new layer of intima formed in response to vascular injury, which consists largely of SMCs, is referred to as neointima.[67]

In rats, there is a migration of undifferentiated "synthetic" SMCs across the internal elastic lamina to form the intima.[67] The formation of the intima occurs in waves that depend upon the time after injury and factors controlling cell replication and migration (i.e, bFGF and PDGF). The matrix is digested by metalloproteinases released by damaged SMCs to make way for the migration of new SMCs. Injury to the epithelium and medial SMCs initiates an initial phase of medial SMC proliferation within the first 24 hours after injury. The first wave is controlled by bFGF released by SMCs that were injured and are dying.[68] Approximately 4 days after the injury, the second wave of SMCs migrate to the luminal surface by crossing the internal elastic lamina.[69] Further replication of these luminal SMCs occurs for weeks to months after the injury, constituting the third wave of intimal proliferation.[70] This phase is followed by a heightened period of responsiveness to hormones and growth factors (i.e., TGF-β, bFGF, and angiotension II) that stimulate the fourth wave of SMC proliferation.[68]

Neointimal cells and endothelial cells produce angiotensin converting enzyme (ACE), which contributes to the degradation of bradykinin. Bradykinin is a potent inhibitor of intima formation, possibly through the release of NO by endothelial cells.[71] The loss of bradykinin, thus, reduces vascular compliance by reducing direct NO-mediated relaxations, and by triggering SMC intimal formation. These basic science findings lead to clinical trials testing the effect of ACE inhibitors on restenosis in humans. The findings were negative, possibly due to major differences between the logic born out of animal models and human production of intima.[71] Nonetheless, there is evidence that ACE inhibitors are advantageous over other antihypertensive agents. For example, there are reports that ACE inhibitors decrease cardiovascular and renal consequences of hypertension, and decrease orthostatic hypertension and the risk of heart failure.[72] Other agents, including somatostatin and heparin analogues, inhibit neointima formation in rats, but once again they are ineffective in altering the course of restenosis in humans.[73] A large part of these clinical failures may reflect the lack of proliferative waves of SMCs following balloon angioplasty in humans, again a difference between animal models and human responses to vascular injury.[71]

Atherosclerotic lesions in humans are reminiscent of intimal changes occurring after vascular lesions in rat models. Atherosclerotic lesions may develop due to local accumulations of glycosamines that promote lipid accumulation.[74] Atherosclerotic intima in humans is characterized by endothelial injury (loss of NO producing cells), or the inactivation of endothelial NO by free radicals, or both.[75] Normally the vessel wall is relaxed due to a steady state production of endothelial NO, but atherosclerosis disrupts endothelial function and impairs this relaxation.

References

1. Lakatta EG: Health disease and cardiovascular aging. In: *Institute of Medicine and National Research Council, Committee on an Aging Society. Health in an Older Society.* Washington, DC: National Academy Press; 73-104, 1985.
2. Lakatta EG: Cardiovascular reserve capacity in older humans. *Aging-Clinical and Exp Res* 6:213-223, 1995.
3. Lakatta EG: Myocardial adaptations in advanced age. *Basic Res Cardiol* 88:125-133, 1993.
4. Cody RJ: Physiological changes due to age: implications for drug-therapy of congestive heart failure. *Drugs and Aging* 3:320-324, 1993.
5. Folkov B, Svanborg A: Physiology of vascular aging. *Physiol Rev* 73:725-764, 1993.
6. Belz GG: Elastic properties and Windkessel function of the human aorta. *Cardiovasc Drugs Ther* 9:78-83, 1995.

7. Rakusan K, Nagai J: Morphometry of arterioles and capillaries in hearts of senescent mice. *Cardiovasc Res* 28:969-972, 1994.
8. Messerli FH: Essential hypertension in the elderly. *Triangle* 24:35-47, 1985.
9. Lakatta EG, Cohen JD, Fleg JL, et al: Hypertension in the elderly: age-related and disease-related complications and therapeutic implications. *Cardiovasc Drugs Ther* 7:643-653, 1993.
10. Marin J: Age-related changes in vascular responses: a review. *Mech Aging Dev* 79:71-114, 1995.
11. Vaitevicius PV, Fleg JL, Engel JH, et al: Effects of age and aerobic capacity on arterial stiffness in healthy adults. *Circulation* 88:1456-1462, 1993.
12. Orlandi A, Mauriello A, Marino B, Spagnoli LG: Age-related modifications of aorta and coronaries in the rabbit: a morphological and morphometrical assessment. *Arch Gerontol Geriat* 17:37-53, 1993.
13. Roman MJ, Pickering TG, Pini R, et al: Prevalence and determinants of cardiac and vascular hypertrophy in hypertension. *Hypertension* 26:369-372, 1995.
14. Cammilleri JP: Structural approach to vascular aging. *Presse Med* 212:1184-1187, 1992.
15. Santilli SM, Stevens RB, Anderson JG, Caldwell MD: The effect of aging on the transarterial wall oxygen gradient. *Ann Vasc Surg* 9:146-151, 1995.
16. Wadsworth RM: Calcium and vascular reactivity in ageing and hypertension. *J Hypertens* 8:975-983, 1990.
17. Epstein FH: Age and the cardiovascular system. *N Engl J Med* 327:1735-1739, 1992.
18. Belmin J, Tedgui A: Aging and the arterial wall. *Med Sci* 9:1068-1078, 1993.
19. Fornieri C, Quaglino D, Mori G: Role of the extracellular matrix in age-related modifications of the rat aorta: ultrastructural, morphometric, and enzymatic evaluations. *Arterioscler Thromb* 12:1008-1016, 1992.
20. Levy BI: Aging in the arterial system. *Presse Med* 21:1200-1203, 1992.
21. Nagasawa S, Handa H, Okumura A, et al: Mechanical properties of human cerebral arteries: effects of age and vascular smooth muscle activation. *Surg Neurol* 12:297-304, 1979.
22. Dollery CM, McEwan JR, Henney AM: Matrix metalloproteinases and cardiovascular disease. *Circ Res* 77:863-868, 1995.
23. Matrisian LM: Metalloproteins and their inhibitors in matrix remodelling. *Trends Genet* 6:121-125, 1990.
24. Sperti G, van Leeuwen RTJ, Quax PHA, et al: Cultured rat aortic vascular smooth muscle cells digest naturally produced extracellular matrix: involvement of plasminogen-dependent and plasminogen independent pathways. *Circ Res* 71:385-392, 1992.
25. Hansson GK, Jonasson L, Seiffert PS, Stemme S: Immune mechanisms in atherosclerosis. *Atherosclerosis* 9:567-578, 1989.
26. Galis ZS, Muszynski M, Suganam K, et al: Cytokine-stimulated human vascular smooth muscle cells synthesize a complement of enzymes required for extracellular matrix digestion. *Circ Res* 75:181-189, 1994.
27. Lindner V, Reidy MA: Proliferation of smooth muscle cells after vascular injury is inhibited by an antibody against basic fibroblast growth factor. *Proc Natl Acad Sci USA* 88:3739-3743, 1991.
28. James TW, Wagner R, White LA, et al: Induction of collagenase and stromelysin gene expression by mechanical injury in vascular smooth muscle-derived cell line. *J Cell Physiol* 157:426-437, 1993.
29. Jiaan DB, Seftel AD, Fogarty J, et al: Age-related increase in an advanced glycation end-product in penile tissue: potential role in erectile dysfunciton. *World J Urol* 13:369-375, 1995.

30. Vlassara H, Striker LJ, Teichberg S, et al: Advanced glycation end-products induce glomerular sclerosis and albuminuria in normal rats. *PNAS* 91:11704-11708, 1995.

31. Ritthaler U, Deng Y, Zhang Y, et al: Expression of receptors for advanced glycation end-products in peripheral occlusive vascular disease. *Am J Pathol* 146:688-698, 1995.

32. Schmidt AM, Hori O, Brett J, et al: Cellular receptors for advanced glycation end-products: implications for induction of oxidant stress and cellular dysfunction in the pathogenesis of vascular lesions. *Arterioscler Thromb* 14:1521-1528, 1994.

33. Lowenson JD, Roher AE, Clarke S: Protein aging: extracellular amyloid formation and intracellular repair. *Trends Cardiovasc Med* 4:3-8, 1994.

34. Pan HY-M, Hoffman RE, Pershe RA, Blaschke TF: Decline in β-adrenergic receptor-mediated vascular relaxation with aging in man. *J Pharmacol Exp Ther* 239:802-807, 1986.

35. Xiao R-P, Lakatta EG: Deterioration of β-adrenergic modulation of cardiovascular function with aging. *Ann Acad Sci* 673:293-310, 1992.

36. Moritoki H, Yoshikawa T, Hisayama T, Takeuchi S: Possible mechanisms of age-associated reduction of vascular relaxation caused by atrial natriuretic peptide. *Eur J Pharmacol* 210:61-68, 1992.

37. White M, Wollmering M, Roden RL, et al: Decreased G-protein functional activity, decreased agonist affinity, and uncoupling of beta-adrenergic receptors from mechanical response with aging in the human heart. *Circulation* 86:766, 1992.

38. Feldman RD, Tan CM, Chorazyczewski J: G-protein alterations in hypertension and aging. *Hypertension* 26:725-732, 1995.

39. Gurdal H, Freidman E, Johnson MD: Effects of dietary restriction on the change in aortic alpha(1)-adrenoceptor mediated responses during aging in Fischer-344 rats. *J Geront* Series A - *Biol Sci* and *Med Sci* 50:B67-B71, 1995.

40. Toda N: Age-related changes in the response to nerve stimulation and catecholamines in isolated monkey cerebral arteries. *Am J Physiol* 260:H1443-H1448, 1991.

41. Benetos A, Huget F, Albaladejo P, et al: Role of adrenergic tone in mechanical and functional properties of carotid artery during aging. *Am J Physiol* 265(suppl 2):H1132-H1138, 1993.

42. Vanhoutte PM, Shepherd JT: Adrenergic pharmacology of human and canine peripheral veins. *Fed Proc* 44:337-340, 1985.

43. Cowen T: Ageing in the autonomic nervous system: a result of nerve-target interactions? A review. *Mech Ageing Dev* 68:163-173, 1993.

44. Buchholz J, Duckles SP: Effect of age on prejunctional modulation of norepinephrine release. *J Pharmacol Exp Ther* 252:159-164, 1990.

45. Murohara T, Yasue M, Ohgushi M, et al: Age related attenuation of the endothelium dependent relaxation to noradrenaline in isolated pig coronary arteries. *Cardiovasc Res* 25:1002-1009, 1991.

46. Moritoki H, Hosoki E, Ishida Y: Age-related decrease in endothelium-dependent dilator response to histamine in rat mesenteric artery. *Eur J Pharmacol* 126:61-67, 1986.

47. Paterno R, Faraci FM, Heistad DD: Age-related changes in release of endothelium derived relaxing factor from the carotid artery. *Stroke* 25:2457-2460, 1994.

48. Shu Y, Scarpace PJ: Forskolin binding sites and G-protein immunoreactivity in rat hearts during aging. *J Cardiovasc Pharmacol* 23:188-193, 1994.

49. La Montagne D, Pohl U, Busse R: Mechanical deformation of vessel wall and shear stress determine the basal release of endothelium-derived relaxing factor in the intact rabbit coronary vascular bed. *Circ Res* 70:123-130, 1992.

50. Gaw AJ, Aberdeen J, Humphrey DP, et al: Relaxation of sheep cerebral arteries by vasoactive intestinal polypeptide and neurogenic stimulation: inhibition by L-N^G monomethyl arginine in endothelium denuded vessels. *Br J Pharmacol* 102:567-572, 1991.
51. Togashi H, Sakuma I, Yoshioka M, et al: Central nervous system action of nitric oxide in blood pressure regulation. *J Pharmacol Exp Ther* 262:343-347, 1992.
52. Bunag RD, Davidow LW: Aging impairs heart rate reflexes earlier in female than male Sprague-Dawley rats. *Neurobiol Aging* 17:87-93, 1996.
53. Vanhoutte PM, Boulanger CM, Mombouli JV: Endothelium-derived relaxing factors and converting enzyme inhibition. *Am J Cardiol* 76:E3-E15, 1995.
54. Ignarro LJ: Biological actions and properties of endothelium-derived nitric oxide formed and released by arteries and vein. *Circ Res* 65:1-21, 1989.
55. Garg UC, Hassid A: Nitric oxide-generating vasodilators and 8-bromo-cyclic guanosine monophosphate inhibit mitogenesis and proliferation of cultured rat vascular smooth muscle cells. *J Clin Invest* 83:1774-1777, 1989.
56. Dinerman JL, Lowenstein CJ, Snyder SH: Molecular mechanisms of nitric oxide regulation: potential relevance to cardiovascular disease. *Circ Res* 73:217-222, 1993.
57. Hynes MR, Duckles SP. Effect of increasing age on the endothelium-mediated relaxation of rat blood vessels in vitro. *J Pharmacol Exp Ther* 241:387-392, 1987.
58. Dohi Y, Kojima M, Sato K, Luscher TF: Age-related changes in vascular smooth muscle and endothelium. *Drugs and Aging* 7:278-291, 1995.
59. Pouregeaud F, Freslon JL: Endothelium function in resistance and coronary arteries of spontaneously hypertensive compared to WKY rats: effects of nitro-L-arginine. In: Sassard J (ed). *Genetic Hypertension*. Vol. 218. Paris: John Libbey Eurotext; 39-41, 1992.
60. Roth GS: Hormone/neurotransmitter action during aging: the calcium hypothesis of impaired signal transduction. *Rev Biol Res Aging* 4:243-252, 1990.
61. Wanstall JC, O'Donnell SR: Influence of age on calcium entry blocking drugs in rat aortae is spasmogen-dependent. *Eur J Pharmacol* 102:282-286, 1989.
62. Dillon JS, Gu XT, Nayler WG: Effect of age and of hypertrophy on cardiac Ca^{2+} antagonist binding sites. *J Cardiovasc Pharmacol* 14:233-240, 1989.
63. Xiao R, Spurgeon HA, O'Connor F, Lakatta EG: Age-associated changes in beta-adrenergic modulation on rat cardiac excitation-contraction coupling. *J Clin Invest* 94:2051-2059, 1994.
64. Hano O, Bogdanov KY, Sakai M, et al: Reduced threshold for myocardial cell calcium intolerance in the rat heart with aging. *Am J Physiol (Heart Circ Physiol)* 38:H1607-H1612, 1995.
65. Velican D, Velican C: Initial thickening in developing coronary arteries and its relevance to atherosclerotic involvement. *Atherosclerosis* 23:345-355, 1988.
66. Chobanian AV, Prescott MF, Haudenschild CC: Recent advances in molecular pathology: the effects of hypertension on the arterial wall. *Exp Molec Pathol* 41:153-169, 1984.
67. Clowes AW, Reidy MA, Clowes MM: Mechanisms of stenosis after arterial injury. *Lab Invest* 49:208-215, 1983.
68. Lindner V, Reidy MA: Proliferation of smooth muscle cells after vascular injury is inhibited by an antibody against basic fibroblast growth factor. *Proc Natl Acad Sci USA* 88:3739-3743, 1991.
69. Clowes AW, Clowes MM, Reidy MA: Kinetics of cellular proliferation after arterial injury. I. Smooth muscle growth in the absence of endothelium. *Lab Invest* 49:327-333, 1983.

70. Clowes AW, Clowes MM, Reidy MA: Kinetics of cellular proliferation after arterial injury. III. Endothelial and smooth muscle growth in chronically denuded vessels. *Lab Invest* 54:295-303, 1986.
71. Schwartz SM, deBois D, O'Brien ERM: The intima: soil for atherosclerosis and restenosis. *Circ Res* 77:445-465, 1995.
72. Israili ZH, Hall WD: ACE inhibitors: differential use in elderly patients with hypertension. *Drugs and Aging* 7:355-371, 1995.
73. Ellis SG, Roubin GS, Wilentz J, et al: Effect of 18- and 24-hour heparin administration for prevention of restenosis after uncomplicated coronary angioplasty. *Am Heart J* 117:777-782, 1989.
74. Camejo G, Olofsson SO, Lopez F, et al: Identification of apo-B-100 segments mediating the interaction of low density lipoproteins with arterial proteoglycans. *Arteriosclerosis* 8:377-388, 1988.
75. Flavahan NA: Atherosclerosis or lipoprotein-induced endothelial dysfunction: potential mechanisms underlying reduction in EDRF/nitric oxide activity. *Circulation* 85:1927- 1938, 1992.

Chapter 5

The Pathophysiology of Vascular Disease by Anatomical Site

Allen W. Averbook, MD
Paul Anain, MD

Atherosclerosis has a predilection for the critical arterial beds: coronary, cerebral, and aortoiliac. Its complications are the major cause of death in North America, as well as in other economically developed societies.[1] Coronary heart disease (CHD) and cerebrovascular disease join cancer as the three leading nontraumatic causes of death in the United States. The development of atherosclerotic lesions follows a variable course dependent on multiple factors.

Anatomical Distribution of Atherosclerotic Lesions

It is quite clear that the bulk of the work in atherosclerotic epidemiology has been concerned with cardiovascular disease, specifically CHD. All of the data compiled to date has demonstrated a common set of precursors to all the major atherosclerotic diseases, whether manifest in the brain, the heart, or peripherally. The relative importance of these different risk factors varies according to the anatomical location and lesion being considered.

Consistent differences in the prevalence and extent of aortic, coronary, and cerebral atherosclerosis have been observed between the Caucasian and African-American populations in New Orleans studied by Strong and Restrepo.[2] Caucasian men developed more extensive fibrous plaques than African-American men in both the aorta and coronary arteries. Conversely, cerebral atherosclerosis was more extensive in African-Americans than in Caucasians in the specimens studied.

DeBakey et al[3] followed the development of atherosclerosis and the course of the disease in human subjects over time. Based on surgical

From: Aronow WS, Stemmer EA, Wilson SE (eds). *Vascular Disease in the Elderly.* Armonk, NY: Futura Publishing Company, Inc., © 1997.

experiences and periodic arteriograms, observations about the distinctive patterns of the disease and their rates of progression were made over several decades. They retrospectively analyzed 13,827 records of patients admitted one or more times between 1948 and 1983 for treatment of atherosclerotic arterial occlusive disease. Five categories of atherosclerotic patterns were used to classify the patients according to the predominant anatomical site or sites of involvement at the time of initial admission:

    I. The coronary arterial bed.
    II. The major branches of the aortic arch.
    III. The visceral arterial branches of the abdominal aorta.
    IV. The terminal abdominal aorta and its major branches.
    V. A combination of two or more of these categories occurring simultaneously.

The analyses performed were based on the assumption that continuity of care necessary for a chronological evaluation of disease progression in each patient was maintained. The study provides a number of interesting and significant observations about the various patterns of atherosclerotic arterial occlusive disease. The data confirms the concept that the occlusive process tends to assume distinctive patterns in the four major arterial beds—the site and distribution of the atherosclerotic disease in each arterial bed being essentially similar. Given that only 5.7% of all patients studied had more than one category of disease on first presentation, the initial clinical manifestation of patients with atherosclerotic occlusive disease tends to reflect predominant involvement of only one of the four categories. Confirming widely held clinical impressions, Category IV distal aorta and branches was the most commonly occurring disease pattern, found in over two fifths of the series, with Categories I (coronary) and II (occurring in almost one third of the series); Category III (abdominal aorta branches) was the least frequent.

Rapid rates of progression (0 to 36 months) were most common in disease of the major branches of the aortic arch (Category II) and terminal aorta (Category IV), whereas moderate (37 to 120 months) and slow (> 120 months) rates of progression were most common in the coronary arterial bed (Category I). The effect of various factors on the development of additional disease was examined by an analysis of variance. The rates of recurrence in the same category or new category did not appear related to sex differences—males and females behaved alike. Age was significant for the development of recurrence in either the same or a new category. The tendency to develop additional disease was greater among younger patients. Increasing age decreased the probability of recurrence; whether this is due to shorter survival times providing less opportunity for recurrence and detection, or to variations in the disease process, remains to be determined.

The interval from initial hospitalization to readmission with a new category was used to classify rates of change in disease. The interval to a new occurrence was shorter in younger patients and longest in Category IV. Gender had no effect on new occurrences, but increasing age significantly decreased the likelihood of new occurrence, as it had for recurrence in the same category.

Patients originally in Category II (branches of the aortic arch) had a somewhat increased tendency to subsequent development of Category IV (terminal aorta) and vice versa. Long-term prognosis of patients who have had surgical intervention obviously depends on the adequacy and the quality of the surgical care, but it is also greatly influenced by the rate of recurrence or progression of the disease. The need for careful and continued follow-up of patients with occlusive arterial disease is evidenced by DeBakey's study which detailed the likelihood of developing a new or recurrent critical lesion. A number of the risk factors for atherosclerosis to be discussed later in this chapter also influence both the patterns and rates of progression of this disease, a factor which was not considered in DeBakey's study and certainly plays a role when evaluating factors predictive of recurrence or progression.

In another study using serial angiography, DeBakey demonstrated that, although taking decades to develop, individual atherosclerotic lesions can progress at a very rapid rate.[4] This is compatible with postmortem examination findings where aortas from patients 65 and older had multiple lesions of several different types and stages within a single segment. They ranged from small focal proliferations of smooth muscle cells to large white fibrous plaques, from fatty spots to large fibrofatty lesions. The cause of death, however, was most often the result of a single specific lesion, progressing rapidly in the course of 1 to 3 years to occlude an artery of critical supply.

The distribution of atherosclerotic plaques in humans tends to be constant and differs from the distribution of fatty streaks. Several major arterial sites are especially prone to developing advanced atherosclerotic lesions, while others are relatively "resistant." The mesenteric, renal, intercostal, and mammary arteries tend to be preserved, while the coronary arteries, carotid bifurcation, infrarenal abdominal aorta, and iliofemoral vessels are particularly susceptible.

Cerebrovascular Disease

Stroke is the third leading cause of death in industrialized countries and a major cause of death in the United States. Each year about 600,000 people in the United States alone suffer a stroke. Of those, greater than 30% result in death and a large number require chronic care. The economic impact and societal burden from this disease process is tremendous.

The most common cause of stroke in the elderly population is atherosclerotic carotid artery disease. The incidence of stroke increases exponentially with age, with studies reporting a one hundredfold increase from the third and fourth decades to the eighth and ninth decades. Ninety-four percent of strokes occur in individuals older than 55 years, while 88% occur among people over the age of 65 years.[5]

Early mapping studies demonstrated that lesions were more common at bifurcations rather than in the straight segments of the coronary and cerebral vasculature.[6,7] Complex and extensive complicated plaques mostly developed within the carotid bifurcation. The distribution of lesions about the bifurcation is probably associated with the particular hemodynamics which exist at the carotid bifurcation. These hemodynamic conditions influence the existing plaques''' overall surface characteristics and contribute to their tendency to ulcerate and embolize.

In a Japanese study of autopsy cases,[8] fatty streaks in the cerebral arteries increased slowly from 1% in the fifth decade to 6.6% in and after the ninth decade of life. Plaque involvement rose rapidly from 7% in the fifth decade. Calcified lesions were first detected in the sixth decade and increased slowly to a maximum of 4.3% after the eighth decade. Ulcerated lesions were found in only eight cases in the ninth decade.

Fabris et al[9] studied 457 patients and found that the prevalence of carotid atherosclerosis was greater in men than in women in all age groups, as was the number of plaques and the severity of vascular narrowing. There was a high prevalence of asymptomatic carotid atherosclerosis in the general population, especially among the very old. Interestingly, the association between risk factors and carotid atherosclerosis was weaker in the elderly than in younger subjects. Nonetheless, risk factors for cerebrovascular disease include age over 55, hypertension (either systolic or diastolic), cigarette smoking, diabetes mellitus, and hypercholesterolemia.

Abdominal Aortic Aneurysm

An abdominal aortic aneurysm (AAA) is defined as a segmental localized dilatation of 50% or greater of the luminal diameter of the aorta. The incidence of AAAs increases with age, and most aneurysms are diagnosed in the sixth and seventh decades of life. In one screening program of men aged 65 to 74 years, the incidence of AAA was 5.4%.[10] Other reported rates in that age group vary from 2% to 5%, but most studies demonstrate a rate reaching 10% in those over 70-years-old. Of note, the incidence of AAAs in the elderly population (age >65) has been increasing over the last 40 years.[11]

In a recent population study, the development of the fibrous plaque of the aorta was seen to be associated with advancing age.[12] In this study, calcified and complicated lesions of the aorta appeared after the age of 40, reaching a peak rate of 42% and 33%, respectively, by the sixth decade; thereafter, only calcified lesions were found in 20% of the cases. This is contrary to the findings of some studies in which calcified and complicated lesions started to appear below 40 years of age, progressing gradually and reaching a rate of 80% after the age of 70 years. Regardless of the actual rate of progression, there is a relationship between aging and the development of fibrous plaques in the aorta.

Most patients with aneurysms have evidence of coexisting atherosclerotic disease and among the risk factors, hypertension has been strongly associated with their development. One study suggested that screening programs should be directed at the population greater than 65 years old with a diastolic blood pressure over 95 mm Hg, given the high incidence of aneurysmal disease in this elderly group.[13] In another study, the effects of aging on aortic morphology in populations with high and low prevalence of hypertension and atherosclerosis was performed via postmortem exam.[14] It was apparent that aging itself had a marked effect on aortic morphology (aortic circumference and intimal thickness) separate from but modified by both hypertension and the presence of atherosclerotic changes. More so, this study suggested that a decrease in tensile strength with advancing age, rather than atherosclerosis alone, is a contributor to the formation of AAAs. Hypertension was an independent contributor to the identified age-related increase in aortic circumference and intimal thickness.

Aneurysm formation may be a later stage of the atherosclerotic degenerative process, but other factors influencing wall strength also play a role. As shown by biochemical studies, decreased quantities of both elastin and collagen are present in the wall of aneurysms as compared to normal aortas.[15] This along with other nutritive changes possibly influenced by the aging process, and other risk factors such as hypertension, may play a role in the development of aneurysmal disease in the elderly population.

Combined Segmental Arterial Disease

In a Chinese retrospective pathological survey,[16] the prevalence of lesions with stenosis greater 50% in the 1,508 aortas examined was highest in the abdominal and lowest in the ascending aorta. The prevalence of lesser stenotic grades was highest in the ascending and lowest in the abdominal aorta. The prevalence of fatty streaks and fibrous plaques was highest in the ascending aorta, while that of complicated lesions was highest in the abdominal aorta. Thus, atherosclerotic lesions were most severe in the abdominal aorta and less so in the thoracic and ascending aorta. Aortic lesions tend to be most prominent around the ostia of its major branches. Although plaques are regularly found in the adult human thoracic aorta, they are often less abundant, more discrete, less complicated, and less calcific than in the abdominal aortic segment of the same individual. Significant occlusive lesions of the thoracic aorta do not develop, and aneurysms of the thoracic aorta are unusual. The infrarenal abdominal aortic segment is particularly prone to early plaque development, occlusive disease, the development of medial atrophy, calcification, and aneurysmal dilatation with mural thrombus formation.

These differences between the thoracic and abdominal aorta may relate to variations in flow rates between the two segments (relatively high flow velocity in the thoracic aorta, and relatively reduced flow rates in the infrarenal abdominal aorta), as well as to the differences in vascular supply; the thoracic aorta has intramural vaso vasorum, whereas the wall of the abdominal aorta is relatively avascular. In contrast to aortic aneurysmal, femoropopliteal, and combined segmental disease, studies have demonstrated that atherosclerotic aortoiliac disease occurs more often in a younger population.[17] Tobacco use may play a critical role in the development of aortoiliac atheromatous disease in the younger population (<60 years old).[18]

In the Japanese study noted earlier,[8] atherosclerosis was more severe in the aorta than in the cerebral arteries of all age groups and this disparity became more conspicuous with age. The involvement of the aorta by atherosclerotic lesions increased linearly with age, from 27.5% in the fifth decade to 68.9% after the age of 80. Most of the increase resulted from the development of plaques which occupied 20.7% of the intimal surface in the sixth decade and more than a third, 36.6%, in the eighth decade. More complex ulcerated and calcified lesions increased gradually to a maximum of about 10% of the intimal surface after the age of 80. The surface involvement of the aorta by fatty streaks remained unchanged in each decade of life.

In general, after the infrarenal aorta and the coronary vessels, the most heavily involved vessels in decreasing order are the popliteal arteries, the descending thoracic aorta, the internal carotids, and the vessels of the circle of Willis; but, there does appear to be a subgroup with more severe atheromatous involvement in the circle of Willis than in the coronary vessels.[19] There is no good explanation for the discrepancies in involvement between the coronary arteries and other aortic branches. Vessels of the upper extremities are usually spared, as are mesenteric arteries and renal arteries, except at their ostia. Differences in hydrostatic pressure and durations in flow rate secondary to varying amounts of physical activity may contribute to the propensity for lower extremity arteries to be more commonly involved by atherosclerotic plaques than vessels of similar size in the upper extremities. Sedentary lifestyles tend to favor low flow rates (secondary to decreased muscular contractions) leading to increased plaque deposition in vessels of the lower extremities and infrarenal abdominal aorta. Other risk factors such as tobacco use and hypertriglyceridemia may also contribute to this pattern of presentation by promoting intra-arterial thrombosis.

The superficial femoral artery is the most commonly involved vessel of the lower extremities, often with multiple stenotic lesions, while the profunda femoris tends to spared. Approximately two thirds of patients with atherosclerotic disease affecting the lower extremity have various combinations of multisegmental disease.[20] The commonly occurring clinical patterns are combined involvement of the aortoiliac and femoral segments, or combined femoral and tibial arterial occlusions. It has been estimated that 3% of this group of patients will have diffuse, extensive involvement of the aorta, iliacs, femorals, and tibial arteries.

Involvement of the deep femoral artery occurs in less than 15% of patients undergoing arterial reconstructive surgery.[21]

Patients with combined segment arterial disease (CSAD) tend to be older than those with localized disease (mean age 64 compared to 56 years) and twice as many patients are diabetic.[22] These patients also have involvement of the coronary and cerebral vessels to a greater degree than patients who have localized aortoiliac disease.[20] Their life expectancy is decreased by approximately 10 years when coronary artery disease (CAD) coexists, and an additional 15 years by diabetes.[23]

Age seems to have a greater influence on the progression of atheromatous changes in the suprapopliteal (large vessel segment) as compared to the more distal vessels. In a study by Crique et al,[24] the prevalence of distal lesions at age 60 or over remained the same (between 10% and 15%), while the prevalence of large vessel involvement increased progressively with age from less than 3% before the age of 60 to 12% at the age of 70 and 22% after the age of 75.

Women with CSAD are older, usually hypertensive (83% versus 23% in women with localized disease) and often have CAD disease (37% versus 0%). Patients with CSAD are more prone to limb-threatening ischemia; patients who have aortoiliac disease and ischemic lesions in the feet will almost always have associated distal arterial stenoses.[25] The deep femoral artery assumes a role of critical importance in patients with CSAD, since the normal anatomy of this artery provides the basis of a rich collateral system that can bypass many levels of iliac, femoral, and popliteal obstruction.[23]

The Framingham Study suggested that hypertension is the principal vascular risk for all the complications of atherosclerosis, including arterial disease of the lower limbs.[26] Because of methodological flaws, it may have underestimated the prevalence of lower extremity arterial disease in the elderly (age >60) population; studies using noninvasive methods have demonstrated a prevalence greater than 20% as compared to Framingham's 2% to 10%.[27] In one study, the prevalence of lower extremity arterial disease in the elderly increased with age, this effect being more pronounced in women than in men, and was associated with a history of current smoking.[28] Lower extremity arterial disease is associated with a four to five relative risk for all-cause mortality and progresses over time, leading to loss of mobility, and gangrene or amputation in over 25% of those affected. Given its greater prevalence in the elderly population, the importance of early recognition of both the disease process and associated risk factors is imperative.

Risk Factors and Atherosclerosis

As already demonstrated, there is a close relationship between age and the incidence and severity of atherosclerosis in both sexes.[16,29,30] Death rates from CHD rise with each decade of life up to age 85. The death rate from CHD among Caucasian males ages 25 to 34 is about 10 in 100,000; between ages 55 to 64, it has increased tenfold to nearly 1,000 in 100,000. It is interesting though that death due to acute myocardial infarction (MI) seems to decline slightly after age 75.

Aortic fatty streaks are present in many children under the age of 3, and in all children over the age of 3. The relationship between the prevalence of atherosclerosis and age may be due to the time required for the lesions to develop, but as pointed out by Tejada and Gore,[29] other factors and the duration of exposure to risk factors possibly accelerate atherogenesis. According to Strong et al,[30] involvement with aortic fatty streaks reaches a maximum during the 25- to 34-year age span, decreasing in extent thereafter, as fatty streaks are gradually replaced by involvement with more advanced lesions. The theory that fatty streaks are precursors of fibrous plaques in all instances remains uncertain.[16]

The early landmark article by Enos et al[31] showed that atherosclerotic changes appear in the coronary arteries years or decades before the age at which CHD becomes a clinically recognized problem. Atherosclerotic lesions in the coronary arteries, some causing narrowing or even occlusion, were present in young men in their twenties and thirties who had no symptoms of CHD. The lesions were commonly located at or near points of bifurcation.

An early study by Strong and McGill[32] demonstrated that coronary atherosclerosis is the significant determinant of CHD in a population, a crucial underlying assumption of many studies which have used the severity of clinically manifested CHD as representative of the severity and extent of atherosclerotic disease. Risk factors for the development of the arterial lesions of atherosclerosis including peripheral vascular and cerebrovascular disease have been shown to be similar to those for clinically overt CHD in both the Framingham Study and other retrospective studies.[33-35]

As early as 1980, a decreasing incidence of coronary atherosclerosis associated with declines in mortality rates from CHD became evident.[36-38] Between 1968 and 1976, CHD mortality decreased 20.7% in adults aged 30 to 74 in the United States.[39] These statistics raised many important questions as to the nature of risk factors and specifically which ones are most important in influencing the development of coronary atherosclerosis. The Minnesota Heart Survey[40] suggested that both preventive efforts and improved medical care had an impact on reducing CHD mortality in the Minneapolis-St. Paul area between 1970 and 1980. Despite these encouraging trends, the death rate for complications of atherosclerosis in the United States is still very high.

While never denying the role that genetic factors must play, epidemiological studies have indicated the possible role of diet, lifestyle, and personal habits as being strongly influential in the pathogenesis and progression of this disease. The downward trend in CHD mortality may be related to the concomitant improvement seen in multiple cardiovascular risk factors.[41]

Risk factors may be independent causal agents, intervening variables, or indicators of other more fundamental associations. The Pooling

Project,[42] which pooled the findings of six major United States studies dealing with several thousand middle-aged American men free of clinical CHD at initial examination, described three principle risk factors: hypercholesterolemia, hypertension, and cigarette smoking. Other important risk factors have emerged, including: diabetes mellitus, male sex, age, obesity, physical inactivity, certain types of behavioral patterns, familial history, hypertriglyceridemia, alcohol consumption, and plasma fibrinogen level. The presence of more than one risk factor for CHD in men aged 30 to 59 had a synergistic effect in the Pooling Project.[43,44] Therefore, when evaluating an individual's risk for atherosclerotic disease, the presence of risk factor clusters correlates with a particularly high risk of CHD.

Sexual and Racial Predisposition

Early population studies hinted at the varying influences of different risk factors that, at the time, were not well defined.[45-47] The Multiple Risk Factor Intervention Trial[48] screening program subsequently demonstrated that the racial differences in CHD mortality between Caucasions and African-Americans may relate to specific risk factor differences between the two racial groups. Results comparing atherosclerotic lesions in 25- to 44-year-old men from Tokyo and New Orleans supported the findings of earlier studies.[49,50] The coronary arteries and abdominal aortas of both African-American and Caucasian men from New Orleans were significantly more involved with raised, atherosclerotic lesions, than those of men from Tokyo. These results parallel the reported differences in mortality from CHD between the two countries. Other studies indicate that atherosclerosis is relatively milder in the Japanese living in Japan than among those living in Hawaii, or Western Caucasians.[47,51-53] These differences in severity of atherosclerosis between men in different geographical locations, but of the same racial stock, demonstrate the important contributions that environmental factors must make in the development and expression of the disease within populations.

Genetics also play a significant role in determining the degree, time course, severity, and anatomical pattern of the atherosclerotic process.[54] The extent to which both environmental and genetic factors each influence the development and expression of atherosclerotic disease is unclear—interaction of both though, is certain.

Male Sex

The association between gender and risk for atherosclerosis is not a trivial one. One of the few prospective studies of a general population that evaluated cardiovascular disease in female as well as male subjects was the Framingham Study.[55] On the average, symptomatic CAD appeared 10 years later in United States women than in men. When basing the comparison on proven MIs, this difference between the sexes was increased to approximately 20 years. Also, the factors that influence the development of raised atherosclerotic lesions seem to act differently in the coronary arteries and in the aorta, as well as in the two sexes.[16,30,45] While the incidence of CHD is much lower in women than in men for each of the four leading risk factors studied in the Framingham Study, the relationship of these risks to the incidence of CHD is at least as strong for women as for men.[56] Interestingly, the sex differential is less apparent in non-Caucasians.[30,45] Sex differences in the extent of atherosclerotic lesions are striking in Caucasians and minimal in African-Americans. These differences are probably related to the influence of other ethnic or racially related risk factors.

Hypertension

Elevated blood pressure, systolic or diastolic, is related to an increased incidence of CHD, as well as to other manifestations of atherosclerotic disease.[53,57-60] It has been strongly associated with CHD after stratification for other risk factors.[58] In the Framingham Study,[57] men aged 45 to 62 with blood pressures exceeding 160/95 had more than five times the incidence of CHD than did normotensive men (BP 140/90 or less). Also, the relationship between blood pressure and the risk of developing CHD was found to be as strong in women as it was in men.

Hypertension is a consistent and powerful contributor to coronary disease with casual blood pressure readings at any age being potent predictors of CHD.[42,55] The controversy persists though, as to which, if either, is individually more influential—systolic or diastolic blood pressure. The traditional teaching that the diastolic measurement is the more important component may not be valid.[60-63] The risk of cardiovascular death increases stepwise with the level of blood pressure beginning at quite low levels. There is a smooth direct linear relationship between the levels of blood pressure and the risk of morbidity and mortality from cardiovascular disease (as well as from other atherosclerotic diseases) over the entire range of values measured under casual conditions; there is no specific critical value above which the risk of atherosclerotic disease increases and below which it decreases (Figure 1).[56]

It is noteworthy then that in the VA Cooperative Study,[61] antihypertensive therapy for diastolic blood pressures exceeding 104 mm Hg was shown to reduce the incidence of strokes and possibly also of CHD, but the benefits of treating mild hypertension, defined as a diastolic blood pressure between 90 and 104 mm Hg, with a subsequent decrease in morbidity and mortality was not demonstrated.[64,65] Whether or not lowering blood pressure in those with mild hypertension will reduce mortality from MIs and coronary disease in general remains unclear, but a recent study has demonstrated that borderline hypertension is clearly

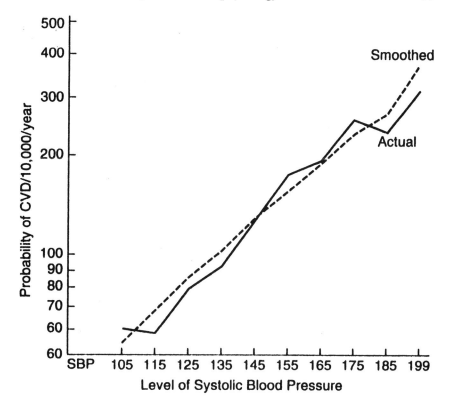

Figure 1. Actual and smoothed probability of cardiovascular disease according to blood pressure (BP) levels in men and women aged 45 to 64 years; the Framingham Study. (Reproduced with permission from Reference 55.)

associated with other risk factors for cardiovascular disease and structural changes of the heart and blood vessels.[66]

As an individual predictor, blood pressure has been found to be more reliable than the level of cholesterol or cigarette smoking, especially after the age of 45. Other risk factors associated with CHD, though, also affect the blood pressure and its prognostic significance. For example, obesity and alcohol intake both cause a significant increase in blood pressure, while regular exercise in men over 20 years old is associated with a decrease in their blood pressure.[67] These interactions must always be considered whenever only a single risk factor is being utilized to detect persons at high risk for cardiovascular disease.

The means by which hypertension induces atherogenesis is unclear. Humoral mediators of blood pressure inducing cellular changes, or the shear stress of the flow of blood at selected anatomical sites within the arterial tree, resulting in focally altered endothelium and the development of atherosclerotic lesions, are both mechanisms that have been proposed. The increased incidence of atherosclerotic vascular disease in the elderly may in part be related to the duration of such effects over the time frame of one's life.

Cigarette Smoking

The risk of cardiovascular death is high in the smoking population (Figure 2). Cigarette smoking has been strongly and independently linked to CHD.[59,60,68] Its association with the extent and character of atherosclerotic peripheral arterial occlusive disease, aortic disease, and cerebrovascular disease is also well documented. In combination with other risk factors, there is a notable synergy yielding increased mortality

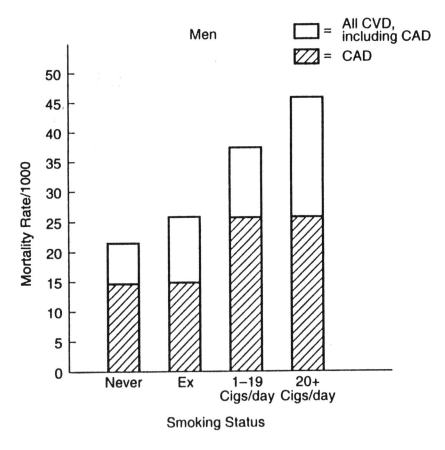

Figure 2. Age-ajusted mortality rates in men after 6 years for coronary artery disease (CAD) and cardiovascular disease (CVD) by smoking status. (Reproduced with permission from Criqui MH: Epidemiology of atherosclerosis: an updated overview. *Am J Cardiol* 57:180, 1986.

from CHD.[69] The association between passive exposure to cigarette smoke and CHD mortality and morbidity is also becoming increasingly apparent.[70]

In the Framingham Study's 30-year follow-up, the risk of having a first-time major coronary event in men who smoke one or more packs of cigarettes per day was two to three times greater than the risk for nonsmokers, especially in younger men (Table 1).[71] At autopsy, the degree of aortic and coronary atherosclerosis has been shown to be greater in smokers than in nonsmokers.[72]

The positive association between cigarette smoking, carotid atherosclerosis, and stroke in men, after controlling for the effect of other risk factors, has been well documented.[73,74] The 1986 Honolulu Heart Program Study[75] firmly demonstrated a strong relationship between cigarette smoking and stroke in men, but it wasn't until two more recently published studies that a significant causal role for cigarette smoking in stroke in middle-aged women was demonstrated; the relative risk for fatal stroke was consistent in magnitude with that reported for men.[76] In both peripheral arterial occlusive disease and CHD, the current number of cigarettes smoked each day is directly related to the risk of development and progression of the disease. A graded dose-response relationship between smoking and cerebrovascular disease has also been well established in both sexes, independent of both age and hypertensive status.[77] Those smoking more than 40 cigarettes per day have nearly a two times greater risk of stroke than those people smoking fewer than 10 cigarettes per day.

The risk of stroke is still high among ex-smokers as compared to nonsmokers, especially in the first 2 years after smoking cessation, although it is lower than that for current smokers (Figure 3). By 2 years after quitting, the risk decreases significantly, and within 5 years after stopping, reverts to the lower levels seen in nonsmokers, a little sooner than that noted in CHD.[77] Through ultrasonography, it has also been demonstrated that the development of carotid atherosclerosis may progress more slowly in people who have quit smoking, as compared to those who continue to smoke, even after taking into account the effect of other risk factors.[78]

Cessation of smoking will also dramatically reduce the rate of cardiovascular death in persons of all ages.[79-82] There is consistent evidence that within 1 year of quitting tobacco, the risk of CHD attributable to smoking drops to approximately 50% that of those who continue to smoke, but the reduced risk only approximates, but never quite equals, that of lifelong nonsmokers, and only after a decade or more according to most studies.[69,83] The cardiovascular risk declines more rapidly than for that of lung cancer or emphysema.[69] The effect of cigarette smoking on both stroke and cardiovascular disease is due predominantly, if not entirely, to current or very recent smoking.[76] This may be a direct manifestation of cigarettes' effect on thrombotic mechanisms.

A definite relationship between cigarette smoking and fibrinogen has been established.[84] Age-adjusted fibrinogen values in the Framing-

Table 1
Risk of Cardiovascular Disease by Cigarette Smoking: 30-Year Follow-Up on the Framingham Study

No. of Cigarettes per Day	Men				Women			
	Age 35–64		Age 65–94		Age 35–64		Age 65–94	
	No. of Events	Age-Adjusted Rate/1000[b]	No. of Events	Age-Adjusted Rate/1000[b]	No. of Events	Age-Adjusted Rate/1000[c]	No. of Events	Age-Adjusted Rate/1000[c]
None	236	12	237	38	276	8	326	26
1–10	47	13	32	36	60	8	35	25
11–20	212	23	43	39	86	10	40	34
21–40	143	21	26	33	33	11	5	12
41–90	27	27	3	81	3	26	0	—
All	665	17	341	38	458	9	406	26

[a] Cardiovascular disease: coronary heart disease, stroke, cardiac failure, peripheral arterial disease.
[b] $p < .001$.
[c] Not significant.
(Reproduced with permission from Reference 71.)

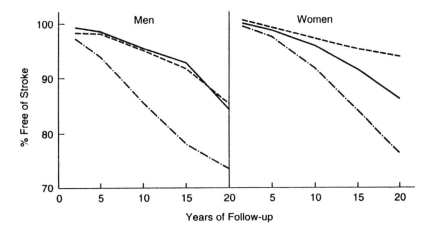

Figure 3. Survival free of stroke in male and female cigarette smokers (**dotted line**), nonsmokers (**solid line**), and former smokers (**dashed line**) aged 60 years, using the Cox proportional hazard regression model. (Reproduced with permission from Reference 77.)

Table 2
Risk of Cardiovascular Disease by Fibrinogen Level and Smoking Status: 14-Year Follow-up on the Framingham Study (Subjects 48 to 80 Years of Age)

	14-Year Age-Adjusted Rate/1000			
	Men		*Women*	
Fibrinogen (mg/dL)	*Nonsmokers[a]*	Cigarette Smokers[b]	*Nonsmokers[b]*	Cigarette Smokers[a]
126–264	318	230	176	213
265–310	295	421	209	165
312–696	397	486	297	343

[a] Trend not significant.
[b] Trend significant at $p < .05$.
(Reproduced with permission from Reference 71.)

ham Study were significantly higher in cigarette smokers than in nonsmokers, and they increased with the amount of tobacco smoked by each sex.[71] The risk of CHD increased with increasing fibrinogen values in both smokers and nonsmokers. There was no evidence of a greater impact in smokers than in nonsmokers (Table 2).

Interestingly, multivariate analysis indicated that fibrinogen had a stronger independent contribution than cigarettes to the occurrence of cardiovascular disease. A direct reversible relationship, though, was suggested, in that fibrinogen values increased in proportion to the amount smoked. The relationship of cigarette smoking to the occurrence of atherosclerotic cardiovascular disease must be attributable, to some extent, to the effect of smoking on fibrinogen levels, which in turn enhances thrombotic tendencies leading to occlusive clinical events. Cigarette smoking exerts both a long-term effect (possibly via an atherogenic mechanism), as well as a short-term triggering effect; it appears to exert this short-term effect by its influence on the incidence of sudden death triggering lethal events in those who already have a compromised coronary circulation.[85] This may occur through a thrombotic or hypoxic mechanism.[83] Nonetheless, cigarette smoking should still be considered an independent risk factor in the development of atherosclerosis, since various chemical components and by-products of tobacco are known to have a direct effect on the cells of the heart, the coronary arteries, and the blood.[83,86-90] The mechanism by which cigarette smoking stimulates atherogenesis is controversial.[83,91-93]

Hyperlipidemia

Multiple prospective population studies have supported the thesis that elevated serum lipid concentrations contribute to the development of atherosclerosis.[59,60,94,95] Populations with relatively high levels of cholesterol have a higher mortality from CHD, and the probability of developing an MI increases in proportion to the plasma cholesterol level. The theory that genetic factors are the predominant determinants of plasma lipids metabolism has not been supported by studies of population groups.[96] The level of plasma cholesterol is measurably influenced by the dietary intake of total calories of cholesterol, saturated fat, and polyunsaturated fat. The hypothesis that increased triglycerides are an independent cause of CHD remains controversial. While some studies initially did not support this relationship, more recent prospective studies do.[97-106]

There are five major groups of cholesterol-bound lipoproteins, each with a different prognostic significance. Of these, elevated low-density lipoprotein (LDL) has the strongest association with coronary disease in both men and women, and high-density lipoprotein (HDL) has an action opposite to that of LDL.[98] Patients with increased LDL-C levels, and particularly increased LDL apolipoprotein B, have the greatest risk of premature atherosclerosis and present the greatest therapeutic challenge.[107] Very low-density lipoprotein (VLDL) is strongly correlated with triglyceride levels.

The development, progression, and regression of atherosclerosis is closely related to the plasma cholesterol level. There is a direct relationship between diet, hyperlipidemia, and the development of CHD.[107] Dietary cholesterol intake from 0 to 600 mg per day correlates closely with plasma cholesterol levels. Interestingly, emigres, from populations with low plasma cholesterol levels to ones in which levels are high, attain cholesterol levels and the associated increased incidence of coronary disease comparable to that of their host populations within a few years of their emigration, as seen in Japanese emigres to the United States.[108]

The North American population's intake of cholesterol has been declining secondary to increasing public awareness, and the polyunsaturate/saturate ratio in dietary fat has been increasing. Concurrently, there has been a definite downward trend in plasma cholesterol levels of adult Americans. These trends have all coincided with a significant reduction (25% to 27%) in CHD mortality among persons 36 to 74 years of age, further supporting the possibility of a causal relationship.[109-111] Dietary therapy can play a major role in reducing CHD events and decreasing progression of coronary atherosclerosis. Dietary modification studies have demonstrated that sustained decreases in serum cholesterol levels of 10% to 20% can be achieved by diet manipulation alone in dissimilar study groups.[94,112,113]

Increased dietary cholesterol usually results in an increase in LDL cholesterol levels, with a lesser increase in HDL cholesterol levels. Serum levels of HDL are inversely related to the risk of coronary disease—the higher the level, the lower the risk of death from heart disease.[98,114-116] In the Framingham Study, HDL cholesterol was a more important predictor of CHD than either total or LDL cholesterol. This was true for both men and women, where for each 1% rise in HDL there was a 2% reduction in the incidence of CAD.[98] More recently, findings have suggested that total LDL and HDL cholesterol levels in men 40 to 69 years of age with and without preexisting cardiovascular disease predict subsequent mortality.[117]

The epidemiological association between increased incidence of atherosclerosis and the increased intake of fat, with concomitant changes in plasma LDL and HDL levels, is very strong. Aside from dietary influences on HDL, alcohol consumption, cigarette smoking, obesity, and exercise may influence the serum level of HDL.[87] Population studies have also shown that HDL levels are increased by alcohol consumption in a dose-response manner, and alcoholics often have very high HDL levels.[118,119] This may explain the protective effect for CHD observed in some studies with moderate alcohol consumption.[120] It is not clear, though, which HDL subfraction is most affected by alcohol.[92,121] One prospective study suggested that with moderate alcohol consumption in middle-aged women, the risks of CHD and ischemic stroke is decreased, but the risk of subarachnoid hemorrhage is increased.[122] This does not imply that drinking heavily is healthy. CHD and related cardiovascular deaths, as well as stroke and hypertension, are more commonly observed with excessive alcohol consumption when compared to those who drink moderately, probably indicating a complex interaction of mechanisms and multiple risk factors.[120]

Many intervention trials have been conducted to determine whether the incidence of CHD can be lowered by reducing total cholesterol, and specifically LDL, with diet and/or drug therapy, and in so doing further strengthen the thesis that there is a relationship between hypercholesterolemia and CHD. Most of the early studies were conducted using a population of middle-aged hypercholesterolemic men, but more recent ones have included an older population and both sexes. The results of these clinical trials are in agreement with predictions from some much longer running epidemiological studies such as the Framingham Study.[123-135] In all of these studies, the reduction of cardiovascular risk was greatest in those patients with the greatest decreases in total cholesterol levels in a graded fashion. In the more recent trials, this risk reduction was shown to apply even to a population of both sexes over the age of 59 and, of great importance, demonstrated a reduction in total mortality with lipid-lowering therapy, something that the earlier studies could not demonstrate.[132,134] These results are now being correlated with angiographically proven slowing and, in some cases, prevention of development of coronary atherosclerosis in both native coronary vessels and saphenous vein bypass grafts.[128,129,131,136] These findings support the argument for aggressive management of lipids in the secondary prevention of ischemic heart disease, although a longer follow-up period is required to truly validate these results.

Results of the major clinical trials of cholesterol lowering are consistent in showing that the greater the degree of cholesterol lowering, the greater the reduction in CHD risk. The results of these studies can be fitted to a regression line relating cholesterol reduction to decreased CHD risk. As a rough rule of thumb, a 1% reduction in cholesterol reduced the risk of developing coronary disease by 2%. Interestingly, in the Helsinki Heart Study,[137] there was a 4% fall in CAD for every 1% fall in cholesterol. This correlated with a 10% rise in HDL levels and an 8% fall in LDL. In the National Heart, Lung, and Blood Institute (NHLBI) Type II Coronary Intervention Study,[128,129] progression of coronary disease was inversely associated with an increase in HDL-C and a decrease in LDL-C levels. Therefore, in men at high risk for CHD with elevated LDL levels, reduction of total cholesterol through a decrease in LDL levels diminishes the incidence of CHD morbidity and mortality.

Many dietary studies give suggestive, but inconclusive results. Changes in recent diet habits that do not represent lifetime patterns may have little overall impact. Development of atherosclerosis occurs over decades, diluting the significance of many studies which analyze diet and other factors over brief intervals. Some authors believe that recent prospective intervention studies have failed to demonstrate statistically significant associations between diet and CHD risk. They feel that reduced mortality from CHD may be due to a reduction in a variety of risk factors not accounted for, including cigarette smoking.[138]

The intervention studies demonstrated that reduction of plasma cholesterol benefits the high-risk population. Yet, most of the attributable cases of CHD in the population arise from people whose cholesterol values are average, not from the few in whom the concentration is conspicuously high. These trials are relevant to cholesterol-lowering dietary changes in the general population.

The incidence of coronary atherosclerosis in a specific population has been found to vary directly with the mean serum cholesterol level,

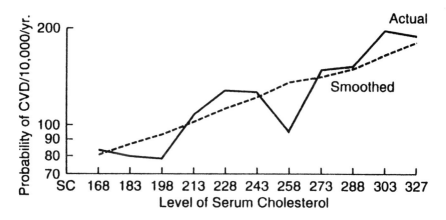

Figure 4. Actual and smoothed probability of cardiovascular disease (CVD) according to serum cholesterol level in men and women aged 45 to 64 years; the Framingham Study. (Reproduced with permission from Reference 55.)

regardless of the population examined.[139] Early on in the Framingham Study[140] in men and women 35 to 44 years of age, serum cholesterol levels of 265 mg/dL or over were associated with a five times higher risk of developing CAD than were those with levels below 220 mg/dL. The Pooling Project[42] supported these findings, suggesting that rates of CHD are relatively constant for cholesterol levels up to 200 to 220 mg/dL, but above this threshold range, the risk for CHD increases as cholesterol concentrations rise.

These findings have been qualified by the Multiple Risk Factor Intervention Trial (MRFIT)[141] which consisted of a large male sample. The unequivocal results were that the relationship between serum cholesterol and CHD is not a threshold one, but rather, a continuously graded one in which the risk of fatal CHD increases with serum cholesterol levels of about 180 mg/dL and greater in a gradual manner (Figure 4). Importantly, the MRFIT has demonstrated an opposite relationship between hemorrhagic stroke and serum cholesterol levels as compared to nonhemorrhagic strokes, which share a similar association with serum cholesterol as does CHD.[142] The basis of the relationship, possibly arising from other intervening variables including hypertension, alcohol consumption, and platelet aggregability, among others, must be considered.

Diabetes Mellitus

The association between diabetes mellitus and an increased incidence of atherosclerosis, MI, atherothrombotic brain infarction, and intermittent claudication is well documented.[56,143] The Framingham Study[144] showed that the risk of cardiovascular disease and death was greater in diabetic women than in men. It appears that risk is mediated in part by the association of diabetes with hypertension and hyperlipidemia, but it is reported that diabetes is an independent risk factor for CHD and stroke.[144,145] The mechanism, though, is poorly understood.

More peripheral arterial, coronary, and cerebrovascular disease develops in diabetics than in nondiabetics. There is a twofold increase in incidence of MI in diabetics as compared with nondiabetics, and an increased tendency toward cerebral thrombosis, intermittent claudication, and an eightfold to one hundred-fiftyfold increased frequency of gangrene of the lower extremity. The difficulty though, arises in trying to differentiate between the contribution of the microvascular changes associated with diabetes mellitus and that of atherosclerosis to the development of these complications.

A relationship between plasma insulin and triglyceride concentrations has been known to exist for some time.[146] There is an increased risk of CHD in persons with hyperinsulinemia associated with elevated plasma triglyceride, low plasma HDL, and elevated blood pressure.[147,148] Plasma insulin level has been shown to be a strong predictor of the HDL_2 cholesterol level in specific populations, suggesting a causal relationship, although this may be more related to the obese rather than the diabetic state.[149] There is no consistency in the studies evaluating whether elevated concentrations of plasma cholesterol and lipoproteins occur in diabetics whose concentrations of blood and urine glucose are carefully regulated. Also, evidence suggests a decreased concentration of HDL levels in diabetics and a high prevalence of hypertension associated with hyperglycemia, raising doubts as to the independent influence that the hyperglycemia of diabetes has on the progression of atherosclerosis.

Obesity and Physical Activity

Obesity is correlated with an increased risk of dying from the clinical complications of atherosclerosis. Obese individuals tend to have severe hyperlipidemia with decreased HDL levels, sedentary lifestyles, hypertension, and diabetes mellitus.[114,150] The Framingham Study, though, suggests that obesity is a risk factor independent of such associations, a finding which has been inconsistently supported in the literature.[151,152] Recent prospective studies have demonstrated the influence of obesity on the development of CHD in women. After controlling for multiple risk factors, being even mildly to moderately overweight increased the risk of coronary disease in middle-aged women.[153] Also, it is upper body obesity rather than total body weight alone that is associated with an increased risk of CHD, possibly through an HDL_2 mechanism.[149] There is little doubt that obese persons have an increased risk for CHD, but obesity is not as consistently predictive of ischemic heart disease risk in Caucasian men as would be expected if it were an independent risk factor.[154] A significant gain in weight may indirectly affect the atherosclerotic process by worsening one or more of the many atherogenic traits with which it has been associated, this effect being more pronounced in Caucasians than African-Americans.[155] Also, the debate as to whether or not obesity paradoxically has a protective effect against cardiovascular disease in persons with hypertension continues to be waged.[156,157]

The loss of substantial body fat through either dieting or exercising alters plasma lipoprotein concentrations favorably, decreases triglyceride levels, and raises HDL and HDL_2 cholesterol levels.[158] This has great significance, given the previously discussed findings of the Helsinki Heart Study. Even without any associated weight loss, the beneficial effect of fitness, if not moderate exercise alone, in decreasing the mortality rate from heart disease, has been demonstrated.[159,160] In the Framingham Study,[161] the most sedentary men had about three times the risk for cardiovascular disease as compared to the 15% most physically active men. There was a trend of improved overall cardiovascular and coronary mortality with increased levels of physical activity at all ages, including the elderly.

Elevations of serum HDL, specifically the protective HDL_2 subfraction, is seen in both weight loss and exercise.[92,150,162,163] This may account for the frequent observation in population studies that higher activity levels appear to be protective against CHD.[164] It is also known that other consequences of physical activity may protect from the effects of ischemic change, including increases in heart volume and mass, development of collaterals, and a decrease in heart rate.

Thrombosis

A thrombotic tendency may also be associated with the development of atherosclerosis as already alluded to in the discussion of cigarette smoking. Moderate alcohol consumption may affect the clotting system and exercise may stimulate fibrinolysis.[165] Certain fish oils may reduce platelet aggregation and exert favorable effects on lipoprotein levels. The omega-3 fatty acids competitively inhibit synthesis of thromboxane A_2 in the membrane of platelets, a vasoconstrictor that promotes platelet aggregation.[166,167] The net effect is decreased platelet reactivity and documented increased bleeding times as is seen in the Eskimos, but the overall effect of the omega-3 fatty acids on hemostasis remains unclear. The antiplatelet effects of fish oils appear to be dose dependent.

Growing evidence points to the interdependence between clotting factors and lipids. Increased blood viscosity and plasma fibrinogen, along with a major fibrinolytic inhibitor alpha2-antiplasmin, have been reported in type II hyperlipoproteinemia.[168] Fibrinogen levels have also been correlated with serum cholesterol.[169] The Framingham Study strongly supports the finding that elevated fibrinogen level is a predictor on the same magnitude, as other well-accepted risk factors for cardiovascular disease and stroke.[170] Arachidonic acid, a stimulator of platelet aggregation, has been noted to be released in greater concentrations from platelets incubated with cholesterol-rich liposomes as compared to cholesterol-poor platelets.[171] The relationships are far from clear, and much research in this area is yet to be done.

Conclusions

The bulk of the work in atherosclerotic epidemiology has been concerned with cardiovascular disease, specifically CHD. The same risk factors, however, apply to cerebrovascular disease, aortoiliac disease, and other forms of peripheral vascular disease. All of the data compiled to date, and specifically the Framingham Study, has demonstrated a common set of precursors to all the major atherosclerotic diseases, whether manifest in the brain, the heart, or peripherally.[56] The relative importance of these different risk factors varies according to the anatomical location and lesion being considered.

Early on Enos et al[31] showed that atherosclerotic changes appear in the coronary arteries years or decades before the age at which CHD becomes clinically recognized. Other studies since have further demonstrated the various patterns of atherosclerotic arterial occlusive disease, confirming the concept that the occlusive process tends to assume distinctive patterns in the four major arterial beds, and that these developmental patterns are based on an interplay between environment and physiological forces.[2-4,6,7,19] The aging process independently and in conjunction with other risk factors plays a role in the various manifestations of atherosclerotic vascular disease.

Atherogenesis is a multifactorial process involving the interaction of blood lipids, metabolism of the arterial wall, and hemodynamic factors. The process increases with age and is influenced by racial, geographical, and dietary factors. Risk factors, including hyperlipidemia, hypertension, diabetes mellitus, obesity, and smoking, determine to what extent the disease will develop. Anatomical distribution of the lesions follows reproducible patterns in most patients, with changes in plaque morphology contributing to the development of complications and symptoms.

Current management favors prevention by minimizing risk factors. It is definitely advantageous to identify and control risk factors in the younger population. It is equally as important, and possibly of greater urgency to do so in the elderly population given the increased likelihood that the atherosclerotic vascular disease process will manifest itself with potentially devastating effects. Kuller et al[172] demonstrated that the prevalence of subclinical atherosclerosis and cardiovascular disease (defined in the study by the presence of specific anatomical or physiological changes in the absence of symptoms, or the presence of unrecognized symptoms by the patient as determined via a questionnaire) was 36% in women and 38.7% in men, and increased with age. The risk factors for subclinical disease were similar to those for clinical disease, suggesting that the older individual with subclinical disease is at very high risk for developing clinical disease.

Given the prevalence, morbidity, and socioeconomic cost of atherosclerotic vascular disease in the elderly population, it is imperative that risk factors be identified early and controlled or reversed. A recognition and understanding of the critical risk factors and appropriate intervention is crucial to preventing development of this disease process as one ages, and preventing progression and recurrence of disease once it has been identified in the elderly patient. Thorough risk factor histories, physical examinations, and vigilant follow-ups looking specifically for stigmata of atherosclerotic vascular disease are, therefore, especially important in this high-risk population.

References

1. Years of Life Lost From Cardiovascular Disease. MMWR 35(42),1986 (Data from CDC Atlanta). Reprinted in *JAMA* 256:2794, 1986.
2. Strong JP, Restrepo C: Coronary and aortic atherosclerosis in New Orleans. *Lab Invest* 39:358, 1978.
3. DeBakey ME, Lawrie GM, Glaeser DH: Patterns of atherosclerosis and their surgical significance. *Ann Surg* 201:115, 1985.
4. The progression of atherosclerosis. *Lancet* i:791-793, 1985.
5. Kawachi I: Epidemiology of stroke: importance of preventive pharmacological strategies in elderly patients and associated costs. *Drugs Aging* 5(4):288-299, 1994.
6. Montenegro MR, Eggen DA: Topography of atherosclerosis in the coronary arteries. *Lab Invest* 18:586, 1968.
7. Solberg LA, Eggen DA: Localization and sequence of development of atherosclerotic lesions in the carotid and vertebral arteries. *Circulation* 43:711, 1971.
8. Sadoshima S, Kurozumi T, Tanaka K, et al: Cerebral and aortic atherosclerosis in Hisayama, Japan. *Atherosclerosis* 36:117, 1980.
9. Fabris F, Zanocchi M, Bo M, et al: Carotid plaque, aging, and risk factors: a study of 457 subjects. *Stroke* 25:1133-1140, 1994.
10. Collin J, Araujo L, Walton J, et al: Oxford screening programme for abdominal aneurysms in men aged 65-74 years. *Lancet* ii:613-615, 1988.
11. Stevens K: The incidence of abdominal aortic aneurysms. BJCP 47(4):208-210, 1993.
12. Maru M: Prevalence of atherosclerosis of the aorta in Ethiopians: a postmortem study. *East Afr Med J* 69:214-218, 1992.
13. Berridge DC, Griffith CDM, Amar SS, et al: Screening for clinically unsuspected aortic aneurysms in patients with peripheral vascular disease. *Eur J Vasc Surg* 3:421-422, 1989.
14. Virmani R, Avollo AP, Mergner WJ, et al: Effect of aging on aortic morphology in populations with high and low prevalence of hypertension and atherosclerosis. *Am J Pathol* 139(5):1119-1129, 1991.
15. Hosoda Y, Kawano K, Yamasawa F, et al: Age-dependent changes of collagen and elastin content in human aorta and pulmonary artery. *Angiology* 35:615-621, 1984.
16. A Coordination Group in China: A pathological survey of atherosclerotic lesions of coronary artery and aorta in China. *Path Res Pract* 180:457, 1985.

17. Cacoub P, Godeau P: Risk factors for atherosclerotic aortoiliac occlusive disease. *Ann Vasc Surg* 7:394-405, 1993.
18. Weiss NS: Cigarette smoking and arteriosclerosis obliterans: prevalence and risk factors. *Br Med J* 1:1379-1381, 1978.
19. Haimovici H: Atherogenesis recent biological concepts and clinical implications. *Am J Surg* 134:174, 1977.
20. Darling RC, Brewster DC, Hallet JW, et al: Aorto-iliac reconstruction. *Surg Clin North Am* 59:565, 1979.
21. Haimovici H: Patterns of arteriosclerotic lesions of the lower extremity. *Arch Surg* 95:918, 1967.
22. Royster TS, Lynn R, Mulcare RJ: Combined aortoiliac and femoropopliteal occlusive disease. *Surg Gynecol Obstet* 143:949, 1976.
23. Samson RH, Scher LA, Veith FJ: Combined segment arterial disease. *Surgery* 97:385, 1985.
24. Criqui MH, Fronek A, Barrett-Connor E, et al: The prevalence of peripheral arterial disease in a defined population. *Circulation* 71:510-515, 1985.
25. Mavor GE: The pattern of occlusion in atheroma of the lower limb arteries: the correlation of clinical and arteriographic findings. *Br J Surg* 43:352, 1956.
26. Stokes J, Kannel WB, Cupples LA, et al: The relative importance of selected risk factors for various manifestations of cardiovascular disease among men and women from 35 to 64 years old: 30 years of follow-up in The Framingham Study. *Circulation* 75(suppl V):V65-V73, 1987.
27. Vogt MT, Wolfson SK, Kuller LH: Lower extremity arterial disease and the aging process: a review. *J Clin Epidemiol* 45(5):529-542, 1992.
28. Newman AB, Sutton-Tyrrell K, Rutan GH, et al: Lower extremity arterial disease in elderly subjects with systolic hypertension. *J Clin Epidemiol* 44(1):15-20, 1991.
29. Tejada C, Gore I: Comparison of atherosclerosis in Guatemala City and New Orleans. *Am J Pathol* 33:887, 1957.
30. Strong JP, Restrepo C, Guzman M: Coronary and aortic atherosclerosis in New Orleans: II. Comparison of lesions by age, sex, and race. *Lab Invest* 39:364,1978.
31. Enos WF, Holmes RH, Beyer J: Coronary disease among United States soldiers killed in action in Korea. *JAMA* 152:1090, 1953.
32. Strong JP, McGill HC Jr: The natural history of coronary atherosclerosis. *Am J Pathol* 40:37, 1962.
33. Solberg LA, Strong JP, Holme I, et al: Stenoses in the coronary arteries: relation to atherosclerotic lesions, coronary heart disease, and risk factors. The Oslo Study. *Lab Invest* 53:648, 1985.
34. Duncan GW, Lees RS, Ojemann RG, et al: Concomitants of atherosclerotic carotid artery stenosis. *Stroke* 8:665, 1977.
35. Bogousslavsky J, Regli F, Van Melle G: Risk factor and concomitants of internal carotid artery occlusion or stenosis. *Arch Neurol* 42:864, 1985.
36. Strong JP, Guzman MA, Tracy RE, et al: Is coronary atherosclerosis decreasing in the U.S.A.? *Lancet* ii:1294, 1979.
37. Strong JP, Guzman MA: Decrease in coronary atherosclerosis in New Orleans. *Lab Invest* 43:297, 1980.
38. Newman WP III, Strong JP, Johnson WD, et al: Community pathology of atherosclerosis and coronary heart disease in New Orleans. *Lab Invest* 44:496, 1981.
39. Stern MP: The recent decline in ischemic heart disease mortality. *Ann Intern Med* 91:630, 1979.
40. Gillum RF, Folsom A, Luepker RV, et al: Sudden death and acute myocardial infarction in a Metropolitan area 1970-1980: the Minnesota Heart Survey. *N Engl J Med* 309:1353, 1983.

41. Sytkowski PA, Kannel WB, D'Agostino RB: Changes in risk factors and the decline in mortality from cardiovascular disease: the Framingham Heart Study. *N Engl J Med* 322:1635, 1990.
42. Final report of the Pooling Project Research Group: Relationship of blood pressure, serum cholesterol, smoking habit, relative weight, and ECG abnormalities to incidence of major coronary events. *J Chron Dis* 31:201, 1978.
43. Stamler J, Beard RR, Connor WE, et al: Report of inter-society commission for heart disease resources: primary prevention of the atherosclerotic diseases. *Circulation* 42:A55, 1970.
44. Criqui MH, Barrett-Connor E, Holdbrook MJ, et al: Clustering of cardiovascular disease risk factors. *Prev Med* 9:525, 1980.
45. Tejada C, Strong JP, Montenegro MR, et al: Distribution of coronary and aortic atherosclerosis by geographic location, race, and sex. *Lab Invest* 18:509, 1968.
46. Strong JP, McGill HC Jr, Tejada C, et al: The natural history of atherosclerosis: comparison of the early aortic lesions in New Orleans, Guatemala, and Costa Rica. *Am J Pathol* 34:731, 1958.
47. Gore I, Hirst AE Jr, Koseki Y: Comparison of aortic atherosclerosis in the United States, Japan, and Guatemala. *Am J Clin Nutr* 7:50, 1959.
48. Neaton JD, Kuller LH, Wentworth D, et al: Total and cardiovascular mortality in relation to cigarette smoking, serum cholesterol concentration, and diastolic blood pressure among black and white males followed up for five years. *Am Heart J* 108:759, 1984.
49. Ishii T, Newman WP III, Guzman MA, et al: Coronary and aortic atherosclerosis in young men from Tokyo and New Orleans. *Lab Invest* 54:561, 1986.
50. Ishii T, Guzman MA, Newman WP, et al: Atherosclerosis in Japan and the USA. *Lancet* i:339, 1984.
51. Stemmermann GN, Steer A, Rhoads GG, et al: A comparative pathology study of myocardial lesions and atherosclerosis in Japanese men living in Hiroshima, Japan, and Honolulu, Hawaii. *Lab Invest* 34:592, 1976.
52. Robertson TL, Kato H, Rhoads GG, et al: Epidemiologic studies of coronary heart disease and stroke in Japanese men living in Japan, Hawaii, and California: incidence of myocardial infarction and death from coronary heart disease. *Am J Cardiol* 39:239, 1977.
53. Sadoshima S, Kurozumi T, Tanaka K, et al: Cerebral and aortic atherosclerosis in Hisayama, Japan. *Atherosclerosis* 36:117, 1980.
54. Neufeld HN, Goldbourt U: Coronary heart disease: genetic aspects. *Circulation* 67:943, 1983.
55. Kannel WB, McGee D, Gordon T: A general cardiovascular risk profile: the Framingham Study. *Am J Cardiol* 38:46, 1976.
56. Gordon T, Kannel WB: Predisposition to atherosclerosis in the head, heart, and legs: the Framingham Study. *JAMA* 221:661, 1972.
57. Kannel WB: Role of blood pressure in cardiovascular disease: the Framingham Study. *Angiology* 26:1, 1975.
58. Szatrowski TP, Peterson AV Jr, Shimizu Y, et al: Serum cholesterol, other risk factors, and cardiovascular disease in a Japanese cohort. *J Chron Dis* 37:569, 1984.
59. Rosenman RH, Friedman M, Straus R, et al: Coronary heart disease in The Western Collaborative Group Study. *J Chron Dis* 23:173, 1970.
60. Rosenman RH, Brand RJ, Sholtz RI, et al: Multivariate prediction of coronary heart disease during 8.5 year follow-up in The Western Collaborative Group Study. *Am J Cardiol* 37:903, 1976.

61. Veterans Administration Cooperative Study Group on Antihypertensive Agents: Effects of treatment on morbidity in hypertension. *JAMA* 202:1028, 1967.
62. Rosenman RH, Sholtz RI, Brand RJ: A study of comparative blood pressure measures in predicting risk of coronary heart disease. *Circulation* 54:51, 1976.
63. Kannel WB, Dawber TR, Sorlie P, et al: Components of blood pressure and risk of atherothrombotic brain infarction: the Framingham Study. *Stroke* 7:327, 1976.
64. Veterans Administration Cooperative Study Group on Antihypertensive Agents: Effects of treatment on morbidity in hypertension: II. Results in patients with diastolic blood pressure averaging 90 through 114 mm Hg. *JAMA* 213:1143, 1970.
65. Taguchi J, Freis ED: Partial reduction of blood pressure and prevention of complications in hypertension. *N Engl J Med* 291:329, 1974.
66. Julius S, Jamerson K, Mejia A, et al: The association of borderline hypertension with target organ changes and higher coronary risk: Tecumseh Blood Pressure Study. *JAMA* 264:354, 1990.
67. Criqui MH, Mebane I, Wallace RB, et al: Multivariate correlates of adult blood pressures in nine North American populations: the Lipid Research Clinics Prevalence Study. *Prev Med* 11:391, 1982.
68. Friedman GD, Dales LG, Ury HK: Mortality in middle-aged smokers and nonsmokers. *N Engl J Med* 300:213, 1979.
69. Fielding JE: Smoking: health effects and control (first of two parts). *N Engl J Med* 313:491, 1985.
70. Svendsen KH, Kuller LH, Martin MJ, et al: Effects of passive smoking in The Multiple Risk Factor Intervention Trial. *Am J Epidemiol* 126:783, 1987.
71. Kannel WB, D'Agostino RB, Belanger AJ: Fibrinogen, cigarette smoking, and risk of cardiovascular disease: insights from the Framingham Study. *Am Heart J* 113:1006, 1987.
72. Robbins JL, Cotran RS, Kumar V: *Pathologic Basis of Disease.* 3rd Ed. Philadelphia: WB Saunders, Co.; 508, 1984.
73. Dyken ML, Wolf PA, Barnett HJM, et al: Risk factors in stroke. *Stroke* 15:1105, 1984.
74. Wolf PA: Cigarettes, alcohol, and stroke. *N Engl J Med* 315:1087, 1986.
75. Abbott RD, Yin Y, Reed DM, et al: Risk of stroke in male cigarette smokers. *N Engl J Med* 315:717, 1986.
76. Colditz GA, Bonita R, Stampfer MJ, et al: Cigarette smoking and risk of stroke in middle-aged women. *N Engl J Med* 318:937, 1988.
77. Wolf PA, D'Agostino RB, Kannel WB, et al: Cigarette smoking as a risk factor for stroke: the Framingham Study. *JAMA* 259:1025, 1988.
78. Tell GS, Howard G, McKinney WM, et al: Cigarette smoking cessation and extracranial carotid atherosclerosis. *JAMA* 261:1178, 1989.
79. Multiple Risk Factor Intervention Trial Research Group: Multiple risk factor intervention trial. *JAMA* 248:1465, 1982.
80. Gordon T, Kannel WB, McGee D: Death and coronary attacks in men after giving up cigarette smoking. *Lancet* ii:1345, 1974.
81. Hermanson B, Omenn GS, Kronmal RA, et al: Beneficial six-year outcome of smoking cessation in older men and women with coronary artery disease: results from the CASS registry. *N Engl J Med* 319:1365, 1988.
82. Rosenberg L, Palmer JR, Shapiro S: Decline in the risk of myocardial infarction among women who stop smoking. *N Engl J Med* 322:213, 1990.
83. Kannel WB, McGee DL, Castelli WP: Latest perspectives on cigarette smoking and cardiovascular disease: the Framingham Study. *J Cardiac Rehab* 4:267, 1984.

84. Wilhelmsen L, Svardsudd K, Korsan-Bengtsen K, et al: Fibrinogen as a risk factor for stroke and myocardial infarction. *N Engl J Med* 311:501, 1984.
85. Dwyer JH, Rieger-Ndakorerwa GE, Semmer NK, et al: Low-level cigarette smoking and longitudinal change in serum cholesterol among adolescents: the Berlin-Bremen Study. *JAMA* 59:2857, 1988.
86. Caro CG, Parker KH, Lever MJ, et al: Effect of cigarette smoking on the pattern of arterial blood flow: possible insight into mechanisms underlying the development arteriosclerosis. *Lancet* ii:11, 1987.
87. Tyroler HA: The Lipid Research Clinics Program Prevalence Study: epidemiology of plasma high density lipoprotein cholesterol levels. *Circulation* (suppl 4)62:, 1980.
88. Davis JW, Davis RF: Acute effect of tobacco cigarette smoking on the platelet aggregate ratio. *Am J Med Sci* 278:139, 1979.
89. Garrison RJ, Kannel WB, Feinleib M, et al: Cigarette smoking and HDL cholesterol. *Atherosclerosis* 30:17, 1978.
90. Renaud S, Blache D, Dumont E, et al: Platelet function after cigarette smoking in relation to nicotine and carbon monoxide. *Clin Pharmacol Ther* 36:389, 1984.
91. Criqui MH, Wallace RB, Heiss G, et al: Cigarette smoking and plasma high-density lipoprotein cholesterol. *Circulation* 62:IV-70, 1980.
92. Haffner J, Appelbaum-Bowden D, Hoover J, et al: Association of high-density lipoprotein cholesterol 2 and 3 with Quetelet, alcohol, and smoking: the Seattle Lipid Research Clinic Population. *CVD Epidemiol Newsletter* 31:20, 1982.
93. Criqui MH, Cowan LD, Tyroler HA, et al: Lipoproteins as mediators for the effects of alcohol consumption and cigarette smoking on cardiovascular mortality: results from The Lipid Research Clinics Follow-up Study. *Am J Epidemiol* 126:629, 1987.
94. Arntzenius AC, Kromhout D, Barth JD, et al: Diet, lipoproteins, and the progression of coronary atherosclerosis. *N Engl J Med* 312:805, 1985.
95. Kushi LH, Lew RA, Stare FJ, et al: Diet and 20-year mortality from coronary heart disease. *N Engl J Med* 312:811, 1985.
96. Motulsky AG, Boman H: Screening for the hyperlipidemias. In: Milunsky A (ed). *The Prevention of Genetic Disease and Mental Retardation.* Philadelphia: WB Saunders, Co.; 306, 1975.
97. Hulley SB, Rosenman RH, Bawol RD, et al: Epidemiology as a guide to clinical decisions: the association between triglyceride and coronary heart disease. *N Engl J Med* 302:1383, 1980.
98. Gordon T, Castelli WP, Hjortland MC, et al: High density lipoprotein as a protective factor against coronary heart disease. *Am J Med* 62:707, 1977.
99. Hulley SB, Rhoads GG: The plasma lipoproteins as risk factors: comparison of electrophoretic and ultracentrifugation results. *Metabolism* 31:773, 1982.
100. Hamsten A, Walldius G, Dahlen G, et al: Serum lipoproteins and apolipoproteins in young male survivors of myocardial infarction. *Atherosclerosis* 59:223, 1986.
101. Cabin HS, Roberts WC: Relation of serum total cholesterol and triglyceride levels to the amount and extent of coronary arterial narrowing by atherosclerotic plaque in coronary heart disease: quantitative analysis of 2,037 five mm segments of 160 major epicardial coronary arteries in 40 necropsy patients. *Am J Med* 73:227, 1982.
102. Newman WP III, Freedman DS, Voors AW, et al: Relation of serum lipoprotein levels and systolic blood pressure to early atherosclerosis: The Bogalusa Heart Study. *N Engl J Med* 314:138, 1986.
103. Castelli WP: The triglyceride issue: a view from Framingham. *Am Heart J* 112:432, 1986.

104. Carlson LA, Bottiger LE: Risk factors for ischaemic heart disease in men and women: results of the 19-year follow-up of the Stockholm Prospective Study. *Acta Med Scand* 218:207, 1985.
105. Aberg H, Lithell H, Selinus I, et al: Serum triglycerides are a risk factor for myocardial infarction but not for angina pectoris: results from a 10-year follow-up of Uppsala Primary Preventive Study. *Atherosclerosis* 54:89, 1985.
106. Lapidus L, Bengtsson C, Lindquist O, et al: Triglycerides—main lipid risk factor for cardiovascular disease in women? *Acta Med Scand* 217:481, 1985.
107. Brunzell JD, Sniderman AD, Albers JJ, et al: Apoproteins B and A-I and coronary artery disease in humans. *Arteriosclerosis* 4:79, 1984.
108. Robertson TL, Kato H, Gordon T, et al: Epidemiologic studies of coronary heart disease and stroke in Japanese men living in Japan, Hawaii, and California: coronary heart disease risk factors in Japan and Hawaii. *Am J Cardiol* 39:244, 1977.
109. Report of the Working Group on Atherosclerosis of the National Heart, Lung and Blood Institute: Arteriosclerosis. Public Health Service NIH Publication No. 82:2035, 1981.
110. Walker WJ: Changing United States life-style and declining vascular mortality: cause or coincidence? *N Engl J Med* 297:163, 1977.
111. United States Department of Health, Education, and Welfare, National Heart, Blood Vessel, Lung, and Blood program: *Fourth report of the director of the National Heart, Lung and Blood Institute.* Washington, D.C., Government Printing Office DHEW Publication No.[NIH] 771170, 1977.
112. Mann JI, Marr JW: Coronary heart disease prevention trials of diet to control hyperlipidemia. In: Miller NE, Lewis B (eds). *Lipoproteins, Atherosclerosis, and Coronary Heart Disease.* Amsterdam: Elsevier/North-Holland Biomedical Press; 197, 1981.
113. Hjermann I, Velve BK, Holme I, et al: Effect of diet and smoking intervention on the incidence of coronary heart disease: report from the Oslo Study Group of a randomised trial in healthy men. *Lancet* ii:1303, 1981.
114. Eder HA, Gidez LI: The clinical significance of the plasma high density lipoproteins. *Med Clin North Am* 66:431, 1982.
115. Castelli WP, Garrison RJ, Wilson PWF, et al: Incidence of coronary heart disease and lipoprotein cholesterol levels. *JAMA* 256:2835, 1986.
116. Miller NE, Thelle DS, Forde OH, et al: The Tromso Heart Study. High-density lipoprotein and coronary heart disease: a prospective case-control study. *Lancet* i:965, 1977.
117. Pekkanen J, Linn S, Heiss G, et al: Ten-year mortality from cardiovascular disease in relation to cholesterol level among men with and without preexisting cardiovascular disease. *N Engl J Med* 322:1700, 1990.
118. Castelli WP, Gordon T, Hjortland MC, et al: Alcohol and blood lipids: the Cooperative Lipoprotein Phenotyping Study. *Lancet* ii:153, 1977.
119. Kuller L, Castelli W: High LDL levels can unmask covert alcoholic. *Skin Allergy News* 11:25, 1980.
120. Kagan A, Yano K, Rhoads GG, et al: Alcohol and cardiovascular disease: The Hawaiian experience. *Circulation* 64:III-27, 1981.
121. Haskell WL, Camargo C, Williams PT, et al: The effect of cessation and resumption of moderate alcohol intake on serum high density-lipoprotein subfractions. *N Engl J Med* 310:805, 1984.
122. Stampfer MJ, Colditz GA, Willett WC, et al: A prospective study of moderate alcohol consumption and the risk of coronary disease and stroke in women. *N Engl J Med* 319:267, 1988.

123. Lipid Research Clinics Program: The Lipid Research Clinics Coronary Primary Prevention Trial results: I. Reduction in incidence of coronary heart disease. *JAMA* 251:351, 1984.
124. Lipid Research Clinics Program: The Lipid Research Clinics Coronary Primary Prevention trial results. II. The relationship of reduction in incidence of coronary heart disease to cholesterol lowering. JAMA 251:365, 1984.
125. Oliver MF, Heady JA, Morris JN, et al: A cooperative trial in the primary prevention of ischaemic heart disease using clofibrate: report from the committee of principal investigators. *Br Heart J* 40:1069, 1978.
126. Coronary Drug Project Research Group: Natural history of myocardial infarction in the Coronary Drug Project: long-term prognostic importance of serum lipid levels. *Am J Cardiol* 42:489, 1978.
127. Canner PL, Berge KG, Wenger NK, et al: Fifteen year mortality in Coronary Drug Project patients: long-term benefit with niacin. *J Am Coll Cardiol* 8:1245, 1986.
128. Brensike JF, Levy RI, Kelsey SF, et al: Effects of therapy with cholestyramine on progression of coronary arteriosclerosis: results of the NHLBI Type II Coronary Intervention Study. *Circulation* 69:313, 1984.
129. Levy RI, Brensike JF, Epstein SE, et al: The influence of changes in lipid values induced by cholestyramine and diet on progression of coronary artery disease: results of the NHLBI Type II Coronary Intervention Study. *Circulation* 9:325, 1984.
130. Frick MH, Elo O, Haapa K, et al: Helsinki Heart Study: primary-prevention trial with gemfibrozil in middle-aged men with dyslipidemia: safety of treatment, changes in risk factors, and incidence of coronary heart disease. *N Engl J Med* 317:1237, 1987.
131. Blankenhorn DH, Nessim SA, Johnson RL, et al: Beneficial effects of combined colestipol-niacin therapy on coronary atherosclerosis and coronary venous bypass grafts. *JAMA* 257:3233, 1987.
132. Kjekshus J, Pedersen TR: Reducing the risk of coronary events: evidence from the Scandinavian Simvastatin Survival Study. *Am J Cardiol* 76(9):64C-68C, 1995.
133. Simes RJ: Prospective meta-analysis of cholesterol-lowering studies: the Prospective Pravastatin Pooling (PPP) Project and the Cholesterol Treatment Trialists (CTT) Collaboration. *Am J Cardiol* 76(9):122C-126C, 1995.
134. Tonkin AM: Disease (LIPID) study after the Scandinavian Simvastatin Survival Study. *Am J Cardiol* 76(9):107C-112C, 1995.
135. Lansberg PJ, Mitchel YB, Shapiro D, et al: Long-term efficacy and tolerability of simvastatin in a large cohort of elderly hypercholesterolemic patients. *Atherosclerosis* 116(2):153-162, 1995.
136. Waters D, Higginson L, Gladstone P, et al: Effects of cholesterol lowering on the progression of coronary atherosclerosis in women: a Canadian Coronary Atherosclerosis Intervention Trial (CCAIT) substudy. *Circulation* 92(9):2404-2410, 1995.
137. Manninen V, Elo MO, Frick MH, et al: Lipid alterations and decline in the incidence of coronary heart disease in the Helsinki Heart Study. *JAMA* 260:641, 1988.
138. Mann GV: Diet-heart: end of an era. *N Engl J Med* 297:644, 1977.
139. Gordon T, Castelli WP, Hjortland MC, et al: Predicting coronary heart disease in middle-aged and older persons: the Framingham Study. *JAMA* 238:497, 1977.
140. McGee D, Gordon T: The results of the Framingham Study applied to four other U.S.-based epidemiologic studies of cardiovascular disease. Washington, D.C. *Government Printing Office DHEW Publication No.*[NIH] 76-1083, 1976.

141. Stamler J, Wentworth D, Neaton JD: Is relationship between serum cholesterol and risk of premature death from coronary heart disease continuous and graded? *JAMA* 256:2823, 1986.
142. Iso H, Jacobs DR Jr, Wentworth D, et al: Serum cholesterol levels and six-year mortality from stroke in 350,977 men screened for the Multiple Risk Factor Intervention Trial. *N Engl J Med* 320:904, 1989.
143. Roehmoldt ME, Palumbo PJ, Whisnant JP, et al: Transient ischemic attack and stroke in a community-based diabetic cohort. *Mayo Clin Proc* 58:56, 1983.
144. Kannel WB, McGee DL: Diabetes and cardiovascular disease: the Framingham Study. *JAMA* 241:2035, 1979.
145. Abbott RD, Donahue RP: Diabetes and the risk of stroke: the Honolulu Heart Program. *JAMA* 257:949, 1987.
146. Reaven GM, Lerner RL, Stern MP, et al: Role of insulin in endogenous hypertriglyceridemia. *J Clin Invest* 46:1756, 1967.
147. Zavaroni I, Bonora E, Pagliara M, et al: Risk factors for coronary artery disease in healthy persons with hyperinsulinemia and normal glucose tolerance. *N Engl J Med* 320:702, 1989.
148. Reaven GM: Role of insulin resistance in human disease. *Diabetes* 37:1595, 1988.
149. Ostlund RE Jr, Staten M, Kohrt WM, et al: The ratio of waist-to-hip circumference, plasma insulin level, and glucose intolerance as independent predictors of the HDL_2 cholesterol level in older adults. *N Engl J Med* 322:229, 1990.
150. Williams PT, Wood PD, Haskell WL, et al: The effects of running mileage and duration on plasma lipoprotein levels. *JAMA* 247:2674, 1982.
151. Hubert HB, Feinleib M, McNamara PM, et al: Obesity as an independent risk factor for cardiovascular disease: a 26-year follow-up of participants in the Framingham Heart Study. *Circulation* 67:968, 1983.
152. Van Itallie TB: Obesity: adverse effects on health and longevity. *Am J Clin Nutr* 32:2723, 1979.
153. Manson JE, Colditz GA, Stampfer MJ, et al: A prospective study of obesity and risk of coronary heart disease in women. *N Engl J Med* 322:882, 1990.
154. Barrett-Connor EL: Obesity, artherosclerosis, and coronary artery disease. *Ann Intern Med* 103:1010, 1985.
155. Patel YC, Eggen DA, Strong JP: Obesity, smoking and atherosclerosis. *Atherosclerosis* 36:481, 1980.
156. Bloom E, Reed D, Yano K, et al: Does obesity protect hypertensives against cardiovascular disease. *JAMA* 256:2972, 1986.
157. Rennie D: Letters: obesity, hypertension, and cardiovascular disease. *JAMA* 257:1598, 1987.
158. Wood PD, Stefanick ML, Dreon DM, et al: Changes in plasma lipids and lipoproteins in overweight men during weight loss through dieting as compared with exercise. *N Engl J Med* 319:1173, 1988.
159. Blair SN, Kohl HW III, Paffenbarger RS Jr, et al: Physical fitness and all-cause mortality: a prospective study of healthy men and women. *JAMA* 262:2395, 1989.
160. Ekelund LG, Haskell WL, Johnson JL, et al: Physical fitness as a predictor of cardiovascular mortality in asymptomatic North American men: the Lipid Research Clinics Mortality Follow-up Study. *N Engl J Med* 319:1379, 1988.
161. Kannel WB, Belanger A, D'Agostino R, et al: Physical activity and physical demand on the job and risk of cardiovascular disease and death: the Framingham Study. *Am Heart J* 112:820, 1986.

162. Hammett F, Saltissi S, Miller N, et al: Relationship of coronary atherosclerosis to plasma lipoproteins. *Circulation* 60:II-167, 1979.
163. Nye ER, Carlson K, Kirstein P, et al: Changes in high density lipoprotein subfractions and other lipoproteins induced by exercise. *Clin Chim Acta* 113:51, 1981.
164. Paffenbarger RS Jr, Hyde RT: Exercise as protection against heart attack. *N Engl J Med* 302:1026, 1980.
165. Williams RS, Logue EE, Lewis JL, et al: Physical conditioning augments the fibrinolytic response to venous occlusion in healthy adults. *N Engl J Med* 302:987, 1980.
166. Thorngren M, Gustafson A: Effects of 11-week increase in dietary eicosapentaenoic acid on bleeding time, lipids, and platelet aggregation. *Lancet* ii:1190, 1981.
167. Knapp HR, Reilly I, Allessandrini P, et al: In vivo indexes of platelet and vascular function during fish oil administration in patients with atherosclerosis. *N Engl J Med* 314:937, 1986.
168. Lowe GDO, Stromberg P, Forbes CD, et al: Increased blood viscosity and fibrinolytic inhibitor in type II hyperlipoproteinaemia. *Lancet* i:472, 1982.
169. Korsan-Bengtsen K, Willhelmsen L, Tibblin G: Blood coagulation and fibrinolysis in a random sample of 788 men 54 years old. *Throm Diath Haemorrh* 28:99, 1972.
170. Kannel W, Wolf PA, Castelli WP, et al: Fibrinogen and risk of cardiovascular disease: the Framingham Study. *JAMA* 258:1183, 1987.
171. Stuart MJ, Gerrard JM, White JG: Effect of cholesterol on production of thromboxane B2 by platelets in vitro. *N Engl J Med* 302:6, 1980.
172. Kuller L, Borhani N, Furberg C, et al: Prevalence of subclinial atherosclerosis and cardiovascular disease and association with risk factors in the cardiovascular health study. *Am J Epidemiol* 139:1164-1179, 1994.

Chapter 6

Risk Factors for Coronary Artery Disease, Peripheral Arterial Disease, and Atherothrombotic Brain Infarction in Elderly Persons

Wilbert S. Aronow, MD

Coronary artery disease (CAD) is the leading cause of death in elderly persons. CAD, peripheral arterial disease (PAD), and atherothrombotic brain infarction (ABI) are more common in elderly persons than in middle-aged persons. This chapter discusses risk factors for CAD, PAD, and ABI in elderly persons.

Coronary Artery Disease

Cigarette Smoking

Findings from the Chicago Stroke Study showed that current cigarette smokers 65 to 74 years of age had a 52% higher mortality from CAD than nonsmokers, ex-smokers, and pipe and cigar smokers.[1] Ex-smokers who had stopped smoking for 1 to 5 years had a similar mortality from CAD as did nonsmokers. The Systolic Hypertension in the Elderly Program pilot project demonstrated that smoking was a predictor of first cardiovascular event and myocardial infarction (MI)/sudden death.[2] At 30-year follow-up of persons 65 years of age and older in the Framingham Heart Study, cigarette smoking was not associated with the incidence of CAD in elderly men and women, but was associated with mortality from CAD in elderly men and women.[3]

In the Honolulu Heart Program, at 12-year follow-up of men aged 65 to 74 years, cigarette smoking was an independent risk factor for nonfatal MI and fatal CAD.[4] The absolute excess risk associated with

From: Aronow WS, Stemmer EA, Wilson SE (eds). *Vascular Disease in the Elderly.* Armonk, NY: Futura Publishing Company, Inc., © 1997.

Table 1
Association of Cigarette Smoking With New Coronary Events, Peripheral Arterial
Disease, and New Atherothrombotic Brain Infarction in Elderly Men and Women

Study	No. of Patients	Mean Age (years)	Mean Follow-Up (months)	Elderly Men Relative Risk	Elderly Women Relative Risk
Incidence of new coronary events[6]	708	82	41	2.5	2.1
Prevalence of PAD[17]	869	82	—	2.4	2.9
Incidence of new ABI[23]	708	82	36	3.5	2.1

PAD = peripheral arterial disease
ABI = atherothrombotic brain infarction

cigarette smoking was 1.9 times higher in elderly men than in middle-aged men. At 5-year follow-up of elderly persons 65 years of age and older in three communities, cigarette smokers were found to have a higher incidence of cardiovascular mortality than nonsmokers.[5] The relative risk for cardiovascular mortality was 2.0 in elderly male smokers and 1.6 in elderly female smokers. The incidence of cardiovascular death in former smokers was similar to those who had never smoked.[5]

At 41-month mean follow-up of 708 elderly persons (516 women and 192 men), mean age 82 years, cigarette smoking was demonstrated to increase the incidence of new coronary events 2.5 times in elderly men and 2.1 times in elderly women (Table 1).[6] Cigarette smoking was found by multivariate analysis to be an independent risk factor for new coronary events in elderly men and in elderly women in this study. At 42-month mean follow-up in a prospective study of 410 elderly patients with hypertension, mean age 81 years, the odds ratio for developing new coronary events was 2.0 in cigarette smokers.[7] It has also been observed that cigarette smoking aggravates angina pectoris and precipitates silent myocardial ischemia in elderly persons with CAD.

In the Coronary Artery Surgery Study registry, patients aged 65 years and older who continued smoking had an increased risk of developing MI or sudden death compared with those who stopped smoking during the year before enrolling in the study.[8] Increasing age did not reduce the beneficial effect of ceasing to smoke found in this study.

Peripheral Arterial Disease

Numerous studies have demonstrated that cigarette smoking is a risk factor for PAD in men and women.[9-16] In a study of 869 elderly persons (244 men and 625 women), mean age 82 years, current cigarette smoking was found to increase the prevalence of PAD 2.4 times in elderly men and 2.9 times in elderly women (Table 1).[17] At 43-month mean follow-up of 291 elderly patients, mean age 82 years, with PAD, multivariate analysis also showed that cigarette smoking was an independent predictor of new coronary events, with a relative risk of 1.62.[18]

Atherothrombotic Brain Infarction

A meta-analysis of 32 studies found that cigarette smoking is a risk factor for ABI in men and women, with a relative risk of 1.9.[19] In the Medical Research Council Trial, the incidence of stroke was 2.3 times higher in cigarette smokers than in nonsmokers.[20] In this study, non-smokers who received propranolol as antihypertensive therapy had a decrease in the incidence of stroke, whereas cigarette smokers did not. At 26-year follow-up in the Framingham Heart Study, cigarette smoking increased the incidence of ABI 1.6 times in men and 1.9 times in women.[21] The incidence of stroke in cigarette smokers who smoked more than 40 cigarettes daily was two times higher than in those who smoked fewer than 10 cigarettes daily. The impact of cigarette smoking did not decrease with increasing age. The risk of stroke was substantially reduced within 2 years of quitting smoking, with the incidence of stroke returning to the level of nonsmokers 5 years after cessation. Elderly persons who quit smoking also have higher cerebral perfusion levels than elderly persons who continue to smoke, but lower cerebral perfusion levels than elderly persons who have never smoked.[22]

At 3-year follow-up in a prospective study of 708 elderly persons, mean age 82 years, current cigarette smoking was demonstrated to increase the incidence of new ABI 3.5 times in elderly men and 2.1 times in elderly women (Table 1).[23] In a study of 1,063 elderly persons, mean age 81 years, cigarette smoking was also found to increase the prevalence of 40% to 100% extracranial internal or common carotid arterial disease 4.2 times.[24]

Recommendations

On the basis of the available data, elderly men and women who smoke cigarettes should be strongly encouraged to stop smoking. In elderly persons, cigarette smoking is a risk factor for CAD, PAD, ABI, and extracranial internal or common carotid arterial disease, as well as other disorders including pulmonary disease and lung cancer. Smoking cessation will reduce mortality from CAD, other cardiovascular disease, and all-cause mortality more than any other risk factor intervention in elderly persons.

Hypertension

Increased peripheral vascular resistance is the cause of systolic and diastolic hypertension in elderly persons. Hypertension as a risk factor

Table 2
Association of Systolic or Diastolic Hypertension With New Coronary Events,
Peripheral Arterial Disease, and New Atherothrombotic Brain Infarction in Elderly
Men and Women

Study	No. of Patients	Mean Age (years)	Mean Follow-Up (months)	Elderly Men Relative Risk	Elderly Women Relative Risk
Incidence of new coronary events[6]	708	82	41	2.0	1.8
Prevalence of PAD[17]	869	82	—	1.7	1.5
Incidence of new ABI[23]	708	82	36	3.6	3.0

PAD = peripheral arterial disease
ABI = atherothrombotic brain infarction

for vascular disease in the elderly is discussed extensively in Chapter 11. Table 2 shows the association of systolic or diastolic hypertension with the incidence of new coronary events, with the prevalence of PAD, and with the incidence of new ABI in our elderly population. In these studies, systolic hypertension in the elderly was diagnosed if the systolic blood pressure was 160 mm Hg or higher on three occasions. Diastolic hypertension in the elderly was diagnosed if the diastolic blood pressure was 90 mm Hg or higher on three occasions. Isolated systolic hypertension in the elderly was diagnosed if the systolic blood pressure was 160 mm Hg or higher on three occasions and the diastolic blood pressure was normal. Isolated systolic hypertension occurred in 51% of 499 elderly patients with hypertension.[7] In a study of 1,414 elderly patients, mean age 82 years, the prevalence of systolic or diastolic hypertension was higher in elderly African-Americans (50%) than in elderly Hispanics (35%) or elderly Caucasians (36%).[25]

The Joint National Committee on Detection, Evaluation, and Treatment of High Blood Pressure recommends as initial drug treatment use of diuretics or beta blockers, because these drugs have been documented to reduce cardiovascular morbidity and mortality in controlled clinical trials.[26] The choice of antihypertensive drug selected as monotherapy should, however, depend on associated medical conditions. For example, elderly patients with hypertension who have had an MI or who have angina pectoris, myocardial ischemia, or compex ventricular arrhythmias should initially be treated with a beta blocker such as propranolol.[27] However, elderly patients with congestive heart failure associated with abnormal or normal left ventricular ejection fraction should receive both a diuretic and an angiotensin-converting enzyme (ACE) inhibitor.[28] In addition, elderly patients with hypertension who have diabetes mellitus or left ventricular hypertrophy (LVH) should initially be treated with an ACE inhibitor.

Left Ventricular Hypertrophy

LVH caused by hypertension or other cardiovascular disease is not only a marker for, but also a contributor to, cardiovascular morbidity and mortality in elderly persons. Patients with electrocardiographic LVH[7,29,32] and echocardiographic LVH[7,30-34] have an increased risk of developing new cardiovascular events (Table 3). In our studies,[7,30] electrocardiographic LVH was diagnosed if the Romhilt-Estes point score was ≥5.[35] In our studies,[7,30,32-34] echocardiographic LVH was diagnosed if the left ventricular mass index exceeded 134 g/m² in men and 110 g/m² in women.[36]

At 4-year follow-up of elderly men and women in the Framingham Heart Study, echocardiographic LVH predicted new coronary events independent of standard coronary risk factors.[31] Echocardiographic LVH was 15.3 times more sensitive in predicting new coronary events in elderly men and 4.3 times more sensitive in predicting new coronary events in elderly women than was electrocardiographic LVH.[31] The relative risk for new coronary events per 50 g/m increase in left ventricular mass/height was 1.67 for elderly men and 1.60 for elderly women.[31]

The 8-year age-adjusted incidence of cerebrovascular events in 447 elderly men in the Framingham Heart Study was 18.4% in the highest quartile of left ventricular mass-to-height ratio and 5.2% in the lowest quartile.[37] The 8-year age-adjusted incidence of cerebrovascular events in 783 elderly women in the Framingham Heart Study was 12.5% in the highest quartile of left ventricular mass-to-height ratio and 2.9% in the lowest quartile. After adjustment for age, sex, and cardiovascular disease risk factors, the hazard ratio for new cerebrovascular events was 1.45 for each quartile increase of left ventricular mass-to-height ratio.

At 27-month mean follow-up of 557 elderly patients, mean age 82 years, patients with echocardiographic LVH had a 2.7 times higher incidence of new coronary events and a 3.7 times higher incidence of new ABI than did patients with normal left ventricular mass index.[32] At 37-month mean follow-up of 360 elderly patients, mean age 82 years, with hypertension or CAD, patients with electrocardiographic LVH had a 1.4 times higher incidence of new coronary events and a 1.7 times higher incidence of new ABI than did patients without electrocardiographic LVH.[30] Patients with echocardiographic LVH had a 2.0 times higher incidence of new coronary events and a 2.8 times higher incidence of new ABI than did patients with normal left ventricular mass index.[30] Echocardiographic LVH was 4.3 times more sensitive in predicting new coronary events and 4.0 times more sensitive in predicting new ABI than was electrocardiographic LVH.[30] At 27-month mean follow-up of 468 elderly patients, mean age 82 years, with heart disease, patients with echocardiographic LVH had a 3.3 times higher incidence

Table 3

Association of Electrocardiographic and Echocardiographic Left Ventricular Hypertrophy With Coronary Events, Peripheral Arterial Disease, and Atherothrombotic Brain Infarction in Elderly Men and Women

Study	Follow-Up	Increased Incidence of Cardiovascular Events					
		ECG LVH			Echo LVH		
		Coronary Events	PAD	ABI	Coronary Events	V Fib or SCD	ABI
Elderly men in Framingham Study[29]	30 years	3.0	1.9	3.2			
Elderly women in Framingham Study[29]	30 years	3.7	2.7	6.5			
406 elderly men in Framingham Study[31]	4 years				1.67*		
735 elderly women in Framingham Study[31]	4 years				1.60*		
557 elderly patients[30]	27 months				2.7		3.7
360 elderly patients with hypertension or CAD[30]	37 months	1.4		1.7	2.0		2.8
468 elderly patients with heart disease[33]	27 months					3.3	
110 elderly patients with chronic atrial fibrillation[34]	—						2.4†
84 elderly blacks with hypertension[7]	37 months	1.5		1.8	3.3		2.8
326 elderly whites with hypertension[7]	43 months	1.4		1.9	2.7		3.3

ECG = electrocardiographic; Echo = echocardiographic; LVH = left ventricular hypertrophy; PAD = peripheral arterial disease; ABI = atherothrombotic brain infarction; V Fib = primary ventricular fibrillation; SCD = sudden cardiac death

* relative risk for new coronary events per 50 g/m increase in left ventricular mass/height

† increased prevalence of thromboembolic stroke

(Adapted with permission from Reference 35.)

of primary ventricular fibrillation or sudden cardiac death than did patients with normal left ventricular mass index.[33]

In 110 elderly patients, mean age 82 years, with chronic atrial fibrillation, the prevalence of echocardiographic LVH was 2.4 times higher in patients with prior thromboembolic stroke than in patients without prior thromboembolic stroke.[34] Logistic regression analysis showed that echocardiographic LVH was an independent predictor of thromboembolic stroke with an odds ratio of 6.6.[34] In 1,283 elderly patients, mean age 81 years, the prevalence of LVH was also 1.36 times higher in patients with hypertension and 40% to 100% extracranial internal or common carotid arterial disease than in patients with hypertension without 40% to 100% extracranial internal or common carotid arterial disease.[38]

At 37-month mean follow-up of 84 elderly African-Americans, mean age 78 years, with hypertension, patients with electrocardiographic LVH had a 1.5 times higher incidence of new coronary events and a 1.8 times higher incidence of new ABI than did patients without electrocardiographic LVH.[7] Hypertensive African-Americans with echocardiographic LVH had a 3.3 times higher incidence of new coronary events and a 2.8 times higher incidence of new ABI than did hypertensive African-Americans with normal left ventricular mass index.[7] At 43-month mean follow-up of 326 elderly Caucasians, mean age 82 years, with hypertension, patients with electrocardiographic LVH had a 1.4 times higher incidence of new coronary events and a 1.9 times higher incidence of new ABI than did patients without electrocardiographic LVH.[7] Hypertensive Caucasians with echocardiographic LVH had a 2.7 times higher incidence of new coronary events and a 3.3 times higher incidence of new ABI than did hypertensive Caucasians with normal left ventricular mass index.[7] Multiple logistic regression analysis in 410 elderly African-Americans and Caucasians with hypertension showed that echocardiographic LVH was an independent risk factor for new coronary events (odds ratio = 3.21) and for new ABI (odds ratio = 4.17).[7] Electrocardiographic LVH was an independent risk factor for new ABI (odds ratio = 2.10), but not for new coronary events.[7]

Physicians should try to prevent LVH from developing or progressing in patients with hypertension or other cardiovascular disease. An appropriate balance between blood pressure, left ventricular mass, and coronary blood flow should be maintained. The effect of different antihypertensive drugs on reduction of left ventricular mass is discussed elsewhere.[39,40] A meta-analysis of 109 treatment studies showed that ACE inhibitors are more effective than other antihypertensive drugs in reducing left ventricular mass.[40]

Decrease of left ventricular mass with antihypertensive drugs does not cause deterioration of left ventricular systolic function, and may improve left ventricular diastolic function. Framingham Heart Study data have shown a reduction of cardiovascular events in patients with regression of LVH.[41] The Cornell group has also observed in patients with uncomplicated hypertension followed for 10.2 years that the devel-

Table 4
Association of Dyslipidemia With New Coronary Events at 41-Month Follow-Up
of 192 Elderly Men and 516 Elderly Women

	Relative Risk of New Coronary Events	
	Men	Women
Serum total cholesterol ≥200 mg/dL	1.6	1.8
Serum total cholesterol ≥250 mg/dL	2.2	2.0
Serum HDL cholesterol <35 mg/dL	1.8	1.5
Serum total cholesterol/HDL cholesterol ≥6.5	2.5	2.0
Serum triglycerides ≥190 mg/dL	1.6*	1.4

* Significant by univariate analysis, but not by multivariate analysis.
(Adapted with permission from Reference 6.)

opment of LVH increases, and the regression of LVH probably decreases, the incidence of new cardiovascular events.[42] However, prospective studies using different types of antihypertensive drugs are necessary to determine whether regression of left ventricular mass leads to a reduction in cardiovascular morbidity and mortality.

Dyslipidemia

Hypercholesterolemia

Serum total cholesterol was an independent risk factor for CAD in elderly men and women in the Framingham Heart Study.[43] Among patients with prior MI in the Framingham Heart Study, serum total cholesterol was most strongly related to death from CAD and to all-cause mortality in patients aged 65 and older.[44]

Serum total cholesterol was an independent predictor of CAD in elderly men in the Honolulu Heart Program[45] and an independent risk factor for mortality from CAD in elderly men and women in a Southern California community.[46] Serum total cholesterol was shown to be a predictor of first cardiovascular event in the Systolic Hypertension in the Elderly Program pilot project.[2] The Kaiser Permanente Coronary Heart Disease in the Elderly Study also found that the excess risk of CAD-related mortality attributed to a high serum total cholesterol increased 5.1 times from age 60 to age 79.[47]

In a retrospective study of 518 elderly persons, mean age 82 years, hypercholesterolemia was associated with CAD in elderly men and in elderly women.[48] In a prospective study of 708 elderly persons, mean age 82 years, at 41-month follow-up, a serum total cholesterol of 200 mg/dL or higher increased the incidence of new coronary events 1.6 times in elderly men and 1.8 times in elderly women (Table 4).[6] In this study, a serum total cholesterol of 250 mg/dL or higher increased the

Table 5

Serum Lipids in 1,246 Elderly Women and 547 Elderly Men With and Without Coronary Artery Disease

	Men		Women	
	CAD (n = 259)	No CAD (n = 288)	CAD (n = 515)	No CAD (n = 731)
Abnormal total cholesterol and abnormal HDL cholesterol	20%	5%	17%	5%
Abnormal total cholesterol and normal HDL cholesterol	36%	25%	50%	44%
Normal total cholesterol and abnormal HDL cholesterol	22%	10%	20%	7%
Normal total cholesterol and normal HDL cholesterol	21%	61%	13%	44%

Abnormal serum total cholesterol = ≥200 mg/dL

Abnormal serum HDL cholesterol = <35 mg/dL

There was a 1.28 times greater probability of having CAD for an increment of 10 mg/dL of serum total cholesterol or serum low-density lipoprotein cholesterol after controlling for other prognostic variables; there was a 2.56 times higher probability of having CAD for a decrement of 10 mg/dL of serum HDL cholesterol after controlling for other prognostic variables.

CAD = coronary artery disease

(Adapted with permission from Reference 49.)

incidence of new coronary events 2.2 times in elderly men and 2.0 times in elderly women (Table 4).[6] Multivariate analysis showed that serum total cholesterol was an independent risk factor for new coronary events in elderly men and in elderly women.[6] In 410 elderly patients, mean age 81 years, with hypertension, serum total cholesterol was also shown to be an independent risk factor for new coronary events.[7]

In a study of 1,246 elderly women and 547 elderly men, mean age 81 years, a serum total cholesterol of 200 mg/dL or higher was present in 56% of elderly men and in 67% of elderly women with CAD (Table 5).[49] A multiple logistic regression model showed that there was a 1.28 times greater probability of having CAD for an increment of 10 mg/dL of serum total cholesterol or of serum low-density lipoprotein (LDL) cholesterol after controlling for other prognostic variables.[49]

There are conflicting data about the association of increased serum total cholesterol with PAD. Some studies show an association of increased serum total cholesterol with PAD (Table 6),[5,9,11,50,51] whereas other studies do not show this association.[13,52,53]

The Framingham Heart Study found no association between serum total cholesterol and ABI in men or women.[9] The Multiple Risk Factor Intervention Trial demonstrated an association between serum total

Table 6
Correlation of Serum Lipids in 1,275 Elderly Women and 559 Elderly Men With and Without Peripheral Arterial Disease and Atherothrombotic Brain Infarction

Study	Independent Serum Lipid Predictors
PAD[50]	1.24 times higher probability of having PAD for a decrement of 10 mg/dL of serum HDL cholesterol after controlling for other prognostic variables.
ABI[50]	1.06 times higher probability of having ABI for an increment of 10 mg/dL of serum total cholesterol after controlling for other prognostic variables; 1.27 times higher probability of having ABI for a decrement of 10 mg/dL of serum HDL cholesterol after controlling for other prognostic variables

PAD = peripheral arterial disease
ABI = atherothrombotic brain infarction
(Adapted with permission from Reference 50.)

cholesterol level and death from nonhemorrhagic stroke in men.[54] In a study of 1,275 elderly women and 559 elderly men, mean age 81 years, an association was observed between serum total cholesterol and ABI in elderly men and in elderly women (Table 6).[53] A multiple logistic regression model showed that there was a 1.06 times greater probability of having ABI for an increment of 10 mg/dL of serum total cholesterol after controlling for other prognostic variables.[53]

Low Serum, High-Density Lipoprotein Cholesterol

The Framingham Heart Study demonstrated that a low serum, high-density lipoprotein (HDL) cholesterol was an independent risk factor for CAD in elderly men and women, and the strength of this association was greater than that for serum total cholesterol.[43] In a prospective study of 708 elderly persons, mean age 82 years, at 41-month follow-up, a low serum HDL cholesterol (<35 mg/dL) increased the incidence of new coronary events 1.8 times in elderly men and 1.5 times in elderly women (Table 4).[6] Multivariate analysis showed that a low serum HDL cholesterol was an independent risk factor for new coronary events in elderly women and men. Multivariate analysis also showed at 43-month follow-up of elderly patients, mean age 82 years, with PAD that a low serum HDL cholesterol was an independent risk factor for new coronary events.[18]

In a study of 1,246 elderly women and 547 elderly men, mean age 81 years, a serum HDL cholesterol less than 35 mg/dL was present in 42% of elderly men and in 37% of elderly women with CAD (Table 5).[49] A multiple logistic regression model showed that there was a 2.56 times greater probability of having CAD for a decrement of 10 mg/dL of serum HDL cholesterol after controlling for other prognostic variables.[49] In this study, a serum HDL cholesterol less than 35 mg/dL with a normal serum total cholesterol was present in 20% of elderly women and in 22% of elderly men with CAD (Table 5).[49] Lavie and Milani[55] also showed that 52 of 212 patients (25%) with CAD had a serum HDL cholesterol less than 35 mg/dL with a normal serum total cholesterol.

Serum HDL cholesterol has been reported to be inversely associated with PAD.[11,50,51,53] In a study of 1,275 elderly women and 559 elderly men, mean age 81 years, an inverse association was observed between serum HDL cholesterol and PAD in elderly men and in elderly women.[53] A multiple logistic regression model showed that there was a 1.24 times higher probability of having PAD for a decrement of 10 mg/dL of serum HDL cholesterol after controlling for other prognostic variables.[53]

In the Framingham Heart Study, there was a tendency for an inverse association of serum HDL cholesterol with ABI in both men and women by univariate and multivariate analysis.[56] However, this association was not statistically significant. Bihari-Varga et al[57] demonstrated an inverse association of serum HDL cholesterol with ABI in men and women. In a study of 1,275 elderly women and 559 elderly men, mean age 81 years, an inverse association was observed between serum HDL cholesterol and ABI in elderly men and in elderly women.[53] A multiple logistic regression model showed that there was a 1.27 times greater probability of having ABI for a decrement of 10 mg/dL of serum HDL cholesterol after controlling for other prognostic variables.[53]

Serum Total Cholesterol/High-Density Lipoprotein Cholesterol

In the Framingham Heart Study, the serum total cholesterol/HDL cholesterol ratio was an independent risk factor for CAD in elderly men and women.[43] The strength of this association was similar to that for serum HDL cholesterol and greater than that for serum total cholesterol.[43] In a prospective study of 708 elderly patients, mean age 82 years, at 41-month follow-up, an increased serum total cholesterol/HDL cholesterol ratio (≥6.5) increased the incidence of new coronary events 2.5 times in elderly men and 2.0 times in elderly women (Table 4).[6] In a study of 1,246 elderly women and 547 elderly men, mean age 81 years, an association was observed between the serum total cholesterol/HDL cholesterol ratio and CAD in elderly men and in elderly women.[49] In a study of 1,275 elderly women and 559 elderly men, mean age 81 years, an association was also observed between the serum total cholesterol/HDL cholesterol ratio and both PAD and ABI in elderly men and in elderly women.[53]

Serum Triglycerides

In the Framingham Heart Study, serum triglycerides were an independent risk factor for CAD in elderly women but not in elderly men.[43]

In a prospective study of 708 elderly patients, mean age 82 years, at 41-month follow-up, hypertriglyceridemia (serum triglycerides ≥190 mg/dL) was associated with an increased incidence of new coronary events in elderly men by univariate analysis, but not by multivariate analysis, and was associated with an increased incidence of new coronary events in elderly women by both univariate and multivariate analysis (Table 4).[6] In a study of 1,246 elderly women and 547 elderly men, mean age 81 years, serum triglycerides were associated with CAD in elderly men and in elderly women by univariate analysis, but not by multivariate analysis.[49]

Increased serum triglycerides have been associated with PAD in some studies,[11,13,51] but not in other studies.[16,50,53] Fowkes et al[50] demonstrated an association between serum triglycerides and PAD by univariate analysis, but not by multivariate analysis. In a study of 1,275 elderly women and 559 elderly men, mean age 81 years, serum triglycerides were associated with PAD in elderly men and in elderly women by univariate analysis, but not by multivariate analysis.[53]

In the Framingham Heart Study, very LDL cholesterol was not associated with ABI in men or women.[56] In a study of 1,275 elderly women and 559 elderly men, mean age 81 years, serum triglycerides were associated with ABI in elderly men and in elderly women by univariate analysis, but not by multivariate analysis.[53]

Clinical Studies

Dayton et al[58] demonstrated at 8.5-year follow-up in a randomized, double-blind, controlled study of 846 men, mean age 66 years, that a diet low in cholesterol and saturated fat and high in polyunsaturated fat caused a 31% decrease in new atherosclerotic events, a 33% reduction in sudden CAD-related mortality, an 18% decrease in total CAD-related mortality, and a 31% reduction in fatal atherosclerotic events, but no significant change in all-cause mortality. Vegetarians aged 65 to 84 years have lower serum total cholesterol levels and CAD mortality rates than do nonvegetarians.[59] In the Stockholm Ischemic Heart Disease Study of survivors of a recent MI, half of the patients were 65 years of age and older.[60] Patients treated with nicotinic acid and clofibrate had a 26% decrease in mortality, with a 28% reduction in mortality for patients older than 60 years.

In the Scandinavian Simvastatin Survival Study, 4,444 men and women with CAD were treated with double-blind simvastatin or placebo.[61] At 5.4-year median follow-up, patients treated with simvastatin had a 35% reduction in serum LDL cholesterol, a 25% decrease in serum total cholesterol, and an 8% increase in serum HDL cholesterol. Patients treated with simvastatin also had a reduction in major coronary events of 34%, in coronary deaths of 42%, and in total mortality of 30%. These decreases in coronary events and total mortality were similar in

Table 7
Association of Diabetes Mellitus With New Coronary Events, Peripheral Arterial
Disease, and New Atherothrombotic Brain Infarction in Elderly Men and Women

Study	No. of Patients	Mean Age (years)	Mean Follow-Up (months)	Elderly Men Relative Risk	Elderly Women Relative Risk
Incidence of new coronary events[6]	708	82	41	1.9	2.0
Prevalence of PAD[17]	869	82	—	2.4	3.0
Incidence of new ABI[23]	708	82	36	3.0	2.3

PAD = peripheral arterial disease
ABI = atherothrombotic brain infarction

men and in women between 60 to 70 years of age and those younger
in age.

Recommendations

The above clinical studies suggest that lipid lowering therapy with
diet or drugs may be able to reduce mortality from CAD in elderly
patients. However, well-designed prospective clinical studies are necessary to answer this important question. Until these studies are available,
dietary therapy is recommended for elderly patients, regardless of age,
and in the absence of other serious or life-limiting illness, such as
cancer, dementia, or malnutrition. If hyperlipidemia persists after 3
months of dietary therapy, hypolipidemic drugs should be considered,
depending on: serum lipid levels; presence or absence of CAD, PAD,
or ABI; presence or absence of other risk factors; and the patient's
overall clinical status. In elderly women, the use of estrogen plus cyclic
micronized progesterone is favored as used in the Postmenopausal Es-
trogen/Progestin Interventions (PEPI) Trial[62] as the initial hypolipidemic drug for treating elevated serum LDL cholesterol and reduced
serum HDL cholesterol levels. Simvastatin would be the drug of choice
for treating a high serum LDL cholesterol level.

Diabetes Mellitus

Diabetes mellitus as a risk factor for vascular disease in the elderly
is discussed extensively in Chapter 12. Table 7 shows the association
of diabetes mellitus with the incidence of new coronary events, with
the prevalence of PAD, and with the incidence of new ABI in our elderly
population. In a study of 1,414 elderly persons, mean age 82 years,

Table 8
Association of Number of Major Risk Factors With Incidence of New Coronary
Events at 41-Month Follow-Up of 192 Elderly Men and 516 Elderly Women

	New Coronary Events	
	Men	Women
0 major risk factors	14%	6%
1 major risk factor	25%	21%
≥2 major risk factors	65%	47%

Major risk factors included cigarette smoking, hypertension, serum total cholesterol ≥200 mg/dL or serum HDL cholesterol <35 mg/dL, and diabetes mellitus

(Adapted with permission from Reference 6.)

the prevalence of diabetes mellitus was significantly higher in elderly African-Americans (27%) than in elderly Caucasians (19%).[25] The prevalence of diabetes mellitus was 24% in elderly Hispanics.

Diabetic patients are more often obese and have higher serum LDL cholesterol and very LDL cholesterol levels and lower serum HDL cholesterol levels than nondiabetics. Diabetics also have a higher prevalence of hypertension and LVH than do nondiabetics. These risk factors contribute to the higher prevalence of CAD, PAD, and ABI in diabetics than in nondiabetics.

Elderly diabetics should be treated with dietary therapy, weight reduction if necessary, exercise, and appropriate hypoglycemic drugs if needed to control hyperglycemia. Other risk factors such as smoking, hypertension, dyslipidemia, obesity, and physical inactivity should be controlled.

Warram et al[63] reported that diabetics had an excess mortality associated with diuretic treatment of hypertension. Beta blockers may prolong and potentiate hypoglycemia and can mask many of the signs caused by hypoglycemia. The drug of choice for treating hypertension in diabetics is an ACE inhibitor.

Number of Major Risk Factors

In a prospective study of 192 elderly men and 516 elderly women, mean age 82 years, at 41-month follow-up, the greater the number of major risk factors, the higher was the incidence of new coronary events in elderly men and in elderly women (Table 8).[6] In our elderly men and women, we have also observed that the greater the number of major risk factors, the higher is the prevalence and incidence of PAD and ABI.

Obesity

The Framingham Heart Study found at 30-year follow-up of men and women aged 65 to 94 years that obesity was a risk factor for CAD in elderly men and women.[43] Disproportionate distribution of fat to the abdomen assessed by the waist-to-hip circumference ratio has also been demonstrated to be a risk factor for cardiovascular disease, mortality from CAD, and total mortality in elderly men and women.[64,65]

In a prospective study of 708 elderly patients, mean age 82 years, at 41-month follow-up, univariate analysis showed that obesity ($\geq$20% above ideal body weight) insignificantly increased the incidence of new coronary events 1.3 times in elderly men and significantly increased the incidence of new coronary events 1.7 times in elderly women.[6] However, multivariate analysis showed that obesity was not an independent risk factor for new coronary events in elderly men and women.

The Framingham Heart Study showed that Metropolitan Life Insurance relative weight was not associated with intermittent claudication in women, but was inversely associated with intermittent claudication in men.[9] In a study of 625 elderly women and 244 elderly men, mean age 82 years, obesity insignificantly increased the prevalence of PAD 1.4 times in elderly men and significantly increased the prevalence of PAD 1.8 times in elderly women.[17]

There are conflicting data correlating relative weight with ABI.[56,66-69] Data from a retrospective study of 535 elderly men and women, mean age 82 years, showed that obesity did not significantly correlate with the prevalence of ABI in elderly men or women.[69] In a prospective study of 708 elderly patients, mean age 82 years, at 3-year follow-up, obesity was not a significant risk factor for new ABI in elderly men, but significantly increased the incidence of new ABI 2.6 times in elderly women.[23]

Obese patients with CAD, PAD, or ABI must undergo weight reduction. Weight reduction is also a first approach to controlling mild hypertension, hyperglycemia, and dyslipidemia before placing patients on long-term drug therapy. Regular aerobic exercise should be used in addition to diet to treat obesity.

Physical Inactivity

Physical inactivity is associated with obesity, hypertension, dyslipidemia, and hyperglycemia. Paffenbarger et al[70] reported that persons aged 65 to 79 with a physical activity index greater than 2,000 kcal/wk have a better survival rate than those with a physical activity index less than 2,000 kcal/wk. Wenger[71] discusses physiological bases for the reduction in habitual physical activity with age. Wenger[71] also discusses studies that suggest that physical activity is beneficial in the prevention of CAD.

The relationship of physical inactivity to ABI is unclear.[56,72,73] The Framingham Heart Study showed an insignificant relationship between physical inactivity and stroke.[56] Paffenbarger found a significant association between physical inactivity and stroke in one study,[72] but not in another study.[73]

Moderate exercise programs suitable for elderly persons include walking, climbing stairs, swimming, or bicycling. Exercise training programs are not only beneficial in preventing CAD,[71] but have also been demonstrated to improve endurance and functional capacity in elderly men with CAD.[74]

Prior Coronary Artery Disease, Peripheral Arterial Disease, and Atherothrombotic Brain Infarction

In a prospective study of 708 elderly patients, mean age 82 years, at 41-month follow-up, prior CAD increased the incidence of new coronary events 2.2 times in elderly men and 2.3 times in elderly women.[6] Multivariate analysis showed that prior CAD was an independent risk factor for new coronary events in elderly men and in elderly women. At 42-month follow-up of 410 elderly patients, mean age 81 years, with hypertension, logistic regression analysis showed that prior CAD was an independent risk factor for new coronary events with an odds ratio of 1.7.[7]

We observed that prior PAD increased the incidence of new PAD in our elderly population. At 43-month follow-up of 291 elderly patients, mean age 82 years, with PAD, multivariate analysis showed that prior CAD was an independent risk factor for new coronary events with a relative risk of 2.7.[18]

Patients with prior ABI or transient cerebral ischemic attacks, have a higher incidence of new ABI.[7,56,67,75] At 45-month follow-up of 949 elderly patients, mean age 82 years, multivariate analysis showed that prior ABI was an independent risk factor for new ABI with a relative risk of 2.1.[75] At 42-month follow-up of 410 elderly patients, mean age 81 years, with hypertension, logistic regression analysis found that prior ABI was an independent risk factor for new ABI with an odds ratio of 2.6.[7]

Coexistence of Coronary Artery Disease, Peripheral Arterial Disease, and Atherothrombotic Brain Infarction

Patients with PAD[18,76,77] or cerebrovascular disease[78-81] are at increased risk for developing new coronary events. The Framingham Heart Study demonstrated that the incidence of stroke was increased two to five times in patients with CAD.[56] In a study of 110 elderly patients, mean age 82 years, with chronic atrial fibrillation, logistic regression analysis also showed that prior MI was an independent predictor of thromboembolic stroke with an odds ratio of 4.84.[34] Table 9

Table 9

Prevalence of Coexistence of Coronary Artery Disease, Peripheral Arterial Disease, and Atherothrombotic Brain Infarction in 1,886 Elderly Patients

	CAD	PAD	ABI
ABI is present	53%	33%	—
PAD is present	58%	—	34%
CAD is present	—	33%	32%

CAD = coronary artery disease
PAD = peripheral arterial disease
ABI = atherothrombotic brain infarction
(Adapted with permission from Reference 81.)

shows the prevalence of coexistence of CAD, PAD, and ABI in a study of 1,306 elderly women and 580 elderly men, mean age 81 years.

Age

The incidence of CAD increases with age in elderly men and in elderly women.[3,6] In a prospective study of 708 elderly men and women, mean age 82 years, at 41-month follow-up, age was an independent risk factor for new coronary events in elderly men and in elderly women.[6] In the Framingham Heart Study, the incidence of PAD[10] and of ABI[56] increased with age in men and in women.

Race

African-American men are 2.5 times as likely to die of stroke as Caucasian men.[82] African-American women are 2.4 times as likely to die of stroke as Caucasian women.[82] Table 10 shows the prevalence of CAD, PAD, ABI, and of CAD, PAD, or ABI in 268 elderly African-Americans, mean age 81 years, in 71 elderly Hispanics, mean age 81 years, and in 1,310 elderly Caucasians, mean age 82 years.[83] The prevalence of CAD was not significantly different in elderly African-Americans, Hispanics, and Caucasians. The prevalence of PAD was significantly higher in elderly African-Americans than in elderly Caucasians. The prevalence of ABI was significantly higher in elderly African-Americans than in elderly Hispanics and Caucasians. The prevalence of CAD, PAD, or ABI was significantly higher in elderly African-Americans than in elderly Hispanics and Caucasians.

Gender

Table 11 shows the prevalence of CAD, PAD, and of ABI in 580 elderly men, mean age 81 years, and in 1,306 elderly women, mean age

Table 10
Prevalence of Coronary Artery Disease, Peripheral Arterial Disease, and
Atherothrombotic Brain Infarction in Elderly African-Americans, Hispanics, and
Whites

	African-Americans (n = 268)	Hispanics (n = 71)	Whites (n = 1,310)
CAD	46%	34%	41%
PAD	29%	24%	23%
ABI	47%	31%	22%
CAD, PAD, or ABI	77%	55%	60%

CAD = coronary artery disease
PAD = peripheral arterial disease
ABI = atherothrombotic brain infarction
(Adapted with permission from Reference 84.)

Table 11
Prevalence of Coronary Artery Disease, Peripheral Arterial Disease, and
Atherothrombotic Brain Infarction in Elderly Men and Women

	Men (n = 580)	Women (n = 1,306)
CAD	47%	41%
PAD	29%	23%
ABI	29%	24%

CAD = coronary artery disease
PAD = peripheral arterial disease
ABI = atherothrombotic brain infarction
(Adapted with permission from Reference 81.)

82 years. The prevalence of CAD, PAD, and ABI was significantly higher in elderly men than in elderly women. In a prospective study of 708 elderly men and women, mean age 82 years, at 41-month follow-up, the incidence of new coronary events was not significantly different in elderly men (33%) than in elderly women (29%).[6] In a prospective study of 708 elderly men and women, mean age 82 years, at 3-year follow-up, the incidence of new ABI was not significantly different in elderly men (13%) than in elderly women (12%).[23]

Meta-analysis of observational studies suggest that postmenopausal women taking estrogen have a 50% reduction in CAD.[62] Studies suggest that the most important mechanism for the decrease of CAD by estrogen is an increase in serum HDL cholesterol.[84,85] In the PEPI Trial,[62] use of conjugated equine estrogen, 0.625 mg per day, plus cyclic micronized progesterone 200 mg per day for 12 days per month caused the most favorable effect on serum HDL cholesterol with no excess risk of endometrial hyperplasia. Until data from prospective studies such as the Women's Health Initiative and the Hormone Estrogen/Progestin Replacement Study are available, conjugated equine estrogen is recommended, 0.625 mg daily, plus cyclic micronized progesterone 200 mg per day for 12 days per month in postmenopausal women who have prior CAD or who are at high risk for developing CAD because of coronary risk factors.

References

1. Jajich CL, Ostfield AM, Freeman DH Jr: Smoking and coronary heart disease mortality in the elderly. *JAMA* 252:2831-2834, 1984.
2. Siegel D, Kuller L, Lazarus NB, et al: Predictors of cardiovascular events and mortality in the Systolic Hypertension in the Elderly Program pilot project. *Am J Epidemiol* 126:385-399 1987.
3. Kannel WB, Vokonas PS: Primary risk factors for coronary heart disease in the elderly: The Framingham Study. In: Wenger NK, Furberg CD, Pitt B (eds). *Coronary Heart Disease in the Elderly.* New York: Elsevier Science Publishing Co, Inc; 60-92, 1986.
4. Benfante R, Reed D, Frank J: Does cigarette smoking have an independent effect on coronary heart disease incidence in the elderly? *Am J Public Health* 81:897-899, 1991.
5. LaCroix AZ, Lang J, Scherr P, et al: Smoking and mortality among older men and women in three communities. *N Engl J Med* 324:1619-1625, 1991.
6. Aronow WS, Herzig AH, Etienne F, et al: 41-month follow-up of risk factors correlated with new coronary events in 708 elderly patients. *J Am Geriatr Soc* 37:501-506, 1989.
7. Aronow WS, Ahn C, Kronzon I, et al: Congestive heart failure, coronary events, and atherothrombotic brain infarction in elderly blacks and whites with systemic hypertension, and with and without echocardiographic and electrocardiographic evidence of left ventricular hypertrophy. *Am J Cardiol* 67:295-299, 1991.
8. Hermanson B, Omenn GS, Kronmal RA, et al: Beneficial six-year outcome of smoking cessation in older men and women with coronary artery disease: results from the CASS registry. *N Engl J Med* 319:1365-1369, 1988.
9. Stokes J III, Kannel WB, Wolf PA, et al: The relative importance of selected risk factors for various manifestations of cardiovascular disease among men and women from 35 to 64 years old: 30 years of follow-up in the Framingham Study. *Circulation* 75(suppl V):V-65-V-73, 1987.
10. Kannel WB, McGee DL: Update on some epidemiologic features of intermittent claudication: the Framingham Study. *J Am Geriatr Soc* 33:13-18, 1985.
11. Pomrehn P, Duncan B, Weissfeld L, et al: The association of dyslipoproteinemia with symptoms and signs of peripheral arterial disease: the Lipid Research Clinics Program Prevalence Study. *Circulation* 73(suppl I):I-100-I-107, 1986.
12. Juergens JL, Barker NW, Hines EA Jr: Arteriosclerosis obliterans: review of 520 cases with special reference to pathogenic and prognostic factors. *Circulation* 21:188-195, 1960.
13. Hughson WG, Mann JI, Garrod A: Intermittent claudication: prevalence and risk factors. *Br Med J* 1:1379-1381, 1978.
14. Schroll M, Munck O: Estimation of peripheral arteriosclerotic disease by ankle blood pressure measurements in a population study of 60-year-old men and women. *J Chron Dis* 34:261-269, 1981.

15. Beach KW, Brunzell JD, Strandness DE Jr: Prevalence of severe arteriosclerosis obliterans in patients with diabetes mellitus: relation to smoking and form of therapy. *Arteriosclerosis* 2:275-280, 1982.
16. Reunanen A, Takkunen H, Aromaa A: Prevalence of intermittent claudication and its effect on mortality. *Acta Med Scand* 211:249-256, 1982.
17. Aronow WS, Sales FF, Etienne F, et al: Prevalence of peripheral arterial disease and its correlation with risk factors for peripheral arterial disease in elderly patients in a long-term health care facility. *Am J Cardiol* 62:644-646, 1988.
18. Aronow WS, Ahn C, Mercando AD, et al: Prognostic significance of silent ischemia in elderly patients with peripheral arterial disease with and without previous myocardial infarction. *Am J Cardiol* 69:137-139, 1992.
19. Shinton R, Beevers G: Meta-analysis of relation between cigarette smoking and stroke. *Br Med J* 298:789-794, 1989.
20. Medical Research Council Working Party: MRC trial of treatment of mild hypertension: principal results. *Br Med J Clin Res* 291:97-104, 1985.
21. Wolf PA, D'Agostino PS, Kannel WB, et al: Cigarette smoking as a risk factor for stroke: the Framingham Study. *JAMA* 259:1025-1029, 1988.
22. Rodgers RL, Meyer JS, Judd BW, et al: Abstention from cigarette smoking improves cerebral perfusion among elderly chronic smokers. *JAMA* 253:2970-2974, 1985.
23. Aronow WS, Gutstein H, Lee NH, et al: Three-year follow-up of risk factors correlated with new atherothrombotic brain infarction in 708 elderly patients. *Angiology* 39:563-566, 1988.
24. Aronow WS, Ahn C, Schoenfeld MR: Risk factors for extracranial internal or common carotid arterial disease in elderly patients. *Am J Cardiol* 71:1479-1481, 1993.
25. Aronow WS, Kronzon I: Prevalence of coronary risk factors in elderly blacks and whites. *J Am Geriatr Soc* 39:567-570, 1991.
26. Joint National Committee on Detection, Evaluation, and Treatment of High Blood Pressure: the fifth report of the Joint National Committee on Detection, Evaluation, and Treatment of High Blood Pressure (JNC V). *Arch Intern Med* 153:154-183, 1993.
27. Aronow WS, Ahn C, Mercando AD, et al: Effect of propranolol versus no antiarrhythmic drug on sudden cardiac death, total cardiac death, and total death in patients ≥62 years of age with heart disease, complex ventricular arrhythmias, and left ventricular ejection fraction ≥40%. *Am J Cardiol* 74:267-270, 1994.
28. Aronow WS, Kronzon I: Effect of enalapril on congestive heart failure treated with diuretics in elderly patients with prior myocardial infarction and normal left ventricular ejection fraction. *Am J Cardiol* 71:602-604, 1993.
29. Kannel WB, Dannenberg AL, Levy D: Population implications of electrocardiographic left ventricular hypertrophy. *Am J Cardiol* 60:85I-93I, 1987.
30. Aronow WS, Koenigsberg M, Schwartz KS: Usefulness of echocardiographic and electrocardiographic left ventricular hypertrophy in predicting new cardiac events and atherothrombotic brain infarction in elderly patients with systemic hypertension or coronary artery disease. *Am J Noninvas Cardiol* 3:367-370, 1989.
31. Levy D, Garrison RJ, Savage DD, et al: Left ventricular mass and incidence of coronary heart disease in an elderly cohort: the Framingham Heart Study. *Ann Intern Med* 110:101-107, 1989.
32. Aronow WS, Koenigsberg M, Schwartz KS: Usefulness of echocardiographic left ventricular hypertrophy in predicting new coronary events and atherothrombotic

brain infarction in patients over 62 years of age. *Am J Cardiol* 61:1130-1132, 1988.

33. Aronow WS, Epstein S, Koenigsberg M, et al: Usefulness of echocardiographic left ventricular hypertrophy, ventricular tachycardia, and complex ventricular arrhythmias in predicting ventricular fibrillation or sudden cardiac death in elderly patients. *Am J Cardiol* 62:1124-1125, 1988.
34. Aronow WS, Gutstein H, Hsieh FY: Risk factors for thromboembolic stroke in elderly patients with chronic atrial fibrillation. *Am J Cardiol* 63:366-367, 1989.
35. Romhilt DW, Estes EH: A point score system for the ECG diagnosis of left ventricular hypertrophy. *Am Heart J* 75:752-758, 1968.
36. Devereux RB, Casale PN, Kligfield P, et al: Performance of primary and derived M-mode echocardiographic measurements for detection of left ventricular hypertrophy in necropsied subjects and in patients with systemic hypertension, mitral regurgitation, and dilated cardiomyopathy. *Am J Cardiol* 57:1388-1393, 1986.
37. Bikkina M, Levy D, Evans JC, et al: Left ventricular mass and risk of stroke in an elderly cohort: the Framingham Heart Study. *JAMA* 272:33-36, 1994.
38. Aronow WS, Kronzon I, Schoenfeld MR: Left ventricular hypertrophy is more prevalent in patients with systemic hypertension with extracranial carotid arterial disease than in patients with systemic hypertension without extracranial carotid arterial disease. *Am J Cardiol* 76:192-193, 1995.
39. Aronow WS: Left ventricular hypertrophy. *J Am Geriatric Soc* 40:71-80, 1992.
40. Dahlof B, Pennert K, Hansson L: Reversal of left ventricular hypertrophy in hypertensive patients: a metaanalysis of 109 treatment studies. *Am J Hypertens* 5:95-110, 1992.
41. Kannel WB, D'Agostino RB, Levy D, et al: Prognostic significance of regression of left ventricular hypertrophy (abstr). *Circulation* 78(suppl II):II-89, 1988.
42. Koren MJ, Savage DD, Casale PN, et al: Changes in left ventricular mass predict risk in essential hypertension (abstr). *Circulation* 82(suppl III):III-29, 1990.
43. Castelli WP, Wilson PWF, Levy D, et al: Cardiovascular risk factors in the elderly. *Am J Cardiol* 63:12H-19H, 1989.
44. Wong ND, Wilson PWF, Kannel WB: Serum cholesterol as a prognostic factor after myocardial infarction: the Framingham study. *Ann Intern Med* 115:687-693, 1991.
45. Benfante R, Reed D: Is elevated serum cholesterol level a factor for coronary heart disease in the elderly? *JAMA* 263:393-396, 1990.
46. Barrett-Connor E, Suarez L, Khaw K-T, et al: Ischemic heart disease risk factors after age 50. *J Chron Dis* 37:903-908, 1984.
47. Rubin SM, Sidney S, Black DM, et al: High blood cholesterol in elderly men and the excess risk for coronary heart disease. *Ann Intern Med* 113:916-920, 1990.
48. Aronow WS, Starling L, Etienne F, et al: Risk factors for coronary artery disease in persons older than 62 years in a long-term health care facility. *Am J Cardiol* 57:518-520, 1986.
49. Aronow WS, Ahn C: Correlation of serum lipids with the presence or absence of coronary artery disease in 1,793 men and women aged ≥62 years. *Am J Cardiol* 73:702-703, 1994.
50. Fowkes FGR, Housley E, Riemersma RA, et al: Smoking, lipids, glucose intolerance, and blood pressure as risk factors for peripheral atherosclerosis compared with ischemic heart disease in the Edinburgh Artery Study. *Am J Epidemiol* 135:331-340, 1992.
51. Beach KW, Brunzell JD, Conquest JD, et al: The correlation of arteriosclerosis obliterans with lipoproteins in insulin-dependent and noninsulin-dependent diabetes. *Diabetes* 28:836-840, 1979.

52. Criqui MH, Browner D, Fronek A, et al: Peripheral arterial disease in large vessels is epidemiologically distinct from small vessel disease: an analysis of risk factors. *Am J Epidemiol* 129:1110-1119, 1989.

53. Aronow WS, Ahn C: Correlation of serum lipids with the presence or absence of atherothrombotic brain infarction and peripheral arterial disease in 1,834 men and women aged ≥62 years. *Am J Cardiol* 73:995-997, 1994.

54. Iso H, Jacobs DR Jr, Wentworth D, et al: Serum cholesterol levels and six-year mortality from stroke in 350,977 men screened for the Multiple Risk Factor Intervention Trial. *N Engl J Med* 320:904-910, 1989.

55. Lavie CJ, Milani RV: National Cholesterol Education Program's recommendations, and implications of "missing" high-density lipoprotein cholesterol in cardiac rehabilitation programs. *Am J Cardiol* 1991;68:1087.

56. Wolf PA, Kannel WB: Controllable risk factors for stroke: preventive implications of trends in stroke mortality. In: Meyer JS, Shaw T (eds). *Diagnosis and Management of Stroke and TIAs.* Reading, Massachusetts: Addison-Wesley; 25-61, 1981.

57. Bihari-Varga M, Szekely J, Gruber E: Plasma high-density lipoproteins in coronary, cerebral and peripheral vascular disease: the influence of various risk factors. *Atherosclerosis* 40:337-345, 1981.

58. Dayton S, Pearce ML, Hashimoto S, et al: A controlled clinical trial of a diet high in unsaturated fat in preventing complications of atherosclerosis. *Circulation* 40(suppl II):II-1-II-63, 1969.

59. Snowdon DA, Phillips PL, Fraser GE: Meat consumption and fatal ischemic heart disease. *Prev Med* 13:490-500, 1984.

60. Carlson LA, Rosenhamer G: Reduction of mortality in the Stockholm Ischemic Heart Disease Secondary Prevention Study by combined treatment with clofibrate and nicotinic acid. *Acta Med Scand* 223:405-418, 1988.

61. Scandinavian Simvastatin Survival Study Group: Randomised trial of cholesterol lowering in 4,444 patients with coronary heart disease: the Scandinavian Simvastatin Survival Study (4S). *Lancet* 344:1383-1389, 1994.

62. The Writing Group for the PEPI Trial: Effects of estrogen or estrogen/progestin regimens on heart disease risk factors in postmenopausal women: The Postmenopausal Estrogen/Progestin Interventions (PEPI) Trial. *JAMA* 1273:199-208, 1995.

63. Warram JH, Laffel LMB, Valsania P, et al: Excess mortality associated with diuretic therapy in diabetes mellitus. *Arch Intern Med* 151:1350-1356, 1991.

64. Kannel WB, Cupples LA, Ramaswami R, et al: Regional obesity and risk of cardiovascular disease. *J Clin Epidemiol* 44:183-190, 1991.

65. Folsom AR, Kaye SA, Sellers TA, et al: Body fat distribution and 5-year risk of death in older women. *JAMA* 269:483-487, 1993.

66. Kagan A, Popper JS, Rhoads GG, et al: Dietary and other risk factors for stroke in Hawaiian Japanese men. *Stroke* 16:390-396, 1985.

67. Dyken ML, Wolf PA, Barnett HJM, et al: Risk factors in stroke: a statement for physicians by the Subcommittee on Risk Factors and Stroke of the Stroke Council. *Stroke* 15:1105-1111, 1984.

68. Paffenbarger RS Jr, Williams JL: Chronic disease in former college students. V. Early precursors of fatal stroke. *Am J Public Health* 57:1290-1299, 1967.

69. Aronow WS, Starling L, Etienne F, et al: Risk factors for atherothrombotic brain infarction in persons over 62 years of age in a long-term health care facility. *J Am Geriatr Soc* 35:1-3, 1987.

70. Paffenbarger RS Jr, Hyde RT, Wing AL, et al: Physical activity, all-cause mortality, and longevity of college alumni. *N Engl J Med* 314:605-613, 1986.

71. Wenger NK: Physical inactivity as a risk factor for coronary heart disease in the elderly. *Cardiol Elderly* 2:375-379, 1994.

72. Paffenbarger RS Jr, Wing AL: Characteristics in youth predisposing to fatal stroke in later years. *Lancet* 1:753-754, 1967.

73. Paffenbarger RS Jr: Factors predisposing to fatal stroke in longshoremen. *Preventive Med* 1:522-527, 1972.

74. Williams MA, Maresh CM, Aronow WS, et al: The value of early outpatient cardiac exercise programs for the elderly in comparison with other selected age groups. *Eur Heart J* 5(suppl E):113-115, 1984.

75. Aronow WS, Ahn C, Schoenfeld M, et al: Extracranial carotid arterial disease: a prognostic factor for atherothrombotic brain infarction and cerebral transient ischemic attack. *NY State J Med* 92:424-425, 1992.

76. Hertzer NR, Beven EG, Young JR, et al: Coronary artery disease in peripheral vascular patients: a classification of 1,000 coronary angiograms and results of surgical management. *Ann Surg* 199:223-233, 1984.

77. Smith GD, Shipley MJ, Rose G: Intermittent claudication, heart disease risk factors, and mortality: the Whitehall study. *Circulation* 82:1925-1931, 1990.

78. Hertzer NR, Young JR, Beven EG, et al: Coronary angiography in 506 patients with extracranial cerebrovascular disease. *Arch Intern Med* 145:849-852, 1985.

79. Chimowitz MI, Mancini GBJ: Asymptomatic coronary artery disease in patients with stroke: Prevalence, prognosis, diagnosis, and treatment. *Stroke* 23:433-436, 1992.

80. Aronow WS, Ahn C, Schoenfeld MR, et al: Prognostic significance of silent myocardial ischemia in patients >61 years of age with extracranial internal or common carotid arterial disease with and without previous myocardial infarction. *Am J Cardiol* 71:115-117, 1993.

81. Aronow WS, Ahn C: Prevalence of coexistence of coronary artery disease, peripheral arterial disease, and atherothrombotic brain infarction in men and women ≥62 years of age. *Am J Cardiol* 74:64-65, 1994.

82. Gillum RF: Stroke in blacks. *Stroke* 19:1-9, 1988.

83. Aronow WS: Prevalence of atherothrombotic brain infarction, coronary artery disease, and peripheral arterial disease in elderly blacks, Hispanics, and whites. *Am J Cardiol* 70:1212-1213, 1992.

84. Bush TL, Barrett-Connor E, Cowan LD, et al: Cardiovascular mortality and non-contraceptive use of estrogen in women: results from the Lipid Research Clinics Program Follow-Up Study. *Circulation* 75:1102-1109, 1987.

85. Gruchow HW, Anderson AJ, Barboriak JJ, et al: Postmenopausal use of estrogen and occlusion of coronary arteries. *Am Heart J* 115:954-963, 1988.

Chapter 7

A Rational Approach to the Sequence of Operations in the Elderly

T.J. Bunt, MD
Jeffrey L. Ballard, MD

The elderly tolerate operations well, but complications poorly.

T.J. Bunt

Introduction

It is frequently and fairly stated that cardiovascular disease is the major cause of death in the "elderly" group; however, it may be equivalently stated that the major reason an individual might live to the ripe age of 75 or 80 is that they do not have significant cardiovascular disease. It just depends on your perspective and which side of the statistic you are looking at, and whether or not you are justifying an intended operation.

For the most part, the elderly can be surgically treated for their vascular disease in much the same fashion as a younger patient. The expected results, particularly in terms of improved longevity and lifestyle, are much the same.[1-17] However, it must also be recognized that morbidity and mortality rates steadily increase with each decade over age 65 and that, not infrequently, an initial problem cascades into a constellation of complications resulting in death.[18] Proper recognition of this increasing morbidity is nowhere more important than in the selection of sequence of operations for an elderly patient with multiple reconstructive problems.

Statement of the Problem

An old vascular axiom wisely states that the current symptoms manifested by any given patient represent only the clinically evident

From: Aronow WS, Stemmer EA, Wilson SE (eds). *Vascular Disease in the Elderly.* Armonk, NY: Futura Publishing Company, Inc., © 1997.

tip of the vascular iceberg. Thus, the experienced vascular surgeon does not focus only on the aneurysm, the transient ischemic attack (TIA), or the rest pain; rather, appropriate time is taken to carefully assess for other, less clinically evident vascular disease, disease that might otherwise prove entirely too clinically evident in the perioperative course. Coexistence of other vascular or cardiovascular disease is thus expected, although there are different coefficients of correlation for each initial clinical presentation.

Recognition of the widespread nature of atherosclerotic vascular disease in the elderly then leads to two successive questions in management that are the focus of this chapter:

1. To what extent should the elderly be screened for variations of concomitant disease when admitted for a given primary disease manifestation?
2. If concomitant disease is indeed uncovered, which should be the order of successive therapeutic interventions?

Screening

Presenting Situation—Abdominal Aortic Aneurysm/Aortic Reconstruction

The patient presenting with the diagnosis of an abdominal aortic aneurysm (AAA) has a distinct risk for associated coronary artery disease (CAD), both symptomatic and occult, a small risk for asymptomatic cerebrovascular disease (CVD), and a high incidence of associated peripheral vascular disease (PVD) of which only a small portion needs direct assessment.

Associated Risk

1. CAD: The association of CAD and AAA is probably the most intensively studied situation of concomitant disease. On average, between 50% and 70% of patients will give clinical evidence of CAD (history of myocardial infarction [MI], angina, electrocardiogram [ECG] evidenced MI, etc.) and about another 15% will have clinically occult, but significant CAD. Recognition of this association has lead to the notion that MI is the single largest factor for both perioperative and long-term mortality in aortic surgery.[19-28]

There are a number of ways to arrive at this conclusion:
   a. The noted high incidence of perioperative myocardial infarction (PMI) after all peripheral vascular operations; average rates for all elective patients run 1% to 2% for carotid endarterectomy (CEA), 3% to 5% for aortic aneurysmorrhaphy and aortic reconstruction (AR), 2% to 3% for femoro-

popliteal bypass, and 5% to 8% for femorotibial revasculari-zation. Lower rates have been published in select series utilizing preoperative cardiac screens, but there are numer-ous historical benchmarks for the frequency of PMI in vascu-lar surgery.[19]

b. The high incidence of triple-vessel CAD in peripheral vas-cular patients (without clinical evidence of CAD) in proto-cols utilizing preoperative cardiac catheterization as a screen; 18% of 100 patients studied by Tomatis et al[24] and 16% of over 1000 studied by Hertzer et al.[21]

c. The high frequency of significant impairment of left ventric-ular function on intensive hemodynamic monitoring; 75% of 130 patients in Cohen et al's series[26] and 54% of 350 patients in the series by Bunt.[19,]

d. The significant incidence of clinically occult, but signifi-cant reduction in ejection fraction to less than 35% of values found on routine screening; 9% in Bunt's series.[19,27]

e. The high frequency of ST segment depression indicating segmental ischemia on routine ST segment monitoring of peripheral vascular patients (38% in McCann's and Clem-ents' series, 64% in Pasternak et al's series).[28,29]

It is our firm belief that the broad purpose of a vascular surgeon is to perform the necessary revascularization with not only minimal operative morbidity and mortality, but also with an eye toward optimal long-term patient mortality and quality of life. A thorough routine screening program should, therefore, not only identify the cardiac dis-ease (especially occult), but should quantitate the effect of CAD on the patient's cardiac reserve and ability to tolerate the proposed opera-tion(s), and, finally, should then predicate changes in patient manage-ment, be it levels of monitoring and/or intensive care, anesthetic choice, or even choice of operation.

2. CVD: The incidence of both symptomatic and asymptomatic CVD in AAA/AR patients is quite small, and the indication for its operative therapy follow the standard guidelines. Routine screening with carotid duplex exam for asymptomatic CVD is not considered mandatory. However, our preference is to per-form preoperative screens in all patients, albeit with the expecta-tion that only 5% to 10% will be shown to actually have signifi-cant disease. In these days of "bean counting," it could easily be argued that the cost of the carotid screening program hardly justifies the limited return, particularly when the incidence of cerebrovascular accident (CVA) post-AAA/AR is diminishingly small, and when no studies exist to show that a prophylactic CEA prior to AAA/AR might lower that small risk. Our justifica-tion for routine screening is more on the line of total patient management for the long-term; if a greater than 75% lesion is

picked up, it is probably in the patient's best interest to have it repaired.[19,30-33]

3. PVD: Routinely performed angiography in aneurysm patients will demonstrate roughly half to have peripheral stenoses. Of these, probably half will currently have symptoms (claudication), indicating either a need for screening or for change in operation to aortofemoral grafting to encompass any inflow stenoses.

Screening with a noninvasive laboratory examination is essentially unwarranted if there are palpable pedal pulses and/or no symptoms warranting intervention. If symptoms are present, and particularly if femoral pulses are decreased or absent, then a screening arterial Doppler exam is useful if no more than a baseline prior to partial or complete correction of the stenoses.

Presenting Situation— Coronary Artery Disease

Associated Risk

1. AAA: There is no established reverse correlation between CAD and AAA. Basically, the chance that a CAD patient will have an unrecognized AAA is that of the routinely screened population (see Chapter 23), or less than 5%. Unless the AAA were large (>5 cm), its presence would not materially affect the planned cardiac procedure. Obviously, a clinically apparent AAA requires complete evaluation on its own merits.

2. CVD: The incidence of symptomatic or asymptomatic CVD in cardiac patients is from 3% to 8%, most of whom will have accompanying symptoms (TIA, CVA) to warrant evaluation.[15,30-32,34-36] Routine duplex screening to uncover this small incidence of asymptomatic high-grade lesions is, therefore, a judgment call. If the positive screen led to sequential or combined CEA and cardiac surgery, and if this could be shown to reduce overall CVA rates, then such screening would clearly be justified. This highly controversial subject with papers supporting both sides of the issue is taken up further in the section *Sequence of Operations* (Table).

Faggioli et al,[36] in 1990, noted on routine duplex exam in 539 patients without cerebral symptoms that only 8.7% had greater than 75% stenosis. However, age greater than 60 was an independent indicator for perioperative CVA during cardiac surgery for asymptomatic carotid lesions greater than 75% stenosis; the CVA rate was 11.3% versus 3.8% (p<0.0005), suggesting that in the older age groups, the risk of the occult tight lesion was significant. Overall, mortality was higher (5.3%) for combined procedures than cardiac procedures alone (1.9%).[36]

Brener et al,[31] in their series of 4047 patients undergoing routine duplex exam, noted only a 3.8% incidence of a greater than 50% carotid

Table
Sequencing of Major Operations with Concomitant Operative Comorbidity

	Presenting Syndrome	Concomitant Disease	Staging—1st
CVI	TIA's/RIND/ CVA with recovery Asymptomatic	A—CAD, stable B—CAD, left main or unstable C—AAA, small D—AAA, >5 cm or symptoms E—Claudication F—Limb salvage	1A—CEA 1B—CABG or combined 1C—CEA 1D—CEA 1E—CEA 1F—CEA 2A—CEA 2B—CABG or combined 2C—CEA 2D—AAA 2E—CEA 2F—Revascularization
AAA	Small >5 cm or symptoms	A—CAD, stable B—CAD, unstable or left main C—TIA's/RIND D—>75% asymptomatic E—Claudication F—Limb salvage	1A—AAA 1B—CABG 1C—CEA 1D—CEA 1E—AAA 1F—Revascularization 2A—AAA 2B—CABG or combined 2C—CEA 2D—AAA 2E—AAA 2F—AAA
PVD	Claudication Limb salvage	A—CAD, stable B—CAD, unstable or left main C—TIA's D—CVA, asymptomatic >75% E—Small AAA F—AAA, >5 cm	1A—Revascularization 1B—CABG 1C—CEA 1D—CEA 1E—Revascularization 1F—AAA 2A—Revascularization 2B—CABG 2C—CEA 2D—Revascularization 2E—Revascularization 2F—AAA

stenosis. Bevens noted a 17% incidence of a greater than 50% carotid stenosis and a 5.9% incidence of stenosis greater than 80% in 1087 patients 65 years and older screened with duplex prior to cardiac surgery; carotid screening for this older age group was, therefore, recommended.[20,31,36] The above studies would, therefore, suggest that duplex screening for carotid disease in the elderly cardiac patient is a worthwhile endeavor.

The theoretic risk for the symptomatic carotid stenosis is that either further embolic phenomena resulting in CVA will occur in the perioperative period, or that thrombosis of the stenotic carotid artery may occur during the relatively low pressure of pump perfusion. The theoretic risk for the asymptomatic (and, therefore, presumably discovered at preoperative screening duplex) stenosis is also essentially that of thrombosis during the cardiac procedure.

3. PVD: Patients with primary CAD have a small, but real associated risk for PVD; the risk for associated PVD is higher if the major risk factors for vascular disease in general (hypertension, smoking history, diabetes) are present, rather than hypercholesterolemia alone. Screening for incidental PVD is not, per se, required in the absence of PVD symptoms; however, a pulse exam should be performed and a baseline noninvasive laboratory examination done if pulses are absent or decreased.

Presenting Situation—Cerebrovascular Disease

Associated Risk

1. CAD: There is a remarkably wide disparity among the many published papers regarding the incidence and signifcance of CAD in CVD patients. It can be stated that the risk of PMI during a CEA is quite small, less than for any other peripheral vascular operation.

   Hertzer et al[22,23] performed routine cardiac catheterization in 506 (288 symptomatic, 218 asymptomatic) carotid patients and found severe correctable CAD in 37% of those with clinical symptoms and 16% of those without clinically evident disease. Yeager et al[40] for the Portland group takes the other extreme, noting no cardiac workup in 224 carotid patients and noting a 4% PMI rate at subsequent CEA. O'Donnell et al[38,39] stratifed the risk of PMI at CEA to be 4% for clinically evident CAD to 2.5% for clinically occult CAD.[22,23,33,38-40]

   Mackey et al[38] noted that 30-day survival after CEA was significantly (p<0.5) decreased for those patients with clinically evident CAD (24% prior MI, 21% angina, 35% abnormal ECGs). They noted only two PMIs in 324 symptomatic patients and none in 290 asymptomatic patients and, therefore, recommended cardiac screening only in symptomatic CAD patients.[38]

   Our view parallels that of Yeager and Mackey, based on our experience with routine screening of 630 elective vascular surgery patients, including 114 prospective CEA patients; there was no demonstrated return on the CAD screening in cardiac asymptomatic carotid patients. We do not perform CAD screening unless significant clinical symptoms of CAD warrant it.

2. AAA: The risk of a clinically apparent AAA would justify complete evaluation on its own merit. The chances of a clinically inapparent AAA would not only be small (<5%), but would not be of clinical importance when an indication for CEA existed. No screen is, therefore, necessary nor indicated.
3. PVD: A patient presenting with CVD symptoms rarely has significant symptoms of PVD. A screen would be indicated only for such significant concomitant symptoms and/or as a baseline in the total evaluation of a patient with clinically less significant, but present evidence of PVD.

Presenting Situation—Peripheral Vascular Disease

Associated Risk

1. CAD: All of the statements regarding the high association of CAD in AAA/AR patients apply equally to those with PVD. There is, in addition, an expected higher perioperative risk for any concomitant significant CAD if the patient is over 70 years old, diabetic, and/or requires a limb salvage procedure.[41,42]
2. CVI: The chance of occult greater than 75% carotid stenosis in a patient presenting with PVD symptoms is about 5%. Gentile et al[37] noted on routine screening of 352 infrainguinal revascularization patients that 12.4% had greater than 60% and 4% had greater than 80% asymptomatic carotid stenoses. We, however, routinely do screening carotid duplexes to fully evaluate the patient's operative and long-term risks.[37]
3. AAA: The major reason for screening for AAA in the PVD patient would be the distinct clinical situation of distal emboli suggesting a proximal aortic source (the blue toe syndrome). Routine screening is otherwise unnecessary. Angiography performed for delineation of a planned operative correction may show direct (obvious aneurysm) or subtle (smooth aortic walls, larger distal than proximal aorta) evidence of the AAA. The finding of the aneurysm by this circuitous route would then lead to decisions both as to its risk for rupture and its role in the current PVD symptoms (emboli).

Determining the Order of Operations

Presenting Situation—Abdominal Aortic Aneurysm

The basic indications for repair of an AAA are:

1. Size greater than 5 cm in a patient expected to survive greater than 1 year, despite concomitant medical comorbidities.

2. Size 3.5 to 5.0 cm in a patient with documented good medical health.
3. Complications, including infection, rupture, leakage, and distal embolism.

There are no firm official recommendations as to an age cutoff on any of these scenarios (a topic taken up elsewhere in this book), but most vascular surgeons add the qualifer of "not elderly" to the small aneurysm category, and would follow rather than operate on a small aneurysm in a patient over age 75. This is based on the statistics generated by Katz et al on detailed analysis of the cost-benefit ratio of small aneurysmorrhaphy; age greater than 75 years shifted the operative mortality significantly enough to outweigh the projected benefit of protection from small aneurysm rupture.[43]

The risk of aortic rupture with large or symptomatic AAAs is the basis for operative intervention and, thus, places aneurysmorrhaphy as the primary operation in most situations. The opposing concept is the theoretic risk of aneurysm rupture in the interval between operations and the related, if mythical, concept that an operation on some other organ system somehow increases the risk for aneurysm rupture.

We are unaware of any research that actually delineates such an increased aortic wall dissolution after other surgery, nor of any paper actually demonstrating that AAAs rupture at a higher rate postoperatively. Anecdotal cases abound, but proof is lacking. It is obvious that some aneurysms are statistically going to rupture in the postdiagnosis pretreatment and in the perioperative time frames. This anecdotal occurrence does not however, necessarily indicate causality.

1. AAA/CAD: Basically, the higher risk situation is handled first. Left main/left main equivalant CAD, unstable angina, and recent MI with destabilization indicate that coronary artery bypass grafting (CABG) be done first. Significant three-vessel CAD with good ejection fraction (EF) is a judgment call; aneurysmorrhapy can be performed if intensive hemodynamic monitoring, volume loading, and coronary vasodilator therapy are included; we and others have demonstrated that MI rates can be appreciably lowered with such management. Conversely, and particularly if the aneurysm is smaller and/or recently diagnosed, one can make a case for elective CABG followed by AAA. This has been the Cleveland Clinic approach with combined cardiac and aneurysmorrhaphy mortality rate less than 5%.[19,21,43]

   AAA with significant CAD and reduced EF (particularly less than 35%), to our mind, would indicate the need for CABG first; this would be based on the ability to improve EF, and impact on both longevity and perioperative PMI rate. We and others have shown that less than 35% EF patients can be nursed through aortic surgery with acceptable PMI and mortality rate; however, the posthospital mortality rate is 30% to 50% in the first year, obviating much of the benefit of AAA repair. This would then indicate that unless the heart can also be repaired, there is little benefit to AAA repair. There is, furthermore, data to indicate that an EF less than 28% and uncorrectable by cardiac repair, constitutes a contraindication to AAA repair, based on prohibitive operative and 6-month mortality.[19,26,27]

Combined aortic and cardiac procedures have also been reported; Mohr et al[46] have noted simultaneous cardiac and AAA repair in 25 patients, 21 of whom had symptoms (9) or CAT scan evidence (12) of impending rupture; another 4 had AR for limb salvage. The PMI rate was 4% and mortality 12%, certainly respectable for these uniquely high-risk situations.[28,44-46]

2. AAA/PVD: The AAA is a life-threatening condition, while PVD is, at worst, a limb threat. Consequently, for any AAA greater than 5 cm, repair of the AAA should be the first operation. If a true limb salvage situation exists, a concomitant (preferably two-team approach) procedure may be done, or the patient can have the secondary revascularization performed 4 to 7 days following AAA repair.

There is a theoretic risk for lymphatic contamination of the aortic graft from the distal septic focus (if present) which might suggest distal bypass, and control of the septic focus should be done first followed by aortic grafting. However, the situation of incurring an infected aortic tube or aortoiliac graft from a distal limb septic source has only been described for synthetic grafts with groin incision. No cases exist of more proximal nongroin incision (aortic tube or aortoiliac grafts), as would be the usual case in AAA repair, becoming infected. Were aortobifemoral bypass grafting (ABFB) to be indicated for AAA repair (as is likely in the clinical combination of AAA/limb salvage), it is a moot point as to which recognized risk for groin-wound graft infection is greater—the distal septic focus or a re-do case involving the same groin incision several weeks later?

The other special situation that might arise is the combination of distal emboli and AAA. Here, the large AAA certainly should go first. In the case of a small embolizing AAA, if the limb threat is severe, one can make a case for doing the necessary distal limb revascularization first and the AAA repair second, based on the perceived low threat of interval aortic rupture. Theoretically, further emboli from the AAA could occur in the interim, so the time interval between operations should be short (5 to 7 days).

3. AAA/CVD: There are no real data for establishing which operation goes first in a patient with both AAA and CVD, and most surgeons simply extrapolate from the CAD/CVD data. Basically, one balances the risk of interval aneurysm rupture versus the possibility of CVA during a major aortic procedure. There is, however, no clear theoretic basis for CVA occurring during AAA repair; sustained hypotension to pump perfusion pressures (60 to 80 mm Hg) is certainly not expected.

Our judgment would be that the aneurysm should be done first if it is greater than 5 cm, unless there are frequent (>3) TIAs referable to the carotid disease or unless there is evidence of global decreased perfusion; e.g., bilateral 90% stenoses or 90% stenosis with contralateral occlusion. In the later situation, we would perform the CEA first to be followed within 24 to 48 hours by elective AAA; furthermore, the patient is kept in a monitored situation during that interval so that if aortic rupture does occur, a speedy repair can be effected.

Finding a single asymptomatic 90% lesion or bilateral, but less than 90% stenoses, or having a history of CVA beyond the past 2 months and an ipsilateral lesion, all would indicate that CEA be done as the secondary procedure.

Presenting Situation— Cerebrovascular Insufficiency

The accepted indications for CEA are currently focal TIAs or CVA/ RIND (reversible ischemic neurological deficit) with significant recovery, and referable to an ipsilateral greater than 50% stenosis with or without documented ulcer. CEA is also recommended for an asymptomatic, greater than 75% lesion in a patient in good health. There are a number of other occasional situations, best covered elsewhere in this book. It is also clearly within the recommendation for CEA that the surgeon have a demonstrated ability to perform the operation with acceptable total CVA/mortality rates, 3% for asymptomatic and 6% for symptomatic situations.

These basic indications apply to the elderly, except for the added qualifer of "not too elderly" for asymptomatic lesions. It has been adequately demonstrated by several authors that CEA is tolerated by and beneficial for even the nonogenarian, and many of these cases were actually done for asymptomatic lesions. However, many vascular surgeons set an arbitrary age limit for prophylactic asymptomatic CEA (usually age 80), considering that the increased mortality of any operation at that age combined with limited actuarial survival, begins to predicate against realizing any prophylactic value of the CEA done for asymptomatic disease.[2,4,7,10,12,14-17]

Associated Risk

1. CAD: In patients presenting with both CAD and CVD, a balance is made between incurring a CVA while correcting the CAD, versus incurring a PMI while correcting the CVD. Comparative morbidity analysis is important, since a perioperative CVA during cardiac surgery carries a mortality equivalent to that of a PMI (20% to 50%), so that both events are similarly disastrous.

   Accepted operative sequencing is based on the projected morbidity of the presenting situation. In the event of stable triple-vessel CAD, the CEA goes first if the patient has symptomatic TIAs or if there is bilateral hypoperfusion, represented by bilateral greater than 90% lesions and/or a greater than 90% stenosis with contralateral occlusion. The rationale for this sequence would be that TIAs are a proven indicator of CVA in CABG series, and that the systemic reduction in perfusion pressures while on cardiac bypass might cause a hypoperfusion CVA in the face of high-grade stenoses.

It is, however, important to note in this regard that Brener could not demonstrate loss of cerebral autoregulation or change in lobar cerebral perfusion during total circulatory arrest and assisted perfusion. Previous studies had resulted in conflicting results, but were performed on nonstenotic carotid arteries.[31] Thus, the concept of a CVA occurring during cardiac surgery based on loss of perfusion through a stenotic vessel during absolute relative hypotension remains an unproven concept.

Barnes et al,[35] in 1985, initially outlined the problem by tracking 63 duplex studied and 44 unstudied carotid bruit patients who had undergone cardiac surgery without prophylactic CEA. Of eight cerebral events perioperative to the cardiac surgery, only one occurred ipsilateral to the carotid stenosis. Of 72 survivors of cardiac surgery, 13.9% had TIAs, but only 1.4% had a CVA on 2-year follow-up versus a 0.8% incidence of TIA in 254 other patients undergoing cardiac surgery without cerebral disease.[35]

Hertzer et al[20] noted a decreased incidence of perioperative CVA if CEA was done either combined with cardiac surgery or as first case; CVA rates were 4.2% for 24 patients who underwent CEA first, 4.7% for 71 combined procedures, and 7.4% for 58 patients who underwent CEA as the second case. The rate of CVA for second procedure CEAs was 2.2% for a 2-week delay, but 11% if there was a greater than 2-week interval.[20] Cambria et al,[47] in 1989, noted no differences in operative mortality (2.0% versus 2.2%) or CVA rate (2.0% versus 0.6%) in 71 combined CEA/cardiac procedures versus 3570 single cardiac procedures.[47]

Brener et al[31] screened 4047 patients with duplex prior to cardiac surgery. Of this group, only 3.8% (153) had a carotid stenosis greater than 50%. The perioperative CVA rate was 1.9% if there was no disease, but 9.2% in those with greater than 50% stenosis. The CVA rate varied from 15.0% in 32 with occluded carotids to 7.4% in 121 with greater than 50% stenoses. Overall, they noted a high rate of cerebral events in patients with carotid stenosis, but could not show that a combined procedure decreased the CVA rate, which was 8.8% for 57 combined procedures, but 6.3% in 64 patients without any carotid reconstruction.[31]

Perler et al[48] developed a mortality predictor index (MPI) for combined procedures based upon the factors of age over 65, male sex, left main disease, congestive heart failure, and bilateral carotid disease. They noted that overall mortality was 2.8% for patients less than 65-years-old, but 22% for patients over age 65; 17% for bilateral stenoses versus 6% for unilateral lesions; and 23% for demonstrated occlusion of the contralateral carotid artery. CVA rates in the small series (63 patients) were 2.4% for an MPI of 0 to 2, but 29% for greater than 3.[48] They, therefore, concluded that it was of questionable benefit to consider combined procedures for elderly patients due to the increased CVA rate.

Our generic recommendations for sequencing would be that the more symptomatic lesion goes first, but if both are highly significant, then a combined procedure is probably the most direct method of management.

2. AAA: Attempts have been made to make a similar case for the aneurysm patient with CVD, as is done for CAD, based on the concept that there is a potential for hypotension during AAA and that a CVA might be engendered. An intellectual dismantling of this hypothesis is, however, not difficult. Severe hypotension less than 80 mm Hg is distinctly uncommon in elective AAA repair with current volume loading and invasive monitoring techniques; furthermore, such hypotension would be expected to be transient and not the sustained systemic hypotension of cardioplegia. Furthermore, CVA is an uncommon complication of either elective or ruptured AAA surgery. Certainly, there is little factual data to suggest that the carotid lesion carries as much risk as it might in a patient facing cardiac surgery. Conversely, AAA rupture following CEA surgery is a statistical event that will be anecdotally observed by any surgeon.

Our recommendation would be that a significantly symptomatic carotid (TIAs, recent RIND) would go first with AAA repair to follow within 24 to 48 hours, and the patient followed in an intensive care situation for the duration. A high-grade stenosis would represent a judgment call: for a smaller aneurysm with presumably smaller interval rupture risk, preliminary CEA would be reasonable. For larger and/or symptomatic AAAs, AAA repair should be done first with sequential CEA at 7 to 10 days.

3. PVD: Sequencing of operations is based on the perception of relative risk. The revascularization should be preceded by CEA for frequent and recent TIAs and/or any 90% lesion. Older CVAs and/or less tightly stenotic lesions can be handled in either order, dependent on the urgency of the limb revascularization.

In most situations, we would do the CEA first, followed within 24 to 48 hours by limb revascularization, based on the concept that stroke carries significantly more morbidity/mortality than limb loss.

Presenting Situation—Peripheral
Vascular Disease

The patient with PVD will present with either disabling claudication or a firm limb salvage situation (pedal sepsis, digit gangrene, rest pain, or ischemic ulcer). The severity of the presenting situation dictates the urgency of revascularization, and by extension, the need for/time for screening of other concomitant disease. In general, claudicators allow complete workup of all related systems, while limb salvage situations require that the revascularization be performed without other screens.

Associated Risks

1. CAD: The tip of the vascular iceberg not uncommonly protrudes at the feet, while the Titanic-sinking occult lesion lurks in the heart.

   The highest rates of PMI are seen with limb salvage operations, particularly bypasses distal to the knee in greater than 70-year-old patients. The 5-year mortality rate for limb salvage situations is similarly much higher (30% to 45%) than for revascularizations done for claudication (10% to 28%).[19,41,42]

   As much as we may recognize this increased PMI and higher MI rate, the presenting limb salvage situation does not usually provide sufficient time to allow for full evaluation of the CAD (e.g., coronary catheterization and CABG) before a proposed limb salvage procedure. Furthermore, there are only anecdotal case histories of simultaneous coronary and distal revascularization procedures in this setting.

   Our opinion would be that for truly urgent limb salvage situations (forefoot gangrene, wet digital gangrene with rest pain, etc.), revascularization be done first. We would forcefully recommend perioperative intensive hemodynamic monitoring and also suggest that follow-up cardiac evaluation be mandatory to identify significant CAD whose eventual correction might decrease the long-term cardiac mortality. Claudication and lesser severity "limb salvage" situations (stable rest pain, ischemic ulcer, dry single digital gangrene) should be screened appropriately for CAD, and correction of life-threatening CAD situations be done first with follow-up peripheral revascularization at 2 to 3 weeks.

2. CVD: A similar case can be made for identification of/correction of significant CVD. Fewer than 5% of PVD patients will demonstrate high-grade (>75%) clinically occult CVD on duplex screening. Furthermore, there is no distinct recognizable risk for perioperative CVA in patients undergoing peripheral revascularization, even when they do have clinical symptoms of CVD.

   Therefore, in general, revascularization would proceed first for true limb salvage situations. For significantly symptomatic CVD, CEA would go first; and for claudicators, we would probably perform the CEA for high-grade asymptomatic stenosis, followed within 24 to 48 hours by peripheral revascularization.

3. AAA: Incidental finding of a large AAA in a patient with PVD presenting symptoms is distinctly uncommon, except for those with clear-cut emboli to the feet in the presence of pulses. Were a patient to present with the combination of AAA and PVD, the severity of symptoms of the latter would dictate the sequence of operations, understanding that, in many cases, correction of both may be possible by aneurysmorrhaphy with ABFB.

Were more distal revascularizations required, the patient would most probably be presenting with a more severe limb salvage situation. Our opinion would be that for a small AAA, peripheral revascularization would be first for both claudication and limb salvage situations. Large AAAs would be repaired first for claudicators or less severe limb salvage situations. The patient with a true severe limb salvage situation should undergo correction of that first, with aneurysmorrhaphy at a convenient interval after appropriate CAD and other medical comorbidity screening.

In some situations, a combined approach may be indicated, usually with a two-team approach. Such operations in the elderly, however, need to be carefully considered in light of their limited cardiac reserve for what may be both increased blood loss and greater physiological insult.

Aortic Reconstruction/Abdominal Aortic Aneurysm and Other Abdominal Surgery

Performance of concomitant aortic and visceral surgery can be thoughtfully appraised as raising two distinct questions of risk.

The first is that the visceral procedure will significantly add to the morbidity and mortality of the aortic procedure. However, no one has shown this to be true for elective aortic surgery cases; for more complex, urgent, or complicated situations, there appears to be an added morbidity, but causality is difficult to prove.[49] It, therefore, seems quite reasonable to state that concomitant visceral procedures are safe if the patient is stable at completion of the aortic procedure, he/she is not at high medical risk, and the additional procedure can be performed quickly without expectation of major blood loss, nor other physiological decompensation, nor significant spillage of contaminated fluids. Conversely, it does not seem reasonable to perform extra procedures in unstable patients, those with high preoperative risk factors, if there is already gross retroperitoneal or intraperitoneal hemorrhage/soiling (e.g., ruptured AAA), nor if there is distinct risk of significant contamination of the field by contaminated fluids (e.g., opening distended/obstructed viscera).

For the elderly, concomitant visceral procedures should be very carefully considered as to real benefit in terms of the expected life span of the patient. Concomitant cholecystectomy, paraesophageal herniorr-hapy, or resection of a renal/adrenal/adnexal tumor are all reasonable, whereas colectomy, gastric resection, or incidental appendectomy certainly would not be.

The second issue of risk is whether or not concomitant visceral surgery increases the risk of aortic graft infection (GIF). This can be answered in a number of ways.

Theoretically, such a GIF might occur from:
a. Direct contamination of the graft by fluids from the opened viscus. This is the basic reason for avoidance of the visceral surgery if such contamination is a real possibility, and is also the reason for thoroughly closing the retroperitoneum and then packing off the aortic graft *prior* to the visceral procedure. In the absence of visualized contamination of these packs during the visceral procedure, there is little objective reason for concern about subsequent aortic GIF.
b. Delayed or secondary bacteria-positive visceral fluid leaks into the free intraperitoneal cavity with secondary graft contamination. Again, although theoretically possible, most anastomotic leaks or biliary (hepatic bed) leaks form well-localized regional collections, and are highly unlikely to form collections/abscesses in continuity with the aortic bed. Most importantly, the known statistics on concomitant aortic and visceral surgery do *not* demonstrate an increased risk of GIF. The only reported case of aortic GIF following concomitant visceral surgery occurred when repairing a ruptured AAA— an inappropriate situation. Or looking at it from the other end of the spectrum, of the 650 cases of published GIF, only a handful can be definitively traced to either prior visceral injury or visceral surgery.[49]
c. Bacteremia from secondary infections that were related to the visceral procedure; this alone is a viable and reasonable theoretic avenue for secondary graft sepsis. The most reasonable suspect situation would be anastomotic leaks from bacterial containing viscera; e.g., obstructed enteric or biliary and colonic resections. Since anastomotic leaks/abscess formation/phlegmons are common enough problems with such procedures performed without vascular grafting, it only seems prudent to avoid the combination.

Finally, of course, there is the possibility of avoiding the whole scenario completely. If one feels that the secondary procedure is necessary and cannot be delayed to a later time frame, then one can always cogitate on alternative vascular reconstructions that fit the problem at hand, but avoid an intraperitoneal grafting procedure: axillofemoral;

thoracofemoral; or retroperitoneal supra-aortic aortofemoral grafts can be entertained, allowing the intraperitoneal visceral procedure to be performed in a place extra-anatomical to the graft.

Summary

A reasonable compromise position regarding concomitant vascular/visceral surgery in the elderly would then seem to be to go ahead with both if the situation is elective, both procedures have firm indications, the patient is not high risk and is stable at completion of the vascular procedure, and there is no significant retroperitoneal clot/hemorrhage remaining. In addition, we would restrict this to concomitant cholecystectomy or noncavitary upper gastrointestinal procedures.

References

1. Baker WH, Munns JR: Aneurysmectomy in the aged. *Arch Surg* 110:513-517, 1975.
2. Benhamow AC, Kieffer E, Tricot JF, et al: Carotid artery surgery in patients over 70 years of age. *Int Surg* 66:199-202, 1981.
3. Chalmers RTA, Stonebridge PA, John TG, Murie JA: Abdominal aortic aneurysm in the elderly. *Br J Surg* 80:1122-1123, 1993.
4. Coyle KA, Smith RB, Salom AA, et al: Carotid endarterectomy in the octogenarian. *Ann Vasc Surg* 8:5:417-420, 1994.
5. Edmunds LH Jr: Resection of abdominal aortic aneurysms in octogenarians. *Ann Surg* 165:453-457, 1967
6. Esselstyn CB Jr, Humphreys AW, Young JR, et al: Aneurysmectomy in the aged? *Surgery* 67:34-39, 1970.
7. Favre JP, Guy JM, Frering V, et al: Carotid surgery in the octogenarian. *Ann Vasc Surg* 85:421-426, 1990.
8. Harris KA, Ameli FM, Lally M, et al: Abdominal aortic aneurysm resection in patients more than 50 years old. *Surg Gynecol Obstet* 162:531-538, 1986.
9. O'Donnell TF, Darling RC, Linton ER: Is 80 years old too old for aneurysmectomy. *Arch Surg* 111:1250-1257, 1976.
10. Ouriel K, Penn TG, Ricotta JJ, et al: Carotid endarterectomy in the elderly patient. *Surg Gynecol Obstet* 162:334-336, 1986.
11. Paty PSK, Lloyd WE, Chang BB, et al: Aortic replacement for abdominal aortic aneurysm in elderly patients. *Am J Surg* 166:191-194, 1993.
12. Pinkerton JA, Ghoekar VR: Should patient age be a consideration in carotid endarterectomy? *J Vasc Surg* 11:650-658, 1990.
13. Robson AJ, Currie IC, Poskitt KR, et al: AAA repair in the over 80s. *Br J Surg* 76:1018-1020, 1989.
14. Rosenthal D, Ruddeman RH, Jones DH, et al: Carotid endarterectomy in the octogenarian: is it appropriate? *J Vasc Surg* 3:782-787, 1986.
15. Schroe H, Suy R, Nevelsteen A: Carotid endarterectomy in patients over seventy years of age. *Ann Vasc Surg* 4:133-137, 1990.
16. Schultz RD, Sterpetti AV, Feldhaus RJ: Carotid endarterectomy in octogenarians and nonagarians. *Surg Gynecol Obstet* 166:245-251, 1988.
17. Treiman RL, Wagner WH, Foray RF, et al: Carotid endarterectomy in the elderly. *Ann Vasc Surg* 6:321-324, 1992.

18. Plecha FR, Bertin VS, Plecha ES, et al: The early results of vascular surgery in patients 75 years of age and older: an analysis of 3529 cases. *J Vasc Surg* 26:769-775, 1985.
19. Bunt TJ: The role of a defined protocol for cardiac risk assessment in decreasing perioperative myocardial infarction in vascular surgery. *J Vasc Surg* 15(4):626-634, 1992.
20. Hertzer NR, Loop FD, Beven EG, et al: Surgical staging for simultaneous coronary and carotid disease: a study including prospective randomization. *J Vasc Surg* 9:455-464, 1989.
21. Hertzer NR, Young JR, Kramer JR, et al: Routine coronary angiography prior to elective aortic reconstruction: results of selective myocardial revascularization in patients with peripheral vascular disease. *Arch Surg* 114:1336-1343, 1979.
22. Hertzer NR, Young JR, Beven EG, et al: Coronary angiography in 506 patients with extracranial cardiovascular disease. *Arch Intern Med* 145:849-852, 1985.
23. Hertzer NR, Beven EG, Young JR, et al: Coronary artery disease in peripheral vascular patients: a classification of 1000 coronary angiograms and results of surgical management. *Ann Surg* 199:223-233, 1984.
24. Tomatis LA, Fierens EE, Verbrugge GP: Evaluation of surgical risk in peripheral vascular disease by coronary arteriography: a series of 100 cases. *Surgery* 71:429-435, 1972.
25. Graor RA, Hertzer NR: Management of coexistent carotid artery and coronary disease. *Stroke* 19:1441-1444, 1988.
26. Cohen JL, Wender R, Maginot A, et al: Hemodynamic monitoring of patients undergoing abdominal aortic surgery. *Am J Surg* 146:174-177, 1983.
27. Kazmers A, Cerqueira MD, Zierler RE: The role of preoperative radionuclide ejection fraction in direct abdominal aortic aneurysm repair. *J Vasc Surg* 8:128-136, 1988.
28. McCann RL, Clements FM: Silent myocardiac ischemia in patients undergoing peripheral vascular surgery: incidence and association with perioperative cardiac morbidity and mortality. *J Vasc Surg* 9:583-587, 1989.
29. Pasternack PF, Grossi EA, Baumann FG, et al: Silent myocardial ischemia monitoring predicts late as well as perioperative cardiac events in patients undergoing vascular surgery. *J Vasc Surg* 16:171-180, 1992.
30. Ahn SS, Baker JD, Walden K, Moore WS: Which asymptomatic patients should undergo routine screening carotid duplex scan? *Am J Surg* 162:180-183, 1991.
31. Brener BJ, Brief BK, Alpert J, et al: A four-year experience with preoperative noninvasive carotid evaluation of 2026 patients undergoing cardiac surgery. *J Vasc Surg* 1:326-338, 1984.
32. Flanigan DP, Shuler JJ, Vogel M, et al: The role of carotid duplex scanning in surgical decision making. *J Vasc Surg* 2:15-25, 1985.
33. Turnipseed WD, Berkoff HA, Belzer FO: Postoperative stroke in cardiac and peripheral vascular disease. *Ann Surg* 192:365-368, 1980.
34. Bornese RW, Liebmann PR, Phyllis B, et al: The natural history of asymptomatic carotid disease in patients undergoing cardiovascular surgery. *Surgery* 90:1075-1083, 1981.
35. Barnes RW, Nix MC, Samsonetti D, et al: Late outcome of untreated asymptomatic carotid disease following cardiovascular operations. *J Vasc Surg* 2:843-849, 1985.
36. Faggioli GL, Cure GR, Ricotta JJ: The role of carotid screening before coronary artery bypass. *J Vasc Surg* 12:724-731, 1990.
37. Gentile A, Taylor CM, Moneta GM, Porter JM: Prevalence of asymptomatic carotid stenosis in patients undergoing infrainguinal bypass surgery. *Arch Surg* 130:900-904, 1995.

38. Mackey WC, O'Donnell TF, Callow AD, et al: Cardiac risk in patients undergoing carotid endarterectomy: impact on perioperative and long-term mortality. *J Vasc Surg* 11:226-232, 1990.
39. O'Donnell TF, Callow AD, Miller C, et al: The impact of coronary artery disease on carotid endarterectomy. *Ann Surg* 198:705-712, 1983.
40. Yeager RA, Moneta GL, McConnell DB, et al: Analysis of risk factors for myocardial infarction following carotid endarterectomy. *Arch Surg* 124:1142, 1989.
41. Bunt TJ, Mohr, JD: Revascularization versus amputation. In: Rutherford RB (ed). Vascular Surgery. 4th Ed. Philadelphia: WB Saunders, Co., 2025-2033, 1995.
42. Bunt TJ: Revascularization or amputation. In: Rutherford RB (ed). *Vascular Surgery*. 4th Ed. 1993.
43. Katz DA, Littenberg B, Cronenwett JL: Management of small abdominal aortic aneurysms: early surgery versus watchful waiting. *JAMA* 268:19:2678-2686, 1992.
44. O'Connor MS, Licina MG, Kraensler EJ, et al: Perioperative management and outcome of patients having cardiac surgery combined with abdominal aortic aneurysm resection. *J Cardio Thor Vasc Surg* 8:519-526, 1994.
45. Vermuelen FGG, Hamerlijnck PHN, DeFauw JJAM, Ernst SMPG: Synchronous operations for ischemic cardiac and cardiovascular disease: early results and long-term follow-up. *Ann Thorac Surg* 53:381-390, 1992.
46. Mohr FW, Falk V, Autschbach R, et al: One stage surgery of coronary arteries and abdominal aorta in patients with impaired ventricular function. *Circulation* 91:379-385, 1995.
47. Cambria RP, Ivarsson BL, Akins CW, et al: Simultaneous carotid and coronary disease: safety of the combined approach. *J Vasc Surg* 9:56-64, 1989.
48. Perler BA, Burdick JF, Minken SL, et al: Should we perform carotid endarterectomy synchronously with cardiac surgical procedures? *J Vasc Surg* 8:402-409, 1988.
49. Bunt TJ: *Vascular Graft Infections*. Mt. Kisco, NY: Futura Publishing Co., Inc.; 1994.

Chapter 8

Evaluation of the Cardiovascular System

James M. Guernsey, MD

The risk of cardiac complication occurring in any adult patient undergoing anesthesia and surgery is of concern. This concern grows as clinical evidence of vascular disease and the age of the patient increase. The ability to predict perioperative cardiac complications, and to make a reasoned judgment of the postoperative quality and quantity of life, is important in determining the role of elective surgery in the treatment of a patient's disease.

Calculation of the risk/benefit ratio of surgical procedures is complicated by frequently changing parameters. These changes occur with the development of new surgical procedures, new nonsurgical treatments used in place of traditional operations, and the increasing life expectancy of elderly patients.

In an attempt to increase the accuracy of accessing cardiac risk, several stratification systems have been developed. Some have been helpful, but have not provided the required specificity.

If all patients are subjected to all tests, then a reasonably accurate prediction of the risk of an adverse perioperative myocardial event can be made.

The ability to predict at least one aspect of outcome is important; however, the evaluation can be invasive and expensive. In this time of fiscal constraint and strict accountability for resource utilization, each patient at risk will not be able to undergo each test. An individual strategy based on the patient's history, physical examination, and the electrocardiogram needs to be developed.

This chapter addresses a group of patients that is rapidly increasing in size; for example, at the end of the next two decades 20% to 25% of United States citizens will be over the age of 65.[1] This growth alone means that this group will need an increased allocation of resources for medical care. A careful evaluation of risk and benefit may be the principal method by which these resources are allocated.

From: Aronow WS, Stemmer EA, Wilson SE (eds). *Vascular Disease in the Elderly.* Armonk, NY: Futura Publishing Company, Inc., © 1997.

The definition of that group of people described as elderly changes as medical and surgical knowledge and skills improve. The cardiovascular system changes with age, by the fragmentation of the elastic lamina and hyperplasia in the intima and media. This leads to stiffness in the heart and vessels with resulting increase in the peripheral resistance. Stress associated with surgery increases the cardiac work and myocardial oxygen demand. Younger patients meet the need for increased cardiac output by increasing the cardiac rate. Elderly patients increase cardiac output by increasing stroke volume by increasing end diastolic volume. This stress-induced need to increase cardiac output in the elderly patient is impaired due to decreased reserve capacity. Covert or compensated cardiac disease may result in decreasing myocardial oxygen supply, leading to myocardial ischemia and cardiac failure.[2] Fifty percent of all postoperative deaths in elderly patients are attributed to heart disease.[2] Several schemes for the detection of compensated or overt myocardial disease in the potential surgical patient that have been used to determine cardiac risk of elective surgery are covered in this chapter.

Evaluation of Cardiac Risk Using the History and Physical Examination

The least invasive and least expensive method to determine the cardiac risks of surgery are those based predominately on the patient's history, physical examination, and routine tests. One of the first such systems was developed by anesthesiologists during the 1950s and 1960s and reported by Dripps and Eckenhoff.[3] The purpose of this work was to examine the role of anesthesia, and various anesthesia techniques and agents in surgical mortality. These studies included over 33,000 patients. A simple system based on the patient's physical status emerged and has survived without significant change for almost 40 years (Table 1).

The strength of this evaluation system is that it is simple, clear, reproducible, and useful. It allows comparison of outcomes of patients undergoing specific anesthesia and surgical procedures in groups of patients with matched physical statuses. One example is comparing the surgical outcome of inguinal hernia repair in a 70-year-old patient with controlled congestive heart failure with that of a healthy 18-year-old. Clearly, the morbidity and mortality in the group with the best physical status will be less than those in the group with poorer physical status. It is interesting that the American Society of Anesthesiologists (ASA) physical status is a significant predicator of outcome in the Veteran's Administration Surgical Quality Improvement Program study's evaluation of the results of various surgical procedures in over 90,000 Veterans Administration patients.[4]

While the ASA system made a major advance in assessment of the overall risk/benefit calculation for patients undergoing surgery, a study by Goldman and associates[5] in 1977 used a multifactorial index to determine the risk of adverse cardiac events during and following surgi-

Table 1
American Society of Anesthesiologists Physical Status Classification

Class	Description
1	Normal healthy person.
2	Patient with mild systemic disease.
3	Patient with severe systemic disease that limits activity, but is not incapacitating.
4	Patient with an incapacitating disease that is a constant threat to life.
5	Moribund patient not expected to survive 24 hours with or without operation.
E	In the evaluation of emergencies, the number is preceded with an E.

(Reproduced with permission from the American Society of Anesthesiologists, 520 N. Northwest Highway, Park Ridge, IL 60068-2573.)

cal procedures with the exclusion of heart operations. This study was done prospectively and included 1001 patients over the age of 40. With the use of multivariate discriminate analysis, nine independent correlates for postoperative cardiac morbidity and mortality were identified (Table 2).[5]

Each correlate was assigned a numerical value. The sums of the correlate numerical values were divided into four groups; the groups were assigned a risk factor and the patients placed into a group based on the sums of the correlates they accumulated. Two other systems for evaluating perioperative risk were developed: The New York Heart Association System[6] which compared patients on the basis of cardiac symptoms during ordinary activity and the Canadian Cardiovascular Society System[7] based on similar criteria. Later, Goldman et al[8] further developed their system by adding a new specific activity scale to increase the reproducibility and validity of assessment of cardiac risk.

Table 2
Risk of Adverse Cardiac Events During and Following Surgical Procedures
(excluding heart operations)

1. S1 gallop or jugular vein distention.
2. Myocardial infarction in the preceding 6 months.
3. Rhythm other than sinus or premature atrial contractions.
4. More than 5 premature ventricular contractions.
5. Intraperitoneal, intrathoracic, or aortic operation.
6. Age greater than 70 years.
7. Important aortic valvular stenosis.
8. Emergency operation.
9. Poor general medical condition.

The development of a single, reproducible, and valid scale is extremely difficult. Those patients being considered who were known to have heart disease were clearly at higher risk than those without heart disease. The group of patients who were normal after routine tests were at low risk, but there remained a significant group of patients whose heart disease was occult and the identification of these patients remained problematic. These studies were also helpful in predicting adverse cardiac events not connected with surgery, and helped to determine the ultimate benefit of a surgical procedure to the quality and quantity of the patient's life. Cardiac stratifications are able to reasonably predict perioperative risk of a defined group of patients with similar findings. However, attempting to define the risk for an individual patient who is neither in the high- nor the low-risk group is a problem. The defining factor is whether or not the patient has silent myocardial ischemia. The most commonly used methods of detecting significant coronary disease and silent ischemia are the exercise stress test, 24-hour ambulatory electrocardiograph, and dipyridamole thallium-201 screening.

Exercise Stress Testing

A patient is judged to be a low cardiac risk if there is no induced myocardial ischemia when the heart rate exceeds 85% of the maximum predicated rate during exercise. Among the limiting factors for this test are that as few as 30% of patients over the age of 65 can achieve the level of stress necessary for a valid test because of physical restrictions, such as degenerative joint disease, previous stroke, muscular weakness, or leg claudication. A small number of patients cannot cooperate secondary to mental conditions. An additional subset of patients have electrocardiograph changes that interfere with the accurate interruption of the exercise electrocardiogram. Gerson et al found that exercise stress testing was not helpful in assessing cardiac risk of potential surgical patients over the age of 40 years.[9]

Twenty-Four Hour Ambulatory Electrocardiograph

This test is available to most elective surgical patients preoperatively, since they meet the electrocardiographic and mobility requirements to complete a valid test. In addition, the electrocardiographic evidence of ischemia may be present at normal heart rates. The value of this test in identifying the preoperative patient with ischemia is arguable, but the evidence that a test that does not reveal ischemia indicates low cardiac risk is strong. Furthermore, important 1- to 2-year prognosis relative to adverse cardiac events not related to surgery in those patients with a positive test is important in the determination of the risk/benefit ratio.[10,11]

Dipyridamole Thallium-201 Screening

Dipyridamole thallium-201 screening is a precise way of evaluating the coronary arteries and discovering areas of the myocardium that do not receive blood flow, and other areas that at first are underperfused, but later show increased flow. Thallium-201 is extracted from the blood and imaging is based on relative coronary flow. Dipyridamole causes coronary blood flow in nonobstructed arteries to increase three to five times without significantly increasing myocardial oxygen demand. This is equivalent to the increased blood flow produced by exercise, but without severe tachycardia.[12,13] This test is available to almost all patients and is safe, but is contraindicated in those with asthma and/or unstable angina. The routine use of aminophylline to reverse the effect of dipyridamole is encouraged. Interpretation of the results of dipyridamole thallium-201 screening varies somewhat between users. This variation of interruption confuses, to some extent, its predictive value. The test is considered positive in demonstrating myocardial ischemia if one or more of following occur:

1. The test demonstrates at least one area of the myocardium corresponding to a reversible defect on delayed thallium screening.
2. The patient complained of chest pain during the test.
3. There was evidence of myocardial ischemia on the continuous electrocardiograph monitoring as interpreted by the cardiologist present.

Dipyridamole thallium-201 screening tests without these findings were considered negative. It is of interest to remember that the imaging is dependent on relative coronary blood flow and if all the vessels are severely diseased, a false-negative result could occur.

There is general agreement on the definition of a positive test, but our experience[14] is that there are two separate findings that make up the usual negative interpretations: 1) normal perfusion without defects, fixed or reversible; and 2) fixed defects.

In our experience,[14] patients in whom normal perfusion is demonstrated have very little risk of adverse perioperative cardiac complications. However, in a group of patients with fixed defects, but otherwise found fit for abdominal aortic surgery, 50% had postoperative cardiac complications. These findings are similar to those of McEnroe et al.[15]

Coronary Arteriography

If accurate knowledge of the anatomy and pathology of the coronary arteries is needed, coronary arteriography is the most accurate way to obtain that information. This procedure has its own risks which need to be balanced by the appropriate benefit. When coronary arteriography is done routinely on patients who require peripheral vascular surgery (including abdominal aortic aneurysms), approximately 30% will be found to have critical coronary artery disease that required coronary artery bypass as treatment.[16] Those patients who successfully undergo myocardial revascularization will have their cardiac risk lowered for subsequent major surgery, and a significant improvement in the quality and quality of life after coronary bypass grafting.

Hertzer et al[17] demonstrated that patients with critical coronary artery disease who underwent major vascular surgery had a surgical mortality of 12%. However, if they underwent coronary artery bypass surgery first, the vascular perioperative surgical mortality was decreased to 1.4%.

Furthermore, the cumulative survival at 5 years was 72% with coronary artery bypass surgery versus 43% without that procedure. If only those patients who have a reperfusable dipyridamole thallium-201 screening test or a fixed defect seen are subjected to coronary arteriography, 60% will be found to have critical coronary disease requiring coronary artery bypass graft.[13,14] A compelling case can be made that it benefits the patient if critical artery disease is diagnosed and treated.

Conclusions

There is no uniform approach to determine cardiac risk in an elderly patient requiring major noncardiac surgery. However, the important work already done to develop cardiac risk stratification leads to the conclusion that such stratification serves to identify the perioperative risk and the cardiac risk with or without surgery. Elderly patients who are being evaluated for cardiac risk can be separated into three risk groups once the patient's history, physical exam, and electrocardiogram have been obtained:

Group 1: those patients with symptomatic cardiac disease = high risk.

Group 2: those patients with a history of myocardial infarction, angina, or electrocardiographic findings consistent with myocardial infarction/myocardial ischemia = unknown risk.

Group 3: those patients without the findings in Group 2 = low risk.

If major, noncardiac surgery is mandatory in a Group 1 patient, standard practice is to optimize cardiorespiratory function prior to surgery. These patients demonstrate that they do not have sufficient cardiac reserve to accommodate increased workload and since operations are associated with increased stress, those whose hearts cannot compensate have a very high cardiac risk. With Group 2, further studies are necessary to detect critical coronary artery disease and they are important if the findings could alter the magnitude of the surgical procedure or the selection of alternate therapies.

Arguably, the most effective test for the majority of such patients is the dipyridamole thallium-201 screening test. If this test is positive, or a fixed perfusion defect is seen, coronary arteriography may be indicated in the hope of finding patients who will benefit from myocardial revascularization. Group 3 patients are not risk free, but the cardiac risk is low, and pursuing further tests is not going to be productive enough to be justified.

The major goal is to treat critical coronary disease effectively so that the cardiac risk is decreased in both the short- (perioperative) and the long-term. Coronary artery bypass grafting procedures are effective in accomplishing that goal, but are expensive and invasive. There are several clinical studies in progress that show real promise that drugs, especially beta blockers, will be as effective as surgery in accomplishing that goal without the procedure and its associated risks or costs.

References

1. US Bureau of the Census: 25 million ages 65-85. *Curr Popul Rep* 922:25, 1980.
2. Evers BM, Townsend CM Jr, Thompson JC: Organ physiology of aging. *Surg Clin North Am* 74:23-39, 1994.
3. Dripps RD, Eckenhoff JE: The role of anesthesia in surgical mortality. *JAMA* 178:261-266, 1961.
4. Khuri SF, Daley J, Henderson W, et al: The National Veterans Administration Surgical Study: risk adjustment for the comparative assessment of the quality of surgical care. *J Am Coll Surg* 180:519-531, 1995.
5. Goldman L, Caldera DL, Nussbaum SR, et al: Multifactorial index of cardiac risk in noncardiac surgical procedures. *N Engl J Med* 297:845-850, 1977.
6. The Criteria Committee of the New York Heart Association, Inc: *Diseases of the Heart and Blood Vessels: Nomenclature and Criteria for Diagnosis.* 6th Ed. Boston: Little, Brown; 1964.
7. Campeau L: Grading of angina pectoris (letters). *Circulation* 54:522, 1975.
8. Goldman L, Hashimoto B, Cook EF, et al: Comparative reproducibility and validity for assessing cardiovascular functional class: advantages of a new specific activity scale. *Circulation* 64:1227-1234, 1981.
9. Gerson MC, Hurse JM, Hertzberg VS, et al: Cardiac prognosis in noncardiac geriatric surgery. *Ann Intern Med* 103:832-837, 1985.
10. Raby KE, Goldman L, Cook EF, et al: Long-term prognosis of myocardial ischemia detected by Holter monitoring in peripheral vascular disease. *Am J Cardiol* 66:1309-1313, 1990.
11. Mangano DT, Browner WS, Hollenberg M, London MJ, et al: Association of perioperative myocardial ischemia with cardiac morbidity and mortality in men undergoing noncardiac surgery. *N Engl J Med* 323:1781-1788, 1990.
12. Makaroun MS, Shuman-Jackson N, Rippey A, et al: Cardiac risk in vascular surgery: the oral dipyridamole-thallium test. *Arch Surg* 125:1610-1613, 1990.
13. Cambria RP, Eagle K: Cardiac screening before abdominal aortic aneurysm surgery: a reassessment. *Semin Vasc Surg* 8:93-102, 1995.
14. Strawn DJ, Guernsey JM: Dipyridamole thallium scanning in the evaluation of coronary artery disease in elective abdominal aortic surgery. *Arch Surg* 126:880-884, 1994.
15. McEnroe CS, O'Donnell TF Jr, Yeager A, et al: Comparison of ejection fraction and Goldman risk factor analysis to dipyridamol thallium-201 studies in one evaluation of cardiac morbidity after aortic aneurysm surgery. *J Vasc Surg* 11:497, 1990.
16. Bayazit M, Gol MK, Battaloglu B, et al: Routine coronary angiography before abdominal aortic aneurysm repair. *Am J Surg* 170:246-250, 1995.

17. Hertzer NR, Young JR, Beven EG, et al: Late results of coronary bypass in patients with infrarenal aortic aneurysms. *Ann Surg* 205:360-367, 1987.
18. Deedwania PC, Carbajal EV, Nelson JR, et al: Anti-ischemic effects of atenolol versus nifedipine in patients with coronary artery disease and ambulatory silent ischemia. *J Am Coll Cardiol* 17:963-969, 1991.
19. Pasternack P, Grossie E, Bauman F: Beta blockade to decrease silent myocardial ischemia during peripheral vascular surgery. *Am J Surg* 158:113-116, 1989.

Chapter 9

Anesthetic Management of the Elderly Patient

Debra E. Morrison, MD
Adrienne Knight, MD
Steven J. Barker, PhD, MD

While it is accepted that the elderly patient is physiologically different from a younger adult, it is difficult to establish the chronology of becoming elderly, since physiological age may not correlate with chronological age as the body senesces.[1]

Rowe and Kahn proposed that persons who age with minimal impairment of physiological function undergo what is known as "successful aging," whereas other persons, who have a deterioration of physiological function, undergo "usual aging,"[2] and challenge health care practitioners to match past gains in life span by improving health span, or maintaining unchanged physiological function as near as possible to the end of life. Surgical intervention to correct derangement of a single organ or organ system or to improve blood flow to an ischemic part of the body is one attempt to meet this challenge of preserving physiological function.

Leslie B. Arey, who taught at Northwestern University Medical School into his nineties, offered to a student this explanation for the longevity of his apparent good health: "I have a well-matched set of organs."[3] Arey, a person who experienced successful aging, was correct: his organs failed in close succession, well past the normal limit of life expectancy.[4]

A physiologically young patient who presents with correctable disease in a single organ might safely be assumed to have an ill-matched set of organs, one of which has a shorter life span than the rest of him/her, but successful intervention may afford him/her successful aging. The failure of one organ early in life may not predict imminent failure of other organs: dominoes, placed on end more than a domino's length apart, will continue to stand after one of their number is toppled over

From: Aronow WS, Stemmer EA, Wilson SE (eds). *Vascular Disease in the Elderly*. Armonk, NY: Futura Publishing Company, Inc., © 1997.

by a careless hand. Knock over just one of a group of dominoes, placed on end less than a domino's length apart, and they'll all fall in sequence.

Within a given body, the aging process may vary from one organ system to another,[1] but approaching the limit of life expectancy, even in the "successfully aged," all organ systems must be assumed to be approaching senescence, and one diseased organ system can be viewed as a "herald organ," or the first domino to fall.

It is difficult to separate the primary effects of aging from the secondary effects of the diseases that accompany aging,[5] but the aged physiology is increasingly vulnerable to those diseases, as well as the interventions of surgeons and anesthesiologists as resilience and reserve diminish. The elderly patient, however functional, must be assumed to have little or no reserve; the system is unforgiving. Function sufficient for a sedentary or even moderately active life may be found to be inadequate during the perioperative period, since patients may not normally be active enough to provoke symptoms. Reduced function can often be demonstrated preoperatively only by stress testing.[6]

Although the vasculature is often treated as a hematologic connective tissue container or conduit (i.e., plumbing), and not as a major organ system in itself, it is a major physiological entity on which other organs depend. Disease of the vasculature presents itself as diseases of organs (or limbs) and the focus is on those organs, but single organ disease caused by poor perfusion is a harbinger of failure of other organs. A clear view of the vascular tree in its entirety would reveal the pattern of disease. The vasculopath may present initially in different ways, but hypertension, renal failure, coronary artery disease (CAD), stroke, claudication, visceral ischemia, and aneurysm are announcements to the suspicious anesthesiologist that the herald organ or organs in question may only be the first domino(es) to fall. Other diseases, such as smoking, diabetes, hypercholesterolemia, hyperlipidemia, and connective tissue/other autoimmune diseases, affect the health of the vasculature, and should arouse suspicion that organs are at risk. Smoking, more often than not one of the afflictions of the elderly patient with vascular disease, also places the patient at risk of pulmonary complications. Chronic alcohol abuse increases a patient's risk of developing adult respiratory distress syndrome (ARDS) as well as liver failure.[7]

Sherwin B. Nuland, a surgeon, eloquently writes that the common thread uniting physiologically elderly patients is "the loss of vitality that comes with starvation and suffocation—as the arteries narrow, so does the margin between life and death. There is less nutriment, there is less oxygen, and there is less resiliency after insult. Everything rusts and crusts until life is finally extinguished. What we call a terminal stroke, or a myocardial infarction (MI), or sepsis is simply a choice made by physicochemical factors we do not yet comprehend, the purpose of which is to bring down the curtain on a performance already much closer to its conclusion than may have been realized, even in an old person who has until then appeared vibrantly healthy."[8] "An octogenarian who dies of MI is not simply a weather-beaten senior citizen with heart disease—he is the victim of an insidious progression that involves all of him, and that progression is called aging. The infarction is only one of its manifestations, which in his case has beaten out the rest, though any of the others may be ready to snap him up should some bright young doctor manage to rescue him in a cardiac intensive care unit."[8] Every physiologically elderly patient can be expected to have "advanced atheromatous disease in the vessels of the heart or the brain, usually in both, even if they exhibit no symptoms that require treatment until the terminal event. One or the other of these vital engines is close to quits, if not from ischemia, then from infection. A ruptured appendix, an acutely infected gallbladder, a perforated peptic ulcer or diverticulum can lead to infection with grave consequences in the elderly patient, despite timely surgical intervention,"[8] whereas a physiologically younger patient would withstand the insult and the intervention with ease.

We have attempted to endow the reader with pessimism and unease at the thought of performing anesthesia and surgery on the physiologically elderly patient. In choosing to operate, the surgeon demonstrates conviction that intervention is the course most beneficial to the patient. The task of the anesthesiologist is to anticipate and possibly prevent a turbulent course. This endeavor requires collaboration between surgeons and anesthesiologists. The frailty of the patient and his/her vasculature must be respected: vascular disease is probably widespread; organ perfusion and viability are threatened; vascular access for monitoring and infusion may be challenging; hemostasis may be difficult to achieve; previously undiagnosed disease may declare itself perioperatively; and surgeons may encounter unexpected difficulties. Communication and respect between surgeons and anesthesiologists is of paramount importance: each should inform the other of crucial events during the perioperative course (new preoperative findings, difficulty in placement of invasive monitors, bleeding, ischemia, change in temperature or urine output, and clamping/unclamping of major vessels). Partnership begins in the preoperative period, and continues until the patient recovers from surgery.

Preoperative Assessment

Preoperatively, in order to determine risk as well as to anticipate problems, the anesthesiologist attempts to determine the extent of the patient's physiological vulnerability using a systems appproach.

Peripheral Vascular: Is hypertension stable and well controlled on appropriate medication? An optimal normal range of blood pressures or an optimal mean for the patient should be determined by repeated measurements under normal awake conditions, and a minimum permissible blood pressure should be established, with demonstrated perfusion of brain, heart, and kidneys.[9,10] Initial treatment for hypertension should not occur under general anesthesia.[9,10]

Cardiovascular: Baseline activity level and exercise capacity, and the consequences of a patient's maximal voluntary effort should be determined by focused questioning. Clearly, only when voluntary effort is limited by cardiac symptoms can history be used to define cardiac-specific exercise capacity. Dyspnea on exertion in a patient with pulmonary disease is a nonspecific finding. The patient limited in activity by musculoskeletal or neurological problems may be unable to exert any significant voluntary effort. Because many patients are limited in activity, and because of the high prevalence of diabetes mellitus in elderly vascular patients, manifestation of CAD is frequently silent.[11] Hertzer et al performed prospective coronary angiograms in 1000 consecutive vascular surgery patients and found that 60% had significant stenosis in at least one coronary artery.[12]

In the absence of overt symptoms, should CAD be aggressively ruled out before vascular surgery? One must weigh risks versus benefits of testing[11] (consider the risk of stroke in coronary angiogram versus the risk of MI in carotid surgery), and whether or not information from the test will be used to modify perioperative care.[11] Assessment of risk may be required to make an informed decision to perform or undergo elective surgery, or to determine the appropriate operation (axillary-femoral bypass versus intra-abdominal aortic reconstruction)[11] or anesthetic plan. Ideally, we would like to know baseline ventricular function, degree of myocardium at risk under the amount of stress the patient may experience perioperatively, and whether there is anything that can or should be done to diminish baseline net risk. Significant dysrhythmias and valve disease are also of concern. Although preoperative intervention may not be appropriate or possible, medical management should be optimized.

Pulmonary: Approximately 70% of vascular patients have a smoking history and up to 50% have clinically apparent chronic obstructive pulmonary disease (COPD).[13] Number of pack-years should be calculated. The elderly patient who smokes is at an increased risk for pulmonary aspiration,[14] and should be evaluated for other risk factors. If pulmonary disease is suspected or evident, it may be appropriate to obtain pulmonary function tests to establish baseline and/or to determine if function can be improved preoperatively by aggressive respiratory therapy. In addition, arterial blood gas measurement will establish normal values for the patient, necessary for maintaining homeostasis intraoperatively and determining readiness for extubation postoperatively.

Renal: Renal function declines with age,[6] and chronic renal insufficiency is present in 5% to 17% of vascular patients.[14-16] Renal impairment may be sufficient to affect drug metabolism. Baseline renal function should be determined and any superimposed acute problems addressed. Diagnostic imaging necessary before most vascular procedures may further compromise renal function. It has been demonstrated that administration of renal dose dopamine (3 µg/kg/min) and crystalloid (5% Dextrose and 0.45% normal saline at 75 to 125 mL/hr) commencing prior to infusion of the contrast agent may limit or prevent further renal impairment by preventing contrast-induced renal vasoconstriction.[17-19] The use of furosemide (a nephrotoxin) and mannitol has not been shown to provide renal protection.[17]

Endocrine: The incidence of diabetes increases with age,[6] and is an independent risk factor for vascular disease[11] as well as increased surgical mortality.[20] Subclinical hypothyroidism, demonstrated by elevated serum thyroid-stimulating hormone (TSH), is found in more than 13% of healthy elderly patients.[6] Endocrine disease should be identified and managed appropriately.

Gastroenterological: Patients should be evaluated for gastroesophageal reflux disease, which increases risk of pulmonary aspiration[14]; peptic ulcer disease, which may be exacerbated by perioperative stress; and hepatic dysfunction, which may affect drug metabolism[6] and can be exacerbated by hypoperfusion.

Hematologic: Patients should be questioned about history of bleeding problems. If appropriate, a baseline prothrombin time/partial thromboplastin time (PT/PTT) and bleeding time should be obtained. Is patient on anticoagulant therapy? If significant blood loss is anticipated, baseline hematocrit should be determined, and options for transfusion should be discussed, including whether or not the patient will accept blood products.

Musculoskeletal: Elderly bones, muscle, and skin may be as fragile and unforgiving as elderly physiology. Patients with osteoporosis, renal osteodystrophy, or rheumatoid arthritis may be at high risk for fractures. Joints may not move freely, which causes problems with positioning, and skin and soft tissue may be friable and vulnerable to pressure ulcers.

Neurological: Baseline neurological status should be assessed and documented preoperatively.

Allergies: History of specific allergic reactions should be elucidated.

Medications: All of the patient's medications should be reviewed, and necessary medication continued through the morning of surgery: cardiac drugs, antihypertensives, pulmonary therapeutics, endocrine replacement, and adjustment of insulin while patient is NPO. Drugs affecting coagulation should be stopped when appropriate by the surgical team. Psychotherapeutics, anxiolytics, and pain medication should be continued, as long as mental status is appropriate and any drug-anesthetic interactions are anticipated.

Surgical and Anesthetic History: Details of prior operations, anesthetics, perioperative course and complications, especially if recent and major, are helpful in estimating physiological reserve.

Labs and Studies: Electrocardiogram (ECG), chest radiograph, CBC, and electrolytes should be supplemented by other labs and studies indicated by history in order to evaluate known or suspected medical problems to create an optimal medical baseline.

Physical Exam: The anesthesia exam is focused, but includes baseline vital signs, height, weight, distribution of weight, neck exam for carotid bruits, airway exam, which includes dentition and neck extension, peripheral pulses, intravenous access, heart and lungs, any deformity or potential problem with monitoring or positioning, and mental and neurological status. The anesthesiologist should establish rapport with the patient and family, anticipating the possibility of a prolonged or complicated perioperative course.

Younger patients tend to be more similar and older patients tend to be more dissimilar, making individualization of the anesthetic technique mandatory.[1] During the preoperative period, once the patient has been evaluated, anesthesiologists and surgeons should discuss details of the planned operation and the anesthetic requirements. Projected length of procedure, site of incision, special positioning, available sites for monitoring, necessity and availabililty of blood products, and contraindications for certain techniques can be weighed against the limitations that the patient's constellation of medical problems place on the interdisciplinary team. The patient should arrive in the operating suite in his/her best possible state of physiological equilibrium to find a coordinated team prepared to maintain that state of equilibrium.

Indications for Monitoring

Nonvarying vital signs during anesthesia predict less postoperative morbidity than varying, unstable vital signs.[20] Monitoring is useful for determining baseline and keeping patient at baseline, allowing as little perturbation perioperatively as possible. Monitors provide an array of overlapping data offering evidence of ventilation and perfusion, and can be utilized to guide manipulation of physiological parameters. Monitoring may allow detection of events which are potentially damaging, and institution of therapy before damage is permanent, maintaining perfusion of vital organs.

Type of Monitoring

Standard monitors are 5-lead ECG (leads II and V), noninvasive blood pressure (NIBP), pulse oximetry (which, in the elderly vasculopath, may not work on poorly perfused digits or ear lobes), temperature, end-tidal carbon dioxide ($ETCO_2$) analysis, and respiratory parameters (inspired oxygen [FiO_2], peak inspiratory pressure [PIP], tidal volume [TV], and respiratory rate [RR]). It is desirable to have end-tidal analysis of anesthetic gases for a general anesthetic, and this is becoming routine. Monitors may also include automatic ST segment analysis, which can be useful in alerting the anesthesiologist to subtle changes in the ECG.[21]

Establishing vascular access may be challenging in elderly patients, and adequate access for necessary infusion of blood must be established before blood loss begins. It may be difficult to place peripheral venous catheters, arterial catheters, and central venous catheters in calcified, brittle, or friable vessels; this may predict corresponding difficulty at the operative site.

An indwelling arterial catheter allows continuous monitoring and adjustment of arterial pressure and provides access for repeated blood draws with minimal risk (of ischemia and infection)[22] if sterilely placed. The transduced waveform can be utilized in some peripheral vascular procedures to determine immediately if there is change in flow to an extremity. If radial arterial access is not possible, a more proximal arterial line (femoral, axillary, or brachial) may be necessary.[22]

In the physiologically elderly patient with diminished resilience and reserve, the benefit of invasive monitoring is more likely to outweigh risks. A pulmonary artery (PA) catheter is indicated to monitor cardiac filling pressures if extensive blood loss or volume shifts are anticipated, or if there is significant cardiac or pulmonary disease.[6]

Central venous pressure (CVP) is not particularly helpful on its own for monitoring left ventricular (LV) function, especially in patients with LV dysfunction,(except as a fluid/blood infusion port, to administer vasoactive drugs, as a trend monitor, or as a conduit for a PA catheter or pacemaker) because the CVP catheter transduces right-sided filling pressures, which may not reflect left-sided pressures. A PA catheter provides useful information: filling pressures; mixed-venous saturation (SvO_2); cardiac output (CO) (including continuous cardiac output [CCO]); and data for calculation of hemodynamic parameters, and is a helpful monitor for myocardial ischemia. It has been reported that elevated AC waves (noncompliant ventricle) or V waves (acute papillary muscle dysfunction) are evident on the PA tracing before ECG changes,[23] although it is not certain that these relationships are consistent.[24] A PA catheter helps to assess intravascular volume status, differentiate cardiogenic from noncardiogenic pulmonary edema and hypoxemia, manage low cardiac output states, manage positive end-expiration pressure (PEEP), and manage vasoactive drugs, thereby adding to the clinical assessment of critically ill patients.[25]

Transesophageal echocardiography (TEE) is a less invasive way to characterize ventricular filling, ventricular function, and detect regional wall motion abnormalities using real time ultrasonographic equipment. TEE can be used to assess global ventricular function, and indirectly, CO, stroke volume (SV), and ejection fraction (EF). It can also measure factors that affect ventricular function such as preload, afterload, and contractility.[21]

A urinary catheter helps in assessment of both preload and renal function. Although renal function can be evaluated in many ways, the most practical means during anesthesia is rate of urinary output. A rate of 0.5 to 1.0 mL/kg/hr is considered adequate.[26] This is a reasonable indicator of renal perfusion, provided there is no coexisting disease.[26] In the vasculopath with underlying hypertension which decreases the effective circulating blood volume (with systemic blood pressure out of proportion to renal perfusion pressure), and diabetes which predisposes to renovascular disease, urine output may not be correlated with renal perfusion. Low urine output may be due to a low circulating blood volume, with poor perfusion to the kidney, or the onset of acute renal failure, but acute renal failure may also be associated with high urine output. Apparent adequate or high urine output may be the result of elevated serum glucose, rather than adequate renal perfusion. Specific gravity and urinary sodium can also be measured in the operating room, in order to evaluate renal function acutely.

Choice of Anesthetic

The restrictions placed on the anesthesiologist by the operation planned and the individual elderly patient's usually complex medical and surgical problems stretch our abilities as clinicians and make the job interesting. After eliminating drugs and techniques that are inappropriate or contraindicated, our challenge is to exploit the remaining possibilities to the fullest in order to preserve homeostasis.

What limitations are placed on technique? The anesthetic approach for the planned procedure is often clearly limited by anatomy: general anesthesia is required for coronary artery bypass graft (CABG); repair of thoracic aortic aneurysm, tracheo-innominate fistula, and suprarenal abdominal aortic aneurysm (AAA), as well as axillary-femoral bypass, visceral revascularization, and other operations that require invasion of the thorax and upper abdomen, although regional techniques may be utilized for postoperative pain control when appropriate. Operations where the incision is made in the neck, lower abdomen, flank, or extremities, such as carotid endarterectomy (CEA), repair of infrarenal AAA, and renal artery or limb revascularization, can and have been done with pure regional or combined techniques. There may be several options and, in some patients, no apparent safe option, but an anesthetic plan is ultimately devised: pure epidural for low abdominal or retroperitoneal incision repair of infrarenal AAA in patient with FEV_1 after bronchodilator therapy of 6.5; repair of femoral artery tear under local in patient in renal failure; leg block for amputation in patient in septic shock; and limited, one-sided hyperbaric spinal for repair of a groin aneurysm. The literature suggests many options for managing the average patient, but we submit that the physiologically elderly patient is never an average patient, and the individual practitioner is forced to devise a unique solution for each patient (Table).

Patients who present to the operating room with significantly altered coagulation are not appropriate candidates for neuraxial anesthesia, because of the remote risk of spinal epidural hematoma (SEH) and the potential for resulting spinal cord injury.[27] If the epidural or spinal (one-shot or continuous) is placed (and any catheter later removed) while coagulation is normal, complications are rare, even though the patient is anticoagulated during the operation. If an epidural catheter is utilized in the postoperative period, and the patient is anticoagulated, neurological status should be periodically evaluated by allowing all but the narcotics to wear off before redosing.[27] The risk, which is low, is in this case usually outweighed by the benefit of regional anesthesia,

Table 1
Random Sample of Preoperative Evaluation of Elderly Patient for Vascular Surgery

DEPARTMENT OF VETERANS AFFAIRS
MEDICAL RECORD (600)
PROGRESS NOTE

IN LIEU OF #509 | *MAR 30, 1996 Page: 1*

ANESTHETIC CLINIC - PROGRESS NOTE

Patient: | Urgency: PRE-OP NOTE
SSN: | Visit date: 03/29/96
Date of Birth: JAN 25,1933 | Age: 63
Ht (inches): 6' | Weight: 230 (lbs)

Operation proposed: Thrombectomy of left arm AV graft
Pre-Op Diagnosis: Esrd, Thrombosed AV Graft
ASA Class: 3-Severe Disturb

** For UA, Hemotology, Blood Chemistry see Health Summary***

Special Info: 63 YO male with HX of ESRD on hemodialysis since 1/96. Pt now with clotted left arm AV graft scheduled for thrombectomy.
PMH: IDDM x 28 yrs (Assoc. with diabetic retinopathy).
HTN x 30 yrs, moderately controlled on meds.
Esrd on HD since 1/96 (dialysis on M,W,F last dialysis on Wed).
Cardiac dysfxn', (Echo 12/92 LA 58 MM, decreased LV FXN, 4 chamber enlargement, MOD TR and MR). TMST 5/93 fixed septal defect.
Atrial fibrillation (chronic, and rate controlled on Digoxin).
Obst. sleep apnea 10/94 (no documented H/O pulmn. htn).
Hepatitis B AB Positive, surface antigen negative.
PSH: S/P Av Graft placement (geta w/o comp.) 2/2/96
NED: CA++ Acetate, Digoxin, Lasix, Diltiazem, Epogen, Zantac, Insulin, Coumodin
ALL: NKDA (per pt.) SOC: Denies TOB/ETOH/Drugs
ROS: Poor exercise tol. Less than two flights due to sob, denies cp.
Some difficulty lying supine felt to be due to claustraphobia and sleep apnea (no gross orthopnea), some pedal edema prior to each dialysis (today pt does not feel SOB or fluid overloaded).

Respiratory system
CXR Normal ?: PENDING
PFT Normal ?:
Pre FEV1:
Pre FVC:
Ex. Tolerance:

PFT Date:
Post FEV1:
Post FVC:

Circulatory System
BP/Pulse: 150/90/78
Ekg Normal:
Comments: PENDING (H/O A FIB.)
Other Test: WBC 8.7, H/H 11.2/32.4, PLT 210, K 4.7, BUN/CR 62/7.8, SGOT 58, PT/PTT 15.6/25.3, CA1 1 7.1, MG 2, ALB 3.3

Physical Exam: Normal
Date:

Central Nervous System
CNS:
Exam Airway: Class 2, from, 3 FB from T to M, mouth 3 FB, no reported losse or chipped teeth. AW exam appears NL. despite H/O sleep apnea
Prev An/Comp:
Specialty:
Staff: Morrison, Debra E
Evaluated by: Foster, Todd Anthony

when indicated. Because significant hemorrhage has been reported in patients undergoing fibrinolytic therapy, however,[27] the potential risk for SEH is greater with infusion of thrombolytic agents such as tissue plasminogen activator, urokinase, or streptokinase, and the use of neuraxial anesthesia may be contraindicated in these patients. Non-neuraxial regional techniques such as peripheral blocks are still viable options.

Regional anesthesia causes blockade, greater than that of general anesthesia, of the surgical stress response.[28] Sympathetic blockade causes a decrease in the release of catecholamines, thereby contributing to a decrease in myocardial oxygen demand. A high neuraxial block with resultant bradycardia and hypotension, can, if they are untreated, decrease coronary perfusion pressure, thus decreasing myocardial oxygen supply, resulting in myocardial ischemia. It is controversial whether an epidural anesthetic, whether alone or with a light general anesthetic, provides better cardiovascular stability than general anesthesia alone.[29] Cardiovascular stability seems most dependent on the skill of the anesthesiologist.

Most studies of regional anesthesia in elderly patients have been done on patients undergoing transurethral resection of the prostate (TURP) and total hip arthroplasty (THA).[30] Advantages in use of regional anesthesia for lower abdominal and lower extremity surgery include: decreased blood loss (the mechanism of which is unknown); sympathectomy, which increases blood flow to lower extremities, especially appropriate for vascular surgery patients; and decreased incidence of deep vein thrombosis (DVT) (because of improved blood flow).[30] The use of straight regional anesthesia in the elderly can be particularly advantageous when used with minimal sedation for intraoperative monitoring of and postoperative preservation of mental status. Potential disadvantages include technical difficulty in placement due to calcification of ligamentous structures, loss of disc height, and difficulty with positioning.

The literature shows no difference in outcome for CEA between general anesthesia or cervical plexus blockade alone.[9] Outcome depends on the skill and speed of the surgeon and the skill of the anesthesiologist in managing hemodynamics. The unsedated or minimally sedated, cooperative and awake patient, with a good cervical plexus block, is the best monitor of cerebral perfusion, allowing serial neurological and mental status exams. Intraoperative cerebral ischemia, however, may be accompanied by loss of patient cooperation, seizures, or apnea, which are, in the setting of an uncontrolled airway, a recipe for disaster. Unfortunately, there is no other monitor that is specific for and highly sensitive to cerebral ischemia under general anesthesia.[9] EEG or regional cerebral blood flow monitoring are not available in all centers; other methods of prevention of cerebral ischemia include shunting of all patients and performing the surgery as fast as possible.[9] Management of these patients includes brain protection by pharmacological and/or hemodynamic measures, avoiding drugs and events that can decrease cerebral blood flow, and avoidance of long-acting agents that can cloud neurological function and delay evaluation.[9] There are many strategies:

The patient with a cervical plexus block combined with a light general anesthetic and short-acting neuromuscular blockade can be hemodynamically very stable intraoperatively, as well as without pain postoperatively. A cervical plexus block without general anesthesia is well tolerated in the right patient. Recall can usually be prevented in either case. An interscalene block of the cervical plexus with distal pressure to push the volume of local anesthetic cephalad should provide an adequate block of the operative site without puncturing the skin near the operative site, with one needle stick, since the neural sheath is continuous from the vertebral foramen to the shoulder. CEA is also done under straight general anesthesia.

General anesthesia and the use of neuromuscular blocking agents cause a restrictive ventilatory defect, resulting in ventilation/perfusion (V/Q) mismatch and poor oxygenation. Under regional anesthesia, the patient can maintain a relatively normal ventilatory pattern.[31] Although there are many investigators who have found no difference in the incidence of postoperative pulmonary complications, the use of epidural anesthesia intraoperatively and analgesia postoperatively can offer an improvement in pulmonary function over general anesthesia with intravenous postoperative analgesia.[32-35] Smoking is a risk factor for both pulmonary disease and vascular disease; therefore, many elderly vascular surgery patients are at risk for pulmonary complications including pneumonia, prolonged intubation, and ventilator dependence. For each patient, a strategy must be developed by the surgical and anesthetic team to minimize these complications. Risks and benefits must be enumerated, and the patient advised of the recommendation. A patient's strong preference or an inability to cooperate may limit options, despite sound reasons for the team's recommendation. An operation lasting many hours may not be tolerated by an awake patient.

General anesthesia provides the advantage of preemptive control of the airway, obviates the need to reassure the patient intraoperatively, allows control of ventilation, and focused attention on control of hemodynamics and prevention of ischemia. We are provided with a nearly complete armamentarium with which to accomplish this in the individual patient.

The potent volatile inhalational agents used in general anesthesia are complete anesthetics. They provide unconsciousness, analgesia, muscle relaxation, and blunt hemodynamic responses to various stimuli. These agents are unique in that they are not "fixed" drugs and, because they are administered via the lungs, the depth of anethesia can be modulated by changes in minute ventilation, fresh gas flow, and inspired concentration of agent. In practice, particularly with the elderly patient, volatile agents are used, not as a complete anesthetic, but to complete a balanced anesthetic technique.

The ideal anesthetic should have a rapid onset of action with predictable and rapid recovery from its effects, and an absence of persistent effect on the brain or other organs after the time of anesthesia. It should be easy to administer, and administration should be guided by clear signs of the depth of anesthesia. It should have a wide safety margin in all patients. Of the potent inhalational anesthetics available (isoflurane, halothane, enflurane, desflurane, and sevoflurane), sevoflurane, one of the two newer agents, is unique in its physical properties in that it has a low solubility compared to the other agents. This allows for a faster induction (not always desirable in the elderly patient), more rapid change in anesthetic depth, and decreased time to emergence. It is reported that patients wake up in half the time as compared with isoflurane, with more rapid return of pre-anesthetic function. Volatile agents can decrease myocardial contractility and cause profound myocardial depression and must be used judiciously in patients who have significant myocardial dysfunction. Sevoflurane does not cause the myocardium to be sensitized to circulating catecholamines as does halothane, and it does not cause a tachycardia with rapid increases in anesthetic concentration like isoflurane and desflurane. It is a respiratory depressant in a dose-dependent fashion; however, when combined with N_2O in a spontaneously breathing patient, TV and arterial CO_2 approach normal. Sevoflurane is expensive compared to the other inhalational agents and there is a risk of by-product formation in the CO_2 absorber when lower fresh gas flows are used, as well as a higher risk of renal toxicity than isoflurane.[6,36] We have found, however, that using sevoflurane, at least in the final hour of a general anesthetic (with narcotics and isoflurane), allows patients to wake up more fully and recover more rapidly.

Propofol is a rapidly acting intravenous anesthetic used for both induction and maintenance of anesthesia. Because metabolism is rapid and complete, the drug can be of benefit when rapid recovery is desired. Like sodium thiopental, it can cause vasodilation, cardiac depression, and hypotension, and the dose must be adjusted appropriately in the elderly population. Studies in patients for CABG using propofol for induction and maintenance demonstrated no difference in hemodynamic parameters as compared to enflurane.[37] It is a useful drug in the elderly population, if used with skill and restraint.

Immobility can be provided by any neuromuscular blocking agent with appropriate onset and duration of action, route of metabolism, and minimal to no undesired side effects. Atracurium and vecuronium are both intermediate-acting nondepolarizing neuromuscular blockers, are both easy to titrate and easy to reverse. Atracurium may cause histamine release, but requires no metabolism. The newer cisatracurium, a more potent isomer of atracurium, causes negligible histamine release, and requires no metabolism. Vecuronium has no side effect profile, and elimination is largely in the bile. Rocuronium is a shorter-acting drug much like vecuronium.

Analgesia can be provided by spinal or epidural narcotics, or by parenteral narcotics. In selected patients where there is no contraindication to use of nonsteroidal anti-inflammatory drugs, ketorolac can be utilized to enhance analgesia without sedation.

Many, but not all, anesthetics also cause vasodilation, resulting in undesired hypotension, which can be treated by infusion of fluids or vasoactive drugs, once adequate depth of anesthesia is established, sufficient to ensure amnesia, analgesia, anesthesia, and adequate muscle relaxation. A general anesthetic may allow greater freedom in managing hemodynamics, but may also require greater skill in managing them well. The general challenge of general anesthesia is maintenance of homeostasis and organ perfusion. Vascular surgery causes changes, often acute, in vascular space (anesthesia, clamping and unclamping of vessels), intravascular volume (blood loss, administration of blood and fluids), and milieu (after unclamping, there is release of by-products of anaerobic metabolism from the ischemic limb, with consequent rise in serum potassium). Vasoconstrictors, vasodilators, inotropes, chronotropes, and other rapid-acting, short-duration vasoactive substances are the true armamentarium of the anesthesiologist, utilized to minimize hemodynamic perturbation to protect organ perfusion and viability.

Extubation Criteria: If severe postoperative deficit in pulmonary function is expected and is a significant percentage of vital capacity, extubation should not be anticipated. The patient with acceptable (this is patient-specific, since some of our patients have FEV_1 of 0.45 to 0.7) pulmonary function should be awake, alert, cooperative, and normothermic. Analgesia should be adequate. The patient should be hemodynamically stable, with appropriate CO and blood pressure on minimal inotropic support, and no onoing blood loss. Return of neuromuscular function and airway protective reflexes should be demonstrable by 5 second head lift, forced vital capacity (FVC) 15 mL/kg, negative inspiratory force greater than -25 cm/H_2O, and gag and swallow reflexes intact. The patient should be able to maintain normal pH (7.35 to 7.45), adequate PaO_2 (70 to 90 mm Hg) on FiO_2 of 40% with 5 cm H_2O CPAP, and respiratory rate of 24 or less.

Fluid Management

The patient who undergoes vascular surgery may experience mild (less than 50% of blood volume), moderate (50% to 100% of blood volume), or massive (greater than 100% of blood volume) hemorrhage, depending on the patient and the type of operation.[38] It is unlikely that most elective vascular surgery patients will experience more than a moderate blood loss. Because blood is potentially infectious, patterns of blood administration have developed whereby a patient must show hemodynamic instability, potential for ongoing blood loss, or inadequate oxygen-carrying capacity before administration of packed red blood cells (PRBCs). Measurement of SvO_2 is helpful in determining adequacy of oxygen-carrying capacity.

There continues to be controversy over crystalloid versus colloid for replacement of intravascular volume in the face of adequate oxygen-carrying capacity, and most studies show no difference in the setting of moderate blood loss.[38] We do not propose to resolve the conflict here, and admit to using crystalloids and/or colloids when appropriate, since patients have different requirements. Each physiologically elderly patient is unique in his/her combination of problems: when the patient is not resilient, it may behoove the anesthesiologist to be so.

When the patient requires massive blood transfusion, consideration must be given to administration of other components present in whole blood, but missing from PRBCs. Patients who undergo massive hemorrhage develop a dilutional thrombocytopenia, as well as a functional thrombocytopenia. Administration of platelets to the clinically bleeding patient is helpful in restoring hemostasis. In the presence of a clinical coagulopathy, a decision must be made quickly to avoid more than necessary delays in administering necessary components, to prevent more bleeding and the need for more blood products.[38]

In order to avoid homologous blood transfusion, autologous blood can be predeposited, blood loss can be decreased by acute preoperative hemodilution, or salvaged blood administered. Even older, sicker patients may, by taking oral iron and erythropoietin, tolerate phlebotomy and regenerate red cell mass prior to surgery. In acute hemodilution, one or more unit(s) of blood is/are drawn off before incision and replaced with crystalloid, with the goal of decreasing the hematocrit to 20% to 30% and reducing the red cell mass lost from the wound. In sick vascular patients, the procedure may not be well tolerated because it acutely diminishes oxygen-carrying capacity.[38] Salvage and reinfusion of autologous blood from the surgical field may decrease the quantity of PRBCs transfused, but introduce the possibility of coagulopathy and increased requirement for platelet transfusion. In all three methods, care must be taken to avoid contamination and misdirection of blood products. None has been shown to be safer for all patients, and each case is unique. The advent of recombinant hemoglobin will add a fourth alternative to homologous blood transfusion.

Control of Body Temperature

Maintaining normal body temperature is another component of strict maintenance of homeostasis. Patients under general anesthesia are unable to autoregulate temperature because of vasodilation and consequent redistribution of blood flow to the periphery, and become poikilothermic, losing heat by radiation, conduction, and convection, to approach the ambient temperature. Patients under regional anesthesia, by vasodilating in the area affected by the block, share this problem to a lesser degree.

Hypothermia impairs coagulation, increases blood viscosity, impairs hepatic function and drug metabolism, depresses CO, and causes ventricular irritability, decreases tissue perfusion, impairs release of oxygen to tissues, increases oxygen consumption, increases systemic catecholamines, increases myocardial oxygen demand, even in the absence of shivering, and is, therefore, to be avoided.[39] It is far easier to maintain body temperature than to rewarm a cold patient. A minimum amount of body surface should be exposed to ambient temperature and, from the moment the patient enters the operating room until the final drape is placed, the operating room should be kept warm if at all possible. The room can safely be cooled for the comfort of the surgical team once the drapes are in place.

Circulating warm water mattresses are often placed under egg-crate mattresses, and do little to help maintain body temperature; they certainly do not contribute to active warming of an adult patient. A considerate nurse will often place a warm sheet on top of the operating table immediately before the patient is moved onto it, a commendable action without significant long-term benefit. Intravenous fluids should be warmed routinely, but conventional fluid warmers are ineffective in preventing heat loss: slow infusion through a conventional warmer allows cooling to take place in the tubing between the warmer and the patient, and rapid infusion does not allow sufficient time for heating. The Level 1® fluid warmer, which effectively warms even rapidly infused fluids by increasing the temperature in proportion to the rate of flow, effectively if expensively prevents delivery of cold fluids; however, fluid infusers, except for the systems frequently used in liver transplant or cardiopulmonary bypass, are not able to contribute significantly to active warming of an already cold patient. Warming and humidifying inspired gases are beneficial, but do not contribute significantly to maintenance of body temperature. Irrigating fluid should absolutely be warmed. The most effective means of maintaining body temperature is a forced air blanket such as the Bair Hugger® because it warms by convection and works well, even if only used on the head and upper body. This is the only effective and practical means of actively warming a patient; other methods only contribute to prevention of heat loss. We often place the blanket before induction and activate the device (at 43°C). The secured inflated blanket does not interfere with induction or surgical prep and can be deflated if necessary for placement of invasive monitors. The forced air temperature can be decreased if core temperature rises above 37°C.

Conclusion

The skill of the anesthesiologist lies in manipulating vascular space and intravascular volume with fluids and vasoactive drugs which are rapidly titratable, maintaining close communication with surgeons to enable anticipation of changes on the surgical field, in order to maintain constant perfusion pressure to vital organs (normal cardiac index, ventricular filling pressures, and systemic vascular resistance), and anticipating and treating perturbations in the intravascular milieu to maintain normal electrolyes, temperature, and oxygen-carrying capacity. Impaired function of major organ systems makes this task more difficult, yet more critical to the survival of the patient with limited reserve.

References

1. McLeskey C: Anesthesia for the geriatric patient. In: Barash PG, Cullen BF, Stoelting RK (eds). *Clinical Anesthesia*. 2nd Ed. Philadelphia: JB Lippincott; 1353-1387, 1992.
2. Rowe JW, Kahn RL: Human aging: usual and successful. *Science* 237:143, 1987.
3. Arey LB: Personal communication, 1985.
4. Wilson LF: Personal communication, 1989.
5. Hazzard WR: The biology of aging. In: Braunwald E, Isselbacher KJ, Petersdorf RG, et al (eds). *Harrison's Principles of Internal Medicine*. 11th Ed. New York: McGraw-Hill; 447-450, 1987.
6. Stoelting RK, Dierdorf SF: Physiologic changes and disorders unique to aging. In: Stoelting RK, Dierdorf SF (eds). *Anesthesia and Coexisting Disease*. 3rd Ed. New York: Churchill Livingstone, Inc.; 631-637, 1993.
7. Moss M, Bucher B, Moore FA, et al: The role of chronic alcohol abuse in the development of acute respiratory distress syndrome in adults. *JAMA* 275:50-54, 1996.
8. Nuland S: *How We Die*. New York: Alfred A. Knopf; 80-81, 1994.
9. Roizen MF: Anesthesia goals for operations to relieve or prevent cerebrovascular insufficiency. In: Roizen MF (ed). *Anesthesia for Vascular Surgery*. New York: Churchill Livingstone, Inc; 103-122, 1990.
10. Michenfelder JD: Anesthesia and surgery for cerebrovascular insufficiency: one approach at the Mayo Clinic. In: Roizen MF (ed). *Anesthesia for Vascular Surgery*. New York: Churchill Livingstone, Inc.; 123-133, 1990.
11. Fleisher LA: Preoperative cardiac evaluation of the patient undergoing major vascular surgery. In: Benumof JL, Hannallah MS (eds). *Anesthesiology Clinics of North America: Anesthesia for Vascular Surgery*. Philadelphia: WB Saunders, Co.; 53-65, 1995.
12. Hertzer NR, Bevan EG, Young JR, et al: Coronary artery disease in peripheral vascular patients: a classification of 1000 coronary angiograms and results of surgical management. *Ann Surg* 199:223, 1984.
13. Lampe GH, Mangano DT: Anesthetic management for abdominal aortic reconstruction. In: Roizen MF (ed). *Anesthesia for Vascular Surgery*. New York: Churchill Livingstone, Inc.; 265-284, 1990.
14. Orkin FK: Morbidity following anesthetic procedures in the perioperative period. In: Roizen MF (ed). *Anesthesia for Vascular Surgery*. New York: Churchill Livingstone, Inc.; 29-58, 1990.
15. Young AE, Sandberg GW, Couch NP: The reduction of mortality of abdominal aortic aneurysm resection. *Am J Surg* 134:585-590, 1977.
16. Diehl JT, Cali RF, Hertzer NR, et al: Complications of abdominal aortic reconstruction: an analysis of perioperative risk factors in 557 patients. *Ann Surg* 197:49-56, 1983.
17. Hall KA, Wong RW, Hunter GC, et al: Contrast-induced nephrotoxicity: the effects of vasodilator therapy. *J Surg Res* 53:317-320, 1992.
18. Schwartz LB, Gewertz BL: The renal response to low-dose dopamine. *J Surg Res* 45:574, 1988.
19. Felder RA, Felder CC, Eisner GM et al: The dopamine receptor in adult and maturing kidney. *Am J Physiol* 257:F315, 1989.
20. Jones RL: Anesthesia risk in the geriatric patient. In: McCleskey CH, Kirby RR, Brown DL, (eds). *Problems in Anesthesia: Perioperative Geriatrics*. Philadelphia: JB Lippincott; 550, 1989.

21. Leung JM: Monitoring in vascular surgery. In: Benumof JL, Hannallah MS (eds). *Anesthesiology Clinics of North America: Anesthesia for Vascular Surgery.* Philadelphia: WB Saunders, Co.; 67-81, 1995.
22. Cohen NH, Brett CM: Arterial catheterization. In: Benumof JL (ed). *Clinical Procedures in Anesthesia and Intensive Care.* Philadelphia: JB Lippincott; 375-389, 1992.
23. Kaplan J, Well P: Early diagnosis of myocardial ischemia using the pulmonary arterial catheter. *Anesth Analg* 60:789-793, 1981.
24. Van Daels VD, Sutherland G, Mitchell M et al: Do changes in PCWP adequately reflect myocardial ischemia during anesthesia? A correlative preoperative hemodynamic, electrocardiographic, and TEE study. *Circulation* 81:865-871, 1990.
25. ASA practice guidelines for pulmonary artery catheterization. *Anesthesiology* 78:380-394, 1993.
26. Cullen DJ: Monitoring of renal function. In: Miller RD (ed). *Anesthesia.* 3rd Ed. New York: Churchill Livingstone, Inc.; 1165- 1184, 1990.
27. Petrovich C: Regional anesthesia and anticoagulation. In: Benumof JL, Hannallah MS (eds). *Anesthesiology Clinics of North America: Anesthesia for Vascular Surgery.* Philadelphia: WB Saunders, Co.; 97-113, 1995.
28. Bonica JJ, Kennedy WF, Akamatsu TJ, et al: Circulatory effects of peridural block. I. Influence of level of analgesia and dose of lidocaine. *Anesthesiology* 33:619-626, 1970.
29. Reitz S, Balfours E, Sorenson MB, et al: Coronary hemodynamic effects of general anesthesia and surgery: modification by epidural analgesia in patients with ischemic heart disease. *Reg Anesth* (suppl 7):s8-s18, 1982.
30. Park WY: Regional versus general anesthesia for patients undergoing vascular surgery. In: Benumof JL, Hannallah MS (eds). *Anesthesiology Clinics of North America: Anesthesia for Vascular Surgery.* Philadelphia: WB Saunders, Co.; 83-96, 1995.
31. Hiljamae H, Stefansson T, Wickstrom I: Influence of anesthetic technique on postoperative pulmonary complications in geriatric patients. *Reg Anesth* (suppl 7):s122-s132, 1982.
32. Baron JF, Bertland M, Barre E, et al: Combined epidural and general anesthesia versus general anesthesia for abdominal aortic surgery. *Anesthesiology* 75:611-618, 1991.
33. Jayr C, Thomas H, Rey, A, et al: Postoperative pulmonary complications: epidural analgesia using bupivicaine and opioids versus parenteral opioids. *Anesthesiology* 78:666-676, 1993.
34. Tuman KJ, McCarthy RJ, March RJ, et al: Effects of epidural anesthesia and analgesia on coagulation and outcome after major vascular surgery. *Anesth Analg* 73:696-704, 1991.
35. Yeager PM, Glass DD, Neff RK, et al: Epidural anesthesia and analgesia in high-risk surgical patients. *Anesthesiology* 66:729- 736, 1987.
36. Brown B, Lerman J, Ebert TJ, et al: The clinical pharmacology of sevoflurane. *Anesth Analg* (suppl 81):s1-s72, 1995.
37. Fragen RJ, Avram MJ: Nonopioid intravenous anesthetics. In: Barash PG, Cullen BF, Stoelting RK (eds). *Clinical Anesthesia.* 2nd Ed. Philadelphia: JB Lippincott; 385-412, 1992.
38. O'Connor MF, Roth S, Roizen MF: Blood transfusion therapy for vascular surgery. In: Roizen MF (ed). *Anesthesia for Vascular Surgery.* New York: Churchill Livingstone, Inc.; 441-463, 1990.
39. Frank SM, Beattie C, Christopherson R, et al: Unintentional hypothermia is associated with postoperative myocardial ischemia. *Anesthesiology* 78:468-476, 1993.

Chapter 10

The Surgical ICU:

Perioperative Management of Elderly Patients Undergoing Vascular Surgery

David H. Wong, PharmD, MD

Intensive care unit (ICU) management of elderly vascular surgery patients, in many ways, is similar to the care of younger patients who undergo vascular surgery, and elderly patients who undergo other types of surgery. What is noteworthy about the perioperative care of elderly vascular surgery patients, is the combination of being elderly and undergoing vascular surgery.

The most specific data regarding elderly vascular surgery patients is available in elderly patients undergoing carotid endarterectomy (CEA). Advanced age has been reported to be a risk factor for complications after CEA.[1-3] Indeed, an exponential increase in mortality with advancing age in patients undergoing CEA has been reported.[4]

Conversely, the morbidity and mortality in patients aged 70 to 85 has been reported to be similar to younger patients undergoing CEA.[5] Recent multicenter studies have reported that age is not a risk factor for complications in patients undergoing CEA.[6,7]

Attempts to reconcile the different findings regarding advanced age as a risk factor for perioperative complications have led to two different hypotheses: 1) advanced chronological age itself is not a risk factor, but advanced physiological age[8] is an independent risk factor for perioperative complications; and 2) the medical problems common in elderly patients are the independent risk factors for perioperative complications.[9]

Elderly patients may be more vulnerable than younger patients for perioperative complications because they may have diminished physiological reserve. Neurologically, elderly patients are more sensitive to sedative hypnotic drugs, have lower anesthetic requirements, and have impaired thermoregulatory vasoconstriction response to hypothermia.

From: Aronow WS, Stemmer EA, Wilson SE (eds). *Vascular Disease in the Elderly*. Armonk, NY: Futura Publishing Company, Inc., © 1997.

Elderly patients are more prone to hypothermia during surgery and anesthesia.[10]

Changes in the cardiovascular system with increasing age include increased mean and increased systolic blood pressure, decreased heart rate, and increased stroke volume. The resting cardiac output is not necessarily decreased. Baroreceptor response is reduced and the vulnerability for orthostatic hypotension is increased.[11] Decreased heart rate may also be accompanied by a decreased, possibly inadequate heart rate response to hypovolemia or hypotension.[12]

Changes in the pulmonary system with increasing age include increased residual lung volume, decreased functional residual capacity, decreased vital capacity (VC), increased dead space, and decreased respiratory protective reflexes. These changes result in decreased PaO_2 at rest. Elderly patients also have impaired responses to hypoxia and hypercapnia, making them more prone to respiratory depression from narcotics and other drugs. Increased sleep apnea events associated with silent myocardial ischemia have been noted in elderly vascular surgery patients.[13] Changes in the renal system include decreased creatinine clearance and fewer glomeruli, even though serum creatinine is unchanged because of reduced muscle mass.

Elderly patients undergoing vascular procedures are essentially patients with age-associated diminished physiological reserves undergoing the stress of a vascular procedure. Elderly patients with diagnosed medical disease have further diminished physiological reserves. If the physiological stress during the perioperative period is greater than the patient's physiological reserve, then a perioperative complication may occur. Therefore, in order to prevent complications, the perioperative management of elderly vascular patients requires the prompt diagnosis and treatment of any physiological derangements. Such intensive monitoring and treatment is most commonly available in the ICU setting. Elderly patients undergoing vascular surgery are routinely admitted to the ICU postoperatively, and occasionally admitted to the ICU preoperatively.

Preoperative ICU Management

Occasionally, elderly patients scheduled to undergo elective vascular surgery may have medical problems severe enough to warrant preoperative ICU evaluation and treatment. A sound perioperative management principle is that patients must be in their best possible physiological condition before undergoing elective surgery. Therefore, patients with chronic illnesses such as hypertension, diabetes, chronic obstructive pulmonary disease (COPD), angina, and dialysis-dependent renal failure must be controlled medically as much as possible; generally, these illnesses should be treatable on an outpatient basis. Hospital admission may be needed for patients with medical problems such as uncontrolled diabetes, acute lung infections, or urinary tract infections.

Preoperative ICU admission may be necessary for treatment of serious medical problems such as acute congestive heart failure, new onset or breakthrough heart arrhythmias, or low cardiac output syndromes. The goal of preoperative ICU stabilization of the cardiac organ system should be a normal mixed venous oxygenation, serum lactate, and normal total body oxygen delivery.[14]

Preoperative hemodynamic evaluation with pulmonary artery catheters has been shown to help assign operative risk and improve the survival of some high-risk elderly patients undergoing operations.[15] In a prospective, randomized trial, Berlauk et al[16] inserted pulmonary artery catheters preoperatively and treated 45 vascular surgery patients to reach the goals of pulmonary capillary wedge pressure (PCWP) from 8 to 15 mm Hg, cardiac index (CI) ≥ 2.8 L/min per m$_2$, and (SVR) ≤ 1100 dyne/sec per cm^{-5}. Although two patients had myocardial infarctions (MIs) during "optimization," the treatment group still had a lower morbidity and mortality than the control group.[16] Of Berlauk's 45 patients, 31 required fluid and/or intravenous (IV) drug infusion intervention to meet the hemodynamic goals. Conversely, Baxter et al inserted pulmonary artery catheters to preoperatively evaluate systemic oxygen delivery in 39 high-risk vascular surgery patients[17] and estimated that only 15% to 20% of patients undergoing major vascular surgery would benefit from preoperative invasive monitoring and optimization. Preoperative ICU admission for hemodynamic treatment may benefit selected patients.

Vascular surgery adds additional stress to the underlying medical problems elderly patients may already have. Vascular operations can stress the cardiac, pulmonary, and renal systems, and potentially can cause neurological damage as well. Vascular surgery may be painful, frequently involves hemorrhage, and frequently involves changes in the coagulation system. The most common operations, CEA, abdominal aortic aneurysm (AAA) resection, and infra-inguinal bypass, pose different challenges to these organ systems; therefore, the perioperative management of each procedure will be discussed separately.

ICU Management of Elderly Patients After Carotid Surgery

CEA is the most common vascular procedure. The most serious complications occurring after CEA are MI, stroke, and death. Patients aged 65 or over undergoing CEA in the 1980s had mortality rates ranging from 2% to 3%, and an incidence of perioperative stroke of 3% to 6%.[3,18]

In 1987, the Committee on Health Care Issues of the American Neurological Association recommended that asymptomatic patients undergoing CEA should have a combined stroke and mortality rate less than 3%; for symptomatic patients, the combined stroke and mortality rate should be less than 6%.[19] A study of 1160 patients undergoing CEA from 1988 to 1990 at 12 different medical centers reported a 1.4%

mortality rate, overall incidence of stroke of 3.4%, and an overall incidence of MI of 2%.[20] A 2.1% incidence of stroke in 2,365 patients undergoing CEA was reported by Riles, et al.[21] More recently, a 30-day mortality rate of less than 1% after CEA has been reported.[22]

Cebul et al have further suggested that symptomatic patients undergoing CEA should have mortality rates less than 1%, with less than a 3% incidence of perioperative stroke, and asymptomatic patients should have a combined mortality and stroke related morbidity less than 2%.[23] Both strokes and MIs after CEA may require ICU care for optimal management.

Neurological Complications: Central and Peripheral Nerve Damage

New neurological deficits may be due to acute cerebrovascular thrombosis, embolism, subarachnoid hemorrhage, vasospasm, hyperreinfusion syndrome, or oversedation. The operating surgeon should be immediately notified whenever there are new neurological deficits. New neurological deficits may be evaluated by taking patients back to the operating room, performing CT scan, arteriography, or ultrasound examination.

If a thrombotic or embolic stroke is diagnosed, administration of nimodipine within 12 hours of the stroke may improve neurological outcome.[24,25] The value of thrombolytic therapy or cytoprotective therapy in acute thrombotic stroke in the nonoperative setting is currently being studied.[24] Thrombolytic therapy is contraindicated if the neurological changes are due to intracerebral hemorrhage. Patients with intracerebral hemorrhage may have symptoms consisting of a progressively worsening headache associated with visual changes, vomiting, or altered mental status.

Altered mental status may also be a sign of cerebral vasospasm. If neurological symptoms are thought to be due to vasospasm, treatment options include hypervolemic (CVP 10 to 12 mm Hg, or PCWP 15 to 18 mm Hg), hyperdynamic (inotrope therapy; or systolic bp 160 to 220 mm Hg), and hemodilution (HCT 30 to 35) therapy. Hypervolemic, hyperdynamic, and hemodilution therapies have been recommended for vasospasm associated with subarachnoid hemorrhage occurring after cerebral aneurysm repair,[26] and cerebral vasospasm after subarachnoid hemorrhage.[27] However, there are no studies regarding the efficacy of this treatment for vasospasm after carotid artery surgery. In elderly patients, pulmonary artery catheterization may be useful in titrating fluid and inotrope therapy and avoiding cardiac complications.

Hyperreinfusion syndrome consists of an ipsilateral headache, followed by focal or generalized seizures. Transient neurological deficits may also occur. Hyperreinfusion syndrome mostly occurs in patients with very high-grade stenoses who undergo CEA. Seizures should be treated symptomatically with benzodiazepines and/or barbiturates.

New neurological deficits are usually related to intraoperative factors,[21] not oversedation. Oversedation does not cause focal neurological deficits. If necessary, oversedation can be excluded as a cause of postoperative neurological change by titrating 100 mcg of naloxone or 0.1 mg of flumazenil at 2- to 3-minute intervals, until a total of 400 mcg naloxone or 1.0 mg flumazenil have been given. Naloxone or flumazenil should be stopped if the patient develops pain or anxiety.

Peripheral nerves may be damaged during CEA. Damage of the hypoglossal nerve or recurrent laryngeal nerve may occur in 5% of patients undergoing CEA.[28] Recurrent laryngeal nerve damage may cause respiratory distress, particularly if there is bilateral recurrent laryngeal nerve damage. Damage to the marginal mandibular nerve (seen as drooping of the corner of the mouth) or superior laryngeal nerve occurs less frequently. Peripheral nerve injuries usually resolve spontaneously.

Cardiac Complications: Hypertension, Hypotension, Myocardial Ischemia, and Myocardial Infarction

Hypertension is the most common problem after CEA that requires drug treatment. However, hypotension or bradycardia may also occur postoperatively. More significant, although fortunately less common, are occurrences of myocardial ischemia and MI. Mortality after CEA is most commonly due to cardiac complications.[5]

Carotid surgery patients may be predisposed to either hypertension or hypotension because there may be two different effects on the carotid baroreceptor and the carotid sinus. Stimulation of the carotid sinus causes decreased heart rate and blood pressure. Inhibition of the carotid sinus nerve causes the opposite effect. During CEA, the carotid baroreceptors may be traumatized, resulting in nerve dysfunction. The dysfunctional carotid baroreceptors then "sense" the arterial blood pressure as being lower than it truly is, resulting in increased central nervous system (CNS) sympathetic tone and increased systemic blood pressure. Conversely, removal of atheromatous plaque over the carotid baroreceptors may allow the carotid baroreceptors to "sense" the true arterial blood pressure whereas before, the baroreceptors sensed the arterial blood pressure through plaques. The newly sensitized barorocoptors then "sense" a higher blood pressure than before, and thereby cause the CNS sympathetic tone to decrease systemic blood pressure, causing hypotension.

Hypertension may occur in 20% of patients undergoing CEA.[29] Postoperative hypertension may be a contributing factor for neurological deficits which develop postoperatively.[30] Although postoperative hypertension after CEA is generally transient, it should be aggressively, yet carefully, treated because it may contribute to the risk of postoperative hemorrhagic stroke. Perioperative hypertension associated with CEA may be transient and labile, and usually resolves within 24 hours. Hypertension should be treated with titratable, fast acting, short duration drugs. Fast acting drugs help treat hypertension faster and help decrease the risk of hemorrhagic stroke. Short duration drugs help avoid the risk of iatrogenic hypotension. In general, an antihypertensive drug should be given by IV infusion. Nitroprusside is the standard drug for this situation. Nitroglycerin, nicardipine, and labetolol infusions are second line choices. The use of sublingual nifedipine, while convenient, should be discouraged.

Significant hypotension after CEA is less common than hypertension and may be associated with bradycardia. The perioperative hypotension associated with CEA usually resolves within 24 hours. Often, hypotension has been significant intraoperatively and a phenylephrine infusion has been started. Postoperatively, all that is necessary is to continue or restart the phenylephrine infusion until the carotid baroreceptors adjust to the new physiological state (when the infusion should be weaned as tolerated). Since phenylephrine is a pure vasoconstrictor without any inotropic effects, it should be weaned as soon as possible when systemic vasodilation (i.e., general anesthesia) is not present. Before phenylephrine therapy is started, the more common causes of hypotension should be excluded (i.e., hypovolemia, acute sedative or narcotic drug administration).

MI occurs in approximately 2% to 3% of patients undergoing CEA[19,31] and is the most frequent cause of postoperative mortality. MI is the most common cause of death within 30 days of operation after CEA. Coronary artery disease (CAD) is very prevalent in patients undergoing CEA; in one prospective study where patients scheduled for CEA underwent coronary angiography, severe CAD was present in 94 of 295 patients (32%), and advanced but compensated CAD was present in 80 of 295 patients (27%).[32] The prevalence of surgically correctable CAD in patients with cerebral vascular disease was 26%.[32] Myocardial ischemia is often silent in the postoperative patients and may be unrelated to changes in heart rate or blood pressure.[33-35] Thus, a heightened index of suspicion should be kept for elderly patients in the postoperative period. Abnormal heart rate and blood pressure should be treated, if present. Real-time ST segment analysis monitoring should be used, if available. New onset of ectopy or abnormal arrhythmias may be the first manifestation of myocardial ischemia. If these events occur, then a 12-lead electrocardiogram (EKG) should be obtained and compared to the respective preoperative EKG. If the EKG has changed, then a rule out MI protocol should be initiated.

Pulmonary Complications

Respiratory muscle function is preserved after CEA, since no abdominal or thoracic incision is made. Routine postoperative pulmonary care (incentive spirometry) should be adequate. If respiratory distress does occur, nonpulmonary causes should be suspected. For example, stridor may be due to vocal cord paresis due to recurrent laryngeal nerve damage and airway obstruction may be due to wound hematoma. Carotid body chemoreceptor dysfunction may be manifested by loss of response to hypoxia or CO_2 retention.

Renal Complications

Fluid shifts are minimal in CEA patients. Fluid requirements due to third spacing are minimal. Unless patients have preexisting renal disease, routine postoperative IV fluids are generally sufficient until the patients' oral intake can be advanced as tolerated.

Pain

Generally, patients have minimal pain after CEA. Morphine sulfate, 1 to 4 mg IV prn every 2 hours, should be adequate.

Hematologic Complications: Bleeding

Bleeding after CEA is usually not severe enough to cause anemia in patients; estimated blood losses (EBL) are usually less than 200 cc.[36] However, the location of the bleeding is significant. Wound hematomas may occur in 1% to 3 % of patients undergoing CEA.[37,38] A wound hematoma can compromise the patient's airway, and a rapidly expanding wound hematoma can be an airway emergency. The patient's thyroid cartilage should be checked for deviation in the direction opposite the operative site. Intubation may be difficult if a large hematoma is present; if an airway cannot be maintained by the patient spontaneously, by mask ventilation, or by intubation, then releasing the patient's sutures and evacuating the wound may be lifesaving.

Miscellaneous

Hypothermia, fluid shifts, and electrolyte shifts should not be problems after CEA. The ICU management of elderly patients after CEA is summarized in Table 1.

ICU Management Elderly Patients After Aortic Reconstructive Surgery

The mortality of patients undergoing aortic reconstructive surgery is significant. A review of 6,488 patients reported an overall mortality of 4% for nonruptured AAA repair.[39] A review of 1,289 European patients

Table 1
Guidelines for ICU Management of Elderly Patients After CEA

Upon arrival in ICU	Review perioperative course; note current HR and BP, SaO$_2$. CNS—Evaluate and document neurological status—ability to move all 4 extremities upon command; see whether voice is hoarse; ask patient to stick out tongue. Compare mental status to preoperative baseline. If a focal neurological deficit is present, notify operating surgeon immediately—consider diagnostic evaluation, e.g., emergency Doppler, CT scan, angiography, or re-operation. Cardiac—Look for any hypertension or hypotension. If present, treat with drug infusion. Pulm—Encourage deep breathing; ensure that airway is clear. Renal—Order maintenance fluids. Heme—Check for hematoma. Pain—Treat pain, if present. Misc—Document dressing is dry. If patient had episode of unstable vital signs or ischemia in the OR, order 12-lead EKG.

First hr. in ICU	CNS—Look for changes in neurological status as above
	Cardiac—Look for hypertension, hypotension, or bradycardia.
	  Treat hypertension with nitroprusside, nitroglycerine.
	  Treat hypotension (if present) with IV fluid; continue/start phenylephrine infusion.
	Pulmonary—Encourage deep breathing; ensure that airway is clear; look for respiratory distress—stridor due to laryngeal nerve paralysis; hematoma-induced airway obstruction.
	Renal—Check urine output hourly; goal is 0.5–1.0 cc/kg/hr.
	Heme—Check for hematoma.
	Pain—Treat pain, if present, with IM or IV narcotics; consider PCA if pain is severe.
	Misc—Compare 12 lead EKG to preoperative EKG; if ischemia changes are present, initiate rule out MI protocol.

(continued)

Table 1 (*continued*)
Guidelines for ICU Management of Elderly Patients After CEA

First 4 hrs in ICU	CNS—Patient should be at pre-procedure neurological baseline. Cardiac—Continue treatment of hypertension or hypotension as needed; try to wean cardiac drug infusion as tolerated. Pulmonary—Encourage incentive spirometry; goal is 15 cc/kg. Renal—as above. Pain—as above. Misc—as above.
First 24 hrs in ICU	CNS—as above. Cardiac—as above. Pulmonary—as above. Renal—as above. Pain—Continue p.r.n. pain relief. Misc—as above.
Patient is ready to be discharged from ICU when:	No neurological deficits have occurred; if neurological deficits have occurred; when they have been evaluated and stabilized. Cardiac—Hemodynamics stable for 8 hours (i.e., overnight) without drug therapy. Pulmonary—Back to preoperative state. Renal—as above. Pain—Controlled on IM or PO medication. Misc—Airway is patent, no bleeding at wound; HCT stable.

ICU = intensive care unit; CEA = carotid endarterectomy; CNS = central nervous system; HR = heart rate; BP = blood pressure; SaO$_2$ = oxygen saturation; EKG = electrocardiogram; MI = myocardial infarction; IV = intravenous; IM = intramuscular; PO = oral; HCT = hematocrit.

revealed a 6.8% mortality for elective repair of infrarenal AAA.[40] The perioperative mortality of patients ≥ 80 years old compares favorably with the results for all patient ages. Petracek et al reported a 5.2% mortality in 38 patients older than 80 years after abdominal aortic aneurysmectomy.[41] O'Hara et al reported a mortality rate of 17% in patients older than 80 years operated from 1984 to 1988, and a mortality rate of 4% in patients older than 80 years operated on from 1989 to 1993.[42] Even if elderly patients and younger patients have similar mortalities after aortic reconstructive surgery, a 4% mortality is still significant. Neurological, cardiac, pulmonary, and renal morbidity may also occur.

Neurological Complications: Spinal Cord Injury

Spinal cord injury after aortic cross-clamping may develop in 0.2% of patients undergoing elective aortic reconstruction.[43,44] The blood supply of the spinal cord is mostly provided by the anterior spinal artery, which is fed by branches from the aorta; the largest is at the T9-T12 level with few collaterals. Risk of spinal cord ischemia is exacerbated by longer cross-clamp times, suprarenal cross-clamping, and low cardiac output states. Evaluation of lower spinal cord neurological function should be done as soon as possible postoperatively. If spinal cord injury is suspected, a thorough neurological exam should be done. The sensory and motor level of neurological dysfunction should be documented. If spinal cord injury has occurred, a similar neurological exam should be repeated daily until the patient's neurological exam is unchanged for 2 or 3 days.

Cardiac Complications: Myocardial Ischemia and Infarction

In one study, 7 of 97 patients (7%) undergoing elective infrarenal aortic aneurysm repair had a postoperative MI.[45] In a study involving 666 patients undergoing AAA repair, 5.2% patients had MI.[46] Cardiac morbidity is common in patients undergoing AAA repair because CAD is very prevalent in these patients. In one prospective study, of 263 patients scheduled for AAA repair who underwent coronary angiography, 93 patients (36%) had severe CAD and 72 patients (29%) had advanced, but compensated CAD.[32]

Cardiac morbidity is the main cause of death in patients undergoing AAA repair.[47,48] Cardiac morbidity in aortic reconstruction patients typically occurs on the second or third postoperative day,[48,49] and is associated with remobilization of interstitial fluid into the intravascular space. Clinical signs and hemodynamic information derived from invasive monitors regarding the patient's intravascular volume status should be observed closely. Invasive pressures and urine output should be recorded hourly. The patient's intravascular volume changes predictably postoperatively. On postoperative days 1 and 2, the patient may still be third spacing and may become relatively hypovolemic; yet on postoperative days 2 and 3, edema fluid may start to mobilize, placing the patient at risk for congestive heart failure. A rough guide of how much fluid may need to be mobilized is the net amount of fluid that had to be administered intraoperatively.

Myocardial ischemia in elderly patients may be manifested by arrhythmia, ectopy, and unaccompanied by angina, particularly in the postoperative period. Myocardial ischemia occurs when the myocardial oxygen demand exceeds the myocardial oxygen supply. Four main factors increase myocardial oxygen demand: 1) tachycardia; 2) increased myocardial wall tension, due to increased preload (increased intravascular volume); 3) increased myocardial wall tension due to increased afterload (hypertension); and 4) increased myocardial contractility.

Catecholamines with beta agonist properties can cause tachycardia, hypertension, and increased myocardial contractility. Plasma catecholamines are elevated after AAA surgery.[50] The use of beta adrenergic blocking drugs has been associated with decreased perioperative MIs after vascular surgery.[51] Since pain can also release catecholamines, adequate pain treatment is important. Another cause of increased myocardial oxygen demand which should be avoided is increased preload (increased intravascular volume).

Another strategy in the treatment of myocardial ischemia is to increase myocardial oxygen supply. Myocardial oxygen supply can be improved by increasing myocardial oxygen delivery (increasing plasma hemoglobin/hematocrit and avoiding hypoxia). Conditions which can decrease myocardial oxygen supply which should be avoided include hypocapnia, hypoxia, and anemia. There is a low threshold for investigating the possibility of an MI in AAA patients. Most AAA patients should have a 12-lead EKG on arrival in the ICU.

Pulmonary Complications: Pneumonia and Respiratory Insufficiency

Pulmonary complications are also common in patients undergoing AAA repair. In one study of 666 patients undergoing AAA repair, 8% patients developed respiratory insufficiency.[46] In another study of 475 patients undergoing aortic reconstructive surgery, 15% developed postoperative pneumonia and 18% developed respiratory insufficiency.[52] In another study of 181 aortic surgery patients, pneumonia occurred in 17 patients (9%) and prolonged intubation occurred in 9 patients (5%).[53]

Patients undergoing AAA repair are at risk for pulmonary complications because of a variety of factors. COPD and smoking are preoperative risk factors. Abdominal incision for AAA decreases functional residual capacity, PaO_2, and VC. Postoperatively, splinting may occur because of incision-induced pain.

Epidural or intrathecal narcotics may improve pulmonary function with less respiratory depression than IV or intramuscular (IM) narcotics. Even if patients have not had an epidural catheter inserted preoperatively or intraoperatively, an epidural catheter inserted postoperatively may still benefit patients postoperatively and even prevent reintubation. If epidural or intrathecal narcotic administration is unavailable, patient-controlled analgesia (PCA) is the next best choice. Adequate pain control must be provided to prevent splinting and maximize tidal volume and VC. Patients with a preoperative $FEV_1 > 1.5$ L and VC > 2.5 L should be able to have a VC > 1 L, and be weaned from the ventilator and extubated within 24 hours postoperatively.

Renal Complications:
Acute Renal Failure

Acute renal failure may develop in 4% to 6 % of patients undergoing aortic reconstructive surgery.[46,48] If the patients have preexisting renal disease, the incidence of acute renal insufficiency has been reported to be 32%.[48] The mortality rate of patients who develop acute renal failure after AAA repair is 32%.[54] Even patients in whom the cross-clamp is applied on the aorta below the renal arteries are at risk for acute renal failure. Postoperatively, urine output should be measured every hour. Prerenal azotemia should be avoided by closely following indicators of intravascular volume, cautiously titrating fluid challenges when the urine output falls below 0.5 cc/kg per hour, and avoiding iatrogenic hypovolemia by overzealous diuresis. Nephrotoxins (e.g., aminoglycosides) in patients with chronic or new onset renal insufficiency also should be avoided. Furosemide can exacerbate renal toxicity and, thus, should be used only when necessary. If urine output remains low, despite an apparently adequate intravascular volume, dopamine at 2 to 3 mcg/kg per minute should be added. Whether dopamine actually increases urine output, increases renal perfusion, or acts as a diuretic is uncertain.[55]

Urine output may appear adequate despite intravascular hypovolemia, if there is an osmotic diuresis (hyperglycemia in a diabetic, IV contrast dye that has been recently given for an angiogram, or mannitol given intraoperatively before aortic cross-clamp). Spontaneous urine output which is greater than the fluid input is a particularly good sign; it demonstrates that the patient is not only starting to mobilize fluid, but that the fluid can be accommodated intravascularly and appropriately excreted.

Once the patient starts to mobilize fluid, generally on the second or third postoperative day, if the patient's intravascular volume status cannot be determined conclusively, a small "test" dose of furosemide (5 to 10 mg IV) may be given, particularly in patients who have been on oral diuretics on a chronic basis. Patients who are hypervolemic will often diurese; patients who are hypovolemic will not.

Pain

Vascular patients with more intense pain may have a greater incidence of postoperative atelectasis.[56] Poor pain control has been associated with an increased incidence of myocardial ischemia after cardiac surgery.[57] Abdominal vascular surgery is even more painful than cardiac surgery.[56] The improved morbidity and mortality with combined epidural/general anesthesia versus plain general anesthesia alone[58] has been attributed to postoperative epidural pain relief.[59] The first analgesic choice is epidural or intrathecal narcotics. If an epidural or intrathecal catheter is unavailable, then PCA should be used.

Hematologic Complications: Blood Loss

Average EBL of 1100 cc[35] and 1756 mL[60] for abdominal aortic aneurysmectomy and 1759 cc for aortobifemoral bypass have been reported.[35] Dilution of platelets and hypothermia may exacerbate surgical hemorrhage. While the exact minimum hematocrit acceptable for any given patient is an individual decision, elderly vascular patients are particularly at risk for myocardial ischemia because of their age and high prevalence of CAD, hypertension, or diabetes. Nelson et al have shown that vascular surgery patients have an increased incidence of myocardial ischemia when their hematocrit is less than 28.[61] Baxter et al studied 39 patients who underwent a variety of vascular procedures and measured hemodynamic and oxygen delivery parameters.[17] They argued that high-risk elderly vascular patients cannot mount a normal cardiac compensatory response to anemia[17,62] and may need hemoglobin levels of 10 to 12 g/dL (i.e., HCT of 30 to 36) to have an adequate oxygen delivery.[17] The decision to transfuse packed red blood cells should be based on each patient's medical condition. Transfusing elderly vascular patients at a higher hematocrit than younger patients should be considered, particularly if signs of hypoperfusion such as myocardial ischemia, myocardial ectopy, metabolic acidosis, or low mixed venous oxygen tension or saturation, are present.

Miscellaneous

Hypothermia may be present in AAA patients at the end of surgery. Shivering related to hypothermia increases global oxygen consumption which may cause myocardial ischemia[63] and mortality.[64] Bush et al reported a 12% mortality rate in abdominal aortic aneurysmectomy patients who were hypothermic (34.5°C) compared to a 1.5% mortality rate in those patients who were normothermic at the end of surgery.[64] The physiological response to hypothermia (vasoconstriction) may render systemic perfusion (as measured by cardiac output) inadequate. Treatment of postoperative hypertension in hypothermic patients may result in vasodilation and sudden severe hypovolemia. In the acute postoperative period (first 1 to 4 hours post-op), as much as 1 L of colloid or 2 to 3 L crystalloid may be needed for fluid replacement. Severe hypothermia can also cause a coagulopathy. In the ICU, a heated air convection blanket is probably the most effective way to warm patients.

Lower extremity ischemia due to embolization of atheroma or thrombus may occur in less than 1% of patients undergoing aortic reconstruction.[65] Emboli of large thrombi can be treated with thrombectomy. Emboli of microthrombi are not treatable.

Ischemia of the bowel is a rare, but highly fatal complication of aortic reconstruction. Bowel ischemia may appear as early as 24 to 36 hours postoperatively. Clinical signs include mucus filled stool followed by bloody diarrhea, and it is usually associated with metabolic acidosis. Diagnostic evaluation may include sigmoidoscopy, arteriography, or reexploration.

Pancreatitis, acalculous cholecystitis, and graft infection are late, but serious complications of aortic reconstruction. The ICU management of elderly patients after aortic reconstruction is summarized in Table 2.

ICU Management of Elderly Patients After Infrainguinal Bypass Surgery

The perioperative mortality for infrainguinal bypass has been reported to range from 3.7% to 7%.[66,67] L'Italien et al reported a perioperative MI rate twice as high as patients undergoing aortic reconstruction; 13% versus 6%.[68] In patients over 80-years-old, an 11%[67] and 12%[69] mortality has been reported. Infrainguinal bypass procedures do not involve abdominal or thoracic incisions, are often done under regional anesthesia, and are associated with less than 300 cc blood loss.[36] Why should elderly patients undergoing infrainguinal bypass procedures have a morbidity that equals[68,70] and mortality rate that equals or even exceeds that of aortic reconstruction surgery? Apparently, patients undergoing infrainguinal bypass procedures have a greater prevalence of underlying cardiac risk factors than other vascular surgery patients.[68] Surprisingly, patients who undergo simple amputation have an even higher 30-day perioperative mortality than patients undergoing infrainguinal bypass.[69]

One way to quantitate the perfusion status of the lower limb preoperatively and postoperatively is to determine the ankle brachial index (ABI). The ABI is the ratio of the systolic blood pressure (or systolic pressure at which the pulse is detected) of the ankle over the brachial artery. A normal ABI is 1. An ABI less than 0.5 indicates ischemia. The postoperative ABI should increase at least 0.15 compared to the preoperative ABI.

Patients who have severe ischemia of the lower extremity also are susceptible to two potentially serious permanent sequelae-compartment syndrome and rhabdomyolysis. Compartment syndrome may result in permanent nerve damage. Rhabdomyolysis may lead to acute renal failure.

Neurological Complications: Compartment Syndrome

When a lower limb that has been severely ischemic has its perfusion restored, the injured muscle may have a capillary leak syndrome. If fluid leaks from the capillaries into a closed space, such as the fascia-lined muscle compartments of the lower extremity, and pressure inside the compartment increases, a compartment syndrome is possible.

Compartment syndrome may be diagnosed clinically or by measuring pressures within the compartment. Neurological signs of compartment syndrome include numbness, pain on palpation, and paresthesia. Diminished pulses and muscle weakness are also signs of compartment syndrome. Loss of sensation, paralysis, and absent pulses are late signs of compartment syndrome. The pressure within the compartment is readily measured by inserting a hollow needle or an IV catheter inside the compartment and connecting it to a standard pressure transducer and monitoring system. A hollow needle is more resistant to kinking, but is harder to secure than an IV catheter. Whether a hollow needle or an IV catheter is used, the pressure reading may be inaccurate due to clots or tissue. An elevated compartment pressure above 30 mm Hg may cause nerve and muscle damage.

The operating surgeon should be notified as soon as compartment syndrome is suspected, because permanent nerve damage may occur if the compartment syndrome lasts for 8 hours or more. Muscle death may begin if the compartment syndrome lasts for 4 hours or more.

Treatment of compartment syndrome is fasciotomy. Some authors have indicated that a fasciotomy should be performed if the compartment pressure is greater than 40 mm Hg or between 30 and 40 mm Hg for 4 hours; however, compartment syndrome may occur even at lower pressures. If the limb has already been severely ischemic at the time of the bypass surgery, prophylactic fasciotomies are sometimes done at that time.

Cardiac Complications

Patients undergoing infrainguinal bypass procedures are at risk for cardiac complications. In one study where vascular surgery patients underwent routine coronary angiography, of 381 patients with lower extremity ischemia, severe CAD was present in 107 patients (28%), and advanced but compensated CAD disease was present in 111 patients

Table 2

Guidelines for ICU Management of Elderly Patients After Aortic Reconstruction

Before arrival in ICU	Set up cardiac output injectate system; have monitor set up for 3 pressure transducers; have forced air warming blanket system available; have supplies for stat laboratories available; have mechanical ventilator available.
Upon arrival in ICU	Review intra-operative course; note current HR, BP, and SaO_2. Ensure a smooth transfer from the transport monitors to the ICU monitors; the patient's HR, BP, and SaO_2 should always be monitored.
	CNS—When patient is awake, evaluate and document neurological status, focusing on lower spinal cord function—ability to move all 4 extremities upon command; If a neurological deficit is present, notify operating surgeon immediately.
	Cardiac—Look for hypertension or hypotension. Treat blood pressure if it not within 20% of pre-op values. Continue drug infusions as needed.
	Measure cardiac output. Calculate SVR. If SVR > 1800, systolic BP > 180, and patient's temp < 35°C, start low dose nitroprusside infusion. Be prepared to give IV fluids to support blood pressure.
	Evaluate pedal pulses, skin temp, and color of both feet.
	Pulm—Extubate when:
	patient is awake and responsive, able to maintain and protect their own airway, weaning criteria are acceptable (VC > 15 cc/kg; TV > 5 cc/kg; NIF more negative than −20 cm H_2O), core temp >36°C, patient is hemodynamically stable, and post-op bleeding is minimal.
	Renal—Order maintenance IV fluids. Note urine output in Foley bag; empty Foley bag.
	Pain—Evaluate pain. If epidural catheter is present; if epidural narcotics were not given, administer epidural narcotic. If no epidural catheter is present and patient has pain, control pain with IV morphine and start PCA.
	Misc—Document dressing is dry.
	Measure core temperature; if temp <35.5°C or patient is shivering, warm patient with forced air warming blanket.
	Obtain mixed venous blood gas; calibrate SvO_2 catheter if present.
	Obtain 12 lead EKG and compare to pre-op EKG. If EKG has new ischemia changes, initiate rule out MI protocol.

(continued)

Table 2 (*continued*)

Guidelines for ICU Management of Elderly Patients After Aortic Reconstruction

First hr. in ICU	CNS—Look for changes in mental and neurological status.
	Cardiac—Look for hypertension, hypotension, metabolic acidosis, low cardiac output, and low mixed venous oxygen.
	Treat hypertension or hypotension.
	Treat hypertension with IV antihypertensive drug.
	Treat hypotension, if present, with IV fluid; titrate fluid according to changes in CVP and PCWP.
	If intravascular volume is adequate, then add inotrope as necessary for hypotension, low cardiac output, or low mixed venous oxygen.
	Pulmonary—Extubate as above.
	If patient is extubated, encourage deep breathing.
	Renal—Measure urine output hourly. Usual goal is 0.5–1.0 cc/kg/hr.
	Misc—Determine whether metabolic acidosis is present or improving.
First 4 hrs. in ICU	CNS—as above.
	Cardiac—Repeat cardiac output and mixed venous oxygen measurements. Repeat SVR calculation; continue treatment of hypertension or hypotension as needed. Try to wean cardiac drug infusion as tolerated.
	Pulmonary—Extubate using same criteria as above.
	If patient is extubated, encourage deep breathing.
	Encourage incentive spirometry with goal of 15 cc/kg.
	Renal—as above.
	Pain—Treat pain with epidural narcotics, if epidural present. Use PCA if epidural or intrathecal narcotics are not possible.
	Misc—By now, patient's temperature should be >36.5°C, metabolic acidosis should be resolving (base deficit should be less than 4 meq/L), BP and HR should be in normal range; cardiac output should be > 2.8 L/min/m^2 with SvO$_2$ > 65%.
	Check labs. Correct electrolyte deficiencies.
	If HCT is lower than last intraoperative HCT, repeat HCT and order PT, PTT, platelet count. Look for signs of intra-abdominal bleeding—soaked dressing, expanding abdomen. Consider what HCT the patient needs for adequate oxygen delivery.
	Repeat ABG.

Table 2 (continued)
Guidelines for ICU Management of Elderly Patients After Aortic Reconstruction

First 24 hrs in ICU (morning after surgery)	CNS—as above.
	Cardiac—
	  Measure cardiac output and mixed venous oxygen again. Calculate SVR again.
	  Wean IV drugs for hypertension, hypotension, low cardiac output, or low SvO2 as tolerated.
	  Remove PA catheter when:
	    cardiac output and SvO_2 are in the normal range without any inotropic drug infusions (except for renal dose dopamine), and intravascular volume status can be readily evaluated without knowing PA_d or PCWP.
	Pulmonary—Extubate using same criteria as above. If patient is extubated, encourage deep breathing, encourage incentive spirometry with goal of 15 cc/kg.
	Renal—Give fluids for signs of hypovolemia—urine output < 0.5—1.5 cc/kg/hr; low CVP or PCWP, or hypotension.
	Pain—Continue epidural or PCA pain relief.
	Misc—If extubated, sit upright in chair; check distal pulses.
	  ABG, electrolyte, and HCT should be normal; if they are not, correct them.

Postoperative Days 2 or 3	CNS—as above.
	Cardiac—Continue weaning drug infusions.
	  PA catheter management as above.
	  Remove CVP when:
	    intravascular volume status can be readily evaluated without knowing CVP, and patient does not need infusion of K^+, phosphate, renal dose dopamine, or blood products.
	Pulmonary—as above.
	Renal—as above.
	Pain—as above. Stop epidural narcotics by 3rd postoperative day and remove epidural catheter. Start PCA. Convert to IM analgesia when PCA morphine use is <24 mg per 24 hours (or equivalent drug and dose).

Table 2 *(continued)*
Guidelines for ICU Management of Elderly Patients After Aortic Reconstruction

Postoperative Day 3, etc.	CNS—as above.
	Cardiac—Look for fluid mobilization. If urine output is less than fluid input, patient has rales, or intravascular filling pressures are elevated, consider diuresis. Test dose of 5–10 mg furosemide may initiate diuresis.
	Remove arterial catheter when:
	  blood pressure is stable without any IV medication.
	  only one or two blood draws are needed within 24 hours.

Patient is ready to be discharged from ICU when:	No CNS deficits have occurred; if neuro deficits have occurred, when they have been evaluated and stabilized. Cardiac hemodynamics stable for 8 hours (i.e., overnight). Pulm—Patient can voluntarily perform incentive spirometry repeatedly to 20 cc/kg or more. Normal ABG on 2–3 L O_2 by simple mask or nasal cannula. Renal—Intravascular volume status is readily determined without invasive catheters. Pain is controlled on IM or PO medication. Misc—HCT stable.

ICU = intensive care unit; HR = heart rate; BP = blood pressure; SaO_2 = oxygen saturation; CNS = central nervous system; SVR = systemic vascular resistance; VC = vital capacity; TV = tidal volume; NIF = negative inspiratory force; IV = intravenous; PCA = patient controlled analgesia; SvO_2 = mixed venous oxygen saturation; EKG = electrocardiogram; MI = myocardial infarction; CVP = central venous pressure; PCWP = pulmonary capillary wedge pressure; HCT = hematocrit; PT = prothrombin time; PTT = partial thromboplastin time; PA = pulmonary artery; PA_d = pulmonary artery diastolic pressure; ABG = arterial blood gas; IM = intramuscular; PO = oral; HCT = hematocrit.

(29%).[32] Diagnosis and management of cardiac problems is similar to that of elderly patients undergoing CEA and AAA repair.

Pulmonary Complications

Infrainguinal bypass procedures are often done under regional anesthesia. If the procedure has been done under general anesthesia, patients should be able to be extubated soon after the procedure is complete, unless there are underlying factors such as COPD, obesity, or aspiration risk. Adequate pain relief and incentive spirometry should be customary and sufficient to prevent pulmonary complications.

Renal Complications: Acute Renal Failure from Rhabdomyolysis

Patients undergoing infrainguinal bypass procedures are at risk for acute renal failure from IV contrast dye from angiography, advanced age, diabetes, and hypertension, but also from acute rhabdomyolysis caused by ischemia of the lower extremity. Skeletal muscle deprived of perfusion for 4 hours is at risk for ischemia and subsequent rhabdomyolysis.[71]

Acute renal failure caused by rhabdomyolysis is a significant cause of morbidity and mortality after lower extremity vascular procedures and may occur in up to 90% of patients undergoing revascularization after acute lower extremity ischemia.[72] In a study of 93 patients with rhabdomyolysis, 51% developed acute renal failure and 32% died. They also found that the incidence of acute renal failure was higher in those patients who had serum creatinine phosphokinase (CPK) greater than 15,000 U/L.[73] Most of the published literature regarding treatment of rhabdomyolysis has been published in patients who developed rhabdomyolysis because of trauma or prolonged immobilization; the basis for treatment of rhabdomyolysis from lower extremity ischemia is extrapolated from these other studies.

Dark brownish urine, a sign of myoglobinuria, may be the first clinical sign of rhabdomyolysis. In rhabdomyolysis, the dark urine is accompanied by normal appearing serum, elevated serum CPK, and normal serum haptoglobin. In hemoglobinuria, the dark urine is accompanied by pink serum, normal serum creatinine phosphokinase enzyme, and decreased serum haptoglobin. The Hematest(R) is positive in both myoglobinuria and hemoglobinuria.[74] If rhabdomyolysis is suspected, the urine should be tested with the Hematest and a serum CPK sample sent. Measure CPK every 8 hours once rhabdomyolysis is diagnosed. After the CPK has peaked, CPK should be measured daily, until the CPK is less than 1000 U/L. Measuring CPK enzymes repeatedly has two benefits: CPK determinations are easier to obtain and quicker to report than myoglobin, and they mark the clinical course of the rhabdomyolysis. Absolute CPK values, however, may be unreliable predictors for the development of renal failure; 35 patients with exercise induced rhabdomyolysis with average CPK values of 40,000 (range 700 to 165,000 U/L) did not develop renal failure.[75] Conversely, another study reported four patients who developed oliguric renal failure with CPK of 1300 to 10,000 U/L.[76]

The main treatment of rhabdomyolysis is vigorous fluid administration of a crystalloid, e.g., Ringer's lactate solution, with resultant diuresis. An absolute minimum of 1 cc/kg per hour with an average urine out put of 1.5 cc/kg per hour should be the goal at all times, until the risk of acute renal failure is over (CPK < 1000 U/L). Since myoglobin is excreted into the urine, urine color is a crude marker for myoglobinuria; urine appearing lighter and more dilute is a sign that muscle breakdown is decreasing.

If adequate crystalloid fluid administration has been done, the patient is well hydrated, and the urine output is still less than 1 cc/kg per hour, consider giving an IV diuretic. Mannitol, 100 mL of a 25% solution (25 gm) IV over 15 to 30 minutes, is probably the preferred diuretic in this situation. Mannitol should be administered over 1 hour if congestive heart failure is a concern. The use of loop diuretics should be avoided; these may acidify the urine which may predispose to precipitation of myoglobin in the kidney tubules.[77] If, for some reason, the patient has a metabolic alkalosis, acetazolamide will correct the metabolic alkalosis and increase urine pH.

The use of IV bicarbonate to alkalinize the urine is controversial.[74,78] The administration of bicarbonate may cause precipitation of calcium salts, particularly in the damaged muscle tissue.[79] Furthermore, the use of bicarbonate to alkalinize the urine may be unnecessary; diuresis itself raises the urine pH toward 7.0.[80] The most sensible way to administer bicarbonate is to give it only if the urine pH is less than 6.5 and the urine output is greater than 1 cc/kg per hour.

Hematologic Complications: Blood Loss, Thrombosis

Average reported blood loss after infrainguinal procedures is less than 300 cc.[36] Postoperative bleeding should be minimal.

Postoperative thrombosis is a significant complication of infrainguinal bypass surgery patients. It is the most common cause of need for reoperation,[81] and 25% of operations involving a femoral artery to a distal artery have been reported to need reoperation.[81] Patients who undergo reoperation for vascular surgery problems have a higher perioperative mortality of 12%.[81] Impaired fibrinolysis appears to be related to postoperative arterial thrombosis.[82] Postoperative epidural narcotic analgesia may help prevent postoperative inhibition of fibrinolysis.[82] Postoperative thrombosis in infrainguinal bypass patients also appears to be related to higher catecholamine levels and the development of postoperative hypertension.[83]

Pain

Controlling the patient's pain can decrease the incidence of hypertension, catecholamine release, and thrombosis.[82] Epidural narcotics should be used if an epidural catheter is present. Otherwise, PCA should be used until the patient's pain requirements are less than 24 mg morphine per day (or an equivalent drug and dose).

The ICU management of elderly patients after infrainguinal bypass surgery is summarized in Table 3.

Summary

ICU care of elderly vascular surgery patients is similar to the care of other vascular surgery patients. With proper patient selection and appropriate perioperative management, elderly vascular surgery patients may have similar perioperative morbidity and mortality as younger patients. Since elderly patients have less physiological reserve than younger patients, elderly patients have a smaller margin for error in their perioperative management. Although no elderly patient should be denied medical treatment based on advanced age alone, wide patient variation means that individual patients may have severe physiological derangements and medical disease. Prevention of morbidity and mortality in elderly vascular patients is best accomplished by avoiding physiological stress, paying meticulous attention to physiological parameters, and expediently treating any abnormal physiological state. ICU care of elderly vascular surgery patients is similar to other patients, only it is more intensive.

References

1. 6Allen BT, Anderson CB, Rubin BG, et al: The influence of anesthetic technique on perioperative complications after carotid endarterectomy. *J Vasc Surg* 19:834-843, 1994.
2. Hertzer NR: Outcome assessment in vascular surgery: results mean everything. *J Vasc Surg* 21:6-15, 1995.
3. Fisher ES, Malenka DJ, Solomon NA, et al: Risk of carotid endarterectomy in the elderly. *Am J Public Health* 79:1617-1620, 1989.
4. Glaser RB: Morbidity and mortality from major vascular surgery. In: Roizen MF (ed). *Anesthesia for Vascular Surgery.* New York: Churchill Livingstone, Inc.; 1-27, 1990.
5. Meyer FB, Meissner I, Fode NC, et al: Carotid endarterectomy in elderly patients. *Mayo Clin Proc* 66:464-469, 1991.
6. Goldstein LB, McCrory DC, Landsman PB, et al: Multicenter review of preoperative risk factors for carotid endarterectomy in patients with ipsilateral symptoms. *Stroke* 25:1116-1121, 1994.
7. Brook RH, Park RE, Chassin MR, et al: Carotid endarterectomy for elderly patients: predicting complications. *Ann Intern Med* 113:747-753, 1990.
8. Goldman L: Cardiac risk assessment in patients with arteriosclerotic vascular disease. In: Kaplan J (ed). *Vascular Anesthesia.* New York: Churchill Livingstone, Inc.;1-20, 1991.

Table 3
Guidelines for ICU Management of Elderly Patients After Infrainguinal Bypass Surgery

Upon arrival in ICU	Review peri-operative course; note current HR and BP, SaO_2.
	 CNS—Evaluate and document neurological status—ability to move all 4 extremities upon command.
	 Cardiac—Look for any hypertension or hypotension. Treat if BP is not within 20% of pre-operative values.
	 Pulm—If patient had general anesthesia, extubate when:
	   patient is awake and responsive, able to maintain and protect their own airway, weaning criteria
	   are acceptable (VC > 15 cc/kg; TV > 5 cc/kg; NIF > −20 cm H_2O), core temp >36°C, patient
	   is hemodynamically stable, and post-op bleeding is minimal.
	 Renal—Order maintenance fluids.
	 Heme—Check of hematoma.
	 Pain—Treat pain, if present. If an epidural catheter is present, administer epidural narcotics. If an
	   epidural catheter is not present, use PCA or prn IM, or prn IV narcotics.
	 Misc—Document dressing is dry. If patient had large changes in vital signs or ischemia in the OR,
	   order 12 lead EKG.

First hr. in ICU	CNS—as above.
	 Cardiac—Look for signs of myocardial ischemia; if present, treat and start rule out MI protocol.
	 Pulmonary—Encourage deep breathing.
	 Renal—Check urine output hourly. Goal is 0.5–1.0 cc/kg/hr.
	 Heme—Check for hematoma.
	 Pain—Treat pain, if present.
	 Misc—If extubated, advance diet as tolerated.
	   Continue chronic medical therapy (diabetes, etc.).
	   Order HCT and electrolytes.
	   Check lower extremity pulses; color and warmth of feet.

(continued)

Table 3 (continued)
Guidelines for ICU Management of Elderly Patients After Infrainguinal Bypass Surgery

First 4 hrs. in ICU	CNS—Patient should be at pre-procedure neurological baseline.
	Cardiac—Treat hypertension or hypotension as needed.
	Pulmonary—Encourage incentive spirometry.
	Renal—as above.
	Pain—Treat pain, if present; provide p.r.n. pain relief.
	Misc—Check HCT, electrolytes, and 12-lead EKG.
	Determine whether HCT adequate for patient.
	Correct electrolyte abnormalities.
	Compare 12-lead EKG to preoperative baseline. If ischemic changes are present on the postoperative EKG, start rule out MI protocol.
First 24 hrs in ICU	CNS—as above.
	Cardiac—as above.
	Pulmonary—as above.
	Renal—as above.
	Pain—Continue prn pain relief.
	Misc—Patient should be back on chronic medical therapy or IV equivalents.
Patient is ready to be discharged from ICU when:	No neurological deficits have occurred; if neurological deficits have occurred, when they have been evaluated and stabilized.
	Cardiac—Hemodynamics stable for 8 hours (i.e., overnight) without drug therapy.
	Pulmonary—Back to preoperative state.
	Renal—Back to preoperative state.
	Pain is controlled on IM or PO medication.
	Misc—Airway is patent, no bleeding at wound. HCT stable. Lower extremity perfusion is stable.

ICU = intensive care unit; CNS = central nervous system; HR = heart rate; BP = blood pressure; SaO_2 = oxygen saturation; EKG = electrocardiogram; MI = myocardial infarction; IV = intravenous; IM = intramuscular; PO = oral; HCT = hematocrit.

9. Dauchot PJ, Lina AA: Geriatric anesthesia. In: Brown DL (ed). *Risk and Outcome in Anesthesia.* 2nd Ed. Philadelphia: JB Lippincott Co.; 535-536, 1992.
10. Kurz A, Plattner O, Sessler DI, et al: The threshold for thermoregulatory vasoconstriction during nitrous oxide/isoflurane anesthesia is lower in elderly than in young patients. *Anesthesiology* 79:465-469, 1993.
11. Stolarek I, Scott PJW, Caird FI: Physiological changes due to age: implications for cardiovascular drug therapy. *Drugs Aging* 1:467-476, 1991.
12. Weitz HH: Noncardiac surgery in the elderly patient with cardiovascular disease. *Clin Geriatr Med* 6:511-529, 1990.
13. Goldman MD, Reeder MK, Muir AD, et al: Repetitive nocturnal arterial oxygen desaturation and silent myocardial ischemia in patients presenting for vascular surgery. *J Am Geriatr Soc* 41:703-709, 1993.
14. Amin DN, Iberti TJ: Use of the surgical intensive care unit in the preoperative preparation of the high-risk patient. *J Cardiothorac Anesth* 4(suppl 1):24-28, 1990.
15. Del Guercio LRM, Cohn JD: Monitoring operative risk in the elderly. *JAMA* 243:1350-1355, 1980.
16. Berlauk JF, Abrams JH, Gilmour IJ, et al: Preoperative optimization of cardiovascular hemodynamics improves outcome in peripheral vascular surgery: a prospective, randomized clinical trial. *Ann Surg* 214:289-299, 1991.
17. Baxter BT, Minion DJ, McCance CL, et al: Rational approach to postoperative transfusion in high-risk patients. *Am J Surg* 166:720-725, 1993.
18. Brook RH, Park RE, Chassin MR, et al: Carotid endarterectomy for elderly patients: predicting complications. *Ann Intern Med* 113:747-753, 1990.
19. Committee on Health Care Issues, American Neurological Association: Does carotid endarterectomy decrease stroke and death in patients with transient ischemic attacks? *Ann Neurol* 22:72-76, 1987.
20. McCrory DC, Goldstein LB, Samsa GP, et al: Predicting complications of carotid endarterectomy. *Stroke* 24:1285-1291, 1993.
21. Riles TS, Imparato AM, Jaocbowitz GR, et al: The cause of perioperative stroke after carotid endarterectomy. *J Vasc Surg* 19:206-216, 1994.
22. Walker MD: Carotid endarterectomy: a little more light at the end of the tunnel (editorial). *Mayo Clin Proc* 67:597-600, 1992.
23. Cebul RD, Whisnant JP: Carotid endarterectomy. *Ann Intern Med* 111:660-670, 1989.
24. Fisher M: Potentially effective therapies for acute ischemic stroke. *Eur Neurol* 35:3-7, 1995.
25. Mohr JP, Orgogozo JM, Harrison MJP, et al: Meta-analysis of nimodipine trials in acute ischemic stroke. *Cerebrovasc Dis* 4:192-203, 1994.
26. McGrath BJ, Guy J, Borel CO, et al: Perioperative management of aneurysmal subarachnoid hemorrhage. Part 2. Postoperative management. *Anesth Analg* 81:1295-1302, 1995.
27. Awad IA, Carter P, Spetzler RF, et al. Clinical vasospasm after subarachnoid hemorrhage: response to hypervolemia hemodilution and arterial hypertension. *Stroke* 18:365-372, 1987.
28. Hertzer N, Feldman B, Bevan E, et al: A prospective study of the incidence of injury to the cranial nerves during carotid endarterectomy. *Surg Gynecol Obstet* 151:781, 1980.
29. Bove EL, Fry WI, Gross WS, et al: Hypotension and hypertension as consequences of baroreceptor dysfunction following carotid endarterectomy. *Surgery* 85:633-637, 1979.
30. Towne JB, Bernhard VM: The relationship of postoperative hypertension to complications following carotid endarterectomy. *Surgery* 88:575-580, 1989.

31. Riles TS, Kopelman I, Imparato AM: Myocardial infarction following carotid endarterectomy: a review of 683 operations. *Surgery* 85:249-252, 1979.
32. Hertzer NR, Beven G, Young JR, et al: Coronary artery disease in peripheral vascular patients: a classification of 1000 coronary angiograms and results of surgical management. *Ann Surg* 199:223-233, 1984.
33. Mangano DT, Hollenberg M, Fegert G, et al: Perioperative myocardial ischemia in patients undergoing noncardiac surgery. I. Incidence and severity during the 4-day perioperative period. *J Am Coll Cardiol* 17:843-850, 1991.
34. Mangano DT, Browner WS, Hollenberg M, et al: Association of perioperative myocardial ischemia with cardiac morbidity and mortality in men undergoing noncardiac surgery. *N Engl J Med* 323:1781-1788, 1990.
35. Ashton CM: Perioperative myocardial infarction with noncardiac surgery. *Am J Med Sci* 308:41-48, 1994.
36. Spence RK, Atabek U, Alexander JB, et al: Preoperatively assessing and planning blood use for elective vascular surgery. *Am J Surg* 168:192-196, 1994.
37. Kunkel JM, Gomez ER, Spebar MJ, et al: Wound hematomas after carotid endarterectomy. *Am J Surg* 148:844-847, 1984.
38. Treiman RL, Coss DV, Foran RF, et al: The influence of neutralizing heparin after carotid endarterectomy on postoperative stroke and wound hematoma. *J Vasc Surg* 12:440-446, 1990.
39. Ernst CB: Abdominal aortic aneurysm. *N Engl J Med* 328:1167-1172, 1993.
40. Akkersdijk GJM, van der Graaf Y, van Bockel JH, et al: Mortality rates associated with operative treatment of infrarenal abdominal aortic aneurysm in The Netherlands. *Br J Surg* 81:706-709, 1994.
41. Petracek MR, Lawson JD, Rhea WG, et al: Resection of abdominal aortic aneurysms in the over-80 age group. *South Med J* 73:579-581, 1980.
42. O'Hara PJ, Hertzer NR, Krajewski LP, et al: Ten-year experience with abdominal aortic aneurysm repair in octogenarians: early results and late outcome. *J Vasc Surg* 21:830-837, 1995.
43. Elliot J, Szilagyi D, Hageman J, et al: Spinal cord ischemia: secondary to surgery of the abdominal aorta. In: Bernhard V, Towne J (eds). *Complications in Vascular Surgery*. Orlando, FL: Grune & Stratton, Inc.;291-310, 1985.
44. Katz N, Blackstone E, Kirklin J, et al: Incremental risk factors for spinal cord injury following operation for acute traumatic aortic transection. *J Thorac Cardiovasc Surg* 81:669-674, 1984.
45. Yeager RA, Weigel RM, Murphy ES, et al: Application of clinically valid cardiac risk factors to aortic aneurysm surgery. *Arch Surg* 12:278-281, 1986.
46. Johnston KW: Multicenter prospective study of nonruptured abdominal aortic aneurysms II. Variables predicting morbidity and mortality. *J Vasc Surg* 9:437-447, 1989.
47. Fine LG, Chairman, Physicians and Scientists, University College, London Medical School: Abdominal aortic aneurysm. *Lancet* 341:215-220, 1993.
48. Diehl JT, Cali RF, Hertzer NR, et al: Complications of abdominal aortic reconstruction: an analysis of perioperative risk factors in 557 patients. *Ann Surg* 197:49-56, 1983.
49. Hertzer NR: Fatal myocardial infarction following abdominal aortic aneurysm resection: 343 patients followed 6 to 11 years postoperatively. *Ann Surg* 192:667-673, 1980.
50. Riles TS, Fisher FS, Schaefer S: Plasma catecholamine concentrations during abdominal aortic aneurysm surgery: the link to perioperative myocardial ischemia. *Ann Vasc Surg* 7:213-219, 1993.
51. Yeager RA, Moneta GL, Edwards JM, et al: Reducing perioperative myocardial infarction following vascular surgery. the potential role of beta blockade. *Arch Surg* 130:869-873, 1995.

52. Cappeller W, Ramirez H, Kortmannn H: Abdominal aortic aneurysm: risk factors and complications and their influence or indication for operation. *J Cardiovasc Surg* 30:572-578, 1989.
53. Calligaro KD, Azurin DJ, Dougherty MJ, et al: Pulmonary risk factors of elective abdominal aortic surgery. *J Vasc Surg* 18:914-921, 1993.
54. Ostri P, Mouritisen L, Jorgensen B, et al: Renal function following aneurysmectomy of the abdominal aorta. *J Cardiovasc Surg* 27:714-718, 1986.
55. Baldwin L, Henderson A, Hickman P: Effect of postoperative low-dose dopamine on renal function after elective major vascular surgery. *Ann Intern Med* 120:744-747, 1994.
56. Puntillo K, Weiss SJ: Pain: its mediators and associated morbidity in critically ill cardiovascular surgical patients. *Nurs Res* 43:31-36, 1994.
57. Mangano DT, Siciliano D, Hollenberg M, et al: Postoperative myocardial ischemia: therapeutic trials using intensive analgesia following surgery. *Anesthesiology* 76:342-353, 1992.
58. Yeager MP, Glass DD, Neff RK, et al: Epidural anesthesia and analgesia in high-risk surgical patients. *Anesthesiology* 66:729-736, 1987.
59. Baron JF, Bertrand M, Barré E, et al: Combined epidural and general anesthesia versus general anesthesia for abdominal aortic surgery. *Anesthesiology* 75:611-618, 1991.
60. Leather R, Shah D, Kaufman J, et al: Comparative analysis of retroperitoneal and transperitoneal aortic replacement for aneurysm. *Surg Gynecol Obstet* 168:387-393, 1989.
61. Nelson AH, Fleisher LA, Rosenbaum SH: Relationship between postoperative anemia and cardiac morbidity in high-risk vascular patients in the intensive care unit. *Crit Care Med* 21:860-866, 1993.
62. Faust RJ: Perioperative indications for red blood cell transfusion: has the pendulum swung too far? *Mayo Clin Proc* 68:512-514, 1993.
63. Frank SM, Beattie C, Christopherson R, et al: Unintentional hypothermia is associated with postoperative myocardial ischemia. *Anesthesiology* 78:468-476, 1993.
64. Bush HL, Hydo LJ, Fischer E, et al: Hypothermia during elective abdominal aortic aneurysm repair: the high price of avoidable morbidity. *J Vasc Surg* 21:392-402, 1995.
65. Weissman C: Postoperative care after major vascular surgery. In: Rodgers M, Stone J, Miller E, Watkins W (eds). *Anesthesiology Report 1: No. 3.* St. Louis: CV Mobsy;304-315, 1989.
66. Shah DM, Darling C, Chang BB, et al: Is long vein bypass from groin to ankle a durable procedure? An analysis of a ten-year experience. *J Vasc Surg* 15:402-408, 1992.
67. Gouny P, Bertrand P, Decaix B, et al: Distal bypass for limb salvage: comparative study in patients below and above 80 years of age. *J Cardiovasc Surg* 35:419-424, 1994.
68. L'Italien GJ, Cambria RP, Cutler BS, et al: Comparative early and late cardiac morbidity among patients requiring different vascular procedures. *J Vasc Surg* 21:935-944, 1995.
69. O'Brien TS, Lamont PM, Crow A, et al: Lower limb ischaemia in the octogenarian: is limb salvage surgery worthwhile? *Ann R Coll Surg Engl* 45:445-447, 1993.
70. Krupski WC, Layug EL, Reilly LM, et al: Comparison of cardiac morbidity between aortic and infrainguinal operations. Study of Perioperative Ischemia (SPI) Research Group. *J Vasc Surg* 15:354-363, 1992.
71. Walker PM: Pathology of acute arterial occlusion. *Can J Surg* 29:340-342, 1986.

72. Wyffels PL, DeBord JR, Marshall JS, et al: Increased limb salvage with intraoperative and postoperative ankle level urokinase infusion in acute lower extremity ischemia. *J Vasc Surg* 15:771-779, 1992.
73. Veenstra J, Smit WM, Krediet RT, et al: Relationship between elevated creatine phosphokinase and the clinical spectrum of rhabdomyolysis. *Nephrol Dial Transplant* 9:637-641, 1994.
74. Reha WC, Mangano FA, Zeman RK, et al: Rhabdomyolysis: need for high index of suspicion. *Urology* 34:292-296, 1989.
75. Sinert R, Kohl L, Rainone T, et al: Exercise-induced rhabdomyolysis. *Ann Emerg Med* 23:1301-1306, 1994.
76. Feinfeld DA, Cheng JT, Beysolow TD, et al: A prospective study of urine and serum myoglobin levels in patients with acute rhabdomyolysis. *Clin Nephr* 38:193-195, 1992.
77. Peacock E: Acute renal failure secondary to nontraumatic rhabdomyolysis. *ANNA J* 19:402-408, 1992.
78. Better OS, Stein JH: Early management of shock and prophylaxis of acute renal failure in traumatic rhabdomyolysis. *N Engl J Med* 332:825-829, 1990.
79. Schulz VE: Rhabdomyolysis as a cause of acute renal failure. *Postgrad Med* 72:145-156, 1982.
80. Knochel JP: Rhabdomyolysis and myoglobinuria. *Annu Rev Med* 33:435-443, 1982.
81. Ng RLH, Davies AH, Magee TR, et al: Early reoperation rates after arterial surgery. *Eur J Vasc Surg* 8:78-82, 1994.
82. Rosenfeld BA, Beattie C, Christopherson R, et al: The effects of different anesthetic regimens on fibrinolysis and the development of postoperative arterial thrombosis. *Anesthesiology* 79:435-443, 1993.
83. Parker SD, Breslow MJ, Frank SM, et al: Catecholamine and cortisol responses to lower extremity revascularization: correlation with outcome variables. *Crit Care Med* 23:1954-1961, 1995.

Chapter 11

Hypertension

William B. Kannel, MD, MPH, FACC

Introduction

Epidemiological studies have shown that the major modifiable cardiovascular risk factors applicable in middle-aged persons remain relevant in the elderly.[1-3] The important identified risk factors in the elderly include systolic blood pressure, cigarette smoking, lipoprotein fractions of cholesterol, blood glucose, weight, physical activity, and alcohol consumption.[3]

Cardiovascular disease accounts for over 50% of all deaths in persons over age 65.[4] More than half of all persons over age 65 have some degree of hypertension requiring medical attention. It is, thus, important to determine whether hypertension is a substantial predisposing factor for the development of cardiovascular disease in the elderly as it is in the middle-aged, and whether the relative risk, risk ingredients, and absolute and attributable risks of elevated blood pressure in the elderly diminish with advancing age. Already at great risk for cardiovascular diease because of their age, the elderly can ill afford a risk factor such as uncontrolled hypertension.

Pathophysiology

Essential hypertension in young adults tends to be as much due to increased cardiac output as to elevated peripheral resistance.[5,6] In older persons with hypertension, cardiac output tends to be normal or impaired, and the arteries stiffen generating a higher systolic pressure and an inverse relationship between age and plasma renin activity because of reduced sympathetic function in old age.[5] Baroreceptor responses are also blunted, making the elderly more prone to episodes of postural hypotension.[6] Because of a tendency toward reduced plasma volume and creatinine clearance, they are more susceptible to diuretic-induced prerenal azotemia.[5,7]

From: Aronow WS, Stemmer EA, Wilson SE (eds). *Vascular Disease in the Elderly.* Armonk, NY: Futura Publishing Company, Inc., © 1997.

Table 1
Systolic Blood Pressure and Diastolic Blood Pressure by Age and Sex
38-Year Follow-Up

Age	Systolic Blood Pressure		Diastolic Blood Pressure	
	Men	Women	Men	Women
35–44	129.4	123.0	83.2	78.5
45–54	133.6	133.7	84.7	82.9
55–64	138.8	141.8	83.7	83.1
65–74	142.1	146.6	80.2	80.1
75–84	143.5	150.7	76.3	77.0
85–94	141.6	149.2	71.8	74.0

Although these age-related pathophysiological phenomena suggest certain preferences for therapy, there are no controlled trial data to support recommendations for the specific therapeutic agents that appear indicated.[5,8] The development of isolated systolic hypertension is attributable to structural alteration of the arterial vasculature leading to decreased compliance and distensibility, resulting in part from decreased elasticity and increased collagen deposition. These vascular changes are often accompanied by left ventricular hypertrophy (LVH) and diastolic dysfunction, increased ventricular mass, and carotid intimal thickening.[9]

Prevalence

The prevalence of hypertension has been estimated to be over 50% among persons age 65 and above.[4,10] The prevalence is higher in elderly women than in elderly men. Because of continuing rise in systolic blood pressure into advanced age, after the diastolic pressure has peaked and begun to fall (Table 1), the prevalence of isolated systolic hypertension rises steeply with age, while the prevalence of diastolic hypertension declines. Some 65% of hypertension is of the isolated systolic variety and is more prevalent in women than men (Figure 1). Beyond age 55, the average systolic blood pressure of women exceeds that of men, whereas the diastolic pressure tends to be similar in the two sexes (Table 1).

Cardiovascular Hazards

Cardiac disease and stroke are the first and third leading causes of death in the United States, and account for most of the mortality and a considerable amount of the disability afflicting the elderly.[4] Hypertension is a common and powerful predisposing factor promoting these cardiovascular events. Hypertension ranks among the major risk factors

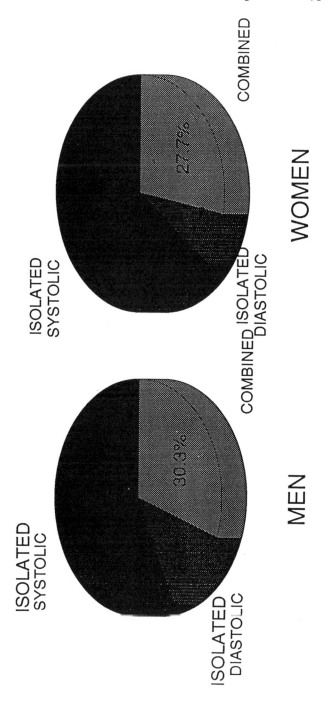

Figure 1. Distribution of hypertensives, ages 65 to 89 years.

for cardiovascular disease in the elderly. Its impact, adjusting for the different units of measurement and range of values, exceeds that of cholesterol and cigarette smoking, and rivals diabetes.[3] Also, the impact of blood pressure is only moderately reduced by adjustment for coexistent risk factors.[3] The impact persists into advanced age and is, in terms of absolute risk, greater in old age than in middle age (Figure 2). Hypertension exacts a greater toll in cardiovascular morbidity and mortality in the elderly because of a greater absolute, excess, and attributable risk.

Hypertension predisposes powerfully to all the major cardiovascular conditions which incapacitate and kill the elderly. Risks of stroke, cardiac failure, coronary heart disease (CHD), and peripheral artery disease are all greatly enhanced by hypertension (Figure 3). The risk ratios, comparing hypertension with normotensive persons, are greatest for cardiac failure and stroke, but in absolute terms, CHD is the most common and most lethal sequela of hypertension (Figure 3).

Blood Pressure Hazards in the Very Old

It has been alleged that hypertension becomes a less potent risk factor in advanced age, possibly because those most suceptible have died prematurely.[11] It has even been claimed that mortality rates may actually be inversely related to blood pressure.[11-14] As a result, the risk benefits of treating very old and frail hypertensive patients have been questioned.[11-15] However, recent meta-analysis indicates that antihypertensive treatment produces a significant 25% reduction in CHD mortality, as well as in stroke events.[16] However, the CHD rate reduction is less than anticipated and less than the stroke rate reduction. Subclinical ischemia and small sample size are likely explanations for the modest influence of treatment on CHD incidence.[17,18] Subclinical myocardial damage may be responsible for an excess mortality reported at low diastolic blood pressure, producing a J-shaped mortality curve.[15,19-22]

Thus, the inverse relationship of blood pressure to mortality in very old people probably reflects either overt or occult poor cardiovascular health.[22] In the Framingham Study, a distinct U-shaped mortality curve was observed in both sexes over age 75 with a substantially increased mortality at systolic blood pressures below 120 mm Hg. This was not observed in subjects free of cardiovascular disease, where a continuous graded effect was noted (Figure 4). Thus, excess mortality reported in aged persons with low blood pressure appears to be a result of poor health and not the low blood pressure itself. Subjects in the Framingham Study who sustained a spontaneous fall in blood pressure after a myocardial infarction (MI) were found to have an excess mortality compared to those who either remained hypertensive or normotensive from before the infarction.[23]

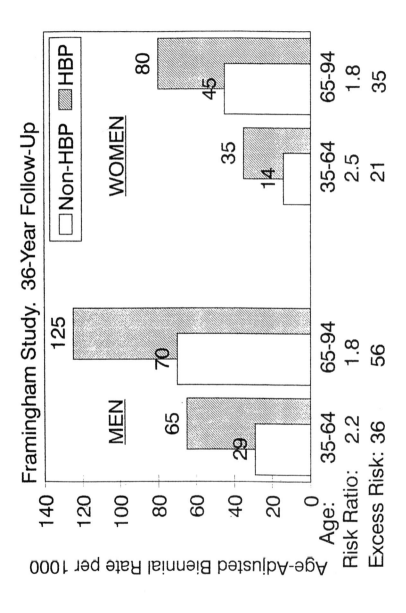

Figure 2. Risk of cardiovascular disease in hypertension by age and sex; a 36-year follow-up in the Framingham Study. HBP = high blood pressure.

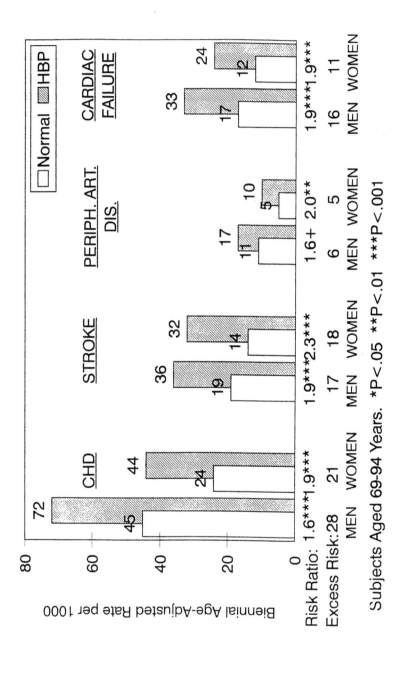

Figure 3. Risk of cardiovascular events by hypertensive status; a 36-year follow-up in the Framingham Study. CHD = coronary heart disease; HBP = high blood pressure.

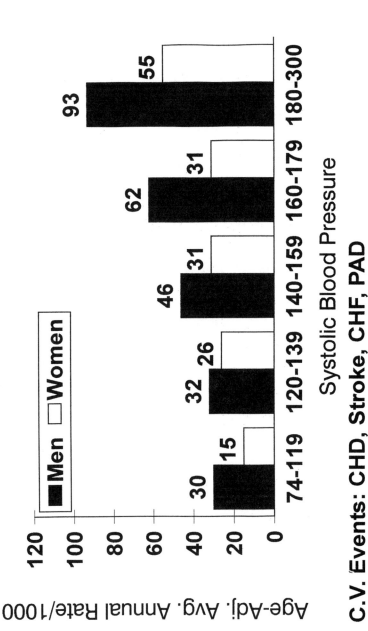

Figure 4. Risk of cardiovascular events by systolic blood pressure in subjects free of cardiovascular disease (men and women ages 65 to 94 years); a 38-year follow-up. CHD = coronary heart disease; CHF = congestive heart failure; PAD = peripheral arterial disease.

Table 2
Risk Factor Adjusted Increment in Risk of Cardiovascular Disease by Systolic
versus Diastolic Blood Pressure According to Age and Sex
Framingham Study: 38-Year Follow-Up

| | Increase per Standard Deviation Increment Blood Pressure Component | | | |
| | Systolic | | Diastolic | |
Age	Men	Women	Men	Women
35–64	40%***	38%***	37%***	29%***
65–94	41%***	25%***	25%***	15%***
***P <.001				

Covariates: Chol., Cig's, Glucose, ECG-LVH. LVH = left ventricular hypertrophy.

Components of Blood Pressure

There is a tenaciously held belief that the adverse sequelae of hypertension derive chiefly from the diastolic blood pressure component. Epidemiological assessment of the impact of the systolic versus the diastolic component of the blood pressure in the Framingham Study and elsewhere provide no support for this fallacious concept.[24] An examination of the increment in risk per standard deviation increase in each blood pressure parameter is greater for systolic than diastolic pressure, and this is particularly true in the elderly (Table 2). The impact of systolic pressure per standard deviation increment does not diminish at all with advancing age in men, whereas the impact of diastolic pressure wanes considerably. In women, there is a greater decline in the impact of the diastolic than systolic pressure with age (Table 2).

In the elderly, risk of cardiovascular sequelae is best determined from the systolic pressure or pulse pressure.[24] Reliance on the diastolic pressure can be misleading. Risk of cardiovascular events increases in a continuous graded fashion with the systolic pressure. The absolute risk is greater in elderly men than women at any blood pressure (Figure 4). Risk gradients are also somewhat steeper in elderly men than they are in elderly women (Table 2).

Comparison of the impacts of each component of blood pressure on the incidence of cardiovascular disease, including systolic, diastolic, mean arterial and pulse pressure, indicates the weakest impact for the diastolic blood pressure (Table 3).[24]

Isolated Systolic Hypertension

Because of the progressive decrease in arterial compliance with advancing age, isolated systolic hypertension is the most common vari-

Table 3
Increase in Risk of Cardiovascular Events per Standard Deviation Increase in
Blood Pressure Parameter
Framingham Study: 30-Year Follow-Up

Pressure Component	Standardized Increment in Risk			
	Men		Women	
	Age: 35–64	65–94	35–64	65–94
Systolic	41%***	51%***	43%***	23%***
Mean arterial	41%***	44%***	42%***	18%***
Pulse pressure	29%***	42%***	36%***	22%***
Diastolic	35%***	30%***	33%***	9%+

+ NS; *** P <.001.

Table 4
Risk of Cardiovascular Events by Pulse Pressure
Framingham Study: 30-Year Follow-Up

Pulse Pressure (mm Hg)	Age-Adjusted Rate Per 1000			
	35–64 Years		65–94 Years	
2–39	9	4	2	17
40–49	13	6	16	19
50–59	16	7	32	22
60–69	22	10	39	25
70–182	33	16	58	32
Reg. Coefficient				
Age-Adj.	.024***	.025***	.024***	.014***
R.F.-Adj.	.018***	.019***	.021***	.010***

***P <.001

ety in the elderly. About two thirds of hypertension in the elderly is of this variety (Figure 1). The chief determinant of this variety of hypertension is a high-normal systolic blood pressure in middle age; one third had prior diastolic blood pressure elevation which disappeared when the arteries become more rigid in advanced age.[25]

This disproportionate rise in systolic blood pressure which occurs in the aged results in a wide pulse pressure. This widening of the pulse pressure is not an innocuous accompaniment of advancing age. Risk of cardiovascular events in both the elderly and middle-aged increases progessively in relation to the pulse pressure (Table 4).

Isolated systolic hypertension is associated with an excess of all the cardiovascular sequelae of hypertension including CHD, stroke, cardiac failure, and peripheral artery disease. Cardiovascular events and mortality are increased two- to threefold.[25]

Table 5
Prevalence of Cardiovascular Disease Coexisting with Hypertension in the Elderly
Framingham Study: Subjects Ages 65–89 Years

	Percent Prevalence	
	Men	Women
Angina	27.4%	27.9%
Myocardial infarction	23.7%	9.4%
Cardiac failure	4.4%	7.9%
Stroke	16.0%	8.9%
Peripheral artery disease	15.9%	10.0%

There has been doubt expressed about the advisability of treating mild diastolic hypertension in the elderly.[26] Controlled trials support recommendations to treat both diastolic and isolated systolic hypertension in the elderly.[5,15] These trials indicate that cardiovascular morbidity and mortality are reduced by treatment, but that the magnitude of the risk reduction in mild hypertension is limited.[16]

Associated Cardiovascular Disease

About half of elderly persons with blood pressures exceeding 140/90 mm Hg will already have overt evidence of cardiovascular disease. Coexistent cardiovascular disease is more commonly found in men than women. Only cardiac failure is more common in hypertensive women than men (Table 5). These associated cardiovascular conditions greatly increase the risk of death and disability in the hypertensive elderly. They also should influence the choice of therapy selected to control the hypertension.

The most common associated condition is CHD, manifested in men, equally as MI or angina, whereas in women angina predominates (Table 5). In men, strokes and peripheral artery disease each occur in about 16% of hypertensive elderly men and about 9% of hypertensive women. Cardiac failure can be expected in 8% of hypertensive women and about 4% of hypertensive men (Table 5).

Indicators of Ischemia

In addition to LVH, hypertension predisposes to other ECG indications of silent myocardial ischemia. A compromised coronary arterial circulation may also be manifested as nonspecific repolarization abnormalities, blocked intraventricular conduction, and MI. MIs in the hypertensive elderly are not only common, but are surprisingly often silent or unrecognized. In the Framingham Study, 49% of MIs in hypertensive women go unrecognized.[18] In order not to overlook these MIs, routine

Table 6
Risk of Cardiovascular Events in the Elderly with ECG-LVH
Framingham Study: 36-Year Follow-Up
Subjects 65–94 Years

Cardiovascular Events	Biennial Age-Adjusted Rate per 1000		Age-Adjusted Risk Ratio	
	Men	Women	Men	Women
Peripheral arterial disease	36	14	3.0**	2.2+
Stroke	71	90	3.1***	4.4***
Cardiac failure	71	84	14.9***	5.4***
Coronary disease	138	94	2.7***	3.0***
Any CV event	234	235	2.8***	4.1***

LVH = left ventricular hypertrophy.

periodic ECG examinations must be carried out at yearly intervals. These infarctions must not be overlooked or taken lightly, as they are associated with a serious prognosis.[18]

Vascular bruits in the carotid and femoral areas in hypertensive persons usually signify diffuse atherosclerosis. They are associated with an increased risk of not only stroke and intermittent claudication, but of CHD as well.[27] All of the foregoing indicators of compromise of the arterial circulation indicate the need for urgent treatment of hypertension and coexistent risk factors.

Structural Remodeling

In hypertension, the risk of adverse events such as cardiac failure, coronary attacks, and strokes are greatly increased when hypertension induces LVH (Table 6). The relative risk tends to decrease with advancing age, but this is offset by a greater absolute risk or excess risk. There is no definable critical degree of hypertrophy which separates compensatory from pathological hypertrophy.[28]

However, morphological studies of the structural remodeling of the hypertensive heart suggest that the quality, as well as the quantity, of myocardium in hypertrophy may be important in conferring risk.[29] Changes in structure observed include remodeling on intramyocardial coronary artorioloc, and a disproportionate accumulation of fibrillar collagen in arteriolar adventitia and interstitial space. There are also microscopic myocardial scars which have replaced necrotic myocytes. The fibrosis observed may be linked to the angiotensin-renin-aldosterone system. Angiotensin-converting enzyme (ACE) may be responsible for regulating local angiotensin II and bradykinin that govern fibroblast collagen turnover. This may represent a wound-healing process gone awry.[29]

Table 7
Prevalence of Other Cardiovascular Risk Factors in Hypertensive Elderly
Framingham Study: Subjects Ages 65–89 Years

	Normotensive (<140/90 mm Hg)		Hypertensive (>140/90 mm Hg)	
Risk Factors	Men	Women	Men	Women
Cholesterol ≥240 mg/dL	21%	44%	51%	51%
HCL-C <35 mg/dL	27%	9%	16%	8%
Diabetes	14%	10%	17%	14%
ECG-LVH	2%	3%	6%	4%
Cig. Smoker	21%	16%	21%	14%
Obesity (MRW ≥130)	20%	23%	22%	32%

MRW = metropolitan relative weight; LVH = left ventricular hypertrophy.

Multivariate Risk

Hypertension in the elderly is seldom an isolated phenomenon. Compared to normotensive persons, the elderly with hypertension have a greater prevalence of coexistent dyslipidemia, diabetes, and obesity (Table 7). These tend to be associated with lipoprotein lipase deficiency and insulin resistance, and have been designated the insulin-resistant syndrome.[30] Each of these metabolically linked conditions independently escalate the risk of hypertension. The blood lipid profile most common in the hypertensive is a high triglyceride, low high-density lipoprotein (HDL), high total cholesterol complex. Hypertensive elderly who have a high total/HDL cholesterol ratio are particularly vulnerable to CHD (Figure 5). The risk of cardiovascular events in hypertensive persons is greatly increased by diabetes, rapid heart rate, high normal blood fibrinogen, and white blood cell count.[31]

Thus, the risk of cardiovascular sequelae of hypertension is variable depending on the burden of coexistent risk factors present (Figure 6). Risk varies over a wide range, making determination of the cardiovascular risk profile mandatory in evaluating the risk, urgency, and nature of treatment required. Risk factors to be ascertained are the same for coronary disease and stroke, except that for the latter, it is necessary to look for atrial fibrillation and other associated overt cardiovascular disease (Figure 6) (Tables 8 and 9).[32]

Cognitive Function

Hypertension itself or its treatment may alter cognition or mood in the elderly. The antihypertensive agents most likely to induce these effects are the centrally acting alpha-adrenergic agonist, b-adrenergic receptor blockers, and the rauwolfia alkaloids. For example, one third of patients taking clonidine and alphamethyldopa will experience adverse

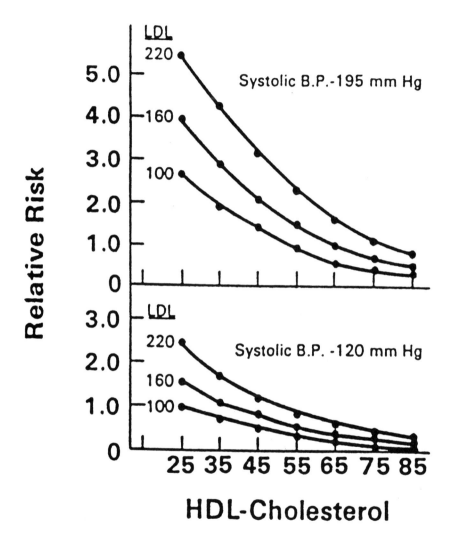

Figure 5. Relative risk of coronary heart disease according to high-density lipoprotein (HDL), low-density lipoprotein (LDL), and systolic blood pressure in men ages 50 to 70 years in the Framingham Study.

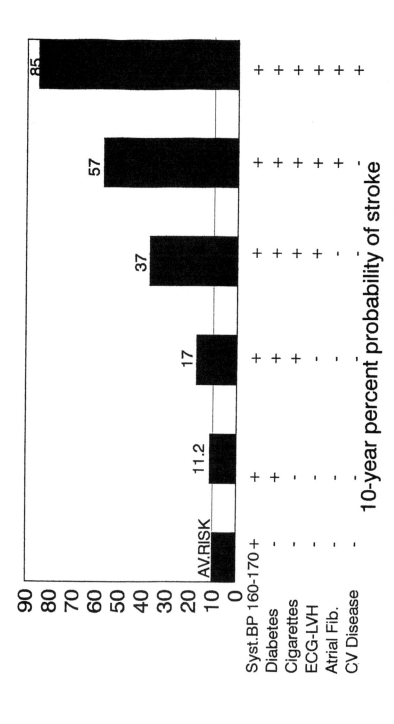

Figure 6. Probability of stroke in mild hypertension by intensity of associated risk factors in men ages 63 to 65 years in the Framingham Study. LVH = left ventricular hypertrophy.

Table 8
Stroke Risk Factor Prediction Chart

1. Find Points for Each Risk Factor

Men

Age	SBP	HYP RX	Diabetes	Cigs	CVD	AF	LVH
54–56 = 0	95–105 = 0	No = 0	No = 0	No = 0	No = 0	No = 0	No = 0
57–59 = 1	106–116 = 1	Yes = 2	Yes = 2	Yes = 3	Yes = 3	Yes = 4	Yes = 6
60–62 = 2	117–126 = 2						
63–65 = 3	127–137 = 3						
66–68 = 4	138–148 = 4						
69–71 = 5	149–159 = 5						
72–74 = 6	160–170 = 6						
75–77 = 7	171–181 = 7						
78–80 = 8	182–191 = 8						
81–83 = 9	192–202 = 9						
84–86 = 10	203–213 = 10						

Women

Age	SBP	HYP RX	Diabetes	Cigs	CVD	AF	LVH
54–56 = 0	95–104 = 0	No = 0	No = 0	No = 0	No = 0	No = 0	No = 0
57–59 = 1	105–114 = 1	If Yes see below	Yes = 3	Yes = 3	Yes = 2	Yes = 6	Yes = 4
60–62 = 2	115–124 = 2						
63–65 = 3	125–134 = 3						
66–68 = 4	135–144 = 4						
69–71 = 5	145–154 = 5						
72–74 = 6	155–164 = 6						
75–77 = 7	165–174 = 7						
78–80 = 8	175–184 = 8						
81–83 = 9	185–194 = 9						
84–86 = 10	196–204 = 10						

If currently under antihypertensive therapy, add the following points depending on SBP level

SBP	95–104	105–114	115–124	125–134	136–144	145–154
Points	6	5	5	4	3	3

SBP	155–164	165–174	175–184	185–194	195–204
Points	2	1	1	0	0

2. Sum Points For All Risk Factors

____ + ____ + ____ + ____ + ____ + ____ + ____ + ____ = ____

Age   SBP   HYP RX   Diabetes   CIGS   CVD   AF   LVH   Point Total

(continued)

Table 8 *(continued)*
Stroke Risk Factor Prediction Chart

3. Look Up Risk Corresponding To Point Total

Men 10 Yr.				Women 10 Yr.			
Pts.	Prob.	Pts.	Prob.	Pts.	Prob.	Pts.	Prob.
1	2.6%	21	41.7%	1	1.1%	21	43.4%
2	3.0%	22	46.6%	2	1.3%	22	50.0%
3	3.5%	23	51.8%	3	1.6%	23	57.0%
4	4.0%	24	57.3%	4	2.0%	24	64.2%
5	4.7%	25	62.8%	5	2.4%	25	71.4%
6	5.4%	26	68.4%	6	2.9%	26	78.2%
7	6.3%	27	73.8%	7	3.5%	27	84.4%
8	7.3%	28	79.0%	8	4.3%		
9	8.4%	29	83.7%	9	5.2%		
10	9.7%	30	87.9%	10	6.3%		
11	11.2%			11	7.6%		
12	12.9%			12	9.2%		
13	14.8%			13	11.1%		
14	17.0%			14	13.3%		
15	19.5%			15	16.0%		
16	22.4%			16	19.1%		
17	25.5%			17	22.8%		
18	29.0%			18	27.0%		
19	32.9%			19	31.9%		
20	37.1%			20	37.3%		

4. Compare To Average 10-Year Risk

Avg. 10 Yr. Prob. By Age

Men		Women	
55–59	5.9%	55–59	3.0%
60–64	7.8%	60–64	4.7%
65–69	11.0%	65–69	7.2%
70–74	13.7%	70–74	10.9%
75–79	18.0%	75–79	15.5%
80–84	22.3%	80–74	23.9%

SBP = systolic blood pressure. HYP RX = under antihypertensive therapy? Diabetes = history of diabetes? CIGS = smokes cigarettes? CVD = history of myocardial infarction, angina pectoris, coronary insufficiency, intermittent claudication, or congestive heart failure? AF = history of atrial fibrillation? LVH = left ventricular hypertrophy on ECG? (Reproduced with permission from *Risk Factor Prediction Kit.* 1990 © American Heart Association.)

Table 9
Coronary Heart Disease Risk Factor Prediction Chart

1. Find Points For Each Risk Factor

Age (If Female)		Age (If Male)				HDL-Cholesterol		Total Cholesterol		Systolic Blood Pressure		Other	
Age	*Pts.*	*Age*	*Pts.*	*Age*	*Pts.*	*HCL-C*	*Pts.*	*Total-C*	*Pts.*	*SBP*	*Pts.*	*Other*	*Pts.*
30	-12	30	-2	57-59	13	25-26	7	139-151	-3	98-104	-2	Cigarettes	4
31	-11	31	-1	60-61	14	27-29	6	152-166	-2	105-112	-1	Diabetic-male	3
32	-9	32-33	0	62-64	15	30-32	5	167-182	-1	113-120	0	Diabetic-female	6
33	-8	34	1	65-67	16	33-35	4	183-199	0	121-129	1	ECG-LVH	9
34	-6	35-36	2	68-70	17	36-38	3	200-219	1	130-139	2		
35	-5	37-38	3	71-73	18	39-42	2	220-239	2	140-149	3	O pts for each NO	
36	-4	39	4	74	19	43-46	1	240-262	3	150-160	4		
37	-3	40-41	5			47-50	0	263-288	4	161-172	5		
38	-2	42-43	6			51-55	-1	289-315	5	173-185	6		
39	-1	44-45	7			56-60	-2	316-330	6				
40	0	46-47	8			61-66	-3						
41	1	48-49	9			67-73	-4						
42-43	2	50-51	10			74-80	-5						
44	3	52-54	11			81-87	-6						
45-46	4	55-56	12			88-96	-7						
47-48	5												
49-50	6												
51-52	7												
53-55	8												
56-60	9												
61-67	10												
68-74	11												

2. Sum Points For All Risk Factors

___ + ___ + ___ + ___ + ___ + ___ + ___ = ___

Age　　HDL-C　　Total-C　　SBP　　Smoker　　Diabetes　　ECG-LVH　　Point Total

NOTE: *Minus Points Subtract From Total.*

(continued)

Table 9 (continued)
Coronary Heart Disease Risk Factor Prediction Chart

3. Look Up Risk Corresponding To Point Total

Pts.	5 Yr.	10 Yr.	Pts.	5 Yr.	10 Yr.	Pts.	5 Yr.	10 Yr.	Pts.	5 Yr.	10 Yr.
≤1	<1%	<2%	10	2%	6%	19	8%	16%	28	19%	33%
2	1%	2%	11	3%	6%	20	8%	18%	29	20%	36%
3	1%	2%	12	3%	7%	21	9%	19%	30	22%	38%
4	1%	2%	13	3%	8%	22	11%	21%	31	24%	40%
5	1%	3%	14	4%	9%	23	12%	23%	32	25%	42%
6	1%	3%	15	5%	10%	24	13%	25%			
7	1%	4%	16	5%	12%	25	14%	27%			
8	2%	4%	17	6%	13%	26	16%	29%			
9	2%	5%	18	7%	14%	27	17%	31%			

4. Compare To Average 10 Year Risk

Age	Women (Probability)	Men (Probability)
30–34	<1%	3%
35–39	<1%	5%
40–44	2%	6%
45–49	5%	10%
50–54	8%	14%
55–59	12%	16%
60–64	13%	21%
65–69	9%	30%
70–74	12%	24%

These charts were prepared with the help of William B. Kannel, M.D., Professor of Medicine and Public Health and Ralph D'Agostino, Ph.D., Head, Department of Mathematics, both at Boston University. (Reproduced with permission from *Risk Factor Kit*, 1990 © American Heart Association.)

effects on mood, sleep, alertness, and cognition. Large doses of reserpine can cause lethargy and depression by depleting central nervous system norepinephrine. However, in the Systolic Hypertension in the Elderly Program (SHEP) trial using diuretic-based therapy, no alteration in cognitive function compared to placebo treatment was noted.[33]

Preventive Implications

The treatment of hypertension in the elderly is clearly justified by its high prevalence in advanced age, the great risk of cardiovascular disease further escalated by hypertension, the rapid aging of the population, and proof of efficacy of treatment.[33] Furthermore, cost-benefit analysis of treating elderly hypertensive persons indicates at least as much advantage in the elderly as in younger hypertensives.[34] Also, studies of the effects of antihypertensive therapy on the quality of life indicate that the elderly tolerate effective doses of antihypertensive agents quite well.[35]

The aggressiveness of treatment justified in those over age 75 is uncertain. There is some evidence to suggest that vigorous reduction of diastolic pressure may be dangerous.[14,36] However, treatment of systolic hypertension at any age appears to be beneficial in either sex.[34,35] There is a suggestion that the greater reported mortality in hypertensive patients with the lowest diastolic pressure may be due to fatal arrhythmias. Signal-averaged ECG abnormality, a risk marker for ventricular arrhythmias, was found to be common in older patients with hypertension who have a low diastolic pressure (under 85 mm Hg).[37] Such data raise questions about too strict control of diastolic pressure in some elderly patients and are consistent with reported J-shaped mortality curves in hypertension.[19,20]

A number of meta-analyses of the effect of treatment of hypertension in patients older than 60 years have been reported, all of which found statistically significant reductions in cardiovascular mortality and strokes, and in overall mortality.[16,38,39] However, they suggest that this benefit may be reduced in the oldest age groups.

In contrast to previously published reports,[16] more recent meta-analysis indicates that antihypertensive treatment produces a significant decrease in CHD mortality in the elderly (odds ratio 0.75). This is of great importance because CHD is the leading cause of death in elderly hypertensive persons.[16] However, the CHD rate is reduced less than that of stroke. Small sample size and subclinical ischemia are possible explanations for this resistance to benefit CHD in persons of all ages with hypertension.[16] Hypertension is known to produce silent ischemia and increase sudden death rates.[16] The hypothesis of a J-shaped curve for CHD mortality in relation to blood pressure is also consistent with the notion that subclinical myocardial damage may be responsible for excess mortality at low diastolic blood pressure.[16]

Practitioners caring for elderly hypertensive patients and wishing to reduce disability of ambulatory patients should attempt to control systolic and diastolic hypertension. However, in the oldest and most ill and frail, treatment may be less effective. Further randomized controlled trials are needed to allow well-founded recommendations for this subgroup of elderly patients.

The elderly with milder degrees of hypertension or a favorable risk profile can be managed with hygienic measures such as weight control, avoidance of salt, alcohol, and cigarettes, and prescription of moderate exercise. These measures can reduce dosage of medications required and also help to correct relevant risk factors. Polypharmacy is a problem in treating elderly hypertensive patients who are often taking sodium-retaining pharmaceuticals such as nonsteroidal anti-inflammatory drugs for arthritis.

There is much to be gained in controlling hypertension of any variety in the elderly, provided appropriate therapy is selected. In the elderly, the quality of the last years of life may be as important as the length of life, and therapy should not compromise the joy of living. However, strokes, heart failure, and coronary attacks should not be the first indication for treatment of hypertension in the elderly.

References

1. Harris T, Cook EF, Kannel WB, Goldman L: Proportional hazard analysis of risk factors for coronary heart disease in individuals aged 65 years or older: the Framingham Heart Study. *J Am Geriatric Soc* 36:1023-1028, 1988.
2. Benfante R, Reed D, Frank J: Do coronary heart disease risk factors measured in the elderly have the same predictive roles as in the middle-aged? Comparison of relative and attributable risks. *Ann Epidemiol* 2:273-282, 1992.
3. Cupples LA, D'Agostino RB: Some risk factors related to the annual incidence of cardiovascular disease and death using pooled repeated biennial measurements: the Framingham Study 30-year follow-up. Sect. 34. *DHHS Pub. No. NIH 83-2703.* Springfield, VA: US Dept. of Commerce, National Technical Information Service; 1987.
4. Chartbook on cardiovascular, lung, and blood disease: morbidity and mortality. *NIH;* US Dept. of Health and Human Services, NHLBI, 1994.
5. Bloomfield RL, Novikov SV, Ferario CM: Hypertension in the elderly. *Am J Geriatric Cardiol* 3:39-44, 1994.
6. Schmieder RE, Frohlich ED, Messerli FH: Pathophysiology of hypertension in the elderly. *Cardiol Clin* 2:235-243, 1986.
7. Houston MC: New insights and new approaches for the treatment of essential hypertension: selection of therapy based on coronary heart disease risk factor analysis, hemodynamic prrofiles, quality of life, and subsets of hypertension. *Am Heart J* 117:911-951, 1989.
8. Zing W, Fergerson RK, Vlasses PH: Calcium antagonists in elderly and black hypertensive patients: therapeutic controversies (review). *Arch Intern Med* 151:2154-2161, 1991.
9. Psaty BM, Furberg CD, Kuller LH, et al: Isolated systolic hypertension and subclinical cardiovascular disease in the elderly. *JAMA* 286:1287-1291, 1992.

10. National High Blood Pressure Education Program Working Group: National High Blood Pressure Education Working Report on Hypertension in the Elderly. *Hypertension* 23:275-285, 1994.
11. Kaplan NM, Lieberman E: *Clinical Hypertension.* 5th Ed. Baltimore: Williams and Wilkins; 5-6, 1990.
12. Langer RD, Graniats TG, Barrett-Connor E: Paradoxical survival in elderly men with high blood pressure. *Br Med J* 29:1356-1358, 1989.
13. Matila K, Haavisto M, Rajala S, Heikinheimo R: Blood pressure and five-year survival in the very old. *Br Med J* (Clin Res Ed) 296:887-889, 1988.
14. Langer RD, Ganiats TG, Barrett-Connor E: Factors associated with paradoxical survival at higher blood pressures in the very old. *Am J Epidemiol* 134:29-38, 1991.
15. Bulpitt CJ, Fletcher AE: Prognostic significance of blood pressure in the very old: implications for treatment decision. *Drugs Aging* 5:184-191, 1994.
16. Insua JT, Sacks HS, Lau T-S, et al: Drug treatment of hypertension in the elderly. *Ann Intern Med* 121:355-362, 1994.
17. O'Kelly BF, Massie BM, Tubau JF, Szlacheic J: Coronary morbidity and mortality, preexisting silent coronary artery disease and mild hypertension. *Ann Intern Med* 110:1017-1026, 1989.
18. Kannel WB, Dannenberg AL, Abbott RD: Unrecognized myocardial infarction and hypertension: the Framingham Study. *Am Heart J* 109:581-585, 1995.
19. Farnett L, Mulrow CD, Linn WD, Lucey CR, Tuley MR: The J-shaped curve phenomenon and the treatment of hypertension: is there a point beyond which pressure reduction is dangerous? *JAMA* 265:485-489, 1991.
20. Cruicksank JM, Throp JM, Zacharias FJ: Benefits and potential harm of lowering high blood pressure. *Lancet* 1:581-584, 1987.
21. Fletcher AE, Bulpitt CJ: Haw far should blood pressure be lowered? *N Engl J Med* 326:251-254, 1992.
22. Sorensen KH, Hilden T: Increased total mortality and decreased functional capacity are associated with low systolic blood pressure among elderly women. *Scan J Prim Health Care* 6:105-110, 1988.
23. Kannel WB, Sorlie P, Castelli WP, Mce D: Blood pressure and survival after myocardial infarction: the Framingham Study. *Am J Cardiol* 45:326-330, 1980.
24. Kannel WB, Dawber JR, McGee DL: Perspectives on systolic hypertension: the Framingham Study. *Circulation* 61:1179-1182, 1980.
25. Wilking SVB, Belanger A, Kannel WB, Steel K: Determinants of isolated systolic hypertension. *JAMA* 260:3451-3455, 1988.
26. Lernfelt B, Landahl S: Is hypertension in the elderly overtreated? *Drugs Aging* 2:469-472, 1992.
27. Kannel WB, McGee DL: Update on some epidemiologic features of intermittent claudication: the Framingham Study. *J Am Geriatric Soc* 33:13-18, 1985.
28. Levy D, Garrison RJ, Savage DD, Kannel WB, Castelli WP: Prognostic implications of echocardiographically determined left ventricular mass in the Framingham Study. *N Engl J Med* 332:1561-1566, 1990.
29. Weber KT, Sun Y, Guarda E: Structural remodeling in hypertensive heart disease and the role of hormones. *Hypertension* 23:869-877, 1994.
30. Reaven GM: Banting Lecture: role of insulin resistance in human disease. *Diabetes* 37:1595-1607, 1988.
31. Kannel WB: Hypertension in the elderly: epidemiologic appraisal from the Framingham Study. *Cardiol Elderly* 1:359-363, 1993.
32. Wolf PA, D'Agostino RB, Belanger AL, Kannel WB: Probability of stroke: a risk profile from the Framingham Study. *Stroke* 22:312-318, 1991.

33. Applegate WB, Berge KG, Black HR, et al: Implications of the SHEP. *Hypertension* 21:335-343, 1993.
34. Hansson L: Future goals for the treatment of hypertension in the elderly with reference to STOP-Hypertension, SHEP, and the MRC trial in older adults. *Am J Hypertens* G(suppl):405-435, 1993.
35. Applegate WB: Managing the older patient with hypertension. *Am J Hypertens* G(suppl)2775-2825, 1993.
36. Langer RD, Criqui MH, Barrett-Connor EL, Klauber MR, Ganiatis TG: Blood pressure change and survival after age 75 years. *Hypertension* 22:551-559, 1993.
37. Shin HH, Sagar KB, Stepniakowski K, Wetherbee JN, Egan BM: Increased prevalence of abnormal signal-averaged electrocardiograms in older patients who have hypertension with low diastolic blood pressure. *Am Heart J* 125:1698, 1993.
38. Leonetti G, Cuspidi C, Fastidio M, Lonati L, Chianca R: Arterial hypertension as a risk factor in the elderly and its treatment. *J Hypertens* 10:53-57, 1992.
39. Celis H, Fagard R, Stassen J, Thijs L, Amery A: The older hypertensive: assessment and treatment. *Neth J Med* 43:566-577, 1993.

Chapter 12

Diabetes Mellitus and Vascular Disease

Edward A. Stemmer, MD

In 1995, in the United States, there were approximately eight million people in whom a diagnosis of diabetes mellitus had been established. The true prevalence of diabetes mellitus is probably twice that number. Almost 750,000 new cases are detected each year.[1] In 1992, there were 50,067 deaths attributed to diabetes mellitus and an additional 100,000 deaths to which diabetes contributed.[2,3] Vascular disease is responsible for approximately 75% of deaths that occur in diabetics. If small vessel disease is included with large vessel disease, 84% of diabetics will have some form of vascular disease if they live 20 years or more after the diagnosis is established. Fifty-four percent of deaths in diabetics are due to cardiac disease, 11% to strokes, and 7% to renal disease. In contrast, in the general population 33% of deaths are due to heart disease, 6.6% to stroke, and 0.5% to renal disease.[3,4] In addition to death, diabetes mellitus, with a 3% prevalence of overt clinical disease, accounts for 30% of those patients with renal failure and half of all nontraumatic amputations.[2] It is the leading cause of blindness in adults older than 30 years of age. Because of its role in the development and severity of one or another type of vascular disease, diabetes is a major threat to health in the United States today. This chapter deals with the unique aspects of vascular disease as it affects diabetics. Other chapters deal with the detection, prevention, and management of the specific vascular diseases.

Historical Highlights

According to Wellman and Volk,[5] the history of diabetes and the search for insulin can be divided into four time periods. The ancient observations of the clinical characteristics of the disease, the diagnostic period when the nature of the disease began to be defined, the period of

From: Aronow WS, Stemmer EA, Wilson SE (eds). *Vascular Disease in the Elderly.* Armonk, NY: Futura Publishing Company, Inc., © 1997.

empiric treatment, and the experimental period.[5] It is clear that ancient peoples were familiar with the salient features of the disease that is known now as diabetes mellitus. Susruta, in an ancient Hindu document (ca. 400 BC), described the diabetic syndrome as characterized by "honeyed urine." The treatment of polyuria, conceivably due to diabetes, is described in the Ebers Papyrus (ca. 1500 BC). The advice given by Cornelius Celsus (53 BC to 7 AD) that diabetics should eat as little as possible foreshadowed a regime of dietary management that was to last into the twentieth century.[6] Nevertheless, the road to the successful management of diabetes mellitus was to be long and tortuous with many false paths taken. Three events, however, stand out as major turning points.

Aretaeus, the Cappadocian, who lived in Alexandria in the first and second centuries AD, is usually given credit for the first systematic description of diabetes. It appeared in his text on the causes and symptoms of acute and chronic diseases. He coined the term *diabetes* (Greek: to pass through) and described the excessive thirst and constant need to urinate, the dry mouth, parched skin, and loss of weight associated with the disease. He noted that the disease was chronic in character, but that the patient died quickly when it was completely established. Over the next 1700 years, numerous observations were made including the fact that the "sweetness" in the urine was sugar.

In 1788, William Cullen added the term *mellitus* (Latin, Greek: honey) to the term *diabetes* to distinguish the disease from diabetes insipidus. It was not until the late 1800s, however, that the pancreas was proven to be responsible for the disease. Until that time, the kidney, brain, blood, stomach, and liver (as well as the pancreas) were thought to be responsible for the diabetic syndrome.[6]

In 1889, Joseph von Mering and Oscar Minkowski, intending to study the role of the pancreas in the digestion and absorption of fats, performed total pancreatectomies in two dogs. Unexpectedly, and within a day, both dogs developed frequent and voluminous urination. A laboratory attendant noted that the urine attracted flies. Minkowski, who had experience with human diabetes, documented that the dogs' urine contained sugar. Minkowski pursued this serendipitous finding over the next 2 years, clearly establishing that a defect in the pancreas was the cause of diabetes mellitus. Laguesse, in 1894, suggested that the "heaps of cells" described by Langerhans in 1869 were the source of an internal secretion, the lack of which produced diabetes mellitus. Jean de Meyer, in 1910, proposed that the as yet unidentified hormone be named insulin when it was discovered.[5,6]

On October 31, 1920, Frederick Banting, an orthopedic surgeon on the faculty at the University of Toronto submitted a plan to isolate insulin to J.J.R. Macleod, the Professor of Physiology at the University of Toronto. Macleod approved the project and assigned a medical student, Charles H. Best, to assist Banting. The initial experiments began on May 17, 1921. On July 20, 1921, the two investigators tested their extract of the pancreas on a pancreatectomized dog named Marjorie. The dog's blood sugar dropped dramatically. In December, 1921, J.B. Collip, a biochemist, was added to the team to purify the extract. On January 23, 1922, the purified extract (Macleod serum) was administered to Leonard Thompson, a 14-year-old diabetic near death in Toronto General Hospital. The patient recovered and lived another 13 years until he died of influenza and pneumonia. The results of the research were presented to the Association of American Physicians in Washington, DC on May 3, 1922. Reaction around the world was almost immediate. The Eli Lilly Pharmaceutical Company began commercial production of insulin. By the end of 1923, the year that Banting and Macleod were awarded the Nobel Prize, insulin was in worldwide use.[7]

Insulin markedly prolonged the life of the diabetic. Several of the patients treated in 1922 lived well into their seventies. As diabetics lived longer, however, their vulnerability to a wide spectrum of complications became apparent. Early death from ketoacidosis was replaced by substantial disabilities and premature death from vascular disease. A cause and effect relationship between diabetes mellitus and vascular disease was not generally recognized until the 1940s.[7,8]

The Diabetic Patient

Diabetes mellitus is clearly a multifactorial and multigenic disease. It has been described as a geneticist's nightmare. Genetic, familial, metabolic, environmental, and immunological factors are involved. Attempts to unravel the relative roles of these factors are confounded by differences in the definition of affected individuals, modification of the expression of the diabetic genotype by environmental effects, and variability in the age of onset of the disease.[9,10] The overall incidence of clinically apparent diabetes mellitus in the United States in 1993 was 2.8 per 1000 population, while the prevalence was 30 per 1000 population.[2] The prevalence of overt diabetes rises with age from approximately 0.18% for persons under age 18 years to an estimated 9.6% for those older than 65 years.[8,11,12]

The World Health Organization (WHO) classifies diabetes mellitus into three major clinical groups: the first consists of individuals meeting the WHO criteria for an established diagnosis of diabetes mellitus; the second, those with an impaired glucose tolerance, but without overt evidence of diabetes, and third, women with gestational diabetes mellitus. The group with established diabetes mellitus is subdided into four categories: those with insulin-dependent diabetes melitus (IDDM), those with noninsulin-dependent diabetes mellitus (NIDDM); those with malnutrition-related diabetes mellitus, and those with "other"types of diabetes mellitus; that is, those with diabetes mellitus due to another underlying disease.[13] Vascular disease associated with IDDM and NIDDM is the subject of this chapter.

Insulin-dependent diabetes mellitus rarely occurs during the first 6 months of life. The incidence of IDDM begins to increase sharply at

9 months of age and continues to rise until age 12 to 14 years after which the incidence begins to decline. The prevalence of diabetes is approximately 1.8 per 1000 school-aged children. Onset of IDDM after the age of 30 years is rare, relative to the incidence of NIDDM. Insulin-dependent diabetes mellitus is characterized by the classic symptoms described by Aretaeus, by the frequent occurrence of ketoacidosis, and by the need to treat the hyperglycemia with insulin. Weight loss is a prominent feature of untreated IDDM. There is little difference in incidence between males and females.[8] The commonest form of insulin-dependent diabetes mellitus is characterized by almost complete destruction of the beta cells in the pancreatic islets. There is a clear and consistent association of IDDM with specific human leukocyte antigen (HLA) loci, as well as with viral infections, thus, indicating that the disease is a result of autoimmune reactions.[12,14,15] As many as 95% of patients with IDDM have a specific set of HLA genes labelled DR3 and DR4. Only 30% of the general population has these genes.[15]

NIDDM accounts for 85% to 90% of diabetes, worldwide. Only 5% to 10% of diabetics 65 years of age or older are survivors of IDDM. NIDDM usually presents in adulthood after a long asymptomatic period. It is characterized by abnormalities of insulin secretion and by resistance of tissues to the action of insulin. Both the incidence and prevalence of NIDDM increase with age. Of the population with NIDDM, 20% develop the disease before the age of 40, 40% between the ages of 40 and 59 years and 40% after the age of 60. The majority of cases have their onset between the third and sixth decades.[8,16,17] Unlike IDDM, there is a marked predominance of women in the distribution of NIDDM, with a much greater incidence in women between the ages of 45 and 64 years (Table 1).[17] Approximately 80% of the NIDDM population is obese. Genetic factors are extremely important in the pathogenesis of NIDDM. In a study conducted in England, concordance of NIDDM among monozygotic twins was over 90% while that for IDDM was 30% to 50%.[18] The incidence of NIDDM among siblings of diabetic parents

Table 1
Incidence of Diabetes Mellitus by Age and by Gender per 100,000 Civilian Noninstitutionalized Population

Groups (years)	Men	Women	Total
0 to 25	Inadeq data	29	14
26 to 44	233	153	192
45 to 54	189	724	466
55 to 64	332	955	661
65 plus	859	941	907
Total	191	337	267

The incidence of diabetes mellitus by age and gender. Depicted is the increasing incidence of diabetes mellitus with age, particularly in the female.

is six times that of a nondiabetic population.[17] In addition to genetic factors, age, obesity, and a sedentary lifestyle are major risks for the development of NIDDM.[19]

Both insulin-dependent diabetics and noninsulin-dependent diabetics suffer similar long-term complications. The majority of these complications are vascular in origin. The incidence and prevalence of the vascular complications increase with duration of the diabetes.

Classification of Vascular Disease

The vascular complications that almost invariably affect diabetics as they age are the result of lesions that progress with time in both the microvasculature and the macrovasculature.

Microvascular disease in the diabetic affects the precapillary arterioles, the capillaries, and the postcapillary venules throughout the body, but it is commonly associated with disease in the retina, kidney, and nervous system. The morphological feature that best characterizes diabetic microangiopathy is thickening of the basement membrane of the capillaries. In most tissues, the basement membrane forms the outer coat of the capillary wall just beyond the endothelium. It consists of fine filaments embedded in a homogeneous matrix composed of proteinaceous material high in carbohydrates.[20,21] Microangiopathy can occur in a variety of collagen diseases, but it is most commonly seen in diabetics. The disease develops in the teenage years of the insulin-dependent diabetic and progresses slowly. Strict management of blood sugar early in the course of IDDM results in a marked reduction in the prevalence of microvascular complications. Retinopathy is reduced by 76%, neuropathy by 60%, and nephropathy by 54%.[19]

Macrovascular disease affects the large and medium-sized arteries. It most commonly occurs in maturity onset diabetics over the age of 25 and rarely produces clinically significant sequelae in children or adolescents. Macrovascular disease results in major complications and death as a result of involvement of the coronary, cerebral, and leg vessels. There is some evidence that the processes responsible for microangiopathy are also factors in the development of macroangiopathy but, in general, the pathology seen in the medium and large arteries of the diabetic is indistinguishable from the atherosclerosis that occurs in the nondiabetic.[22,23] There is speculation that the hyperinsulinism and increased serum glucose found in NIDDM may have a direct role in the production of atherosclerotic disease in the adult diabetic. If so, it would help to explain the observation that diabetics have a higher risk for coronary arterial disease (CAD) than do nondiabetics with comparable risk factors.[23] The incidence of macroangiopathy increases with the duration of diabetes, but does not appear to be related to the severity of the diabetes. Unlike microvascular disease, there is little evidence that strict control of the blood sugar will slow the development of macroangiopathy or decrease its complications. Also, there may be additional genetic factors responsible for the increased prevalence of atherosclerosis in the diabetic. Support for this view was given in 1984 by Mandrup-Poulson et al, who reported that a genetic marker linked to the incidence of atherosclerosis was present proximal to the human insulin gene.[24]

Characteristics of Vascular Disease in the Diabetic

Although the macroangiopathy that occurs in diabetics is morphologically indistinguishable from the atherosclerosis that occurs in nondiabetics, the clinical manifestations of vascular disease that occur in the diabetic are uniquely different. Vascular disease occurs earlier in life in the diabetic, is more extensive, differs in distribution, and increases in prevalence as the duration of diabetes increases. Diabetic women have the same frequency of vascular disease at any age as do diabetic men. Vascular disease has a poorer prognosis in the diabetic and is more likely to result in inoperable CAD, amputation, and premature death. The increased prevalence of atherosclerosis in the diabetic is due almost entirely to occlusive disease. Except for the microaneurysms associated with retinal disease, aneurysmal disease does not appear to be more common in the diabetic than in the nondiabetic.

Age of Onset

Below 20 years of age, renal failure is the most common cause of death in the diabetic. From 20 to 39 years of age and thereafter, cardiovascular disease is the most common cause of death in the diabetic. By contrast, in the general population, accidents are the most common cause of death between the ages of 5 and 44 years. Cardiovascular disease does not become the number one cause of death in the general population until after the age of 45 years.[3,25] Dry and Hines reported that arteriosclerosis is 11 times more frequent in diabetics than in controls and develops about 10 years earlier in the diabetic.[26,27] Leland and Maki reported that symptomatic CAD can develop in 20- and 30-year-old diabetics who have been diabetic for 20 years or more.[28] Warren and LeCompte after reviewing the literature current at the time of their publication noted that there was general agreement that diabetics are more likely to develop atherosclerosis at an earlier age and in a more severe form than nondiabetics.[29] The increased frequency of CAD is particularly striking among women.[28]

Prevalence

Using the presence of claudication as an index of the presence of peripheral vascular disease (PVD), the prevalence of vascular disease in diabetics between the ages of 45 and 74 years is four to six times greater than in the nondiabetic population, even when corrections are made for risk factors other than diabetes.[17,23] Vascular disease does not spare the female. Juergens et al noted that in a series of patients with onset of vascular disease before the age of 60 years, only 8% were women.[30] Kannel, analyzing the results of the Framingham Study, and Ganda, describing macrovascular disease, reported that the female to male ratio in diabetics with vascular disease approaches 1 at any age.[31,32] The probable explanation of this observation is the markedly higher incidence of diabetes in women between the ages of 45 and 64 years.[17] Eighty-four percent of diabetics who live longer than 20 years after a clinical diagnosis of diabetes is established will have some form of vascular disease, predominantly CAD.

Distribution and Extent of Disease

As involvement of the vasculature with atherosclerosis is traced from the abdominal aorta to the lower leg, there is a steadily increasing percentage of patients who are diabetic. Although the absolute incidence of aortoiliac disease in diabetics is higher than in nondiabetics, the relative incidence in diabetics is about half that in nondiabetc patients, reflecting the greater involvement of the distal circulation in diabetic. Gensler et al reported that 13.4% of atherosclerotic lesions occurred in the aortiliac region in diabetics, while 25% of atherosclerotic lesions occurred in the aortoiliac region in nondiabetics.[33] Eleven percent to 17% of patients undergoing aortoilio-femoral reconstruction are clinical diabetics (who constitute about 3% of the total population).[34-36] Mavor in a series of 104 patients found the profunda femoris artery (PFA) spared in all instances. He did not specify how many of the 104 patients were diabetic.[37] In the diabetic, not only is the orifice of the PFA diseased in one third of patients with PVD, but 75% of diabetics with disease at the orifice have disease in the distal segments of the PFA as well.[38] The relative incidence of femoropopliteal disease in the diabetic and nondiabetic is essentially the same. Vascular occlusion is limited to arteries of the leg in about 25% of nondiabetic patients with vascular disease, but less than 5% of diabetic patients with vascular disease. Involvement of only a single vessel below the trifurcation occurs in 65% of nondiabetic patients, but only 31% of diabetic patients. Conversely, occlusion of two or three vessels below the bifurcation occurs in 69% of diabetics with PVD, but only 35% of nondiabetics. The peroneal artery is the vessel most frequently spared in the diabetic.[39] Sixty-five to 75% of patients undergoing tibioperoneal reconstruction are clincial diabetics.

Prognosis of Diabetics with Vascular Disease

Diabetics not only have a higher incidence and prevalence of vascular disease, they also have a higher rate of complications from the disease and a higher mortality that is largely due to the vascular disease.

Hertzer et al,[40] in 1984, reviewed a series of 1000 coronary arteriograms performed in patients being considered for peripheral vascular surgery. There were 170 clinical diabetics in the group. Severe, inoperable CAD was found in 12.4% of the diabetics, but only 4.8% of the nondiabetics. Above the age of 60, the incidence of severe, inoperable CAD rose in both groups, reaching 16% in diabetics and 6.5% in nondiabetics (Table 2).[40] In autopsy series, myocardial infarction (MI) is found two to five times more often in diabetics than in nondiabetics.

Rosenblatt et al demonstrated in a series of 150 patients selected for peripheral vascular reconstruction that diabetics did at least as well as nondiabetics in terms of graft patency and prevention of limb loss.[41] Nevertheless, in the diabetic population as a whole, the rate of amputation is higher and the long-term survival lower than in nondiabetics. Silbert and Zazeela,[42] in 1958, described the natural history of PVD in 1198 patients over a period of 15 years. No vascular reconstructive procedures were performed in this group of patients. There were 399 diabetics and 799 nondiabetics in the group. Thirty-four percent of diabetics required amputation as contrasted to only 8% of the nondiabetics. Ten percent of the nondiabetics were dead 10 years after the onset of PVD; 33% were dead 15 years after the onset of PVD. The corresponding figures for diabetics were 38% and 69%, respectively.[42] Even after peripheral vascular surgery was well established, limb loss in the diabetic remained higher than in the nondiabetic. In a review of amputations performed in multiple hospitals during the late 1970s, Most and Sinnock reported that lower extremity amputations were performed 15 times more frequently in diabetics than in nondiabetics.[43] The rate of amputations performed in both diabetics and nondiabetics rose with increasing age. Below the age of 45, the number of amputations limited to the toes was greater than the number of leg amputations. Above age 45, and particularly above age 65, leg amputations were more frequent (Table 3).[43] Since 1979 when 79,000 amputations were performed in the United States, the number of amputations performed per year has risen steadily in spite of the general availability of periph-

Table 2

Percentage Severe Inoperable CAD in Patients with PVD Diabetics Compared with Nondiabetics

Age Group	Diabetics	Nondiabetics	Total
Less than 50	0.0	1.7	1.4
50 to 59	5.0	1.4	2.0
60 plus	16.0	6.5	8.1
Total	12.4	4.8	6.1

CAD = coronary artery disease; PVD = peripheral vascular disease

The percentage of patients with peripheral vascular disease (PVD) who have severe, inoperable coronary artery disease (CAD). The unique vulnerability of the diabetic is depicted.

Table 3
Distribution of Amputations in Diabetics Percentage at Each Level Within Each
Age Group

Group (years)	Toe	Foot	Leg
0 to 44	56.5	6.8	36.7
45 to 64	39.9	6.5	53.6
65 Plus	24.4	3.2	72.4
Total	30.5	4.4	65.1

Source: Selected states, 1976–1978
The percentage of amputations that occur at each of three levels of the lower extremity. Depicted is the progressively higher level with increasing age.

eral vascular reconstruction. In 1985, 115,000 amputations were performed (31,000 above knee, 29,000 below knee, 12,000 foot, and 43,000 toe amputations). Complications of diabetes are responsible for 50% to 66% of all nontraumatic amputations. Diabetics tend to undergo minor amputations more frequently than do their nondiabetic counterparts. Approximately 40% of diabetics who present with gangrene will have the process limited to the toes.[41,44]

The life expectancy of diabetics at any age and in either sex is lower than that of the general population. However, the later in life that diabetes makes its clinical appearance, the less it affects survival. For example, the median survival of female diabetics in whom the diagnosis is established before age 30 years is 25 years less than that of the general female population. For female diabetics in whom the diagnosis is established between the ages of 30 and 49 years, median survival is 12 years less than the general female population. Female diabetics with onset of the disease between the ages of 50 and 69 years have a median survival five years less than the general female population. After age 70 at diagnosis, survival in female diabetics is shortened by only 2 years. Male diabetics follow the same pattern, although the differences in survival are not as great prior to age 70 years and disappear after age 70.[45] Fifty-four percent of deaths in diabetics are due to cardiac disease in contrast to 33% in nondiabetics. Less than 1% of deaths in diabetics are directly the result of gangrene.[4]

Intermittent Claudication

Intermittent claudication is a term first used by a veterinarian, Vouley, in 1831, to describe a condition of limping in the horse.[46] It is the symptom that most often calls attention to the presence of vascular disease. As the studies of Criqui have shown, however, claudication as an index of the presence of vascular disease markedly underestimates the true prevalence of PVD, particularly in the elderly.[47] Intermittent claudication is characterized by crampy pain in the leg muscles. The pain develops after exercise and is relieved within 10 minutes by rest (the "Rose criteria"). Leg pain at rest is not considered to be claudication.[46,47] The level of claudication (calf, thigh, buttock) provides a clue to the level of arterial disease. The superficial femoral and popliteal arteries are the sites of occlusion most frequently associated with intermittent claudication (36% and 22%, respectively). Arteriosclerotic disease in the aorta and the common iliac arteries are of themselves much less frequently responsible for claudication (2% and 4%, respectively). About a fourth of patients with claudication have diffuse or multilevel disease.[48] Since diabetics have a strong predilection for more distal sites of involvement as well as more diffuse disease, it would not be unexpected to find that diabetics have a higher incidence of claudication than do nondiabetics. In the Framingham Study, in the group aged 45 to 74, the incidence of claudication per 100,000 population was 1260 in men and 840 in women. In contrast, the incidence in nondiabetic males was 330 and in nondiabetic females, 130. This resulted in relative risk ratios for diabetics of 4.2 for men and 5.0 for women.[31]

Intermittent claudication is generally believed to be a relatively benign symptom of PVD because of the low frequency with which tissue necrosis, gangrene, or amputation occurs in these patients. The classic study which led to this belief was performed in 1962 by Boyd of Manchester, England. In his study, he reported a 10-year follow-up of 1476 patients who presented with intermittent claudication, but without gangrene or pregangrenous conditions. At 5 years, 7% of the group had undergone amputations. At 10 years, 12% had undergone amputations for an average annual amputation rate of 1.4%. The survival rate of the patients in the study approximated that of a population 10 years older. No mention is made of the number of diabetics in the study population, and neither was the severity of claudication graded.[48] In a 1970 report from the Framingham Study, 162 patients with intermittent claudication were followed for an average of 8.3 years. During that time, only four patients progressed to major amputations, with three additional patients suffering loss of one or more toes.[49] Imparato et al,[50] in 1973, described the fate of 104 patients with intermittent claudication followed for an average of 2.5 years. Only 5.8% progressed to amputation for an average annual rate for amputation of 2.3%. Again, no mention is made of the number of diabetics in the series, but Imparato did grade the severity of claudication as mild (symptoms occurring after walking more than two blocks), moderate (one to two blocks), or severe [one block or less). Fifteen percent of those with severe claudication required amputation. However, 6 (27%) of the 22 patients whose claudication worsened during the period of observation required amputation. Another 6 patients in this group of 22 underwent successful revascularization when their claudication worsened.[50] As late as 1987, it was stated that the risk of amputation in patients with intermittent claudication averaged about 1%. The author did comment that of the one third of the patients whose symptoms worsened, most were either diabetics or tobacco users.[51]

As early as 1961, it was recognized that intermittent claudication in diabetics is not the relatively benign disease that it appears to be in nondiabetics. Schadt et al[52] followed 422 patients (collected from 1939 to 1948) for 9 years after the onset of intermittent claudication. Sixty-four of the patients were diabetics; 40 of the entire group were women. In the nondiabetic group, the ratio of men to women was 12 to 1, while in the diabetic group, the ratio of men to women was 4 to 1, reflecting the relatively higher incidence of PVD in diabetic women. None of the patients underwent revascularization. During 9 years of follow-up, 5.4% of the nondiabetics developed ischemic ulceration, compared with 12.5% of the diabetics; 9.2% of the nondiabetics developed gangrene of an extremity, compared with 39.6% of the diabetics; 7.3% of the nondiabetics underwent amputation, compared with 27.1% of the diabetics; 59.1% of the nondiabetics were alive at the end of the 9 years, compared to 37.9% of the diabetics. Schadt et al[52] commented that arterial reconstructive surgery for prophylaxis against gangrene and amputation was probably not indicated in nondiabetics, but such prophylaxis would be justified in diabetics. The reports of increased complications associated with intermittent claudication and decreased survival in the diabetic with PVD have continued well into the era of widely available vascular reconstructive procedures.

In 1985, Jonason and Ringqvist[53] reported a study of 47 diabetic patients followed for 6 years for intermittent claudication. They compared the outcomes in this group of patients with the outcomes of 225 nondiabetic patients who had also been followed for 6 years for intermittent claudication (the "control" group). Six of the diabetics (13%) underwent reconstructive surgery, five because of the development of rest pain and/or gangrene. Thirteen of the 224 nondiabetics (5.8%) underwent arterial reconstruction, all for disabling claudication. Six (13%) of the diabetics required amputation, including two of the six who had undergone vascular reconstruction. The amputation rate in the nondiabetics was 0.5%. Only 50% of the diabetics were alive at the end of the 6-year observation period, in contrast to 74% of the nondiabetics. These authors, like those in 1961, recommended that more aggressive treatment would be appropriate in diabetics with intermittent claudication in an effort to decrease the complications and disability associated with their vascular disease. Both Schadt et al,[52] in 1961, and Jonason et al,[53] in 1985, noted that peripheral vascular reconstruction would not improve survival statistics in diabetics since the mortality observed was rarely due to PVD itself.[52-54]

It is important to realize that even though claudication is the most common presenting symptom of PVD in a general population, the diabetic may present with rest pain, tissue loss, or gangrene as the first manifestation of PVD. Even when diabetics do present with claudication as the initial symptom, it is often of shorter duration than in nondiabetics, and progresses more often and more rapidly to more serious sequelae of ischemia. In Schadt et al's study,[52] 95% of nondiabetics presented with intermittent claudication as their predominant symptom. Only 10% had ulceration or gangrene at the time a diagnosis of PVD was established. In contrast, over 50% of the diabetics in the series presented with ischemic ulceration, gangrene, or neuropathy.[52,55] The average duration of symptoms in diabetics was 15.5 months, while that in the nondiabetics was 27.8 months.[52] Steer et al,[56] reviewing a group of 332 patients, found that the incidence of gangrene with or without rest pain was almost twice as high in diabetics as in nondiabetics.[56]

Because of the continuing high amputation rate in diabetics even when arterial reconstruction is performed, and because of the consistently low survival rate of diabetics with or without vascular surgery, physicians are often reluctant to recommend vascular reconstruction early in the course of PVD in diabetics. The results of delaying operation until it is unavoidable are amputation, decreased mobility of the patient, and impaired quality of life. The limited mobility of these patients often results in their withdrawal from an active role in society and an accelerated deterioration in their mental status, particularly in elderly patients. Preservation of a functional extremity may be the key event in preserving a functional, independent individual. For the reasons given above, the onset of claudication in a diabetic patient should not be taken lightly and should be treated aggressively. Cost-benefit considerations associated with limb preservation are addressed in Chapter 21 dealing with occlusive disease below the inguinal ligament.

Coronary Arterial Disease

In 1994, a report based on data from the Coronary Artery Surgery Study (CASS) Registry described the clinical features of 2160 patients aged 65 years or older treated for symptomatic CAD. Three hundred seventeen patients were diabetics; 1843 were nondiabetics. When compared with the nondiabetic group, the diabetics had higher grades of angina, a higher number of coronary arterial occlusions, more frequent three-vessel disease, and a higher incidence of unstable angina. The diabetics developed more frequent congestive heart failure (CHF) and left ventricular hypertrophy (LVH). They were found to have a higher incidence of elevated systolic blood pressure and a greater incidence of associated PVD. Diabetic patients were more likely to be women and were more likely to have never smoked cigarettes.[57] Leland and Maki,[28] describing patients being followed in the Joslin Clinic, noted that the frequency of CAD is much increased in the diabetic, that the disease is more advanced, that the increase in CAD is particularly striking among women, and that the disease affects younger people than does CAD among nondiabetics.[28] Leland, in a clinical study of 98 diabetic patients in their seventh decade of life reported that after diabetes had been present for 5 years, 15% of the patients were found to have CAD. When diabetes had been present for 10 years or more, 33% of the patients had clinically apparent CAD.[58] Aronow,[59] in a review of 1654 patients aged 62 years or older, reported a prevalence of CAD of 41%. Stearns, in an autopsy study using injection techniques, found significant CAD in 74% of diabetics and 37% of nondiabetics.[60] Leland commented that more than a third of diabetics with nephropathy and an average age of 34 years were found to have silent, high-grade, coronary obstructive disease when they presented to the Joslin Clinic.[58] As described earlier in this chapter, Hertzer et al[40] found that severe, inoperable CAD was present in 16% of diabetics over the age of 60, but only 6.5% of nondiabetics of the same age (Table 2). Aronow,[61] in a study of 192 men and 516 women aged 62 to 98 years (mean 82 years), reported that the relative risk of new coronary events within 41 months was twice as high in diabetics as in nondiabetics.[61] Over the age of 40, CAD is eight times more common in diabetic women than in nondiabetic women. As is the situation in PVD, diabetes neutralizes the benefits of female gender.[58]

MI secondary to CAD occurs in 13.2% of diabetics over the age of 65, but in only 2.9% of nondiabetics of the same ages.[17] Forty-two percent of diabetics report having had no pain during an acute MI (although only 5% are entirely asymptomatic). Thirty-nine percent of acute MIs in diabetics are clinically unrecognized. The corresponding percentages for nondiabetics are: 6% without chest pain; none entirely asymptomatic; and 22% clinically unrecognized.[62,63] Mortality following an acute MI is reported to be between 24% and 40% in diabetics, in contrast to 18% to 19% in nondiabetics. Poor control of hyperglycemia results in an even higher mortality in diabetics (87% if the blood glucose was over 400 mg/dL at the time of MI. In a 1980 study of mortality following MI in 64 diabetic patients 60 to 70 years old, women suffered a mortality of 37% compared with 12% in men. There was an equal distribution of MIs between the sexes.[28] In 1993, Donahue et al[64] described a series of 4109 patients with acute who MI were followed for 12 years after hospital discharge. During the 12 years of follow-up, the relative risk of dying was 1.56 times higher for diabetic men than for nondiabetic men, and 1.57 times higher for diabetic women than for nondiabetic women.[64] Thus, CAD is not only more common in diabetics than in nondiabetics, it results in a greater number of acute MIs in diabetics. It is associated with poorer short-term and long-term survivals following acute MI.

In the CASS series of 1260 patients aged 65 years or older treated for CAD, diabetics had a poorer long-term survival than did nondiabetics. At 5, 10, and 14 years, the respective survivals were: diabetics, 62.6%, 39.4%, and 21.1%; nondiabetics, 74.8%, 55.4%, and 34.5%.[57]

Considering the severe adverse effects that the presence of diabetes mellitus has on the prevalence and outcome of CAD, do the benefits of revascularization outweigh the risks and costs of treatment, particularly in the elderly?

Leland[58] remarked that coronary artery bypass surgery (CABG) results in a marked decrease or elimination of angina pectoris in 70% to

90% of both diabetic and nondiabetic patients. Vogt et al[68] analyzed the outcome of CABG, percutaneous translumnal angioplasty (PTCA), or medical management in 98 patients aged 70 years or older. Twenty-seven percent of the entire series were diabetics. The authors noted that patients undergoing CABG have consistently better outcomes than those managed by PTCA or medication. Outcomes in the diabetic cohort were not specifically addressed.[65] Barzilay et al[57] reported the outcome of medical or surgical management for 2160 patients aged 65 years or older with symptomatic CAD. Three hundred seventeen of the patients were diabetics. All were enrolled in the CASS Registry. He found that diabetic patients treated surgically had better survivals at 5, 10, and 14 years than did diabetic patients treated medically. Over the 14-year time span, the diabetics treated by CABG enjoyed a 44% reduction in the risk of dying, a result almost identical to that observed for the entire group of elderly patients treated surgically. Diabetics undergoing CABG had a 50% chance of living 10 years. Diabetics treated medically had a 25% chance of living 10 years. Barzilay did not specifically discuss operative mortality in his article, but other CASS reports identify a 7.9% operative mortality for the group 70 years of age or older. Barzilay makes the comment that, based on his analysis, diabetes as a risk factor is as powerful as smoking, age, or CHF.[57] Gehlot et al[66] described the results of CABG in 170 patients 70 years of age or older. Twenty-two (12.9%) of the group were diabetic. Thirty-day or hospital mortality was 2.9% overall; 2.1% for elective surgery; 3.1% for urgent procedures, and 11.1% for emergency operations. While female gender and preoperative hypertension correlated with increased mortality, the presence of diabetes had no significant effect on outcome.[66] Curtis et al[67] described the determinants of operative mortality for CABG in 668 patients 70 years of age or older. One hundred forty-eight (22%) of the patients were diabetic. Operative mortality overall (30-day and hospital) was 5.2%: 4.2% in the 600 patients aged 70 to 79 years; 14.7% in the 68 patients aged 80 years or older. Diabetes was not a significant risk factor for hospital mortality (p=0.916). Again, female gender was a significant risk factor for hospital mortality (9.0% versus 4.0% for males, p=0.006).[67] Peterson et al[68] described the results of CABG in 24,461 Medicare patients 80 years of age or older. There were 2152 diabetics in the study (8.8 %). Thirty-day mortality in the entire series of octagenarians was 10.5%. Three-year survival was 71.2%. (For comparison, the authors noted that the operative mortality for the 65- to 70-year-old Medicare cohort was 4.3%, with a 3-year survival of 86.9%). Diabetes was not a significant predictor of 30-day mortality, but was for 3-year survival (odds ratios 0.93% and 1.17%, respectively). Once more, female gender was an independent predictor of higher 30-day and 3-year mortalities (odds ratios 1.19% and 1.18%, respectively). According to Weintraub and his colleagues, as quoted by Peterson,[68] 82% of octagenarians with severe baseline angina who are alive 3 years following operation remain asymptomatic. Peterson gives the costs for CABGs in octagenarians as being 21% higher than for younger patients.[68] Kaul et al[69] reported the outcomes in 310 patients aged 80 years or older who had undergone either CABG or PTCA. The difference in mortality between CABG and PTCA was not statistically significant. Diabetes mellitus was not a significant predictor of increased hospital mortality.[69]

The characteristics of diabetics with CAD mimic those of diabetics with PVD. Compared with nondiabetics, the atherosclerotic disease in both sites in diabetics occurs earlier in life, is more extensive, is more likely to result in infarction or gangrene, does not spare the female, and is associated with a shorter life expectancy. Nevertheless, diabetics, even elderly diabetics, fare as well with operation as do nondiabetics. In the case of CAD, operation markedly prolongs survival when compared with medical management and to some degree with PTCA. It is important to recognize that waiting for a surgical procedure to become urgent or emergent will result in a substantially higher hospital mortality, particularly in the older patient. The variation between series in the percentage of diabetics in the group undergoing surgery (8.8% to 22%) suggests a persisting reluctance to perform major surgery in diabetics, particularly elderly diabetics.

Cerebrovascular Disease

Currently, 400,000 to 500,000 individuals in the United States suffer new, nonfatal strokes each year. There are approximately 170,000 to 200,000 deaths due to stroke each year in the United States.[70,71] About 20% of stroke victims die within 14 days of suffering a stroke. An additional 15% die within 1 year of the stroke. Within 5 years of the incident, 45% of stroke victims are dead. Fifty percent of these deaths result from recurrent stroke(s), whereas 30% of the deaths result from MI. Almost 90% of first strokes in both men and women occur after the age of 55. Forty percent of first strokes in men and 47% of first strokes in women occur at age 74 or beyond. Ninety-four percent of deaths from cerebrovascular disease occur in those 75 years of age and older. A slight preponderance of deaths from cerebrovascular disease is seen in men from ages 35 through 74. Above 75 years, however, almost twice as many women die from stroke as do men.[72]

Survivors of a stroke suffer significant disabilities. Thirty percent of individuals will recover normal function after a stroke, but the other 70% will have functional deficits. Thirty-six percent of survivors following a stroke will be able to return to work; 29% will require aid in daily living; 16% percent will require aid in ambulation; 10% will require institutionalization, and 4% will require total custodial care.[73]

Risk factors for a stroke are: an elevated serum cholesterol, cigarette smoking, diabetes mellitus, LVH by ECG, and systolic or diastolic hypertension. If none of the risk factors is present, individuals have a risk of stroke of 1 per 1000 population per year. If hypertension is present, the risk of stroke rises to 6 per 1000 population per year. If all six risk factors are present, the risk of stroke increases to 36 per 1000 population per year.

In the Framingham study, severe extracranial carotid arterial disease (75% to 100% stenosis) was present in 3% of 1189 patients aged 66 to 93 years.[74] In a study conducted by Aronow et al,[75] severe extracranial carotid arterial disease was present in 4% of 1063 patients aged 60 to 101 years.[75] Kannel,[76] reporting results of the Framingham Study noted that in a population 45 to 74 years old, the incidence of stroke was 2.7 times higher in male diabetics than in male nondiabetics. In females, the ratio was 3.8 to 1.[76] In addition, the mortality from stroke was 2.5 times greater in diabetics than in nondiabetics.[76]

Drielsma et al,[77] in 1988, presented a study of 780 patients with stroke and prestroke conditions. Eighty (10.3%) were diabetics. Eighty-two percent of the diabetic population and 83% of the nondiabetic population were men. The mean age of both groups was 65 years. Seventy-six percent of the diabetics were symptomatic at presentation, as were 82% of the nondiabetics. Stroke, as the presenting symptom, was seen more frequently in diabetics than in nondiabetics (37.7% versus 23.9%). Transient ischemic attacks (TIAs), as the presenting symptom, were seen more often in nondiabetics than in diabetics (48.1% versus 18%). An ipsilateral TIA preceded the stroke in 13.8% of nondiabetics, but in only 8.7% of diabetics. Vertebrobasilar insufficiency was the presenting symptom in 44.3% of symptomatic diabetics, but only 27.9% of symptomatic nondiabetics. The method of diabetic control made little difference to the mode of presentation. Drielsma et al found no difference in the frequencies of various plaque types between diabetics and nondiabetics, but diabetics treated with insulin had marked differences from nondiabetics in the morphology of the plaques. Associated PVD was present in 38.8% of diabetics compared with 28.6% of nondiabetics (p<0.05).[77]

Pullicino et al[78] investigating the incidence of stroke following an acute MI in 148 diabetics and 297 nondiabetics found that stroke was more common in diabetics than in nondiabetics (7% versus 3%, p=0.020). A history of a previous stroke, preinfarction hypertension and postinfarction hypotension were risk factors for stroke in diabetics following an acute MI.[78]

Thus, carotid arterial disease in diabetics mimics the pattern of macrovascular disease elsewhere in the diabetic. Carotid arterial disease is more frequent in the diabetic than in the nondiabetic, is more likely to involve other cerebral vessels, and is more often associated with PVD. It does not spare the diabetic female, is more likely to present at a more advanced level of disease, and is more likely to result in death than in the nondiabetic. TIAs are less likely to precede a stroke than in the nondiabetic. A more detailed description of the medical and surgical treatment of cerebrovascular disease will be presented in other chapters. Suffice it to say that, like diabetics who present with intermittent claudication and angina pectoris, diabetics who present with signs or symptoms of cerebrovascular insufficiency need to be treated aggressively if serious impairment of function and excessive mortality are to be avoided.

Comments and Overview

In the opening chapter of this book, the statement was made that currently available techniques of medical and surgical management of vascular disease can, if applied, prolong life, increase its quality, and make it more active. Appropriate management of the diabetic can even prevent disease that would otherwise result in disability and death. It is clear from the data presented in this chapter that diabetes mellitus is a major threat to the life, limb, and function of a sizeable segment of the population in the United States. Reduction in the prevalence of the more severe complications of diabetes mellitus by the year 2000 was established as one of the 22 objectives for the United States by the Department of Health and Human Services in September, 1990.[2]

Adult onset diabetes or type II diabetes represents a greater threat to life, limb, and function than do other forms of diabetes, for two reasons. First, it is by far the most common form of diabetes and, second, it typically has a long, "prediabetic" period during which severe microvascular and macrovascular complications can develop before the clinical presence of diabetes is recognized. In fact, the initial presentation of clinical diabetes may be by way of one of its major complications. It has been estimated that for every individual with clinically apparent diabetes, there is another in whom the clinical diagnosis is yet to be established.

Strict control of blood sugar has been shown to markedly reduce the incidence of complications of microvascular disease (retinopathy, neuropathy, and neuropathy) in diabetics, particularly young diabetics. The role of strict management of the blood sugar in controlling complications from macrovascular disease is still unsettled. Hyperinsulinism and borderline hyperglycemia can be present for one or two decades before overt diabetes is recognized. Studies conducted in the general population have shown that during this prediabetic period, there is an increasing incidence of CAD associated with the gradually increasing levels of serum glucose.[22,23,79] When compared with standard management of blood sugar, the use of intensive insulin therapy to control hyperglycemia in type II diabetics has been found to substantially increase the frequency of major cardiovascular events in these patients (4% versus 25% at 27 months).[80]

The majority of amputations in diabetics are precipitated by relatively minor injuries to their feet, sometimes as a result of ill advised "bathroom" procedures performed by a patient with eyesight impaired by diabetes. Simple measures, such as formal educational sessions with diabetics, can halve the incidence of amputations. Yet, as of 1993, only 43% of diabetics were provided with this education, a growth of only 10% since 1983.[81]

An awareness of the higher incidence of serious implications of intermittent claudication in diabetics and a more aggressive use of elective peripheral vascular reconstruction in these patients can further reduce the amputation rate. Earlier operation would also avoid the higher morbidity and mortality associated with urgent and emergent attempts at last ditch limb salvage. Certainly, a major amputation in the diabetic can start a sequence of events that begins with loss of mobility and ends with death.

The knowledge that diabetics with extracranial carotid arterial disease present less often with TIAs and more often with strokes than do nondiabetics can lead to better surveillance for cerebrovascular disease in diabetics and elective surgical intervention before a disabling, crippling, or fatal stroke occurs.

An appreciation that "silent" CAD is more frequent in diabetics, that their survival following an MI is lower than that of nondiabetics, and that diabetics undergoing elective coronary arterial revascularization have twice the likelihood of living 10 years than do diabetics treated nonoperatively, can lead to earlier operation in these patients. It is worth emphasizing that current surgical studies have demonstrated that diabetes mellitus is not associated with a statistically significant risk for increased postoperative in-hospital mortality. Age, gender, and the need for urgent operation *are* significant predictors of an increased operative mortality.

Clearly, appropriate management of diabetics and of the vascular disease found in these patients can prolong life, increase its quality, render it more active and, in addition, markedly decrease the incidence of complications associated with this increasingly prevalent disease.

References

1. Eastman R: Prevalance of diabetes increasing in U.S. *Surg Rounds* 19:32, 1996.
2. Diabetes and chronic disabling conditions. In: *Healthy People 2000: National Health Promotion and Disease Prevention Objectives.* Washington, DC: US Government Printing Office; 73, 1991.
3. Parker SL, Tong T, Bolden B, et al: Table 6: Reported deaths; 10 leading causes of death by age and sex, United States, 1992. In: Murphy GP (ed). *A Cancer Journal for Clinicians.* New York: Lippincott-Raven Publishers; 16, 1996.
4. Entmacher PS, Krall LP, Kranczer SN: Diabetes mortality from vital statistics. In: Marbel A, Krall LP, Bradley RF, et al (eds). *Joslin's Diabetes Mellitus.* 12th Ed. Philadelphia: Lea and Febiger; 278-297, 1985.
5. Wellman KF, Volk BW: Historical review. In: Volk BW, Wellman KF. *The Diabetic Pancreas.* New York: Plenum Press; 1-14, 1977.
6. Krall LP, Levine R, Barnett D: The history of diabetes. In: Kahn CR, Weir GC (eds). *Joslin's Diabetes Mellitus.* 13th Ed. Philadelphia: Lea and Febiger; 1-52, 1994.
7. Bliss M: Who discovered insulin? In: Bliss M: *The Discovery of Insulin.* Chicago: University of Chicago Press; 31-36, 1982.
8. Kuller LH, Laporte RE, Orchard TJ: Diabetes. In: Last JM (ed). *Public Health and Preventive Medicine.* 12th Ed. Norwalk, CT: Appelton-Centure-Crofts; 1225-1238, 1986.

9. Thompson JS, Thompson MW: Overview. In: Thompson JS, Thompson MW: *Genetics in Medicine.* 3rd Ed. Philadelphia: WB Saunders, Co.; 331-347, 1980.

10. Rotter JI, Anderson CE, Rimoin DL: Genetics of diabetes mellitus. In: Ellenberg M, Rifkin H (eds). *Diabetes Mellitus: Theory and Practice.* New York: Medical Examination Publishing Co.; 481-503, 1983.

11. Blaum CS, Halter JB: Diabetes in the elderly: choosing the right path. *Fed Pract* 12(5):12-23, 1995.

12. Warram JH, Rich SS, Krolewski AS: Epidemiology and genetics of diabetes mellitus. In: Kahn CR, Weir GC (eds). *Joslin's Diabetes Mellitus.* 13th Ed. Philadelphia: Lea and Febiger; 201-215, 1994.

13. Bennett PH: Definition, diagnosis, and classification of diabetes mellitus and impaired glucose tolerance. In: Kahn CR, Weir GC (eds). *Joslin's Diabetes Mellitus.* 13th Ed. Philadelphia: Lea and Febiger, 193-200, 1994.

14. Eisehbarth GS, Ziegler AG, Colman PA: Pathogenesis of insulin-dependent (type I) diabetes mellitus. In: Kahn CR, Weir GC (eds). Joslin's Diabetes Mellitus. 13th Ed. Philadelphia: Lea and Febiger; 216-239, 1994.

15. Kraus S: New clues to diabetes. *Stanford Med* 2:26-29, 1985.

16. Weir GC, Leahy JL: Pathogenesis of noninsulin-dependent (type II) diabetes mellitus. In: Kahn CR, Weir GC (eds). *Joslin's Diabetes Mellitus.* 13th Ed. Philadelphia: Lea and Febiger; 240-264, 1994.

17. Herman WH, Teutsch SM, Geiss LS: Closing the gap: the problem of diabetes mellitus in the United States. *Diabetes Care* 8:391-406, 1985.

18. Barnett AH, Eff C, Leslie RDG, et al: Diabetes in identical twins: a study of 200 pairs. *Diabetologia* 20:87-93, 1981.

19. Fradkin J: Editorial: the challenge of managing NIDDM in the elderly. *Fed Pract* 12(5):11, 1995.

20. Osterby R: Basement membrane morphology in diabetes mellitus. In: Ellenberg M, Rifkin H (eds). *Diabetes Mellitus: Theory and Practice.* New York: Medical Examination Publishing Co.; 323-341, 1983.

21. McMillan DE: Pathophysiology of diabetic macro- and microvascular disease. In: Ellenberg M, Rifkin H (eds). *Diabetes Mellitus: Theory and Practice.* New York: Medical Examination Publishing Co.; 343-359, 1983.

22. Keen H, Jarrett RJ: Macroangiopathy: its prevalence in asymptomatic diabetes. *Adv Metabolic Disorders* (suppl)2: 3-9, 1973.

23. Chait A, Bierman EL: Pathogenesis of macrovascular disease in diabetics. In: Kahn CR, Weir GC (eds). *Joslin's Diabetes Mellitus.* 13th Ed. Philadelphia: Lea and Febiger; 648-664, 1994.

24. Mandrup-Poulson T, Mortensen SA, Meinertz H, et al: DNA sequences flanking the insulin gene on chromosome 11 confer risk of atherosclerosis. *Lancet* 1:250-252, 1984.

25. *Health United States, 1993, U.S. Department of Health and Human Services. Table 31.* Hyattsville, MD: Public Health Service; 99-100, 1994.

26. Dry TJ, Hines EA, Jr: The role of diabetes in the development of degenerative vascular disease: with special reference to the incidence of retinitis and peripheral neuritis. *Ann Intern Med* 14:1893-1902, 1941.

27. Joslin EP, Root HF, White P, et al: *The Treatment of Diabetes Mellitus.* 7th Ed. Philadelphia: Lea and Febiger; 783, 1940.

28. Leland OS, Maki PC: Heart disease and diabetes mellitus. In: Marble A, Krall LP, Bradley RF, et al (eds). *Joslin's Diabetes Mellitus.* 12th Ed. Philadelphia: Lea and Febiger; 553-582, 1985.

29. Warren S, LeCompte PM, Legg MA: *The Pathology of Diabetes Mellitus.* 4th Ed. Philadelphia: Lea and Febiger; 178-187, 1966.

30. Juergens JL, Barker NW, Hines EA, Jr: Arteriosclerosis obliterans: review of 520 cases with special reference to pathogenic and prognostic factors. *Circulation* 21:188-195, 1960.
3l. Kannel WB, McGee DL: Diabetes and vascular disease: the Framingham study. *JAMA* 241:2035-2038, 1979.
32. Ganda OP: Pathogenesis of macrovascular disease including the influence of lipids. In: Marble A, Krall LP, Bradley RF, et al (eds). *Joslin's Diabetes Mellitus.* 12th Ed. Philadelphia: Lea and Febiger; 217-250, 1985.
33. Gensler SW, Haimovici H, Hoffert P, et al: Study of vascular lesions in diabetic, nondiabetic patients. *Arch Surg* 91:617-622, 1965.
34. Crawford ES, Bonberger RA, Glaeser DH, et al: Aortoiliac occlusive disease: factors influencing survival and function following reconstructive operation over a twenty-five-year period. *Surgery* 90:1055-1067, 1981.
35. Brewster DC, Darling RC: Optimal methods of aortoiliac reconstruction. *Surgery* 84:739-748, 1978.
36. Malone JM, Moore WS, Goldstone J: The natural history of bilateral aortofemoral bypass grafts for ischemia of the lower extremities. *Arch Surg* 110:1300-1306, 1975.
37. Mavor GE: Pattern of occlusion in atheroma of lower limb arteries. *Br J Surgery* 43:352-354, 1956.
38. Haimovici H: Reconstruction of the profunda femoris artery. In: Haimovici H: *Vascular Surgery Principles and Techniques.* New York: McGraw-Hill; 480-492, 1976.
39. Haimovici H: Arteriographic patterns of atherosclerotic occlusive disease of the lower extremity. In: Haimovici H: *Vascular Surgery Principles and Techniques.* New York: McGraw-Hill; 240-263, 1976.
40. Hertzer NR, Beven EG, Young JR, et al: Coronary artery disease in peripheral vascular patients: a classification of 1000 coronary angiograms and results of surgical management. *Ann Surg* 199:223-233, 1984.
41. Rosenblatt MS, Quist WC, Sidaway AN, et al: Results of vein graft reconstruction of the lower extremity in diabetic and nondiabetic patients. Surg Gynecol Obstet 171:331-335, 1990.
42. Silbert S, Zazeela H: Prognosis in arteriosclerotic peripheral vascular disease. *JAMA* 166:1816-1821, 1958.
43. Most RS, Sinnock P: The epidemiology of lower extremity amputations in diabetic individuals. *Diabetes Care* 6:87-91, 1983.
44. Gutman M, Kaplan 0, Skornik Y, et al: Gangrene of the lower limbs in diabetic patients: a malignant complication. *Am J Surg* 154:305-308, 1987.
45. Krolewski AS, Warram JH, Christlieb AR: Onset, course, complications, and prognosis of diabetes mellitus. In: Marble A, Krall LP, Bradley RF, et al (eds). *Joslin's Diabetes Mellitus.* 12th Ed. Philadelphia: Lea and Febiger; 251-276, 1985.
46. Harris R: Occlusive diseases of arteries in old age. In: Harris R: *The Management of Geriatric Cardiovascular Disease.* Philadelphia: JB Lippincott; 269-289, 1970.
47. Criqui MH, Fronek A, Barret-Connor E, et al: The prevalence of peripheral arterial disease in a defined population. *Circulation* 71:510-515, 1985.
48. Boyd AM: The natural course of arteriosclerosis of the lower extremities. Proc R Soc Med 55:591-596, 1962.
49. Kannel WB, Skinner JJ, Schwartz MJ, et al: Intermittent claudication: incidence in the Framingham Study. *Circulation* 41:875-893, 1970.
50. Imparato AM, Kim G, Davidson T: Intermittent claudication: its natural course. *Surgery* 78:795-799, 1975.
51. Kuritzky L: Intermittent claudication. *Resid and Staff Phys* 33(7):65-85, 1987.

52. Schadt DC, Hines EA JR, Juergens JL, et al: Chronic atherosclerotic occlusion of the femoral artery. *JAMA* 175:937-940, l961.

53. Johason T, Ringqvist I: Diabetes mellitus and intermittent claudication: relation between peripheral vascular complications and location of the occlusive atherosclerosis in the legs. *Acta Med Scand* 218:217-221, 1985.

54. Jonason T, Ringqvist I: Factors of prognostic importance for subsequent rest pain in patients with intermittent claudication. *Acta Med Scand* 218:27-33, 1985.

55. Juergens JL, Bernatz PE: Atherosclerosis of the extremities (arteriosclerosis obliterans, atherosclerosis obliterans, ASO). In: Juergens JL, Spittel JA, Jr (eds). Textbook of Peripheral Vascular Disease. Philadelphia: WB Saunders, Co.; 253-293, 1980.

56. Steer HW, Cuckle HS, Franklin PM: The influence of diabetes mellitus upon peripheral vascular disease. *Surg Gynecol Obstet* 157:64-72, 1983.

57. Barzilay JI, Kronmal RA, Bittner V: Coronary artery disease and coronary artery bypass grafting in diabetic patients aged ≥65 years (Report from the Coronary Artery Surgery Study [CASS] Registry). *Am J Cardiol* 74:334-339, 1994.

58. Leland OS Jr: Diabetes and the heart. In: Kozak GP (ed). *Clinical Diabetes Mellitus*. Philadelphia: WB Saunders, Co.; 302-316, 1981.

59. Aronow WS: Prevalence of atherothrombotic brain infarction, coronary artery disease, and peripheral arterial disease in elderly Blacks, Hispanics, and Whites. *Am J Cardiol* 70:1212-1213, 1992.

60. Stearns S, Schlesinger JM, Rudy A: Incidence and clinical significance of coronary artery disease in diabetes mellitus. *Arch Intern Med* 80:463-469, 1947.

61. Aronow WS: Coronary disease in the elderly: what factors increase risk? How to predict the influences of gender, race, and increasing age. *J Crit Illness* 8(I):59-74, 1993.

62. Bradley RF, Schonfeld A: Diminished pain in diabetic patients with acute myocardial infarction. *Geriatrics* 17:322-331, 1962.

63. Margolis JR, Kannel WS, Feinleib M, et al: Clinical features of unrecognized myocardial infarction—silent and asymptomatic: Eighteen-year follow-up: the Framingham Study. *Am J Cardiol* 32:1-8, 1973.

64. Donohue RP, Goldberg RJ, Chen Z, et al: The influence of sex and diabetes mellitus on survival following acute myocardial infarction: a community-wide persepctive. *J Clin Epidemiol* 46(3):245-252, 1993.

65. Vogt AR, Funk M, Remetz M: Comparison of symptoms, functional ability, and health perception of elderly patients with coronary artery disease managed with three different treatment modalities. *Cardiovasc Nursing* 30(5):33-38, 1994.

66. Gehlot AS, Santamaria JD, White AL, et al: Current status of coronary artery bypass grafting in patients 70 years of age and older. *Aust N Z J Surg* 65:177-181, 1995.

67. Curtis JJ, Walls JT, Boley TM, et al: Coronary revascularization in the elderly: determinants of operative mortality. *Ann Thorac Surg* 58:1069-1072, 1994.

68. Peterson ED, Cowper PA, Jollis JG, et al: Outcomes of coronary artery bypass graft surgery in 24,461 patients aged 80 years or older. *Circulation* 92(suppl II)(9):85-91, 1995.

69. Kaul TJ, Fields BL, Wyatt DA, et al: Angioplasty versus coronary artery bypass in octagenarians. *Ann Thorac Surg* 58:1419-1426, 1994.

70. Heart disease and stroke. In: *Healthy People 2000: National Health Promotion and Disease Prevention Objectives*. Washington, DC: US Printing Office; 392-413, 1991.

71. The nations health: age groups. In: *Healthy People 2000: National Health Promotion and Disease Prevention Objectives*. Washington, DC: United States Printing Office; 9-27, 1991.

72. Boring CC, Squires TS, Tong T, et al: Mortality, 10 leading causes of death, by age group and sex, United States, 1990. In: Murphy GP (ed). *A Cancer Journal for Clinicians*. New York: JB Lippincott; 14-15, 1994.
73. Cohen JR: Cerebral vascular disease. In: Cohen JR. Vascular Surgery for the House Officer. 2nd Ed. Baltimore, MD: Williams & Wilkins; 68-80, 1992.
74. O'Leary DH, Anderson KM, Wolf PA, et al: Cholesterol and carotid atherosclerosis in older persons: the Framingham Study. *Ann Epidemiol* 2:147-153, 1992.
75. Aronow WS, Ahn C, Schoenfeld MR: Risk factors for extracranial internal or common carotid arterial disease in elderly patients. Am J Cardiol 71:1479-1481, 1993.
76. Kannel WB: Recent findings of the Framingham Study. *Resid and Staff Phys* 24(1):56-71, 1978.
77. Drielsma RF, Burnett JR, Gray-Weale AC, et al: Carotid artery disease: the influence of diabetes mellitus. *J Cardovasc Surg* 29:692-696, 1988.
78. Pullicino PM, Xuereb M, Aguilina J, et al: Stroke following acute myocardial infarction in diabetics. *J Intern Med* 231(3):287-293, 1992.
79. Krolewski AS, Warram JH: Epidemiology of late complications of diabetes. In: Kahn CR, Weir GC (eds). *Joslin's Diabetes Mellitus*. 13th Ed. Philadelphia: Lea and Febiger; 605-619, 1994.
80. Hurley D: Intensive insulin therapy may pose a risk in diabetics with heart disease. *Cardiology* 5(6)1-16, 1994.
81. Priority area 17: Diabetes and chronic disabling conditions. Figure 18: Proportion of people with diabetes who have taken formal patient education: United States, 1983-1993, and the year 2000 target for objective 17.14a. In: *Healthy People 2000 Review 1994*. Hyattsvile, MD: US Department of Health and Human Services; 101-102, 1995.

Chapter 13

Medical Management of Carotid Arterial Disease

Wilbert S. Aronow, MD

Atherosclerosis may cause extracranial internal or common carotid arterial disease (ECAD). Significant ECAD may cause cerebral ischemia or infarction by decreasing blood flow distal to a stenotic carotid artery, by distal propagation of thrombus, or by arterial to arterial embolism from the site of carotid stenosis or ulceration. Hemodynamically obstructive plaques lead to cerebrovascular events. Atheroembolic emboli from the carotid bifurcation to intracranial arteries may cause cerebrovascular events.[1,2] Intraplaque hemorrhage may contribute to embolization from the plaques.[3,4] Mural plaques growing in a crescentic configuration along the wall of the carotid bifurcation cause more cerebrovascular symptoms than do plaques that maintain a nodular configuration.[5]

Diagnosis of Extracranial Carotid Arterial Disease

The noninvasive procedure of choice for evaluating ECAD is carotid duplex ultrasonography.[6] Pulsed echo or B-mode ultrasonography shows an anatomical image of the carotid artery, and pulsed Doppler ultrasonography shows changes in carotid blood flow.[6] The sensitivity of carotid duplex ultrasonography in diagnosing ECAD is 85%.[6] The specificity of carotid duplex ultrasonography in diagnosing ECAD is 90%. Carotid duplex ultrasonography can diagnose hemodynamically significant ECAD, differentiate between high-grade stenosis and total occlusion, and diagnose carotid ulcers, plaques, and plaque hemorrhages.[6] Carotid duplex ultrasonography is recommended in patients with neck bruits, in patients with prior stroke or symptomatic transient cerebral ischemic attacks (TIA) in the distribution of the carotid circulation, and in patients with vertigo, diplopia, or syncope. However, ca-

From: Aronow WS, Stemmer EA, Wilson SE (eds). *Vascular Disease in the Elderly.* Armonk, NY: Futura Publishing Company, Inc., © 1997.

rotid angiography is the reference standard diagnostic test for evaluating ECAD and is recommended before performing carotid endarterectomy.[6]

Prevalence of Extracranial Carotid Arterial Disease

Bilateral carotid duplex ultrasonography was performed in 1,275 persons, mean age 81 years (range 60 to 101), in a long-term health care facility.[7] This group included 906 women and 369 men. Bilateral carotid duplex ultrasonograms were obtained with an Interspec XL machine using a 7.5 MHz transducer with combined two-dimensional, real-time, and pulsed or high-pulse frequency Doppler capabilities. The severity of internal or common carotid atherosclerotic obstruction was semi-quantified by using conventional Doppler criteria: maximal velocity (V_{max}) <0.8 m/s = <40% arterial luminal diameter reduction; V_{max} 0.80 to 1.75 m/s = 40% to 80% reduction; V_{max} >1.75 m/s = 80% to 99% reduction; and V_{max} 0m/s (no Doppler signal on at least two separate tests) = 100% reduction.

Table 1 shows that 16% of the 1,275 elderly persons had 40% to 100% ECAD. Forty percent to 100% ECAD was present in 67 of 369 elderly men (18%), and in 135 of 906 elderly women (15%) (difference not significant). This study also showed that elderly patients with 40% to 100% ECAD had a higher prevalence of valvular aortic stenosis than did elderly patients with no significant ECAD.[7]

In the Framingham Study, 50% to 100% ECAD was diagnosed by bilateral carotid duplex ultrasonography in 8% of 1,189 elderly persons aged 66 to 93 years.[8] Severe ECAD with 75% to 100% stenosis was present in 3% of this elderly population.[8]

Caplan et al[9] demonstrated that ECAD occurred more often in Caucasians with atherothombotic brain infarction (ABI) than in African-Americans with ABI. African-Americans with ABI had a predominance of intracranial vascular lesions.[9] Heyman et al[10] also showed in patients with ischemic stroke that African-Americans had a higher frequency

Table 1
Prevalence and Severity of 40% to 100% Extracranial Carotid Arterial Disease in 1,275 Elderly Men and Women

% of Diameter Reduction of Carotid Arteries	% of Patients
0 to 39%	84%
40% to 79%	12%
80% to 100%	4%
40% to 100%	16%

(Adapted with permission from Reference 7.)

Table 2
Prevalence of 40% to 100% Extracranial Carotid Arterial Disease in Elderly
African-Americans, Hispanics, and Whites

	African-Americans (n = 204)	Hispanics (n = 42)	Whites (n = 817)
ECAD	14%	17%	17%
ECAD if prior ABI	15%	31%	33%

ECAD = extracranial carotid arterial disease
ABI = atherothrombotic brain infarction
(Adapted with permission from Reference 11.)

of occlusive disease of the intracranial arteries, whereas Caucasians were more likely to have occlusive disease of the extracranial arteries.

In a study of 204 elderly African-Americans, mean age 80 years, 42 elderly Hispanics, mean age 80 years, and 817 elderly Caucasians, mean age 81 years, the prevalence of ABI was 50% in elderly African-Americans, 31% in elderly Hispanics, and 24% in elderly Caucasians.[11] The prevalence of 40% to 100% ECAD was similar in elderly African-Americans (14%), elderly Hispanics (17%), and elderly Caucasians (17%). However, in elderly patients with prior ABI, the prevalence of 40% to 100% ECAD was 15% in elderly African-Americans, 31% in elderly Hispanics, and 33% in elderly Caucasians (Table 2).[11] Therefore, the higher prevalence of prior ABI in the elderly African-Americans in this study was due to a higher frequency of occlusive disease of the intracranial arteries.

Risk Factors for Extracranial Carotid Arterial Disease

Cigarette Smoking

Numerous studies have demonstrated that cigarette smoking is a strong risk factor for ECAD.[12-20] Candelise et al[12] found by multivariate analysis in 462 patients that cigarette smoking was the only risk factor showing a strong association with the angiographic extracranial atherosclerosis score. In a study of 306 elderly men and 757 elderly women, mean age 81 years, 40% to 100% ECAD was observed in 175 patients (16%).[19] Table 3 shows that the most powerful risk factor for ECAD by multivariate analysis in this study was current cigarette smoking, with an odds ratio of 4.002.[19] Tell et al[16] found in 1,692 African-American and Caucasian men and women who had B-mode ultrasonography of the carotid arteries that the difference in mean carotid plaque thickness was smaller between past smokers and nonsmokers than between current smokers and nonsmokers. Their data suggest a slower rate of progression of carotid atherosclerosis in patients who quit smoking com-

Table 3
Risk Factors for 40% to 100% Extracranial Carotid Arterial Disease in 1,063
Elderly Persons, Mean Age 81 years

Risk Factor	Odds Ratio
Cigarette smoking	4.002*
Serum total cholesterol	1.014*
Serum HDL cholesterol	0.982*
Diabetes mellitus	1.684*
Prior coronary artery disease	1.572*
Age	1.017
Hypertension	1.193†
Sex	0.876
Obesity	0.837
Serum triglycerides	0.999†

* Significant prognostic variable for ECAD in the multivariate logistic regression models.
† Significant by univariate analysis, but not by multivariate analysis.
ECAD = extracranial carotid arterial disease
(Adapted with permission from Reference 19.)

pared with patients who continued to smoke. On the basis of the available data, patients with ECAD should be strongly encouraged to stop smoking.

Dyslipidemia

Ford et al[13] demonstrated by multivariate analysis in 121 patients, mean age 62 years, who had cerebral angiography that serum high-density lipoprotein (HDL) cholesterol (inverse association) and serum total cholesterol/HDL cholesterol ratio were risk factors for carotid bifurcation atherosclerosis. This group of investigators also found by multivariate analysis in 376 patients who had B-mode ultrasonography that serum HDL cholesterol (inverse association) was a risk factor for ECAD.[14] In the Rotterdam Elderly Study, only 13 of 954 persons (1%) had 50% or greater ECAD.[17] In this study, reduced serum HDL cholesterol was a risk factor for ECAD. In the San Daniele Project Study, multivariate analysis showed that serum HDL cholesterol protected against ECAD.[18] Two studies with B-mode ultrasound evaluation for ECAD found after multivariate analysis that both a low serum HDL cholesterol and an increased serum low-density lipoprotein (LDL) cholesterol predicted the extent of ECAD.[21,22]

The association between ECAD and serum total cholesterol and HDL cholesterol measured 8 years before carotid duplex ultrasonography and concurrently was investigated in 1,189 elderly persons aged 66 to 93 years in the Framingham Study.[8] There was a strong association in both elderly women and men between the severity of ECAD and the serum total cholesterol measured 8 years before the carotid studies. There was a strong association in women, but not in men between the severity of ECAD and the serum HDL cholesterol (inverse association) measured 8 years before the carotid studies and concurrently.

In a study of 175 elderly persons, mean age 81 years, with 40% to 100% ECAD, and 888 elderly persons, mean age 81 years, with no significant ECAD, multivariate analysis showed that serum total cholesterol (odds ratio = 1.014) and serum HDL cholesterol (inverse association; odds ratio = 0.982) were risk factors for ECAD (Table 3).[19] Serum triglycerides were a risk factor for ECAD by univariate analysis, but not by multivariate analysis in this study. On the basis of the available data, low serum HDL cholesterol and increased serum total cholesterol and LDL cholesterol, but not increased serum triglycerides would be considered risk factors for ECAD in elderly patients.

In the Cholesterol Lowering Atherosclerosis Study, 24 patients randomized to treatment with diet plus colestipol and niacin therapy, and 22 patients randomized to treatment with diet plus placebo had carotid ultrasound studies with matching cervical angiograms performed at baseline, and at 2 and 4 years after randomization.[23] Patients treated with colestipol plus niacin had a progressive decrease in common carotid intima-media thickness at 2 years and at 4 years, whereas patients treated with placebo had an increase in common carotid wall thickness. Decreased serum levels of apolipoprotein B and increased levels of serum HDL cholesterol and apolipoprotein C were significant predictors of carotid wall thinning.

In the Asymptomatic Carotid Artery Progression Study, 919 men and women, mean age 62 years (range 40 to 79 years), with early carotid atherosclerosis, moderately increased LDL cholesterol levels, and no symptomatic cardiovascular disease, were randomized to lovastatin only (231 patients), to lovastatin plus warfarin (229 patients), to warfarin only (229 patients), or to placebo (230 patients).[24] At 34-month follow-up, lovastatin caused a reduction in LDL cholesterol level, slowed the progression of mean intimal-medial thickness of the common carotid arteries, and reduced mortality and major cardiovascular events in men and women with early carotid atherosclerosis.

In the Pravastatin, Lipids, and Atherosclerosis in the Carotid Arteries Study, 151 patients with coronary artery disease (CAD) were randomized to treatment with pravastatin (75 patients) or placebo (76 patients) for 3 years.[25] At 3-year follow-up, patients treated with pravastatin had a reduction in serum total cholesterol, a decrease in serum LDL cholesterol, an increase in serum HDL cholesterol, a 12% decrease in progression of the mean maximum intimal-medial thickness of the carotid arteries, a 35% decrease in intimal-media thickness progression in the common carotid arteries, a decrease in fatal and nonfatal myocardial infarction (MI), and a reduction in any fatal event plus nonfatal MI.

The major cause of death in elderly patients with ECAD is a new coronary event. In the Scandinavian Simvastatin Survival Study, 4,444 men and women with CAD were treated with double-blind simvastatin or placebo.[26] At 5.4-year median follow-up, patients treated with simvastatin had a 35% decrease in serum LDL cholesterol, a 25% reduction in serum total cholesterol, and an 8% increase in serum HDL cholesterol. Patients treated with simvastatin also had a decrease in major coronary events of 34%, in coronary deaths of 42%, and in total mortality of 30%. These reductions in coronary events and total mortality were similar in men and in women between 60 to 70 years of age and younger.

On the basis of the available data, elderly patients with ECAD and increased serum total cholesterol and LDL cholesterol levels and low serum HDL cholesterol levels should be treated with diet, plus a drug such as simvastatin,[26] pravastatin,[25] or lovastatin,[24] to slow progression of ECAD and to reduce cardiovascular events and total mortality.

Hypertension

Hypertension is the most powerful risk factor for ABI in elderly patients.[27] In a prospective study of 708 elderly men and women, mean age 82 years, at 3-year follow-up the incidence of new ABI increased 3.6 times in elderly men with hypertension and was increased 3.0 times in elderly women with hypertension.[27]

Numerous studies have demonstrated by univariate analysis that hypertension is a risk factor for ECAD.[15, 17,19,28-31] However, multivariate analysis showed that hypertension was a risk factor for ECAD in some studies,[14,21] but not in other studies.[12,19] In the study by Crouse et al,[14] coronary stenosis was excluded as an independent variable from the multivariate analysis. In a study of 1,063 elderly men and women, mean age 81 years, hypertension was a risk factor for 40% to 100% ECAD by univariate analysis, but not by multivariate analysis (Table 3).[19] The variable of hypertension became nonsignificant when the variable prior CAD was entered into the multivariate logistic regression model which included 11 independent variables. Harrison and Wilson[32] also found in an angiographic study that the effect of hypertension on ECAD was small.

These data lead one to conclude that the association between hypertension and ABI is not merely due to an association between hypertension and ECAD. Other factors including intracranial arterial disease and left ventricular hypertrophy (LVH) contribute to the association between hypertension and ABI.

Many studies have demonstrated that anithypertensive therapy reduces the incidence of ABI in elderly patients with hypertension.[33-38] Therefore, elderly patients with hypertension, with and without ECAD, should be treated with antihypertensive drugs to reduce the incidence of ABI.

Left Ventricular Hypertrophy

LVH is a strong independent risk factor for ABI in elderly men and women.[39-42] In a prospective study of 410 elderly patients, mean age 81

Table 4
Prevalence of Hypertension and of Echocardiographic Left Ventricular
Hypertrophy in 1,283 Elderly Patients With and Without 40% to 100%
Extracranial Carotid Arterial Disease

	40% to 100% ECAD	*0% to 39% ECAD*
Hypertension	55%	44%
LVH if hypertension	76%	56%
Hypertension with LVH	42%	24%

LVH = left ventricular hypertrophy
ECAD = extracranial carotid arterial disease
(Adapted with permission from Reference 31.)

years, with hypertension, at 42-month follow-up, multivariate analysis showed that echocardiographic LVH was the most powerful independent risk factor for ABI with an odds ratio of 4.17.[41] The Framingham Heart Study showed in 447 elderly men and in 783 elderly women at 8-year follow-up that after adjustment for age, sex, and cardiovascular disease risk factors, the hazard ratio for new cerebrovascular events was 1.45 for each quartile increase of left ventricular mass-to-height ratio.[42]

Roman et al[43] demonstrated that persons with echocardiographic LVH were twice as likely to have carotid atherosclerosis. In a study of 372 elderly men and 911 elderly women, mean age 81 years, 40% to 100% ECAD was present in 16% of the elderly patients.[31] In this study, the prevalence of hypertension with LVH was 1.75 times higher in patients with 40% to 100% ECAD (42%) than in patients with 0% to 39% ECAD (24%) (Table 4).[31] The association between LVH and 40% to 100% ECAD may contribute to the high incidence of ABI in elderly patients with LVH.

On the basis of the available data, antihypertensive drugs should be used to reduce left ventricular mass. A meta-analysis of 109 treatment studies found that angiotensin-converting-enzyme (ACE) inhibitors are more effective than other antihypertensive drugs in decreasing left ventricular mass.[44] However, prospective studies using different types of antihypertensive drugs are necessary to determine whether regression of left ventricular mass causes a decrease in ABI.

Diabetes Mellitus

Diabetes mellitus increases the incidence of ABI in elderly patients. In a prospective study of 708 elderly men and women, mean age 82 years, at 3-year follow-up, the incidence of new ABI was increased 3.0 times in elderly men with diabetes mellitus and 2.3 times in elderly women with diabetes mellitus.[27] Some studies,[15,19,29] but not all,[14,18] have shown an association between diabetes mellitus and ECAD. In a study of 1,063 elderly men and women, mean age 81 years, diabetes mellitus was a risk factor for 40% to 100% ECAD by multivariate analysis with an odds ratio of 1.684 (Table 3).[19]

Elderly diabetics should be treated with diet, weight loss if necessary, exercise, and appropriate hypoglycemic drugs, if necessary, to control hyperglycemia. Other risk factors such as smoking, dyslipidemia, hypertension, obesity, and physical inactivity should be controlled. The drug of choice for treating hypertension in elderly diabetics is an ACE inhibitor.

Prior Coronary Artery Disease

Craven et al[45] demonstrated that the B-mode score (extent of carotid atherosclerosis) was strongly and independently associated with CAD in patients older than 50 years. In a study of 1,063 elderly men and women, mean age 81 years, prior CAD was an independent risk factor for 40% to 100% ECAD by multivariate analysis with an odds ratio of 1.572 (Table 3).[19]

Obesity, Sex, and Age

Obesity is not a risk factor for ECAD.[14,15,19] Sex is also not a risk factor for ECAD.[7,14,15,19] In a study of 1,275 elderly patients, mean age 81 years, 40% to 100% ECAD was present in 47 of 369 men (18%) and in 135 of 906 elderly women (15%) (difference not significant).

However, age is a risk factor for ECAD.[14,18] In a population of 1,063 elderly persons, mean age 81 years, multivariate analysis showed that age was a marginal risk factor for ECAD (p value = 0.06) with an odds ratio of 1.017 (Table 3).[19]

Plasma Homocysteine

In a study of 418 elderly men and 623 elderly women, ages 67 to 96, from the Framingham Heart Study, after adjustment for age, sex, serum HDL cholesterol, systolic blood pressure, and smoking status, the odds ratio for ≥25% ECAD measured by carotid duplex ultrasonography was 2.0 for persons with the highest plasma homocysteine levels as compared with those with the lowest levels.[46] After adjustment for sex, age, and other risk factors, plasma levels of folate and pyridoxal-5'-phosphate (the coenzyme form of vitamin B_6) and the level of folate intake were inversely associated with ECAD. On the basis of these data, a randomized, controlled clinical trial should be performed evaluating the effect of homocysteine-lowering vitamin therapy on ABI in elderly patients with increased plasma homocysteine levels and ECAD.

Mitral Annular Calcium and Protuding
Atheromas of Aortic Arch

Mitral annular calcium (MAC) is a risk factor for thromboembolic stroke and TIA.[47-50] In a prospective study of 928 elderly men and women, mean age 82 years, the prevalence of MAC was 1.4 times higher in patients with 40% to 100% ECAD (67%) than in patients without significant ECAD (47%).[49] In this study, at 45-month follow-up, the incidence of new thromboembolic stroke was 2.2 times higher in elderly patients with MAC than in elderly patients without MAC. The incidence of new thromboembolic stroke was 4.6 times higher in elderly patients with 40% to 100% ECAD and MAC than in elderly patients with no significant ECAD and no MAC.[49] The incidence of new TIA was 3.1 times higher in elderly patients with MAC than in elderly patients without MAC.[49] The incidence of new TIA was 8.0 times higher in elderly patients with 40% to 100% ECAD and MAC than in elderly patients with no significant ECAD and no MAC (Table 5).[49] In a study of 1,159 elderly patients in the Framingham Heart Study, at 8-year follow-up, the incidence of new cerebrovascular events was increased 2.7 times in elderly patients with MAC than in elderly patients without MAC.[50]

Using transesophageal echocardiography, Demopoulos et al[51] showed that protruding atheromas of the aortic arch were present in 17 of 45 patients (38%), mean age 70 years, with ≥50% ECAD and stroke or TIA within 6 weeks and in 7 of 45 control patients (16%) with a recent cerebral event, but without significant ECAD. Mobile protruding atheromas of the aortic arch which have the greatest potential for causing thromboembolic stroke were present in 6 of 45 patients (13%) with ≥50% ECAD, and in 1 of 45 control patients (2%). Therefore, in addition to MAC, protruding atheromas of the aortic arch may represent another etiology for thromboembolic stroke in elderly patients with significant ECAD.

Table 5

Incidence of New Thromboembolic Stroke and of New Cerebral Transient Ischemic Attack at 45-Month Follow-Up in 928 Elderly Patients With and Without 40% to 100% Extracranial Internal or Common Carotid Arterial Disease and With and Without Mitral Annular Calcium

	New TE Stroke	New TIA
ECAD and MAC	51%	8%
ECAD and no MAC	33%	6%
No ECAD and MAC	24%	3%
No ECAD and no MAC	11%	1%

TE = thromboembolic

TIA = transient ischemic attack

ECAD = extracranial carotid arterial disease

MAC = mitral annular calcium

(Adapted with permission from Reference 49.)

Symptoms and Signs

Patients with ECAD may be asymptomatic. However, they have an increased incidence of new ABI or new TIA at follow-up.[49,52-57] New ABI is diagnosed if the patient develops a sudden, focal neurological deficit lasting longer than 24 hours in the absence of a known source of embolism, bloody cerebrospinal fluid, known hypercoagulable conditions, or other diseases causing focal brain deficits.[49] ABI is diagnosed if the documented focal neurological deficit lasts longer than 24 hours and leaves residual or no residual focal neurological deficit. A careful neurological examination will show signs of a focal neurological deficit that conforms to the typical vascular distribution of an ABI. ABI should also be confirmed by computerized axial tomography or by a magnetic resonance imaging scan. TIA is diagnosed if the patient develops transient (<24 hours), contralateral (to the ECAD) hemiparesis or hemianesthesia, or transient ipsilateral blindness or visual field defect.[49] Symptoms suggestive of TIA due to ischemia caused by significant ECAD include recurrent unilateral weakness, recurrent unilateral sensory loss, dysarthria, transient monocular blindness, dysphasia, and rarely, homonymous hemianopsia.

Carotid Bruit

Systolic cervical bruits are associated with significant ECAD, transmitted systolic murmurs from aortic stenosis or dilation of the ascending aorta, hyperdynamic states such as thyrotoxicosis, fever, and anemia, tortuosity of the carotid vessels, and venous hums. Compression of the jugular vein low in the neck will obliterate a venous hum. In examining for carotid bruits, the physician should avoid causing a murmur by compressing the carotid artery. Carotid bruits are heard loudest in the midcervical region, whereas transmitted systolic murmurs are heard loudest at the base of the neck. The cross-sectional area of the carotid arterial lumen needs to be reduced by one half to two thirds for a carotid bruit to be heard. A systolic cervical bruit was detected in 43 of 64 elderly patients (67%) with 40% to 100% ECAD.[58]

In persons aged 50 to 84 years, free of stroke in the Framingham Heart Study, the age adjusted 2-year incidence of stroke was 3.6 times higher in women and 2.1 times higher in men with an asymptomatic carotid bruit than in women and men without a carotid bruit.[59] In a Mayo Clinic study, the incidence of ABI by actuarial analysis at 5 years was 7.5% in 566 patients, mean age 65 years, with an asymptomatic carotid bruit and 2.4% in 428 patients, mean age 64 years in a population-based cohort without a carotid bruit and free of cerebrovascular symptoms.[60] Therefore, patients with an asymptomatic carotid bruit in this study were 3.1 times more likely to develop ABI than those without a carotid bruit.[60]

Incidence of New Atherothombotic
Brain Infarction and Transient Cerebral
Ischemic Attack

Chambers and Norris[52] followed in a prospective study 500 asymptomatic patients, mean age 64 years, with cervical bruits. At 23-month follow-up, 22 of 113 patients (19%) with 75% to 100% ECAD (19 of whom had carotid endarterectomy) developed new ABI or TIA, 9 of 157 patients (6%) with 30% to 74% ECAD developed new ABI or TIA, and 5 of 230 patients (2%) with 0% to 29% ECAD developed new ABI or TIA.

Norris et al[30] followed in a prospective study 696 asymptomatic patients, mean age 64 years, with ECAD for 41 months. The annual percent rate of ABI was 3.3% for patients with 75% or greater ECAD, 1.3% for patients with 50% to 74% ECAD, and 1.3% for patients with less than 50% ECAD. The annual percent rate of TIA alone was 7.2% for patients with 75% or greater ECAD, 3.0% for patients with 50% to 74% ECAD, and 1.0% for patients with less than 50% ECAD.

In a prospective study of 949 elderly patients, mean age 82 years, 37 patients (4%) had 80% to 100% ECAD, 113 patients (12%) had 40% to 79% ECAD, and 799 patients (84%) had 0% to 39% ECAD.[57] The average annual incidence of new ABI was 37% at 2-year follow-up in elderly patients with 80% to 100% ECAD, 9% at 40-month follow-up in elderly patients with 40% to 79% ECAD, and 4% at 47-month follow-up in elderly patients with 0% to 39% ECAD (Table 6).[57] At follow-up, the average annual incidence of new TIA alone was 3% in elderly patients with 80% to 100% ECAD, 2% in elderly patients with 40% to 79% ECAD, and 1% in elderly patients with 0% to 39% ECAD (Table 7).[57]

Multivariate analysis showed that after controlling for other prognostic variables, patients with 80% to 100% ECAD have a 6.4 times higher chance of developing new ABI and an 8.0 times higher probability of developing new TIA alone than patients with 0% to 39% ECAD

Table 6

Incidence of New Atherothrombotic Brain Infarction in Elderly Patients With and Without Extracranial Carotid Arterial Disease

	No. of Patients	Follow-Up (months)	Average Annual Incidence of ABI
80% to 100% ECAD	37	24	37%
40% to 79% ECAD	113	40	9%
0% to 39% ECAD	799	47	4%

ABI = atherothrombotic brain infarction

ECAD = extracranial carotid arterial disease

(Adapted with permission from Reference 57.)

Table 7
Incidence of New Transient Cerebral Ischemic Attack Alone in Elderly Patients
With and Without Extracranial Carotid Arterial Disease

	No. of Patients	Follow-Up (months)	Average Annual Incidence of TIA Alone
80% to 100% ECAD	37	24	3%
40% to 79% ECAD	113	40	2%
0% to 39% ECAD	799	47	1%

TIA = transient ischemic attack
ECAD = extracranial carotid arterial disease
(Adapted with permission from Reference 57.)

(Table 8).[57] Patients with 80% to 100% ECAD have a 2.5 times higher probability of developing new ABI and a 2.8 times higher chance of developing new TIA alone than patients with 40% to 79% ECAD (Table 8).[57] Patients with 40% to 79% ECAD have a 2.5 times higher chance of developing new ABI and a 2.8 times higher probability of developing new TIA alone than patients with 0% to 39% ECAD (Table 8).[57] After controlling for other prognostic variables, patients with prior ABI have a 2.1 times higher probability of developing new ABI and a 1.9 times higher chance of developing new TIA alone than patients without prior ABI. Age was an independent prognostic variable for new ABI (relative risk = 1.04) and male sex an independent prognostic variable for new TIA alone (relative risk = 1.04).

Most strokes occur in patients without significant ECAD.[11,61] Although significant ECAD increased the incidence of new ABI or TIA

Table 8
Relative Risk for New Atherothrombotic Brain Infarction and Transient Cerebral Ischemic Attack Alone in Elderly Patients With and Without Extracranial Carotid Arterial Disease

	Relative Risk	
	New ABI	New TIA Alone
80% to 100% ECAD compared with 0% to 39% ECAD	6.4	8.0
80% to 100% ECAD compared with 40% to 79% ECAD	2.5	2.8
40% to 79% ECAD compared with 0% to 39% ECAD	2.5	2.8

ABI = atherothrombotic brain infarction
TIA = transient ischemic attack
ECAD = extracranial carotid arterial disease

alone, in a prospective study of 949 elderly patients,[57] 141 of 213 cerebrovascular events (66%) developed in elderly patients with no significant ECAD.[57]

In a prospective study of 208 elderly patients, mean age 81 years, with 40% to 100% ECAD, 69 patients (33%) had silent myocardial ischemia detected by 24-hour ambulatory electrocardiograms.[62] At 42-month follow-up, multivariate analysis showed that after controlling for other prognostic variables, patients with prior ABI have a 2.5 times higher probability of developing new ABI than those without prior ABI, and that patients with silent myocardial ischemia have a 2.1 times higher chance of developing new ABI than those without silent ischemia. Silent myocardial ischemia was an independent risk factor for new ABI in this study. This probably reflects that silent myocardial ischemia is a marker for more advanced or more significant atherosclerotic disease rather than a causal factor for ABI.

Incidence of New Coronary Events

Chambers and Norris[52] followed in a prospective study 500 asymptomatic patients, mean age 64 years, with cervical bruits. At 23-month follow-up, the incidence of new coronary events was 26% in patients with 75% or greater ECAD, 12% in patients with 30% to 74% ECAD, and 6% in patients with 0% to 29% ECAD (Table 9).

Norris et al[30] followed in a prospective study 696 asymptomatic patients, mean age 64 years, with ECAD for 41 months. The annual rate

Table 9
Incidence of New Coronary Events in Patients With and Without Extracranial Carotid Arterial Disease

	No. of Patients	Follow-Up	Incidence of New Coronary Events
Chambers and Norris[52]		23 months	
0% to 29% ECAD	230		6%
30% to 74% ECAD	157		12%
≥75% ECAD	113		26%
Norris et al[30]		Annual rate	
0% to 49% ECAD	303		2.7%
50% to 75% ECAD	216		6.6%
>75% ECAD	177		8.3%
Aronow and Schoenfeld[63]		45 months	
40% to 100% ECAD with CAD	87		80%
0% to 39% ECAD with CAD	314		60%
40% to 100% ECAD with no CAD	63		44%
0% to 39% ECAD with no CAD	485		27%

ECAD = extracranial carotid arterial disease

Table 10
Prognostic Variables for New Coronary Events in 161 Elderly Patients With
Extracranial Carotid Arterial Disease

Variables	Relative Risk
Silent ischemia	3.9
Prior ECAD	2.3
Serum HDL cholesterol	0.95
Cigarette smoking	1.9

ECAD = extracranial carotid arterial disease
(Adapted with permission from Reference 64.)

of new coronary events was 8.3% for patients with greater than 75% ECAD, 6.6% for patients with 50% to 75% ECAD, and 2.7% for patients with 0% to 49% ECAD (Table 9).[30]

Aronow and Schoenfeld[63] followed in a prospective study 949 elderly patients, mean age 82 years, for 45 months. The incidence of new coronary events was 80% for elderly patients with 40% to 100% ECAD with CAD, 60% for elderly patients with 0% to 39% ECAD with CAD, 44% for elderly patients with 40% to 100% ECAD with no CAD, and 27% for elderly patients with 0% to 39% ECAD with no CAD (Table 9). In elderly patients with no prior CAD, the incidence of new coronary events was 1.6 times higher in elderly patients with 40% to 100% ECAD than in elderly patients with no significant ECAD.[63] These studies[30, 52, 63] and others[53-55,59] demonstrated that new coronary events are the major cause of death in patients with significant ECAD.

In a prospective study of 161 elderly patients, mean age 81 years, with 40% to 100% ECAD, silent myocardial ischemia was detected by 24-hour ambulatory electrocardiograms in 56 of 161 patients (35%).[64] At 43-month follow-up, the incidence of new coronary events in elderly patients with prior CAD was 1.4 times higher in patients with silent ischemia (92%) than in patients without silent ischemia (67%). The incidence of new coronary events in patients with no prior CAD was 2.6 times higher in patients with silent ischemia (78%) than in patients without silent ischemia (30%). Table 10 shows that independent risk factors for new coronary events in elderly patients with 40% to 100% ECAD were: 1) silent myocardial ischemia (relative risk = 3.9); 2) prior CAD (relative risk = 2.3); 3) serum HDL cholesterol (inverse association), (relative risk = 0.95); and 4) cigarette smoking (relative risk = 1.9).

Antiplatelet Drugs

Risk factors for ECAD and CAD should be treated in elderly patients with significant ECAD as previously discussed. A meta-analysis by the Antiplatelet Trialists' Collaboration included 145 randomized trials of antiplatelet versus control therapy in about 70,000 high-risk patients and about 30,000 low-risk patients, and 29 randomized comparisons between antiplatelet regimens in about 10,000 high-risk patients.[65] By 3 years, about 40 vascular events (stroke, MI, or vascular death) were prevented per 1000 patients treated with aspirin. In patients with stroke or TIA, aspirin reduced the risk of nonfatal stroke by 25%. Aspirin was equally effective in reducing stroke, MI, or vascular death in doses ranging from 30 mg to 1,300 mg per day. The efficacy of aspirin versus ticlodipine was similar.

A comparison of high-dose aspirin (1,200 mg daily) versus medium-dose aspirin (300 mg daily)[66] and of medium-dose aspirin (283 mg per day) versus low-dose aspirin (30 mg per day)[67] also showed no differences among the different aspirin doses in causing reduction of stroke, MI, and vascular death in patients after a minor stroke or TIA. However, a 900 mg daily dose of aspirin has been shown to slow carotid plaque growth more than did 50 mg daily dose.[68] Additional studies are needed to determine the optimal dose of aspirin necessary to slow carotid plaque growth. Until the results of these studies are available, an aspirin dose of 325 mg daily is recommended.

On the basis of the available data, I would not use the antiplatelet drugs sulfinpyrazone or dipyridamole alone or in combination with aspirin to prevent ABI or TIA, MI, or vascular death in patients with significant ECAD.[65] However, 250 mg of ticlopidine hydrochloride two times per day may be used to decrease the risk of fatal or nonfatal ABI in patients with significant ECAD who are unable to tolerate aspirin therapy or who develop cerebrovascular events on aspirin therapy.[69]

References

1. Thiele BL, Young JV, Chikos PM, et al: Correlation of arteriographic findings and symptoms in cerebrovascular disease. *Neurology* 30:1041-1046, 1980.
2. Moore WS, Hall AD: Importance of emboli from carotid bifurcation in pathogenesis of cerebral ischemic attacks. *Arch Surg* 101:708-711, 1970.
3. Imparato AM, Riles TS, Mintzer K, et al: The importance of hemorrhage in the relationship between gross morphologic characteristics and cerebral symptoms in 376 carotid artery plaques. *Ann Surg* 197:195-203, 1983.
4. Lusby RJ, Ferrell LD, Ehrenfeld WK, et al: Carotid plaque hemorrhage: its role in production of cerebral ischemia. *Arch Surg* 117:1479-1488, 1982.
5. Weinberger J, Ramos L, Ambrose JA, et al: Morphologic and dynamic changes of atherosclerotic plaque at the carotid artery bifurcation: sequential imaging by real time B-mode ultrasonography. *J Am Coll Cardiol* 12:1515-1521, 1988.
6. Health and Public Policy Committee, American College of Physicians: Diagnostic evaluation of the carotid arteries. *Ann Intern Med* 109:835-837, 1988.
7. Aronow WS, Kronzon I, Schoenfeld MR: Prevalence of extracranial carotid arterial disease and of valvular aortic stenosis and their association in the elderly. *Am J Cardiol* 75:304-305, 1995.
8. O'Leary DH, Anderson KM, Wolf PA, et al: Cholesterol and carotid atherosclerosis in older persons: the Framingham Study. *Ann Epidemiol* 2:147-153, 1992.

9. Caplan LR, Gorelick PB, Hier DB: Race, sex, and occlusive cerebrovascular disease: a review. *Stroke* 17:648-655, 1986.
10. Heyman A, Fields WS, Keating RD: Joint study of extracranial arterial occlusion: VI. Racial differences in hospitalized patients with ischemic stroke. *JAMA* 222:285-289, 1972.
11. Aronow WS, Schoenfeld MR: Prevalence of atherothrombotic brain infarction and extracranial carotid arterial disease, and their association in elderly blacks, Hispanics, and whites. *Am J Cardiol* 71:999-1000, 1993.
12. Candelise L, Bianchi F, Galligoni F, et al: Italian multicenter study on reversible cerebral ischemic attacks: III. Influence of age and risk factors on cerebrovascular atherosclerosis. *Stroke* 15:379-382, 1984.
13. Ford CS, Crouse JR III, Howard G, et al: The role of plasma lipids in carotid bifurcation atherosclerosis. *Ann Neurol* 17:301-303, 1985.
14. Crouse JR III, Toole JF, McKinney WM: Risk factors for extracranial carotid artery atherosclerosis. *Stroke* 18:990-996, 1987
15. Aronow WS, Schoenfeld MR, Paul P: Risk factors for extracranial internal or common carotid arterial disease in persons aged 60 years and older. *Am J Cardiol* 63:881-882, 1989.
16. Tell GS, Howard G, McKinney WM, et al: Cigarette smoking cessation and extracranial carotid atherosclerosis. *JAMA* 261:1178-1180, 1989.
17. Bots ML, Breslau BJ, Briet E, et al: Cardiovascular determinants of carotid artery disease: the Rotterdam Elderly Study. *Hypertension* 19:717-720, 1992.
18. Prati P, Vanuzzo D, Casaroli M, et al: Prevalence and determinants of carotid atherosclerosis in a general population. *Stroke* 23:1705-1711, 1992.
19. Aronow WS, Ahn C, Schoenfeld MR: Risk factors for extracranial internal or common carotid arterial disease in elderly patients. *Am J Cardiol* 71:1479-1481, 1993.
20. Tell GS, Polak JF, Ward BJ, et al: Relation of smoking with carotid artery wall thickness and stenosis in older adults: the Cardiovascular Health Study. *Circulation* 90:2905-2908, 1994.
21. Rubens J, Espeland MA, Ryu J, et al: Individual variation in susceptibility to extracranial carotid atherosclerosis. *Arteriosclerosis* 8:389-397, 1988.
22. Salonen R, Seppanen K, Rauramaa R, et al: Prevalence of carotid atherosclerosis and serum cholesterol levels in Eastern Finland. *Arteriosclerosis* 8:788-792, 1988.
23. Blankenhorn DH, Selzer RH, Crawford DW, et al: Beneficial effects of colestipol-niacin therapy on the common carotid artery: two- and four-year reduction of intima-media thickness measured by ultrasound. *Circulation* 88:20-28, 1993.
24. Furberg CD, Adams HP, Applegate WB, et al: Effect of lovastatin on early carotid atherosclerosis and cardiovascular events. *Circulation* 90:1679-1687, 1994.
25. Crouse JR III, Byington RP, Bond MG, et al: Pravastatin, lipids, and atherosclerosis in the carotid arteries (PLAC-II). *Am J Cardiol* 75:455-459, 1995.
26. Scandinavian Simvastatin Survival Study Group: Randomised trial of cholesterol lowering in 4444 patients with coronary heart disease: the Scandinavian Simvastatin Survival Study (4S). *Lancet* 344:1383-1389, 1994.
27. Aronow WS, Gutstein H, Lee NH, et al: Three-year follow-up of risk factors correlated with new atherothrombotic brain infarction in 708 elderly patients. *Angiology* 39:563-566, 1988.
28. Duncan WG, Lees RS, Ojemann RG, et al: Concomitants of atherosclerotic carotid artery stenosis. *Stroke* 8:665-669, 1977.
29. Bogousslavsky J, Regli F, Van Melle G: Risk factors and concomitants of internal carotid artery occlusion or stenosis: a controlled study of 159 cases. *Arch Neurol* 42:864-867, 1985.

30. Norris JW, Zhu CZ, Bornstein NM, et al: Vascular risks of asymptomatic carotid stenosis. *Stroke* 22:1485-1490, 1991.
31. Aronow WS, Kronzon I, Schoenfeld MR: Left ventricular hypertrophy is more prevalent in patients with systemic hypertension with extracranial carotid arterial disease than in patients with systemic hypertension without extracranial carotid arterial disease. *Am J Cardiol* 76:192-193, 1995.
32. Harrison MJG, Wilson LA: Effect of blood pressure on prevalence of carotid atheroma. *Stroke* 14:550-551, 1983.
33. National Heart Foundation of Australia Study: Treatment of mild hypertension in the elderly: report by the management committee. *Med J Austr* 2:398-402, 1981.
34. Amery A, Birkenhager W, Brixko P, et al: Mortality and morbidity results from the European Working Party on High Blood Pressure in the Elderly Trial. *Lancet* 1:1349-1354, 1985.
35. Coope J, Warrender TS: Randomised trial of treatment of hypertension in elderly patients in primary care. *Br Med J* 293:1145-1151, 1986.
36. Dahlof B, Lindholm LH, Hansson L, et al: Morbidity and mortality in the Swedish Trial in Old Patients with Hypertension (STOP-Hypertension). *Lancet* 338:1281-1285, 1991.
37. MRC Working Party: Medical Research Council trial of treatment of hypertension in older adults: principal results. *Br Med J* 304:405-412, 1992.
38. SHEP Cooperative Research Group: Prevention of stroke by antihypertensive drug treatment in older persons with isolated systolic hypertension: final results of the Systolic Hypertension in the Elderly Program (SHEP). *JAMA* 265:3255-3264, 1991.
39. Aronow WS, Koenigsberg M, Schwartz KS: Usefulness of echocardiographic left ventricular hypertrophy in predicting new coronary events and atherothrombotic brain infarction in patients over 62 years of age. *Am J Cardiol* 61:1130-1132, 1988.
40. Aronow WS, Koenigsberg M, Schwartz KS: Usefulness of echocardiographic and electrocardiographic left ventricular hypertrophy in predicting new cardiac events and atherothrombotic brain infarction in elderly patients with systemic hypertension or coronary artery disease. *Am J Noninvas Cardiol* 3:367-370, 1989.
41. Aronow WS, Ahn C, Kronzon I, et al: Congestive heart failure, coronary events, and atherothrombotic brain infarction in elderly blacks and whites with systemic hypertension and with and without echocardiographic and electrocardiographic evidence of left ventricular hypertrophy. *Am J Cardiol* 67:295-299, 1991.
42. Bikkina M, Levy D, Evans JC, et al: Left ventricular mass and risk of stroke in an elderly cohort: The Framingham Heart Study. *JAMA* 272:33-36, 1994.
43. Roman MJ, Pickering TG, Schwartz JE, et al: Association of carotid atherosclerosis and left ventricular hypertrophy. *J Am Coll Cardiol* 25:83-90, 1995.
44. Dahlof B, Pennert K, Hansson L: Reversal of left ventricular hypertrophy in hypertensive patients: a metaanalysis of 109 treatment studies. *Am J Hypertens* 5:95-110, 1992.
45. Craven TE, Ryu JE, Espeland MA, et al: Evaluation of the associations between carotid artery atherosclerosis and coronary artery stenosis: a case-control study. *Circulation* 82:1230-1242, 1990.
46. Selhub J, Jacques PF, Bostom AG, et al: Association between plasma homocysteine concentrations and extracranial carotid-artery stenosis. *N Engl J Med* 332:286-291, 1995
47. Aronow WS, Koenigsberg M, Kronzon I, et al: Association of mitral anular calcium with new thromboembolic stroke and cardiac events at 39-month follow-up in elderly patients. *Am J Cardiol* 65:1511-1512, 1990.

48. Boston Area Anticoagulation Trial for Atrial Fibrillation Investigators: The effect of low-dose warfarin on the risk of stroke in patients with nonrheumatic atrial fibrillation *N Engl J Med* 323:1505-1511, 1990.

49. Aronow WS, Schoenfeld MR, Gutstein H: Frequency of thromboembolic stroke in persons ≥60 years of age with extracranial carotid arterial disease and/or mitral anular calcium. *Am J Cardiol* 70:123-124, 1992.

50. Benjamin EJ, Plehn JF, D'Agostino RB, et al: Mitral annular calcification and the risk of stroke in an elderly cohort. *N Engl J Med* 327:374-379, 1992.

51. Demopoulos LA, Tunick PA, Bernstein NE, et al: Protruding atheromas of the aortic arch in symptomatic patients with carotid artery disease. *Am Heart J* 129:40-44, 1995.

52. Chambers BR, Norris JW: Outcome in patients with symptomatic neck bruits. *N Engl J Med* 315:860-865, 1986.

53. Hennerici M, Hulsbomer HB, Rautenberg W, et al: Spontaneous history of asymptomatic internal carotid occlusion. *Stroke* 17:718-722, 1986.

54. Bogousslavsky J, Despland PA, Regli F: Asymptomatic tight stenosis of the internal carotid artery: long-term prognosis. *Neurology* 36:861-863, 1986.

55. Ford S, Frye JL, Toole JF et al: Asymptomatic carotid bruit and stenosis: a prospective follow-up study. *Arch Neurol* 43:219-222, 1986.

56. Schoenfeld MR, Aronow WS, Paul P: A prospective study of the neurologic outcome of carotid stenoses amongst the elderly. *J Cardiovasc Tech* 8:117-120, 1989.

57. Aronow WS, Ahn C, Schoenfeld M, et al: Extracranial carotid arterial disease: a prognostic factor for atherothrombotic brain infarction and cerebral transient ischemic attack. *NY State J Med* 92:424-425, 1992.

58. Schoenfeld MR, Aronow WS, Paul P: Are systolic cervical bruits clinically significant findings in the elderly? *J Cardiovasc Ultrasonog* 6:269-271, 1987.

59. Wolf PA, Kannel WB, Sorlie P, et al: Asymptomatic carotid bruit and risk of stroke: The Framingham Study. *JAMA* 245:1442-1445, 1981.

60. Wiebers DO, Whisnant JP, Sandok BA, et al: Prospective comparison of a cohort with asymptomatic carotid bruit and a population-based cohort without carotid bruit. *Stroke* 21:984-988, 1990.

61. Schoenfeld MR, Aronow WS, Paul P: Are strokes more likely to result from severe carotid atherosclerotic stenoses? If not, why not? *Angiology* 39:720-724, 1988.

62. Aronow WS, Ahn C, Mercando AD, et al: Association of silent myocardial ischemia with new atherothrombotic brain infarction in older patients with extracranial internal or common carotid arterial disease with and without previous atherothrombotic brain infarction. *J Am Geriatr Soc* 43:1272-1274, 1995.

63. Aronow WS, Schoenfeld MR: Forty-five-month follow-up of extracranial carotid arterial disease for new coronary events in elderly patients. *Coronary Artery Dis* 3:249-251, 1992.

64. Aronow WS, Ahn C, Schoenfeld MR, et al: Prognostic significance of silent myocardial ischemia in patients >61 years of age with extracranial internal or common carotid arterial disease with and without previous myocardial infarction. *Am J Cardiol* 71:115-117, 1993.

65. Antiplatelet Trialists' Collaboration: Collaborative overview of randomized trials of antiplatelet therapy: I. prevention of death, myocardial infarction, and stroke by prolonged antiplatelet therapy in various categories of patients. *Br Med J* 308:81-106, 1994.

66. UK-TIA Study Group: United Kingdom Transient Ischaemic Attack (UK-TIA) aspirin trial: interim results. *Br Med J* 296:316-320, 1988.

67. The Dutch TIA Trial Study Group: A comparison of two doses of aspirin (30 mg vs 283 mg a day) in patients after a transient ischemic attack or minor ischemic stroke. *N Eng J Med* 325:1261-1266, 1991.
68. Ranke C, Hecker H, Creutzig A, et al: Dose-dependent effect of aspirin on carotid atherosclerosis. *Circulation* 87:1873-1879, 1993.
69. Hass WK, Easton JD, Adams HP Jr, et al: A randomized trial comparing ticlopidine hydrochloride with aspirin for the prevention of stroke in high-risk patients. *N Engl J Med* 321:501-507, 1989.

Chapter 14

Carotid Endarterectomy in the Elderly

Samuel Eric Wilson, MD
Patrick Yoon, MD

Carotid endarterectomy is commonly performed for prophylaxis against stroke in patients with severe atherosclerotic stenosis of the internal carotid artery. The prevalence of this procedure in the United States peaked at 103,000 operations in 1984, dropping to 70,000 in 1989.[1,2] The number of patients undergoing endarterectomy is now increasing, after long-standing controversy regarding its effectiveness was settled by the results of several large scale clinical trials, including the North American Symptomatic Carotid Endarterectomy Trial (NASCET), the European Carotid Surgery Trial (ECST), the Veterans Administration Cooperative Studies 309 and 167 (VA 309 and 167), and the Asymptomatic Carotid Atherosclerosis Study (ACAS).[3-7] Although these trials confirmed the efficacy of carotid endarterectomy for both symptomatic and asymptomatic patients with severe carotid stenosis, the procedure must be performed with acceptable perioperative morbidity and mortality rates in order for patients to derive benefit. However, morbidity and mortality varies; the combined mortality and stroke morbidity in the European study was 7.5% compared to 5.6% in the VA 309 study.[4,5] In asymptomatic disease, the mortality and morbidity is lowest as seen in the ACAS study with a total of 2.3%.[7] The frequency in performing carotid endarterectomy also varies, by as much as threefold between areas within the United States, and by as much as twentyfold between the United States and Great Britain.[1] With the variation in both mortality/morbidity, as well as the different rates of operation, special consideration is required in evaluation of older patients undergoing this procedure. Accordingly, in managing older patients with carotid stenosis, whether symptomatic or asymptomatic, the referring physicians and surgeons must have assurance that the symptoms warrant operation,

From: Aronow WS, Stemmer EA, Wilson SE (eds). *Vascular Disease in the Elderly.* Armonk, NY: Futura Publishing Company, Inc., © 1997.

or that the patients' risk status is good enough to recommend operation for stenosis without symptoms.

The elderly population has the highest risk for developing stroke, and among those over 65, the annual death rate from stroke is some 394 per 100,000 population.[8] Moreover, the elderly is the fastest growing segment in our society; from 1995 to 2005, there will be a projected increase of 24% in the age group over 75 (from 14.7 million to 18.3 million).[8] In carefully selected elderly patients, carotid endarterectomy may provide prophylaxis against stroke. However, because older patients are already at greater risk for perioperative mortality and morbidity, one must be discriminating in choosing elderly patients who are fit enough to undergo carotid endarterectomy. With careful selection, one may achieve acceptably low operative mortality and morbidity rates in the elderly, even comparable to the 4.3% and the 2.3% of the VA 167 and ACAS studies, in which the patients' mean ages were 64.1 and 67 years, respectively.[6,7]

Indications

The indications for carotid endarterectomy in the elderly should generally follow those recognized for the population at large. Specific indications for endarterectomy were finally established in relatively recent years (considering the procedure has been performed since the 1960s).[3-7] Carotid endarterectomy prevents subsequent ipsilateral stroke in symptomatic patients with internal carotid stenosis over 70%. Indications have generally been accepted to include hemispheric symptoms, namely transient ischemic attack (TIA), reversible ischemic neurological deficit (RIND), small completed stroke, amaurosis fugax, or stroke in progress in carefully selected patients. Nonhemispheric symptoms, such as dizziness, vertigo, or headache, should be viewed with caution. For patients with hemispheric symptoms, the benefits of operation are clear; subsequent stroke rates for surgically versus medically treated patients were found to be 7.7% versus 19.4% at 11.9 months for stenosis greater than 50% (VA 309); 10.3% versus 16.8% at 36 months for stenosis greater than 70% (ECST); and 9% versus 26% at 24 months for stenosis greater than 70% (NASCET).[3-5] For patients with significant carotid stenosis but without symptoms, selection must be somewhat more restricted. After several other studies failed to conclusively prove the benefits of surgery, the ACAS trial established that for asymptomatic patients with stenosis greater than 60%, surgery reduces the risk of ipsilateral stroke provided that operative morbidity and mortality are held to less than 3%.[7,8]

Special Considerations for Elderly Patients

For elderly patients, the difference in indications for carotid endarterectomy must be tempered by the increased operative risk. Another concern is that older patients have fewer years of life left and, therefore, less to gain from the procedure, especially when weighed against peri-operative mortality. However, the life expectancy of older patients should not be underestimated. As of 1990, the remaining life expectancy was 10.9 years at age 75 and 8.3 years at age 80, so it is clear that elderly patients stand to gain from the procedure if the surgical risk is acceptably low. In fact, the fit patient at age 80 may have a longer life expectancy than a patient 20 years younger who has risk factors such as heavy tobacco use or diabetes mellitus.[9]

Older patients tend to have significant concomitant morbidity; therefore, surgical judgment must be refined. The incidence of diabetes mellitus, congestive heart failure (CHF), chronic obstructive pulmonary disease (COPD), and hypertension all increase with age.[10,11] Moreover, prior myocardial infarction (MI), associated with higher operative risk if within the previous 6 months, is prevalent in 10% of men and 5% of women over 65 years.[11] Older patients have been shown to have higher operative mortality and morbidity after other cardiovascular pro-cedures, including coronary artery bypass graft and peripheral vascular reconstruction[12-14] MI, along with postoperative stroke, constitutes the majority of postcarotid endarterectomy mortality. Carotid endarterec-tomy, angina, CHF, COPD, hypertension, and MI experienced within the previous 6 months, were all correlated with an increase in incidence of postoperative MI after carotid endarterectomy.[12] The increase in oper-ative risk in the elderly may not only be due to concomitant disease; age over 70 itself as an independent risk factor was correlated with postoperative MI for a wide variety of major surgical procedures.[12,15]

The risks and benefits of surgery for elderly patients with asymp-tomatic carotid stenosis and significant concomitant disease pose a major challenge to surgical judgment. On the one hand, operative mor-tality and morbidity should be kept to less than 3% considering the patient is asymptomatic; on the other hand, significant medical condi-tions may push the risk of postoperative MI, stroke, or death to 7%.[12] Among patients of the Cleveland Vascular Registry, the overall com-bined mortality and morbidity rates for carotid endarterectomy fell somewhere in between, with 4.3% for patients younger than 75 and 5.5% for those over 75.[13]

The decision is further complicated by the prevalence in the elderly of cerebrovascular disease due to other etiologies, such as lacunar infarct or vertebrobasilar disease. Lacunar infarct has been shown not to be due to carotid embolization, but rather to intracerebral small vessel vasculopathy.[16] The presence of vertebrobasilar disease can result in such symptoms as dysarthria, dysphagia, diplopia, nystagmus, visual field defects, hoarseness, ataxia, and even syncope.[17] Combinations of these symptoms may not be due to carotid disease, and distinguishing the two etiologies can be confusing. For nonhemispheric symptoms, Ouriel et al suggested that endarterectomy may actually be indicated if ocular pneumoplethysmography (OPG) indicates a hemodynamically significant carotid lesion.[18] Nonhemispheric symptoms, such as vertigo, lightheadedness, and blurry vision in these patients were presumably due to generalized hypoperfusion rather than embolus.

Preoperative evaluation of elderly patients must be performed carefully because of the increased surgical risk due to concomitant disease, and the prevalence of symptoms caused by cerebrovascular disease other than classic carotid bifurcation stenosis or plaque.

Review of the Literature

Thirteen studies of carotid endarterectomy in the elderly, published between 1981 and 1994, have been reviewed and the pertinent results from each detailed in Table 1.[13,19-30] Age cutoffs for defining elderly patients varied among the studies (70-, 75-, or 80-years-old). Among those studies which also included a series of younger patients below the age cutoff, none showed a statistically significant difference between younger and older patients in either mortality or postoperative stroke. The results analyzed in these studies are corroborated by others which failed to find any correlation between age and mortality/morbidity following carotid endarterectomy.[31,32] However, when the individual studies are grouped by the age cutoff (>70, >75, >80) used to define *elderly*, there is a statistically significant increase in combined mortality and morbidity for the over 75 group (Table 2). No increase in risk for the elderly was found when greater than 70 or 80 was used as a cutoff.

The failure of individual studies to find a difference in mortality and morbidity rates between younger and older patients has been attributed to various factors. Several studies, rather than being comprehensive in nature, are reports from individual referral centers with uniform surgical techniques and wise patient selection by a limited number of surgeons who have great familiarity with performing the procedure. An additional, though no less important, factor is the inherent difference between carotid endarterectomy and other surgical procedures. Loftus et al cited the relatively less postoperative pain involved in endarterectomy, resulting in decreased postoperative respiratory impairment and pulmonary complications.[25] Morgan et al postulated that surgery in the head and neck region, in general, poses less of a threat to elderly patients than does surgery in other regions of the body.[33] These arguments may well explain the consistently low surgical risk for elderly patients undergoing carotid endarterectomy relative to other surgical procedures. It appears that several other risk factors play a more significant role than does age in postoperative morbidity and mortality. Sundt et al found a much higher death rate, often as high as 10%, among those patients operated for stroke in progress, multiple MI, or daily TIA; these patients were also found to sustain a prolonged postoperative recovery.[12]

Although some reports show a significant decrease in mortality and morbidity rates over the years the individual study was conducted, no significant change over time was observed to correlate with publication dates when all studies are considered (Table 3). Presumably, this

Table 1
Summary of Carotid Endarterectomy Morbidity and Mortality Rates in Younger Versus Elderly Patients

			Study Size		Morbity		Mortality		Morbidity + Mortality		
Author	Year	Cutoff	Young	Elderly	Young	Elderly	Young	Elderly	Young	Elderly	Significant Difference?
Benhamou	1981	>70		220		8 (3.6)		8 (3.6)		16 (7.3)	
Brott	1984	>70	307	124	32	5 (4.0)	8 (2.6)	4 (3.2)	40 (13)	9 (7.3)	No
		>80	412	19	36 (8.7)	1 (5.3)	12 (2.9)	0 (0)	48 (11.7)	1 (5.3)	No
Courbier	1985	>75		76		2 (2.6)		1 (1.3)		3 (3.9)	
Plecha	1985	>75	5220	782	94 (1.8)	17 (2.2)	77 (1.5)	18 (2.3)	171 (3.3)	35 (4.5)	No
Ouriel	1986	>75	393	77	12 (3.1)	3 (3.9)	2 (0.5)	0 (0)	14 (3.6)	3 (3.9)	No
Rosenthal	1986	>80	1008	90	20 (2.0)	4 (4.4)	6 (0.6)	2 (2.2)	26 (2.6)	6 (6.7)	No
Schultz	1988	>80		116		1 (0.9)		2 (1.7)		3 (2.6)	
Loftus	1988	>70		53		1 (1.9)		0 (0)		1 (1.9)	
Schroe	1990	>70	483	222	20 (4.1)	7 (3.2)	8 (1.7)	3 (1.4)	28 (5.8)	10 (4.5)	No
Pinkerton	1990	>75	560	125	2 (0.4)	0 (0)	5 (0.9)	1 (0.8)	7 (1.3)	1 (0.8)	No
Meyer	1991	>70		749		23 (3.1)		10 (1.3)		33 (4.4)	
		>75		265		10 (3.8)		4 (1.5)		14 (5.3)	
		>80		56		3 (5.4)		0 (0)		3 (5.4)	
Treiman	1992	>80		183		3 (1.6)		3 (1.6)		6 (3.3)	
Coyle	1994	>80	992	79	26 (2.6)	0 (0)	16 (1.6)	1 (1.3)	42 (4.2)	1 (1.3)	No

Morbidity indicates postoperative stroke ipsilateral to endarterectomy. For morbidity and mortality, percentages are shown in parentheses. *Young* and *Elderly* refer to patients below and above the age cutoff for each particular study. *Study Size* indicates number of procedures performed. None of the differences in combined morbidity and mortality rates between young and elderly patients were statistically significant ($p < 0.05$).

Table 2
Carotid Endarterectomy Morbidity and Mortality: Studies Grouped by Age Cutoff

Age Cutoff	No. of compiled	Total No. of Young Patients	Total No. of Elderly Patients	Morbidity		Mortality		Morbidity + Mortality	
				Young	Elderly	Young	Elderly	Young	Elderly
>70	5	790	1368	52 (6.6)	44 (3.2)	16 (2.0)	25 (1.8)	68 (8.6)	69 (5.0)
>75	5	6173	1325	108 (1.7)	32 (2.4)	84 (1.4)	24 (1.8)	192 (3.1)	56 (4.2)
>80	6	2412	543	82 (3.4)	12 (2.2)	34 (1.4)	8 (1.5)	116 (4.8)	20 (3.6)

Number of compiled studies totals to >13, because several studies listed results by more than one age cutoff. Italicized figures indicate statistical significance.

Table 3
Carotid Endarterectomy Morbidity and Mortality by Year of Study Publication

5-Year	Number of Studies Compiled	Total Procedures	Morbidity	Mortality	Morbidity + Mortality
1981–85	4	6729	158 (2.3)	116 (1.7)	274 (4.1)
1986–90	6	3127	70 (2.2)	29 (0.9)	99 (3.2)
1991–95	3	2003	52 (2.6)	30 (1.5)	82 (4.1)

may be because of the wide variation among studies in how many years were reviewed retrospectively.

Conclusion

Age over 65 was once considered a high-risk threshold for performing carotid endarterectomy. Over the last 20 years, the age limit for successful carotid endarterectomy has been extended progressively higher; in fact, many reports fail to show significant difference in perioperative mortality and morbidity rate between younger and older patients. Age itself should not be the sole discriminating factor in weighing the value of the procedure for clear-cut symptoms or high-grade asymptomatic stenosis. Nevertheless, one must still be more selective in choosing which elderly patients are eligible to undergo carotid endarterectomy. To minimize mortality and morbidity in elderly patients, the clinical workup must be performed more carefully, and operative risk factors such as previous stroke and myocardial disease identified. If these caveats are followed, prevention of ischemic or embolic stroke can greatly enhance the quality of life for this enlarging segment of our population.

References

1. Cebul RD, Whisnant JP: Carotid endarterectomy. *Ann Intern Med* 111:660-670, 1989.
2. Easton JD, Wilterdink JL: Carotid endarterectomy: trials and tribulations. *Ann Neurol* 35:5-17, 1994.
3. North American Symptomatic Carotid Endarterectomy Trial Collaborators: Beneficial effect of carotid endarterectomy in symptomatic patients with high-grade carotid stenosis. *N Engl J Med* 325:445-453, 1991.
4. European Carotid Surgery Trialist's Collaborative Group: MRC European Carotid Surgery Trial: Interim results for symptomatic patients with severe (70%-99%) or with mild (0%-29%) carotid stenosis. *Lancet* 337:1235-1243, 1991.
5. Mayberg MR, Wilson SE, Yatsu F, et al: Carotid endarterectomy and prevention of cerebral ischemia in symptomatic carotid stenosis. *JAMA* 266:3289-3294, 1991.
6. Hobson RW II, Weiss DG, Fields WS, et al: Efficacy of carotid endarterectomy for asymptomatic carotid stenosis. *N Engl J Med* 328:221-227, 1993.

7. Executive Committee for the Asymptomatic Carotid Atherosclerosis Study: Endarterectomy for asymptomatic carotid artery stenosis. *JAMA* 273:1421-1428, 1995.
8. Moore WS, Barnett HJM, Beebe HG, et al: Guidelines for carotid endarterectomy. *Circulation* 91:566-579, 1995.
9. US Bureau of the Census: *Statistical Abstract of the United States.* 114th Ed. Washington, DC: Department of Commerce; 24,88,95, 1994.
10. Chalfin DB, Nasraway SA II: Preoperative evaluation and postoperative care of the elderly patient undergoing major surgery. *Clin Ger Med* 10:51-70, 1994.
11. Weitz HH: Noncardiac surgery in the elderly patient with cardiovascular disease. *Clin Ger Med* 6:511-529, 1990.
12. Sundt TM, Sandok BA, Whisnant JP: Carotid endarterectomy: complications and preoperative assessment of risk. *Mayo Clin Proc* 50:301-306, 1975.
13. Plecha FR, Bertin VJ, Plecha EJ, et al: The early results of vascular surgery in patients 75 years of age and older: an analysis of 3259 cases. *J Vasc Surg* 2:769-774, 1985.
14. Kuan P, Bernstein SB, Ellestad MH: Coronary artery bypass surgery morbidity. *J Am Coll Cardiol* 3:1391-1397, 1984.
15. Goldman L, Caldera DL, Nussbaum SR, et al: Multifactorial index of cardiac risk in noncardiac surgical procedures. *N Engl J Med* 297:845-850, 1977.
16. Tegeler CH, Shi F, Morgan T: Carotid stenosis in lacunar stroke. *Stroke* 22:1124-1128, 1991.
17. Donayre CE, Wilson SE, Hobson RW II: Extracranial carotid artery occlusive disease. In: Veith FJ, Hobson RW, Williams RA, et al (eds). *Vascular Surgery: Principles and Practice.* 2nd Ed. New York: McGraw-Hill; 649-664, 1994.
18. Ouriel K, Ricotta JJ, Green RM, et al: Carotid endarterectomy for nonhemispheric cerebral symptoms: patient selection with ocular pneumoplethysmography. *J Vasc Surg* 4:115-118, 1986.
19. Benhamou AC, Kieffer E, Tricot JF, et al: Carotid artery surgery in patients over 70 years of age. *Int Surg* 66:199-202, 1981.
20. Brott T, Thalinger K: The practice of carotid endarterectomy in a large metropolitan area. *Stroke* 15:950-955, 1984.
21. Courbier R, Ferdani M, Reggi M: Carotid stenosis: surgery after 75 years. *Int Angiol* 4:295-299, 1985.
22. Ouriel K, Penn TE, Ricotta JJ, et al: Carotid endarterectomy in the elderly patient. *Surg Gyn Obstet* 162:334-336, 1986.
23. Rosenthal D, Rudderman RH, Jones DH, et al: Carotid endarterectomy in the octogenarian: is it appropriate? *J Vasc Surg* 3:782-787, 1986.
24. Schultz RD, Sterpetti AV, Feldhaus RJ: Carotid endarterectomy in octogenarians and nonagernarians. *Surg Gyn Obstet* 166:245-251, 1988.
25. Loftus CM, Biller J, Godersky JC, et al: Carotid endarterectomy in symptomatic elderly patients. *Neurosurgery* 22:676-680, 1988.
26. Schroe H, Suy R, Nevelsteen A: Carotid artery endarterectomy in patients over seventy years of age. *Ann Vasc Surg* 4:133-137, 1990.
27. Pinkerton JA, Gholkar VR: Should patient age be a consideration in carotid endarterectomy? *J Vasc Surg* 11:650-658, 1990.
28. Meyer FB, Meissner I, Fode NC, et al: Carotid endarterectomy in elderly patients. *Mayo Clin Proc* 66:464-469, 1991.
29. Treiman RL, Wagner WH, Foran RF, et al: Carotid endarterectomy in the elderly. *Ann Vasc Surg* 6:321-324, 1992.
30. Coyle KA, Smith RB III, Salam AA, et al: Carotid endarterectomy in the octogenarian. *Ann Vasc Surg* 8:417-420, 1994.

31. Richardson JD, Main KA: Carotid endarterectomy in the elderly population: a statewide experience. *J Vasc Surg* 9:65-73, 1989.
32. Brook RH, Park RE, Chassin MR, et al: Carotid endarterectomy for elderly patients: predicting complications. *Ann Intern Med* 113:747-753, 1990.
33. Morgan RF, Hirata RM, Jaques DA, et al: Head and neck surgery in the aged. *Am J Surg* 144:449-451, 1982.

Chapter 15

Clinical Characteristics and Diagnosis of Coronary Artery Disease in Older Patients

Donald D. Tresch, MD
Wilbert S. Aronow, MD

Coronary artery disease (CAD) is one of the most common disorders in older people, and autopsy studies show that at least 70% of older patients demonstrate CAD.[1,2] In many of these older patients, the findings of coronary atherosclerosis is coincidental with the patients free of CAD symptoms. The majority of older patients with CAD, however, have clinically manifested the disease much earlier in life, although in some older patients, this disease is clinically silent until the eighth or ninth decade of life. Despite this high prevalence of CAD and the presence of clinical manifestations, the disease unfortunately may not be diagnosed or is misdiagnosed in many older persons. In other older patients, the disease is not diagnosed until death, which in a percent of older persons, is sudden; or the diagnosis is not made until the disease is end stage with the older patient's symptoms refractory to therapy. Failure to correctly diagnose CAD in older patients may be due to the difference in clinical manifestation of the disease in this age group compared to younger patients. Such differences may reflect a difference in the disease processes between older and younger patients, or it may be related to the superimposition of normal aging change, plus the presence of concomitant disease, which may mask the usual clinical findings.

Myocardial Ischemia

Typical exertional angina pectoris is commonly the first manifestation of CAD in young and middle-aged patients, and is usually easily recognized. This may not be the case in older patients with CAD. Due

From: Aronow WS, Stemmer EA, Wilson SE (eds). *Vascular Disease in the Elderly.* Armonk, NY: Futura Publishing Company, Inc., © 1997.

to limited physical activity, many older persons do not experience exertional angina, despite the presence of severe CAD. In older patients, angina pectoris frequently occurs at rest and is described as less severe and less distressful than in younger patients with CAD. Due to this atypical presentation, plus the high prevalence of other disorders which cause chest pain, the diagnosis of CAD is often missed, and the chest pain is attributed to other etiologies. For example, myocardial ischemia presenting as shoulder or back pain may be misdiagnosed as degenerative joint disease, or, if the pain is located in the epigastric area, it may be ascribed to peptic ulcer disease. Nocturnal or postprandial epigastric discomfort that is burning in quality is often attributed to hiatus hernia or esophageal reflux, instead of CAD.

Instead of typical exertional angina, myocardial ischemia in older patients is commonly manifested as dyspnea. In many older patients, the dyspnea may be exertional and is thought to be related to a transient rise in left ventricular end-diastolic pressure, due to acute ischemia superimposed on diminished ventricular compliance. Diminished left ventricular compliance occurs secondary to normal aging changes and is accentuated by the presence of other cardiac diseases, such as hypertension which is so common in older patients.[3,4] In other older patients, myocardial ischemia is manifested as acute left ventricular failure with pulmonary edema. Siegel and associates[5] reported on a group of elderly patients (mean age 69 years) with CAD whose manifestation of the disease was acute pulmonary edema. The majority of patients were without angina and many were without a prior history of CAD; however, 90% had a past history of hypertension. Angiographically, the majority of patients had three-vessel CAD, although left ventricular systolic function was only moderately depressed with a mean ejection fraction of 43%. Over 60% of these patients were treated with interventional therapy (coronary bypass surgery or percutaneous transluminal angioplasty), and long-term prognosis was excellent. Similar findings have been reported in other studies of acute pulmonary edema due to CAD.[6-8] The majority of patients are usually elderly, have a past history of hypertension, and demonstrate multivessel coronary disease with usually only moderate impairment of systolic left ventricular function.

In a study of elderly patients with CAD, Tresch and associates[9] studied the initial manifestations of CHD in those who underwent coronary angiography. The mean age of the group was 71 years, with some of the patients over the age of 80 before the onset of symptoms. The initial manifestation in the majority of patients was ischemic chest pain with 34% of the patients sustaining an acute myocardial infarction. In 8% of these elderly patients, the initial manifestation was acute heart failure unassociated with an acute myocardial infarction. On cardiac catheterization, the majority of the patients demonstrated multivessel disease, although left ventricular systolic function was good; only 9% of the total patients had an ejection fraction of less than 35%. Comparing these findings to a group of patients younger than 65 years with CAD, it was found that younger patients more commonly sustained an acute myocardial infarction as the initial manifestation of CAD, were less likely to present with heart failure, and had less multivessel coronary disease.

Cardiac arrhythmias may be a manifestation of myocardial ischemia and is not an uncommon problem in elderly patients with CHD. Sudden death as an initial manifestation of CHD increases with age.[10,11] In the Tresch et al study,[9] approximately 14% of the older patients demonstrated arrhythmias as the initial manifestation of CHD and 2% of the patients experienced out-of-hospital cardiac arrest. As in younger patients with CAD who sustained out-of-hospital cardiac arrest, the majority of older patients demonstrate multiple vessel disease with abnormal systolic dysfunction; however, the arrest will not usually be associated with an acute myocardial infarction. Atrial fibrillation is not a common isolated finding of CAD in older patients. In the Framingham Study,[12] CAD was responsible for 8% of the cases of chronic atrial fibrillation; myocardial infarction was associated with an increased risk of 1.8 in men and 2.1 in women of developing chronic atrial fibrillation.

Silent or asymptomatic ischemia occurs frequently in patients with CAD, regardless of the patient's age. Some investigators have reported silent ischemia to be more common than symptomatic ischemia and to increase with age. In their study of the initial manifestations of CAD, Tresch and associates[9] reported 15% of the older patients (70 years or older) were asymptomatic, and silent myocardial ischemia was detected by exercise stress testing during a preoperative evaluation. In a study of very old (mean age 83 years) nursing home residents, Aronow and associates[13] demonstrated silent myocardial ischemia by Holter monitoring in 21% of the patients who had documented underlying heart disease. Similar findings were reported by Hedblad and associates[14] in a study of 394 elderly Swedish patients (mean age 68 years); Holter monitoring findings of silent ischemia were found in 36% of the patients.

Myocardial Infarction

As with myocardial ischemia, a percentage of patients with myocardial infarction may be completely asymptomatic (silent), or they may be so vague that the symptoms are not recognized by the patient or physician as an acute myocardial infarction. The Framingham Heart Study[15,16] found that in the general population approximately 25% of myocardial infarctions diagnosed by pathological Q waves on electrocardiogram were clinically unrecognized, and of these, 48% were truly silent. The incidence was noted to increase with age, with 42% of infarctions clinically silent in males aged 75 to 84 years. In women, the proportion of silent or unrecognized myocardial infarctions was greater than in men, but the incidence was unaffected by increasing age. Other studies[17-24] have also reported a high prevalence of silent or unrecognized myocardial infarction in older persons, with some studies reporting as high as 60% of infarctions being unrecognized or silent in very old persons (Table 1). Importantly, most studies indicate that the incidence of new coronary events, including recurrent infarction, ventricular fibrillation, and sudden death, is similar in elderly patients with either recognized or unrecognized infarction.[15,24]

The reason for the frequent absence of chest pain in elderly patients with CAD is unclear. Various speculations have included: 1) mental deterioration with inability to verbalize a sensation of pain; 2) better myocardial collateral circulation related to gradual progressive coronary artery narrowing; and 3) a decreased sensitivity to pain due to aging changes. Another theory has suggested that the increase in silent myocardial ischemia and infarction in elderly patients with CAD is related to increased levels of, or receptor sensitivity to, endogenous opioids.[25] This explanation does not appear likely, since studies have demonstrated similar response in B-endorphin levels to exercise in both elderly and younger subjects,[26] and animal studies show a decrease in opioid receptor responsivity with advancing age.[27]

Symptoms, when present, in elderly patients with an acute myocardial infarction may be extremely vague and, as with myocardial ischemia, the diagnosis may be missed. Numerous studies[28-35] have demonstrated the atypical features and the wide variability of symptoms in elderly patients with acute myocardial infarction (Table 2). In an early study, Rodstein[32] found that approximately 30% of elderly nursing home residents who sustained an acute myocardial infarction were without any symptoms referable to heart disease. In 40% of the patients, classic chest or neck pain was absent, but symptoms such as dyspnea, syncope, vertigo, or abdominal pain were common. In the 1960s, Pathy[31]

Table 1
Prevalence of Incidence of Silent or Unrecognized
Q-Wave Myocardial Infarction in Elderly Patients

Study	# of Pts	Age (years)	Unrecognized or Painless MI No.	Percent
Rodstein[32]	52	>60	16	31
Aronow et al[18]	115	>64	78	68
Aronow[21]	110	>62	23	21
Vokonas et al[16]	199 (men)	>65	65	33
	162 (women)	>65	58	36
Muller et al[19]	46 (men)	>65	14	30
	67 (women)	>65	34	51
Nadelmann et al[20]	115	>75	50	43

MI = myocardial infarction
(Adapted with permission from Reference 22.)

Table 2
Prevalence of Chest Pain, Dyspnea, and Neurological Symptoms Associated with
Acute Myocardial Infarction in Elderly Patients

	# of Pts	Age (yrs)	Chest Pain no.	Chest Pain %	Dyspnea no.	Dyspnea %	Neuro-logical Symptoms no.	Neuro-logical Symptoms %
Rodstein[32]	52	>60	15	29	a		a	
Pathy[31]	387	>65	75	19	77	20	126	33
Tinker[34]	87	74*	51	59	19	22	14	16
Bayer et al[29]	777	76*	515	66	329	42	232	30
Aronow[21]	110	>62	24	22	38	35	20	18
Wroblewski[35]	96	84*	19	20	57	59	14	15

a = symptom present, but number and percentage not stated
* = mean age
(Adapted with permission from Reference 22.)

reported similar findings. Patients older than 80 years who sustained an acute myocardial infarction commonly presented with dyspnea or neurologic symptoms, such as acute confusion, stroke, or vertigo, rather than with typical chest pain. Both Rodstein and Pathy emphasized the importance of suspecting an acute myocardial infarction in elderly persons who demonstrate unexplained behavior changes, acute signs of cerebral insufficiency, or dyspnea. More recent studies[21,29,33,35] have also stressed the importance of atypical presentations in elderly patients with acute myocardial infarction, and some studies have suggested that dyspnea may be more common than chest pain as the presenting symptom. In the Multicenter Chest Pain Study,[33] the clinical presentation of acute myocardial infarction was compared in 1615 patients aged over 65 years and 5109 patients aged below 65 years. Due to the decreased prevalence of some typical features (e.g., pressure-like pain), it was found that the initial symptoms and signs had a lower predictive value for diagnosing acute myocardial infarction in elderly patients compared to younger patients. In another prospective study, Wroblewski and associates[35] reported that only 20% of older patients in a Swedish geriatric hospital manifested chest pain at the onset of acute myocardial infarction, whereas 70% complained of dyspnea.

Diagnostic Techniques

Resting Electrocardiogram

The resting electrocardiogram may be used in elderly patients to diagnose myocardial infarction or ischemia, whether silent or symptomatic. Electrocardiographic type of acute myocardial infarction has been noted to be different in older patients, compared to younger patients.[36-39] Krumholz and associates[36] in a study of thrombolytic therapy found that only 31% of infarction patients 75 years or older upon admission to an emergency department demonstrated electrocardiographic findings of ST segment elevation or new pathological Q waves. Similar findings were reported by Tresch and associates[37]; approximately 40% of acute infarctions in patients 70 years or older were classified as non-Q wave infarctions, compared to 25% of the infarctions in patients less than 70 years of age.

In addition to being beneficial in diagnosing CAD, electrocardiographic findings may be predictive of future coronary artery events, including death. In a study of older nursing home patients, in whom resting electrocardiographic findings were assessed as predictors of mortality and new coronary events, Aronow[40] found that at 37 months mean follow-up, older patients (mean age 82 $\pm$ 8 years, range 62 to 103) with ischemic ST segment depression $\geq$ 1.0 mm on the resting electrocardiogram, were 3.1 times more likely to develop new coronary events (myocardial infarction, primary ventricular fibrillation, or sudden cardiac death) than older patients with no significant ST segment depression. Older patients with an ischemic ST segment depression of 0.5 to 0.9 mm on the resting electrocardiogram were 1.9 times more likely to develop new coronary events than older patients with no significant ST segment depression. In another study of older nursing home patients, Aronow[41] found resting electrocardiographic findings of electronic pacemaker rhythm, atrial fibrillation, premature ventricular complexes, left bundle branch block, nonspecific intraventricular conduction defect, and type II second-degree atrioventricular block were also associated with a higher incidence of new coronary events in older patients with CAD, than in patients without these arrhythmias or conduction abnormalities.

Numerous studies have documented that older patients with electrocardiographic left ventricular hypertrophy have an increased incidence of new cardiovascular events. In the Framingham Heart Study,[42] men and women 65 to 94 years of age with electrocardiographic left ventricular hypertrophy had an increased incidence of coronary events, atherothrombotic brain infarction, congestive heart failure, and peripheral arterial disease, compared to subjects without left ventricular hypertrophy. Similar results were reported by Aronow and associates.[43] Older nursing home patients with hypertension or CAD and electrocardiographic left ventricular hypertrophy had an increased incidence of new coronary events and atherothrombotic brain infarctions at 37 months mean follow-up. The increased incidence of cardiovascular morbidity was not different between black and white older nursing home patients who had hypertension and demonstrated electrocardiographic findings of left ventricular hypertrophy.

Exercise and Pharmacological Stress Testing

Exercise stress testing using electrocardiogram, isotope perfusion scintigraphy, radionuclide ventriculography, or echocardiography may be used to diagnose CHD in both asymptomatic and symptomatic older patients. Some investigators have reported exercise stress testing to be more sensitive, but less specific for CAD in older patients, compared to younger patients. Newman and Phillips[44] demonstrated exercise stress testing in patients 65 years of age or older to have sensitivity of 85%, a specificity of 56%, and a positive predictive value of 86% for diagnosing CAD. Similar findings were found in a study by Hlatley and associates[45] with a sensitivity of 84% and a specificity of 70% reported for exercise stress testing in patients 60 years or older.

In contrast to the findings of Newman and Hlatley,[44,45] other investigators have not found findings of exercise stress testing in older patients to be different that those found in younger patients. Martinez-Caro and associates,[46] using symptom-limited upright bicycle exercise testing found, in patients 65 years or older, a sensitivity of 62% and a specificity of 93% for the exercise electrocardiogram in diagnosing CAD, findings similar to those usually found in younger patients.

Besides the usefulness of stress testing in diagnosing CAD in older persons, stress testing may be beneficial as a prognostic marker of future coronary events in older patients. The demonstration of exercise-induced ischemic ST segment depression, ventricular arrhythmias, or inadequate blood pressure response have all been found to be associated wtih poor prognosis in older patients following an acute myocardial infarction.[47,48]

In older patients who, due to musculoskeletal disorders or general debilitation, are unable to perform exercise, intravenous dipyridamole-thallium has been found to have high sensitivity and specificity in diagnosing CHD.[49] Recently, the pharmacological dobutamine-echocardiographic stress test has been shown to be an alternative to dipyridamole-thallium in diagnosing CHD in older patients who cannot exercise. The sensitivity and specificity of dobutamine-echocardiography stress testing is similar to other types of stress testing and is as safe in older patients, as in younger patients.[50,51] Recent studies[50] have found dobutamine-echocardiography stress testing to be useful and safe in stratifying older post-myocardial infarction patients into high-and low-risk groups, including those older patients treated with thrombolytic therapy.

Ambulatory Electrocardiography (Holter Monitoring)

Ambulatory electrocardiographic monitoring (AEM) is useful in the detection of transient cardiac arrhythmias and myocardial ischemia. Such applications are particularly applicable in older patients in whom

CAD is so prevalent and for whom resultant arrhythmias and myocardial ischemia are major clinical problems.

The presence of underlying heart disease is the most important consideration in the evaluation of patients in reference to the significance of arrhythmias as a predictor of future cardiac events. Numerous studies[52-56] have demonstrated ventricular arrhythmias to be an independent predictor of future cardiac events, including sudden death, in older patients with underlying heart disease (Table 3). The risk of future cardiac events increases when ventricular arrhythmias occur in combination with left ventricular dysfunction or left ventricular hypertrophy. In contrast, most studies[52,53,56-58] have failed to demonstrate a correlation between arrhythmias and future cardiac events in healthy older patients without underlying heart disease (Table 3).

Ischemic electrocardiographic ST-T changes demonstrated on AEM correlate with transient abnormalities in myocardial perfusion and ventricular dysfunction. The changes may be associated with symptoms or may be completely asymptomatic, which is referred to as silent ischemia. Silent ischemia is a frequent occurrence and is predictive of future cardiac events including mortality in patients with CAD. Such findings have been reported in both middle-aged and older patients (Table 4).[13,14,56,59-63] A 21% prevalence of silent ischemia as detected by AEM, was reported by Aronow and Epstein[13] in a study of older nursing home patients, mean age 82 years, who had documented underlying heart disease; this compared with only a 5% prevalence in nursing home patients without heart disease. Nursing home patients with CAD had a prevalence of silent ischemia twice that found in patients with other forms of heart disease. Over a 26-month follow-up, 65% of patients with CAD and 33% of patients with other forms of heart disease who demonstrated silent ischemia on AEM had new cardiac events, compared with 32% and 18% patients, respectively, without silent ischemia. In another study of older nursing home patients,[60] the prevalence of silent ischemia was noted to increase significantly in patients with left ventricular ejection fraction of less than 50%, compared with patients with normal ejection fraction (50% or more); an abnormal ejection fraction, as well as silent ischemia, was found to be an independent predictor of new cardiac events. When both variables were present, the incidence of future coronary events markedly increased; 94% of nursing home patients who demonstrated both silent ischemia and abnormal ejection fraction had new cardiac events during a 40-month mean follow-up period.

The combination of silent myocardial ischemia and ventricular arrhythmias as a predictor of future coronary events has also been studied by Aronow and Epstein[59] in their older nursing home population. As expected, ventricular arrhythmias were common in patients with silent ischemia, and both findings were highly predictive of future cardiac events in this older population. Eighty-four percent of the patients with the combination of silent ischemia and complex ventricular arrhythmias had a cardiac event at a mean follow-up of 37 months,

Table 3

Relationship of Ventricular Arrhythmias to Future Cardiac Events in Older Patients

Study	No. of Patients	Mean Age (yrs)	Cardiac Status	Variable	Mean Follow-Up Period	Incidence of Cardiac Events
Fleg[57]	98	69	Healthy*	VPCs, VT	120 mos	No correlation.
Kirkland[58]	30	79	Healthy*	VPCs	29 mos	No correlation.
Aronow[54]	843	82**	Heart disease	Complex VA	39 mos	Approximately 2× incidence in patients with complex VA.
	104		No heart disease	Complex VA	39 mos	No correlation.
Aronow[52]	391	82**	Heart disease	Complex VA, VT, & LVEF	24 mos	Greater than 2× incidence in pts with complex VA or VT. 3× incidence in patients with abnormal LVEF. Greater than 7× incidence in pts with abnormal LVEF and complex VA or VT.
	76		No heart disease	Complex VA, VT & LVEF	24 mos	No correlation.
Aronow[53]	468	82**	Heart disease	Complex VA, VT & LVH	27 mos	3× incidence of SCD or VF in pts with complex VA, VT, or LVH. 7× incidence of SCD or VF in pts with LVH and complex VA or VT.
	86		No heart disease	Complex VA	27 mos	No correlation.

* see text for definition of healthy; ** age of total patients, including patients without heart disease.

LVEF = left ventricular ejection fraction; LVH = left ventricular hypertrophy; SCD = sudden cardiac death; VA = ventricular arrhythmias; VPC = ventricular premature beat; VT = ventricular tachycardia; VF = ventricular fibrillation.

(Adapted with permission from Reference 22.)

Table 4
Relationship of Silent Ischemia to Future Cardiac Events in Older Patients

Study	No. of Patients	Mean Age (yrs)	Cardiac Status	Variable	Mean Follow-up Period	Incidence of Cardiac Events
Fleg[57]	98	69	No heart disease	SI*	120 mos	Approximately 4× incidence in patients with SI.
Aronow[13]	534	82**	Heart disease	SI	26 mos	Greater than 2× incidence in patients with SI.
	92		No heart disease	SI	26 mos	No correlation.
Aronow[60]	393	82	CAD or systemic hypertension	SI & LVEF	40 mos	2× incidence in patients with SI. Greater than 2× incidence in patients with abnormal LVEF. Greater than 3× incidence in patients with SI and abnormal LVEF.
Aronow[59]	404	82	CAD or systemic hypertension	SI, complex VA & VT	37 mos	2× incidence in patients with SI or complex VA. 4× incidence in patients with SI and complex VA. 1.7× incidence in patients with VT. 2.5 × incidence in patients with SI and VT.
Hedblad[14]	394	68	CAD or no CAD	SI	43 mos	4.4× greater risk of MI in patients with SI. Risk increased 16× in patients with SI and CAD.

* included patients with ≥1 mm upsloping ST-segment depression; ** age of total patients, including patients without heart disease; CAD = coronary artery disease; LVEF = left ventricular ejection fraction; MI = myocardial infarction; SI = silent ischemia; VA = ventricular arrhythmias; VT = ventricular tachycardia.

(Adapted with permission from Reference 22.)

compared with only 21% of the patients with neither silent ischemia nor complex ventricular arrhythmias.

As in Aronow's studies, Hedblad and associates[14] found ischemia detected on AEM to be highly predictive of cardiac events in older Scandinavian men, age 68 years. A 4.4-fold increased risk of coronary events was found in men without documented CAD who demonstrated myocardial ischemia on AEM. The relative risk of coronary events increased sixteenfold in the men with CAD. Fleg and Kennedy,[57] in a study of healthy older subjects, which did not demonstrate a correlation between arrhythmias and future cardiac events, did find approximately a fourfold increase in cardiac events in the older persons who demonstrated silent ischemia on AEM; two of the three patients in their study who died suddenly demonstrated silent ischemia and ventricular tachycardia on AEM. Such findings suggest, as in Aronow's study,[59] that the combination of silent ischemia and ventricular arrhythmias in older patients may be a potent indicator of increased cardiac risk.

Silent ischemia detected by AEM has been used in the assessment of patients undergoing noncardiac surgery. Such use of AEM may be especially beneficial in older patients, who frequently are at high surgical risk and may not be able to undergo preoperative exercise stress testing because of concomitant illness. Raby and associates[64] studied 176 patients who underwent 24-hour AEM before noncardiac surgery. Eighteen percent of the patients demonstrated ischemia on AEM, which in the majority of cases was asymptomatic, and the perioperative ischemia was highly predictive of postoperative cardiac events. The sensitivity of preoperative ischemia for postoperative cardiac events in these patients was 92%, the specificity 88%, the predictive value of a positive result 38%, and the predictive value of a negative result 99%. Multivariant analyses demonstrated preoperative ischemia to be the most significant correlative of postoperative cardiac events. The authors concluded that the absence of preoperative ischemia on AEM indicates a very low risk for postoperative cardiac events. Thirty-eight percent of the patients in this study were older than 69 years, and preoperative ischemia was found to be more prevalent in these older patients compared with the younger patients.

In follow-up study, Raby and associates[65] assessed the significance of intraoperative and postoperative ischemia, in addition to preoperative ischemia, detected on AEM in relationship to postoperative cardiac events in patients undergoing peripheral vascular surgery. The mean age of the patients was 67 years, and 37% were 70 years or older. As in their previous study, the authors found preoperative ischemia to be the most important predictor of postoperative cardiac events. Preoperative ischemia also strongly correlated with intraoperative and postoperative ischemia, and perioperative ischemia commonly preceded clinical cardiac events.

Echocardiography

Echocardiography can be a useful procedure in the assessment of older patients with CAD. Detection of regional wall abnormalities, acute myocardial ischemia, left ventricular aneurysm, cardiac thrombus, left main CAD, left ventricular hypertrophy, left ventricular function, and cardiac chamber size is possible with echocardiography. Such findings are useful in diagnosing CAD, and may also be useful in predicting future cardiac events and long-term prognosis in elderly patients.[52,53,66,67] Aronow and associates[66] in studies of older nursing home patients found left ventricular ejection fraction measured by echocardiography to be the most important prognostic variable for mortality in older patients with heart failure associated with CAD. Patients with heart failure and depressed systolic left ventricular ejection fraction were found to have a worse prognosis than patients with heart failure and normal systolic ejection fractions. Echocardiographic left ventricular hypertrophy has also been found to be a predictor of future cardiac events in both middle-aged and older patients with CHD.[43,52,68-70] The Framingham Heart Study[70] found echocardiographic left ventricular hypertrophy to be predictive of coronary events independent of standard risk factors in older patients with CAD. Echocardiographic left ventricular hypertrophy was 15.3 times more sensitive in predicting coronary events in older men and 4.3 times more sensitive in predicting coronary events in older women than electrocardiographic ventricular hypertrophy. In studies of very old nursing home patients with CAD, Aronow and associates[53,69] reported similar findings. Older nursing home patients with echocardiographic left ventricular hypertrophy had at least two times higher incidence of new coronary events at follow-up than patients without echocardiographic left ventricular hypertrophy. The incidence of new atherothrombotic brain infarction, heart failure, and sudden death was also found to be higher in older nursing home patients with CAD or hypertension and echocardiographic left ventricular hypertrophy, than in patients without left ventricular hypertrophy, regardless if CAD or hypertension were present.

Summary

Although CAD is very prevalent in older persons, the disease is often undiagnosed or misdiagnosed, which may be related to its different clinical manifestations in this age group, compared to younger patients with the disease. Instead of typical chest pain, myocardial ischemia or infarction in older patients may commonly be manifested as dyspnea or acute heart failure. In other older persons, myocardial ischemia or infarction may be silent, with the patient completely asymptomatic even though electrocardiographic findings of ischemia or infarction are present. Some older patients with acute myocardial infarction present with neurological symptoms, such as mental confusion or cerebrovascular accidents. Because of these atypical presentations and wide variability of symptoms, physicians have to be highly suspicious of the presence of myocardial ischemia or acute myocardial infarction in older patients who demonstrate an unexplained acute change in their physical condition. Diagnostic procedures, such as resting electrocardiography, stress testing, AEM, and echocardiography, can be very beneficial in diagnosing CAD in older patients, as well as in predicting future coronary events. The use of these diagnostic procedures need to be considered in the evaluation of older patients in whom CAD is suspected.

References

1. McKeown F: *Pathology of the Aged.* London: Butterworths; 44-45, 1965.
2. Monroe RT: *Diseases in Old Age.* Cambridge, MA: Harvard University Press; 1951.
3. Tresch DD, McGough MF: Heart failure with normal systolic function: a common disorder in older people. *J Am Geriatr Soc* 43:1035-1042, 1995.
4. Bonow RO, Udelson JE: Left ventricular diastolic dysfunction as a cause of congestive heart failure. *Ann Intern Med* 117:502-509, 1992.
5. Siegel R, Clemens T, Wingo M, Tresch DD: Acute heart failure in elderly: another manifestation of unstable "angina." *J Am Coll Cardiol* 17:149A, 1991.
6. Clark LT, Garfein OB, Dwyer EM: Acute pulmonary edema due to ischemic heart disease without accompanying myocardial infarction. *Am J Med* 75:332-336, 1983.
7. Dodek A, Kassebaum DG, Bristow JD: Pulmonary edema in coronary artery disease without cardiomegaly: paradox of the stiff heart. *N Engl J Med* 286:1347-1350, 1972.
8. Kunis R, Greenberg H, Yeoh CB, et al: Coronary revascularization for recurrent pulmonary edema in elderly patients with ischemic heart disease and preserved ventricular function. *N Engl J Med* 313:1207-1210, 1985.
9. Tresch DD, Saeian K, Hoffman R: Elderly patients with late onset of coronary artery disease: clinical and angiographic findings. *Am J Geriatr Cardiol* 14-25, 1992.
10. Kannel WB, Schatzkin A: Sudden death: lesions from subsets in population studies. *J Am Coll Cardiol* 141B-149B, 1985.
11. Elveback LR, Connelly DC, Kurland LT. Coronary heart disease in residents of Rochester, Minnesota. II. Mortality, incidence, and survivorship, 1950-1975. *Mayo Clin Proc* 56:665-672, 1981.
12. Kannel WB, Wolf PA: Epidemiology of atrial fibrillation. *In:* Folk RH, Podrid PJ (eds). *Mechanisms of Management.* New York: Raven Press; 81-92, 1992.
13. Aronow WS, Epstein S: Usefulness of silent myocardial ischemia detected by ambulatory electrocardiographic monitoring in predicting new coronary events in elderly patients. *Am J Cardiol* 62:1295-1296, 1988.
14. Hedblad B, Juul-Moller S, Svensson K, et al: Increased mortality in men with ST segment depression during 24-hour ambulatory long-term ECG recording: results from prospective population study "Men Born in 1914," from Malmo, Sweden. *Eur Heart J* 10:149-158, 1989.
15. Kannel WB, Abbott RD: Incidence and prognosis of unrecognized myocardial infarction: an update on the Framingham Study. *N Engl J Med* 311:1144-1147, 1984.
16. Vokonas PS, Kannel WB, Cupples LA: Incidence and prognosis of unrecognized myocardial infarction in elderly: The Framingham Study (abstr). *J Am Coll Cardiol* 11:51A, 1988.

17. Roseman MD: Painless myocardial infarction: a review of the literature and analysis of 220 cases. *Ann Intern Med* 41:1-7, 1956.
18. Aronow WS, Starling L, Etienne F, et al: Unrecognized Q-wave myocardial infarction in patients older than 64 years in a long-term health-care facility. *Am J Cardiol* 56:483, 1985.
19. Muller RT, Gould LA, Betzu R, Racek T, Pradeep V: Painless myocardial infarction in the elderly. *Am Heart J* 119:202-204, 1990.
20. Nadelmann J, Frishman WH, Ooi WL, et al: Prevalence, incidence, and prognosis of recognized and unrecognized myocardial infarction in persons aged 75 years or older: the Bronx Aging Study. *Am J Cardiol* 66:533-537, 1990.
21. Aronow WS: Prevalence of presenting symptoms of recognized acute myocardial infarction and of unrecognized healed myocardial infarction in elderly patients. *Am J Cardiol* 60:1182, 1987.
22. Tresch DD, Aronow WS: Recognization and diagnosis of coronary artery disease in elderly. In: Tresch DD, Aronow WS (eds). *Cardiovascular Disease in Elderly.* New York: Marcel Dekker, Inc.; 285-304, 1994.
23. Yano K, MacLean CJ: The incidence and prognosis of unrecognized myocardial infarction in the Honolulu, Hawaii Heart Program. *Arch Intern Med* 149:1528-1532, 1989.
24. Sigurdsson E, Thorgeirsson G, Sigvaldason H, Sigfusson N: Unrecognized myocardial infarction: epidemiology, clinical characteristics, and the prognostic role of angina pectoris: the Reykjavik Study. *Ann Intern Med* 122:96-102, 1995.
25. Ellestad MH, Kuan P: Naloxone and asymptomatic ischemia: failure to induce angina during exercise testing. *Am J Cardiol* 54:982-984, 1984.
26. Hatfield BD, Goldfarb AH, Sporzo GA, Flynn MG: Serum beta-endorphin and affective response to graded exercise in young and elderly men. *J Gerontol* 42:429-431, 1987.
27. Morley JE: Neuropeptides, behavior and aging. *J Am Geriatr Soc* 34:52-61, 1986.
28. Uretskyu BF: Symptomatic myocardial infarction without chest pain. *Am J Cardiol* 40:498-503, 1977.
29. Bayer AJ, Chadha JS, Farag RR, Pathy MSJ: Changing presentation of myocardial infarction with increasing old age. *J Am Geriatr Soc* 23:263-266, 1986.
30. MacDonald JB: Presentation of acute myocardial infarction in the elderly: a review. *Age Ageing* 13:196-204, 1980.
31. Pathy MS: Clinical presentation of myocardial infarction in the elderly. *Br Heart J* 29:190-199, 1967.
32. Rodstein M: The characteristics of non-fatal myocardial infarction in the aged. *Arch Intern Med* 98:84-90, 1956.
33. Solomon CG, Lee TH, Cook EF, et al: Comparison of clinical presentation of acute myocardial infarction in patients older than 65 years of age to younger patients: the Multicenter Chest Pain Study Experience. *Am J Cardiol* 63:772-776, 1989.
34. Tinker GM: Clinical presentation of myocardial infarction in the elderly. *Age Ageing* 10:237-240, 1981.
35. Wroblewski M, Mikulowski P, Steen B: Symptoms of myocardial infarction in old age: clinical case, retrospective and prospective studies. *Age Ageing* 15:99-104, 1986.
36. Krumholz HM, Friesinger GC, Cook EF, Lee TH, Rouan GW, Goldman L: Relationship of age with eligibility for thrombolytic therapy and mortality among patients with suspected acute myocardial infarction. *J Am Geriatr Soc* 42:127-131, 1994.
37. Tresch D, Aufderheide T, Brady W: Significance of prehospital chest pain, thrombolytic therapy, and mortality in elderly and younger patients. *J Am Coll Cardiol* 23:432A, 1994.

38. Weaver WD, Litwin PE, Martin JS, et al: Effect of age on use of thrombolytic therapy and mortality in acute myocardial infarction. *J Am Coll Cardiol* 18:657-662, 1991.
39. Nicod P, Gilpin E, Dittrich H, et al: Short- and long-term clinical outcome after Q wave and non-Q wave myocardial infarction in a large patient population. *Circulation* 79:528-536, 1989.
40. Aronow WS: Correlation of ischemic ST-segment depression on the resting electrocardiogram with new cardiac events in 1,106 patients over 62 years of age. *Am J Cardiol* 64:232-233, 1989.
41. Aronow WS: Correlation of arrhythmias and conduction defects on the resting electrocardiogram with new cardiac events in 1,153 elderly patients. *Am J Noninvas Cardiol* 5:88-90, 1991.
42. Kannel WB, Dannenberg AL, Levy D: Population implications of electrocardiographic left ventricular hypertrophy. *Am J Cardiol* 60:851-931, 1987.
43. Aronow WS, Koenigsberg M, Schwartz KS: Usefulness of echocardiographic and electrocardiographic left ventricular hypertrophy in predicting new cardiac events and atherothrombotic brain infarction in elderly patients with systemic hypertension or coronary artery disease. *Am J Noninvas Cardiol* 3:367-370, 1989.
44. Newman KP, Phillips JH: Graded exercise testing for diagnosis of coronary artery disease in elderly patients. *South Med J* 81:430-432, 1988.
45. Hlatley MA, Pryor DB, Harrell FE Jr, Califf RM, Mark DB, Rasati RA: Factors affecting sensitivity and specificity of exercise electrocardiography: multivariate analysis. *Am J Med* 77:64-71, 1984.
46. Martinez-Caro D, Alegria E, Lorente D, Azpilicueta J, Colaburg J, Ancin R: Diagnostic value of stress in the elderly. *Eur Heart J* 5(suppl E):63-67, 1984.
47. Glover DR, Robinson CS, Murray RG: Diagnostic exercise testing in 104 patients over 65 years of age. *Eur Heart J* (suppl E):59-61, 1984.
48. Saunamaki KI: Early postmyocardial infarction exercise in subjects 70 years or more of age: functional and prognostic evaluation. *Eur Heart J* 5(suppl E):93-97, 1984.
49. Lam JYT, Chaitman BR, Glaenzer M, et al: Safety and diagnostic accuracy of dipyridamole-thallium imaging in the elderly. *J Am Coll Cardiol* 11:585-589, 1988.
50. Carlos ME, Smart SC, Tresch DD: Benefits and safety of dobutamine stress echocardiography in elderly. *Clin Res* 42:357A, 1994.
51. Polderman D, Fioretti PM, Boersma E, et al: Dobutamine-atropine stress echocardiography in elderly patients unable to perform an exercise test: hemodynamic characteristics, safety, and prognostic value. *Arch Intern Med* 154:2681-2686, 1994.
52. Aronow WS, Epstein S, Koenigsberg M, Schwartz KS: Usefulness of echocardiographic abnormal left ventricular ejection fraction, paroxysmal ventricular tachycardia, and complex ventricular arrhythmias in predicting new coronary events in patients over 62 years of age. *Am J Cardiol* 61:1349-1351, 1988.
53. Aronow WS, Epstein S, Koenigsberg M, Schwartz KS: Usefulness of echocardiographic left ventricular hypertrophy, ventricular tachycardia and complex ventricular arrhythmias in predicting ventricular fibrillation or sudden cardiac death in elderly patients. *Am J Cardiol* 62:1124-1125, 1988.
54. Aronow WS, Epstein S, Mercando AD: Usefulness of complex ventricular arrhythmias detected by 24-hour ambulatory electrocardiogram and by electrocardiograms with one-minute rhythm strips in predicting new coronary events in elderly patients with and without heart disease. *J Cardiovasc Technol* 10:21-25, 1991.

55. Ruderman W, Weinblatt E, Goldberg JD, et al: Ventricular premature beats and mortality after myocardial infarction. *N Engl J Med* 297:750-757, 1977.
56. Tresch DD: Diagnostic and prognostic value of ambulatory electrocardiography monitoring in older patients. *J Am Geriatr Soc* 43:66-70, 1995.
57. Fleg JL, Kennedy HL: Long-term prognostic significance of ambulatory electrocardiographic findings in apparently healthy subjects >60 years of age. *Am J Cardiol* 70:748-751, 1992.
58. Kirkland JL, Lye M, Faragher EB, dos Santos AGR: A longitudinal study of the prognostic significance of ventricular ectopic beats in the elderly. *Gerontology* 29:199-201, 1983.
59. Aronow WS, Epstein S: Usefulness of silent ischemia, ventricular tachycardia, and complex ventricular arrhythmias in predicting new coronary events in elderly patients with coronary artery disease or systemic hypertension. *Am J Cardiol* 65:511-512, 1990.
60. Aronow WS, Epstein S, Koenigsberg M: Usefulness of echocardiographic left ventricular ejection fraction and silent myocardial ischemia in predicting new coronary events in elderly patients with coronary artery disease or systemic hypertension. *Am J Cardiol* 65:811-812, 1990.
61. Gottlieb SO, Weisfeldt ML, Ouyang P, et al: Silent ischemia as a marker for early unfavorable outcomes in patients with unstable angina. *N Engl J Med* 314:1214-1219, 1986.
62. Gottlieb SO, Gottlieb SH, Achuff SC, et al: Silent ischemia on Holter monitoring predicts mortality in high-risk postinfarction patients. *JAMA* 259:1030-1035, 1988.
63. Gottlieb SO, Weisfeldt ML, Ouyang P, et al: Silent ischemia predicts infarction and death during 2-year follow-up of unstable angina. *J Am Coll Cardiol* 10:756-760, 1987.
64. Raby KE, Goldman L, Creager MA, et al: Correlation between preoperative ischemia and major cardiac events after peripheral vascular surgery. *N Engl J Med* 321:1296-1300, 1989.
65. Raby KE, Barry J, Creager MA, et al: Detection and significance of intraoperative and postoperative myocardial ischemia in peripheral vascular surgery. *JAMA* 268:222-227, 1992.
66. Aronow WS, Ahn C, Kronzon I: Prognosis of congestive heart failure in elderly patients with normal versus abnormal left ventricular systolic function associated with coronary artery Disease. *Am J Cardiol* 66:1257-1259, 1990.
67. Setaro JF, Soufer R, Remetz MS, Perlmutter RA, Zaret BL: Long-term outcome in patients with congestive heart failure and intact systolic left ventricular performance. *Am J Cardiol* 69:1212-1216, 1992.
68. Aronow WS, Ahn C, Kronzon I, Koenigsberg M: Congestive heart failure, coronary events, and atherothrombotic brain infarction in elderly blacks and whites with systemic hypertension and with and without electrocardiographic and electrocardiographic evidence of left ventricular hypertrophy. *Am J Cardiol* 67:295-299, 1991.
69. Aronow WS, Koenigsberg M, Schwartz KS: Usefulness of echocardiographic left ventricular hypertrophy in predicting new coronary events and atherothrombotic brain infarction in patients over 62 years of age. *Am J Cardiol* 61:1130-1132, 1988.
70. Levy D, Garrison RJ, Savage DD, Kannel WB, Castelli WP: Left ventricular mass incidence of coronary heart disease in an elderly cohort: the Framingham Heart Study. *Ann Intern Med* 110:101-107, 1989.

Chapter 16

Medical Therapy of Stable and Unstable Angina in the Elderly

Harold G. Olson, MD
Wilbert S. Aronow, MD

Coronary artery disease (CAD) is a major cause of morbidity and mortality in elderly patients. The clinical prevalence of CAD in the elderly is estimated at approximately 20%.[1] However, autopsy data suggest that significant CAD may be present in the elderly, but that it is clinically silent. The autopsy prevalence of CAD in persons age 60 years or greater is approximately 50%.[2,3] Importantly, approximately half of all deaths in persons age 65 years or greater is directly related to CAD.[4,5] Studies indicate that angina pectoris is usually the initial clinical manifestation of CAD in the elderly.[6] However, it should be emphasized that angina pectoris in the elderly may be clinically atypical when compared to angina pectoris in younger patients. For example, instead of chest pain, elderly patients may describe angina as dyspnea on exertion, excessive fatigue, palpitations, dizziness, or syncope. Nevertheless, the management of angina pectoris in the elderly is similar to that of younger patients. This chapter reviews the medical management of chronic stable angina pectoris, and unstable angina pectoris, especially as it relates to elderly patients. Before proceeding with this discussion, some general comments about the aging heart are worthwhile.

Table 1 lists the changes which occur within the cardiovascular system as a result of the aging process. The elderly patient is particularly prone to adverse hemodynamic effects from tachycardia because left ventricular hypertrophy (LVH) and abnormalities of ventricular relaxation are commonly observed in the aging heart.[7,8] For example, during exercise, with its attendant increase in heart rate, left ventricular filling pressure may rise more rapidly and to a higher level in the elderly patient as compared to a younger patient. Thus, the elderly patient's exercise capacity may be more limited by the symptom of dyspnea than the exercise capacity of the younger patient. Moreover, this may explain why

From: Aronow WS, Stemmer EA, Wilson SE (eds). *Vascular Disease in the Elderly.* Armonk, NY: Futura Publishing Company, Inc., © 1997.

Table 1
1. Decrease in resting and exercise heart rates.
2. Decrease in maximal cardiac output.
3. Decreased responsiveness to catecholamines.
4. Increase in left ventricular mass and wall thickness.
5. Slowed and delayed diastolic left ventricular filling (impaired ventricular relaxation).
6. Increased arterial stiffness.
7. Cardiac valves may be affected by fibrous thickening and calcific deposits.
8. Reduction of pacemaker activity from pacemaker cell drop out.
9. Fibrosis of conduction system leading to heart block.
10. Deposition of senile amyloid which may affect the coronary arteries, conduction system, or myocyte.

dyspnea, and not chest pain, is a common angina equivalent in the elderly patient. Accordingly, control of heart rate should be a fundamental goal in the treatment of the elderly patient with heart disease. Change in elastin and collagen properties of the peripheral blood vessels lead to a decrease in arterial compliance and an increase in peripheral resistance. The net effort is an increase in afterload. This is clinically manifested as hypertension, especially systolic hypertension, in the elderly patient.[9] In addition to these changes, the older heart is less responsive to catecholamine stimulation, has a longer duration of contraction, has more LVH, and has more coronary atherosclerosis when compared to a younger heart.[9]

General Measures

The diagnosis of CAD can be made by a careful history, physical examination, echocardiogram (ECG), noninvasive testing (treadmill studies, nuclear stress testing, stress echocardiography), and, in some cases, by coronary angiography. After the diagnosis of CAD is established, one should look for and correct factors that could induce and aggravate myocardial ischemia. These potential reversible factors are listed in Table 2.

It is a well-known fact that diastolic and especially systolic blood pressure increase with age. Importantly, systolic hypertension (systolic blood pressure of 160 mm Hg or greater) is commonly found in the elderly.[10] In addition, the level of systolic pressure in the elderly patient is a better predictor of cardiac risk when compared to the level of diastolic pressure.[11] Furthermore, studies indicate that the prevalence of LVH, as determined by ECG or echocardiography, increases with age.[12,13] LVH has been correlated with increased risk for cardiovascular complications, such as arrhythmias, congestive heart failure (CHF), and sudden death.[12-14] It is likely that the LVH seen in the elderly is in part related to the increased incidence of systolic hypertension. It is

Table 2

1. Uncontrolled hypertension.
2. Uncorrected valvular heart disease (i.e., aortic stenosis).
3. Arrhythmias (i.e., atrial fibrillation).
4. Congestive heart failure.
5. Anemia
6. Hyperthyroidism
7. Obesity

noteworthy that large randomized controlled clinical trials assessing medical therapy in elderly patients with hypertension, including elderly patients with isolated systolic hypertension, have shown that control of blood pressure is associated with an improved prognosis.[15-17] Accordingly, control of blood pressure in elderly patients with CAD and angina will not only improve the symptoms of angina, but will also improve the patient's prognosis. Calcific aortic stenosis is the most frequent valvular heart disease seen in the elderly.[9] The cardinal symptoms of aortic stenosis include angina, syncope, and those associated with left ventricular failure, such as dyspnea, orthopnea, and paroxysmal nocturnal dyspnea. This important diagnosis may be frequently missed because the systolic murmur of aortic stenosis is too faint to be heard on physical examination of the elderly patient. Thus, if one suspects underlying aortic stenosis, one should obtain an echocardiogram (ECG). Replacement of the aortic valve will relieve the symptom of angina in the patient with hemodynamically significant aortic stenosis.

It is a well-known fact that hyperthyroidism can be masked in the elderly and, thus, be difficult to diagnose. In the elderly patient with unexplained weight loss, heat intolerance, persistent sinus tachycardia, atrial fibrillation, or cryptic CHF, occult hyperthyroidism should be considered. Thyroid function studies should be ordered, and if hyperthyroidism is found it should be treated accordingly.

After these reversible factors have been corrected, the patient should be evaluated for the traditional coronary risk factors. Whenever possible, an attempt should be made to modify these existing coronary risk factors. Perhaps the single most important coronary risk factor, which if corrected improves not only the well-being of the patient, but also improves the patient's prognosis, is the total cessation of cigarette smoking. It is notable that in some patients, cigarette smoking can even attenuate the antianginal effects of the drugs used to treat angina pectoris. Of importance, it is not too late to stop smoking; studies show that even in the elderly patient, the total discontinuation of smoking improves prognosis.[18] Elderly patients with CAD and angina pectoris, who are free of other life-threatening diseases such as cancer, should be considered for aggressive lipid-lowering therapy. Multiple lipid-lowering trials have shown an approximate 40% reduction in cardiac events (death, myocardial infarction [MI], unstable angina pectoris, or need for bypass surgery, or percutaneous transluminal coronary angioplasty [PTCA]) in patients treated with aggressive lipid-lowering protocols compared to patients treated with less intensive lipid-lowering therapy.[19,20] The recent Scandinavian Simvastatin Trial convincingly showed that cholesterol reduction results in a decrease in both cardiovascular and noncardiovascular mortality. Compared to placebo, patients randomized to a HMG-CoA reductase inhibitor (Simvastatin) had a 30% decrease in total mortality, a 42% decrease in CAD mortality, and a 27% decrease in coronary revascularization.[21] Despite the fact that there are no large randomized controlled trials of lipid-lowering therapy in the elderly, subgroup analysis of data from clinical trials seem to show that patients greater than 65 years enjoy the same clinical benefits from cholesterol reduction as patients younger than 65 years. Thus, a reasonable goal for lipid management in the elderly patient with documented CAD should be to lower the total cholesterol to less than 200 mg/% and low-density lipoprotein (LDL) levels to less than 100 mg/%, while maintaining high-density lipoprotein (HDL) levels greater than 40 mg/%.[22] If this cannot be achieved by diet alone, drug therapy should be considered. Drug therapy includes the bile acid sequestrants, fibrates, niacin, Probucol, and the HMG-CoA reductase inhibitors. However, bile acid sequestrants are difficult to use in the elderly because of their side effects, namely bloating, flatulence, and constipation.

In addition, the bile acid sequestrants can bind with many drugs and minerals, such as thiazides, warfarin, acetaminophen, levothyroxine, magnesium, iron, zinc, and fat-soluble vitamins, which are commonly taken by the elderly patient. Niacin (nicotinic acid) is useful for all types of hyperlipidemia, except hyperchylomicronemia. Niacin reduces cholesterol, triglycerides, LDL, and is the only drug available to show a decrease of Lp(a), a lipoprotein correlated with increased risk for CAD.[23] Importantly, niacin increases HDL cholesterol, which seems to act to retard the atherosclerotic process.[19] Niacin, however, is fraught with many undesirable side effects which include flushing, hepatitis, propensity to precipitate attacks of gout, and worsening of insulin resistance. These side effects make the drug difficult to use in the elderly patient.

Thus, we have found that the HMG-CoA reductase inhibitors, because of their paucity of any major side effects, are the ideal antilipid drugs for the elderly patient. Side effects, which occur rarely and are reversible, include sleep disturbances, myopathic syndromes, and hepatitis. Patients on HMG-CoA reductase inhibitors should have their liver enzymes monitored and, if myopathic symptoms occur, serum creatine phosphokinase levels should be obtained.

Elderly patients with angina should be started and maintained on aspirin therapy, 162 to 324 mgm/d. Large randomized controlled studies have shown that aspirin therapy decreases the incidence of MI and stroke at follow-up.[24,25] It is recommended that elderly patients be given enteric-coated aspirin because this formulation seems to produce less gastrointestinal tract toxicity. Postmenopausal women should be considered for estrogen or estrogen-progestin replacement therapy. Studies indicate that postmenopausal females on estrogen replacement have a significantly lower incidence of CAD than females not taking replacement hormones.[26] Although hormonal replacement therapy does not exert a direct antianginal effect, it may slow the progression of coronary atherosclerosis by its effect on lipids and endothelial cell function and, thus, improve prognosis. Because estrogen therapy may increase the risk of carcinoma of the endometrium and breast, one has to consider estrogen therapy cautiously.

Finally, elderly patients should be encouraged to exercise on a daily basis. Studies indicate that in elderly patients with CAD who undergo an exercise program, there is an improvement in exercise capacity and psychosocial well being.[27] A simple walking program of 30 minutes, three to four times a week, has been recommended by the American Heart Association in the comprehensive risk reduction for patients with CAD.[28]

Drug Therapy for Angina Pectoris

The elderly patient is particularly prone to adverse drug reactions. This is in part due to the aging process itself. Drug absorption, drug distribution, protein binding of drugs, hepatic metabolism, and renal function may significantly differ in the elderly patient as compared to the younger patient. In addition, the elderly patient is more likely to be exposed to polypharmacy because of concurrent illnesses, which increases the risk for significant drug interactions to occur. Accordingly, it is best to abide by the maxim when considering drug therapy in the elderly: "Start low and go slowly."

The operating principle of drug therapy in patients with angina pectoris is to relieve and prevent myocardial ischemia. Myocardial ischemia occurs when nutrient myocardial blood flow, rich in oxygen content (myocardial oxygen supply) does not match myocardial oxygen demand. The result of this mismatch leads to intramyocardial metabolic changes followed by myocardial mechanical changes, such as diastolic dysfunction and systolic dysfunction, and finally by the perception of angina pectoris by the patient. The pharmacological action of antianginal drugs is to favorably alter myocardial oxygen supply, or myocardial demand, or both, so that myocardial supply matches myocardial oxygen demand. Three classes of drugs are available for the treatment of angina pectoris; these include the nitrates, the beta blockers, and the calcium-entry blockers.

Nitrates

In 1867, Brunton published the first report on the efficacy of amyl nitrate in the treatment of angina pectoris.[29] Since then, the nitrates have been considered the cornerstone in drug management of angina pectoris. The mechanisms of action of the nitrates have been extensively studied. Nitrates vasodilate veins, arteries, and arterioles. Following their entry into the blood stream, the nitrates gain access into vascular smooth muscle, whereby several chemical conversions occur. The end point of these chemical conversions is formation of nitric oxide (NO) or a nitrosothiol derivative. NO, through the guanylate cyclase system, triggers relaxation of vascular smooth muscle resulting in vasodilation.[30,31] It is interesting to note that NO is the so-called endothelial-derived relaxing factor (EDRF) which seems to be deficient in atherosclerotic vessels.[32,33] Accordingly, nitrates can theoretically be considered as NO donors, thereby restoring some of the vasodilating properties of the atherosclerotic coronary arteries.

Nitrates primarily relieve or prevent myocardial ischemia by reduction in myocardial oxygen demand and increase in myocardial oxygen supply. Nitrates reduce myocardial oxygen demand by reduction in myocardial wall tension. Myocardial wall tension is determined by intracardiac volume and systolic blood pressure. The nitrates' vasodilatory action on the venous capacitance system results in a redistribution of blood volume toward the splanchnic and mesenteric circulations. This results in a decrease in venous return and a reduction in intracardiac volume.[34] The vasodilation of both veins and arterioles results in a lowering of systolic pressures. The drop in systolic pressure by the nitrates may result in activation of the sympathetic nervous system. This activation could cause an increase in heart rate and myocardial conductility, which would result in an increase in myocardial oxygen demand. However, it should be pointed out that in most cases, the drop in myocardial wall tension induced by nitroglycerin outweighs the effects on myocardial oxygen consumption by the increase in heart rate and contractility so that the net effect is an overall reduction in myocardial oxygen demand.

The effect of nitrates on myocardial oxygen supply is complex. Studies indicate that by decreasing myocardial oxygen demand, nitrates may actually decrease overall coronary blood flow. However, in the patients with obstruction in their coronary arteries, nitrates may improve regional coronary blood flow by their vasodilatory action on the epicardial coronary vessels, as well as the collaterals coronary vessels.[35] Brown et al[36] showed that nitrates have the capacity to dilate coronary arteries at the site of atherosclerotic obstruction, which allows for an increase in both resting and reserve coronary blood flow to occur. Furthermore, nitrates by reducing left ventricular blood volume lower left ventricular end diastolic pressure. This hemodynamic effect creates the setting for a larger coronary perfusion pressure gradient to occur, with the net result of better subendocardial coronary perfusion.[37]

Finally, studies indicate that nitrates have an antiplatelet effect which may decrease the risk of sudden cessation of coronary blood flow to occur in a region of the myocardium from intracoronary platelet thrombi.[38]

Clinically, nitrates are safe and generally well tolerated. Contraindications for nitrate therapy include severe hypotension, especially when associated with hypovolemia, increased intracranial pressure, and in those patients with a known hypersensitivity to nitrates. The major side effects of nitrates are hypotension, flushing, and headache. Hypotension may manifest itself as dizziness to frank syncope. Typically, symptoms occur within minutes after administration of a sublingual preparation of nitrate, and from 30 minutes to 2 hours after oral ingestion of a nitrate. Risk factors associated with nitrate-induced hypotension include initial dosing of the nitrate, high doses of nitrates, hypovolemic state (i.e., diuretic usage), autonomic dysfunction, and in the setting of other vasodilator usage such as angiotensin-converting enzymic (ACE) inhibitors, calcium channel blockers, and other antihypertensive drugs.

Elderly patients are particularly prone to the hypotensive effects of the nitrates. The two mechanisms proposed to explain this phenomenon include: 1) the elderly heart is more preload sensitive due to age-related diastolic ventricular relaxation abnormalities; and 2) impaired age-related baroreceptor function.[39] Accordingly, when nitrates are used in the elderly patient, it is best to start with the lowest dose and titrate the dose slowly upward until clinical efficacy is demonstrated. The patient should be instructed to sit down when taking sublingual nitroglycerin. If the patient experiences symptomatic hypotension, he or she should be told to lie down and elevate their legs. With these measures, blood pressure will return to baseline within minutes and no further treatment is indicated. A rare form of nitrate-induced hypotension, which is a variant of neurocardiogenic syncope is seen in the patients with acute coronary syndromes. This form of nitrate-induced hypotension manifests itself as sudden hypotension and bradycardia following the ingestion of a nitrate. Treatment includes elevation of the legs, fluids, and atropine. Interestingly, this form of nitrate-induced hypotension may not recur after a later challenge of nitrate. Thus, nitrates are not contraindicated in patients who have had this form of nitrate-induced hypotension.

Headache is a common side effect of nitrates. The headache may range from a mild frontal headache to a severe throbbing headache, resembling a migraine attack. The headache may be associated with nausea and vomiting. The mechanism for the headache is thought to be due to nitrate-induced vasodilation of extracranial and intracranial arteries.[40] Approximately half of all patients receiving nitrate therapy will experience nitrate-induced headache. However, clinical experience indicates that if the nitrates are maintained, the headaches will lesson due to the development of nitrate tolerance. Accordingly, the best clinical approach to the nitrate headache issue is to start with the lowest nitrate dosage possible and increase slowly as clinically indicated. If at any time headaches occur, the dose of nitrate should be lowered if possible and then maintained for at least 1 week for tolerance to occur before discontinuing the nitrate. The nitrate-induced headache can be managed with mild analgesics. For example, the patient can take acetaminophen or 80 mg of aspirin with each dose of nitrate. However, if the patient continues to have headaches after 1 week of continuous nitrate therapy, it is unlikely that nitrates can be used on a chronic basis. Accordingly, these patients should be considered for alternative antianginal therapy.

Nitrate tolerance is another issue that impacts nitrate therapy. Studies indicate that continuous 24-hour nitroglycerin infusions, transdermal patches, regimens of isosorbide dinitrate administration four times a day, and long-acting sustained-released nitrate preparations are associated with some degree of nitrate tolerance.[41] The proposed mechanisms for nitrate tolerance include: 1) depletion of sulfhydryl groups, which are needed for the conversion of nitrates to NO; 2) activation of counter-regulatory neurohormones, such as catecholamines, plasma renin, angiotensin, and arginine vasopressin, which result in vasoconstriction and fluid retention; and 3) increased intravascular blood volume.[41]

Studies indicate that the best approach for the prevention of nitrate tolerance is to avoid continuous exposure to the nitrates and to allow for a 12- to 14-hour nitrate-free interval. Studies show that the administration of oral isosorbide dinitrate twice or three times a day is less likely to promote nitrate tolerance than oral isosorbide dinitrate given four times a day.[42] Patients using transdermal nitroglycerin patches should wear them either during the day or during the night, but not both time intervals, thus allowing for a 12-hour nitrate-free period.[43] It should be emphasized that patients who have frequent angina attacks should be covered with an additional antianginal drug, such as beta blocker or calcium entry blocker drug during these nitrate-free intervals. This additional antianginal drug prevents anginal attacks and protects the patient against any rebound myocardial ischemia, which may occur after abrupt nitrate withdrawal.[44] Nitrate-free intervals are not considered, whatsoever, in patients being treated with continuous intravenous nitroglycerin for acute coronary syndromes. If nitrate tolerance develops in these patients, the nitrate infusion is increased and other antianginal agents are administered. Finally, high-dose intravenous infusion of nitroglycerin has been associated with methemoglobinemia, heparin resistance, and Wernicke's encephalopathy.[45] Table 3 lists the nitrate preparation, their dosages, and pharmacokinetics.

Short-Acting Nitrates

The least expensive preparation and the treatment of choice for the acute attack of angina pectoris is sublingual nitroglycerin. The onset of action of sublingual nitroglycerin is rapid, usually within 2 minutes after drug administration. The usual dose is 0.3 to 0.6 mgm. An individual dose can be repeated every 5 minutes for a total of three doses. If symptoms persist, the patient is advised to seek medical attention. The patient should always carry nitroglycerin so that a spontaneous angina attack can be promptly treated. Furthermore, the patient should be

Table 3
Commonly Used Nitrate Preparations

Medication	Recommended Dose	Onset of Action	Peak Action	Duration of Action
Short-Acting Nitrates Used for Treatment of an Angina Attack for Angina Prophylaxis				
Sublingual N troglycerin	0.3–0.6 mg	2–5 minutes	4–8 minutes	10–30 minutes
Aerosol Nitroglycerin	0.4 mg	2–5 minutes	2–5 minutes	10–30 minutes
Buccal Nitroglycerin	1–3 mg	2–5 minutes	4–10 minutes	$^{1}/_{2}$–5 hours
Long-Acting Nitrates Used for Angina Prophylaxis				
Oral Isosorbide Dinitrate	5–40 mg	15–30 minutes	15–60 minutes	3–6 hours
Sublingual and Chewable Isosorbide Dinitrate	2.5–10 mg	3–15 minutes	30–45 minutes	1–2 hours
Oral Isosorbide Dinitrate SR	40 mg	30–60 minutes	45–120 minutes	6–10 hours
Oral Nitroglycerin	2.5–13 mg	30–45 minutes	45–120 minutes	2–8 hours
Oral Erythrityl Tetranitrate	10 mg	30 minutes	80–120 minutes	3–6 hours
Oral Isosorbide Mononitrate	5–60 mg	30 minutes	variable	6–12 hours
Nitroglycerin Ointment 2%	7.5–30 mg	2–5 minutes	30–120 minutes	3–8 hours
Transdermal Nitroglycerin Patch	5–15 mg	30–60 minutes	60–180 minutes	8–12 hours

instructed to assume a sitting position when taking nitroglycerin in order to obviate excessive hypotension which could lead to syncope. Because nitroglycerin tablets are light sensitive, they should be stored in dark containers. The sensation of burning or tingling under the tongue from a nitroglycerin tablet usually indicates to the patient that he has bioactive nitroglycerin. However, to ensure optimal bioavailability of nitroglycerin, nitroglycerin tablets should be renewed every 6 months.

Oral nitroglycerin spray is an excellent short-acting nitroglycerin preparation, especially for the elderly patient with angina pectoris. It is dispensed in metered aerosolized doses of 0.4 mgm of nitroglycerin. It should be emphasized that the metered dose of nitroglycerin spray can be slightly less than an equivalent dose of a nitroglycerin tablet. Therefore, two puffs of aerosol may be necessary to abort or prevent an angina attack. The advantages of nitroglycerin spray over nitroglycerin tablets are: 1) the aerosolized dose of nitroglycerin may be more rapidly and more completely absorbed than a sublingual nitroglycerin tablet; and 2) the nitroglycerin spray is easier to administer when compared to a nitroglycerin tablet. This is particularly important in the elderly patient who may have impaired motor skills and visual acuity. The major disadvantage of nitroglycerin spray is the cost, which exceeds that of sublingual nitroglycerin tablets.

Other short-acting nitroglycerin preparations available include chewable and sublingual isosorbide dinitrate. Both these preparations have a slightly slower onset of action and a longer duration of action when compared to nitroglycerin tablets or spray. Accordingly, they should be only used in the prevention of angina attack and not in the definitive treatment of an attack.

Long-Acting Nitrates

The fundamental goal of using long-acting nitrates is to extend the duration of anti-ischemic effect of the nitrate and, thus, prevent angina attacks. The usual duration of action of a sublingual nitroglycerin is from 15 to 30 minutes. The currently available long-acting nitrate preparations can provide anti-ischemic protection for 2 to 12 hours after administration. Oral isosorbide dinitrate has been the oral long-acting nitrate preparation of choice for years. Its major disadvantage is its low bioavailability, which is due to first pass hepatic metabolism. This, however, can be overcome in part by increasing the dose of the drug. One should start with 10 mgm by mouth two or three times a day, and then increase slowly to 20 to 40 mgm, two or three times a day. The final dose will be determined by clinical efficacy in the absence of adverse side effects, such as headache and or hypotension. Clinical experience and studies suggest that a dose of 30 mgm or greater of isosorbide dinitrate is usually necessary to extend the anti-ischemic effect of the drug to that greater than 3 hours duration.[46]

Recently, isosorbide-5-mononitrate has been approved for use in the treatment of angina pectoris. Isosorbide-5-mononitrate is the active metabolite of isosorbide dinitrate and is completely bioavailable in that it does not undergo first pass hepatic metabolism. The slow release formulation can be given once daily with anti-ischemic protection for up to 12 hours, without the development of nitrate tolerance.

Nitroglycerin ointment 2% which can be applied to the skin is an excellent long-acting nitrate. By having nitroglycerin absorbed directly into the blood stream from the skin, the transdermal nitroglycerin delivery system avoids the first pass liver metabolism. Nitroglycerin patches, which are now very inexpensive, can be used in place of the ointment and, thus, avoid the patient's clothing from being stained by the ointment preparation. This property improves patient compliance. Nitroglycerin patches are useful in the elderly for the following reasons. First, elderly patients are commonly taking multiple drugs. Nitroglycerin patches decrease the number of pills that the patient is taking. Second, elderly patients commonly have CHF with bowel edema, which may result in malabsorption of orally administered nitrate preparations.

The Beta Blockers

The beta blockers are an important class of drugs used in the management of angina pectoris. Their major pharmacological action is to compete with endogenous catecholamines for the beta adrenergic receptor. The hemodynamic effects of this competitive inhibition of the beta adrenergic receptor is a decrease in heart rate, reduction in blood pressure, and a decrease in contractility. Furthermore, these hemodynamic effects are most evident in the setting of increased sympathetic tone and/or adrenal medulla stimulation, which occur during exercise or emotional stress. The beta blockers anti-ischemic action is primarily the result of its reduction in myocardial oxygen demand. The beta blockers may also improve myocardial oxygen supply by slowing the heart rate and extending the duration of diastole, the time interval wherein the majority of coronary blood flow occurs. Additionally, studies show that beta blockers may have a beneficial effect on coronary blood flow in ischemic areas of myocardium by redistributing blood flow from the subepicardium to the subendocardium. Finally, by shifting the oxygen-hemoglobin curve to the right, beta blockers potentially increase oxygen delivery to the myocardium.[47,48]

Beta blockers may, however, augment myocardial ischemia by the following mechanisms. First, beta blockers may block the vasodilator capacity of epicardial coronary arteries by unopposed alpha constriction, which could induce coronary vasospasm and reduce coronary blood flow. Second, beta blockers may, in some patients, increase ventricular volumes, which could increase in wall tension and myocardial oxygen consumption. Fortunately, the favorable effects of beta blockers on reduction in myocardial oxygen consumption outweigh these potential hazards, and beta blockers have proven to be very useful in the management of angina pectoris in most patients.

In addition to its antianginal effects, beta blockers may also improve prognosis in coronary artery patients who have suffered an MI. The Norwegian Multicenter Study Group showed that survivors of MI treated with timolol had both a reduction in mortality and reinfarction at follow-up when compared to patients treated with placebo.[49] These data have been confirmed in other large clinical trials using other beta blockers. Recently, Aronow et al[50] performed a randomized-controlled trial of propranolol versus placebo in 245 older persons, mean age 81 years. Sixty-four percent of these patients had a history of a prior MI. In that study, patients randomized to propranolol had a 47% significant reduction in sudden cardiac death, 37% significant reduction in total cardiac death, and a 20% insignificant reduction in total death when compared to patients randomized to placebo.[50]

Table 4 shows the commonly used beta blockers. The beta blockers are classified by cardioselectivity, duration of action, membrane stability activity, intrinsic sympathetic activity, and lipophilic properties. Cardioselective beta blockers, such as metoprolol and atenolol, which at usual doses only block the $beta_1$ receptor, are less likely to induce bronchospasm, when compared to the nonselective beta blockers such as propranolol. Lipophilic beta blockers, such as propranolol and metoprolol, are rapidly absorbed from the gastrointestinal tract and are metabolized by the liver. The elimination half-life of lipophilic beta blockers tends to be short, which dictates the requirement that multiple doses of the drug be given during a 24-hour period to ensure continuous beta blocker coverage. Finally, lipophilic beta blockers readily cross the blood brain barrier (BBB) which may result in central nervous system side effects such as mood changes and sleep disturbance.

Table 4
Commonly Used Beta Blockers in Treatment of Angina Pectoris

Drug/General Brand	Cardioselectivity (Relative B_1 Selectivity)	Intrinsic Sympathetic Activity	Lipophilic Properties	Usual Daily Dose
Propranolol	0	0	high	10–40 mg/qid
Propranolol LA	0	0	high	40–240 mg/qd
Atenolol	+	0	low	25–100 mg/qd
Metoprolol	+	0	moderate	25–100 mg/bid
Metoprolol (ER)	+	0	moderate	50–200 mg/qd
Timolol	0	0	low	10–20 mg/bid
Acebutolol	+	+	low	200 mg/bid
Pindolol	0	+	moderate	5–20 mg/bid
Nadolol	0	0	high	40–160 mg/qd
Labetalol	0	0	low	100–600 mg/bid

Hydrophilic beta blockers, such as atenolol, tend to have a long elimination half-life, which allows once-a-day dosing. They are predominately excreted by the kidney which necessitate reduced dosing in patients, especially the elderly with reduced renal function. Hydrophilic beta blockers do not readily cross the BBB and theoretically are less likely to induce central nervous system side effects.

Beta blockers with intrinsic sympathetic activity (ISA) may be useful in patients who have low-resting heart rates, depressed atrioventricular (AV) conduction, or reduced myocardial contractility. The ISA property of these beta blockers prevents further slowing of the heart rate, depression of AV conduction, and myocardial contractility in low sympathetic tone states, such as during sleep or at rest. However, it should be emphasized that the beta blockers with ISA have not been shown to reduce the incidence of sudden death in patients following MI, a finding which has been found in all beta blockers studied which do not have ISA. Accordingly, the use of beta blockers with ISA in patients following MI is not recommended.

Labetalol is a unique nonselective beta blocker with alpha receptor-blocking properties. The combination of beta blockade plus alpha blockade results in a greater fall in blood pressure than beta blockade alone. Thus, this drug may be useful in patients with angina and severe hypertension. However, it should be used very cautiously in the elderly patient who may experience a heightened response to alpha blockade. Other beta blockers which have vasodilatory action, such as carvedilol and bucindolol, are being extensively studied. There are encouraging reports that indicate that these novel beta blockers are useful in improving symptoms and prognosis in patients with CHF.[51]

Beta blockers affect lipid metabolism mainly through an increase in serum triglycerides and a slight reduction in serum HDL cholesterol levels. Beta blockers have no effect on serum LDL or total cholesterol levels.[52] The long-term effects of beta blocker-induced lipid changes are unknown and are currently under investigation.

Beta blockers are contraindicated in the clinical setting of bronchospasm, hypotension, severe sinus bradycardia, second-degree or three-degree AV block (unless a pacemaker is in place), decompensated CHF, and hypoglycemia-prone diabetes mellitus. With exclusion of these patients, beta blockers are generally well tolerated, even in the elderly. In a large randomized study which compared propranolol versus placebo for arrhythmia management in a large elderly population (mean age 81 years), 11% of patients taking propranolol had adverse effects which required discontinuation of therapy.[50] The common undesirable side effects of beta blockers are fatigue, symptomatic bradycardia or heart block, central nervous system disturbances such as depression, hallucinations, insomnia and nightmares, bronchospasm, heartburn, diarrhea, constipation, exacerbation of CHF, hypoglycemia, skin rash, sexual dysfunction, intermittent claudication, and Raynauds phenomenon.

It should be emphasized that beta blockers should not be abruptly discontinued in the ambulatory patient. Studies show that a sudden, abrupt withdrawal of beta blockers in patients receiving chronic therapy may rarely lead to a precipitation of an acute ischemic syndrome such as unstable angina or even MI.[53] The mechanism for this phenomenon is thought to be the result of hypersensitivity of the beta receptors. Accordingly, if one wishes to discontinue beta blockers in a patient on chronic therapy, the beta blocker should be tapered slowly and then discontinued. During this period, the patient should be told to reduce his or her activity which may excessively increase sympathetic activity, i.e., exercise or emotional stress. Furthermore, during the period of beta blocker tapering, the patient should be covered with another antianginal agent such as a long-acting nitrate or a nondihydropyridine calcium channel blocker, or both.

Finally, studies have shown that LVH is an independent risk factor for MI and death.[12,13]

Beta blockers have been shown to cause regression of LVH, as assessed by ECG with or without associated reduction in blood pressure.[54] Whether this favorable impact on LVH will be translated in improved prognosis is currently being studied.

Calcium Channel Blockers

The calcium ion plays an important role in the regulation of both myocardial and vascular smooth muscle contraction and relaxation, and in sinus node function and AV node conduction of the heart. The calcium channel blockers block the calcium channels on the cell membrane, which results in a decrease in the availability of intracellular calcium. The decrease in intracellular calcium results in a myriad of effects; the most important for our discussion are: 1) a decrease in vasoconstriction of the coronary, peripheral, and pulmonary vasculative; 2) a decrease in myocardial contractility; 3) a depression of sinus node activity; and 4) a slowing of AV node conduction. The calcium channel blockers are useful anti-ischemic drugs and, hence, antianginal drugs because they decrease myocardial oxygen demand and improve myocardial oxygen supply. The calcium channel blockers decrease myocardial oxygen demand by decreasing blood pressure and myocardial contractility. Nondihydropyridine calcium channel blockers, such as diltiazim and varapamil, further decrease myocardial oxygen demand by slowing the heart rate through their action on the sinus node. Calcium entry blockers can improve coronary blood flow and myocardial oxygen supply by vasodilating epicardial coronary vessels. The vasodilatory property of the calcium blockers make them the drugs of choice in the treatment of pure vasospastic angina (so-called Prinzmetal angina). They are also useful in the treatment of mixed angina, an angina syndrome which is the result of both a fixed coronary obstruction and the vasomotion of the coronary vasculature upon the obstruction. The

mixed angina syndrome is manifested clinically as a constantly changing angina threshold; the patient may have an excellent exercise tolerance one day, while another day, the patient will have angina while
walking only two blocks.

The calcium channel blockers have traditionally been classified
into four groups, which are chemically quite distinct. These four groups
include the dihydropyridines, verapamil, diltiazem, and bepridil. Table
5 shows the commonly used calcium channel blockers.

Nifedipine, which is a first-generation dihydropyridine, is a potent
coronary and peripheral artery vasodilator with negative inotropic properties. Although in vitro studies have shown that nifedipine will block
both the sinoatrial (SA) and AV nodes, the lower dose used in clinical
practice usually does not have this effect. In fact, the reflex sympathetic
discharge which results from the hypotension induced by nifedipine
increases heart rate and ameliorates the negative inotropic properties
of the drug. Furthermore, the intense vasodilation of the peripheral
coronary circulation may result in a coronary steal phenomenon, which
could result in worsening of angina. It has been suggested that 10%
to 20% of patients taking short-acting nifedipine have an increased
incidence of angina. This potential for worsening in angina by nifedipine use occurs in patients with severe three-vessel CAD and in patients
with acute ischemic syndromes.[55] Accordingly, we recommend that if
one wishes to use a short-acting nifedipine for the treatment of angina,
one should add a beta blocker to counteract the heightened sympathetic
tone which occurs following nifedipine administration.

Recently, a new formulation of nifedipine has been released for
the treatment of angina. This sustained release preparation of nifedipine
utilizes a unique gastrointestinal therapeutic system (GITS), which compared to the short-acting nifedipine preparation, results in less sympathetic nervous system activation. Nevertheless, even with this once-a-

Table 5
Commonly Used Calcium Entry Blockers in the Treatment of Angina Pectoris

Drug	Potential for SA Node and AV Node Depression*	Potential for Depression of Myocardial Contractility*	Usual Adult Oral Dosage
Nifedipine	0	0 to +	10–30 mg/tid
Nifedipine XL	0	0 to +	30–90 mg/qd
Nicardipine	0	0 to +	20–30 mg/tid
Amlodipine	0	0	2.5–10 mg/qd
Felodipine	0	0	2.5–20 mg/qd
Diltiazem	++	+	30–90 mg/tid
Diltiazem CD	++	+	120–300 mg/qd
Verapamil	++	++	40–120 mg/tid
Verapamil SR	++	++	120–240 mg/qd

day long-acting nifedipine preparation, one should still consider combining it with a beta blocker.

A major limitation of the nifedipine preparation is the high incidence of peripheral edema, which can occur in 10% to 30% of patients during chronic therapy. In addition, the side effect of syncope is not a rare phenomenon.

The second-generation dihydropyridines, amlodipine and felodipine, have a long duration of action and can be given once a day. In addition, these dihydropyridines have a greater vascular selectivity and less negative inotropy when compared to nifedipine. Accordingly, they can be given to patients with left ventricular dysfunction. These calcium channel blockers have no clinical effect on the SA or AV nodes. It must be emphasized that these dihydropyridines should be used cautiously in the elderly. One should start with the lowest possible dose (i.e., 2.5 mg of felodipine a day) and increase the dose if indicated very slowly, always watching for untoward side effects. In the elderly patient, amlodipine and felodipine blood levels can reach very high levels due to prolonged elimination half-lives. Accordingly, these drugs should be used very cautiously, or not at all, in the elderly patient.

Verapamil dilates both systemic and coronary arteries, has a negative inotropic effect of the myocardium, and is a potent inhibitor of SA node depolarization and AV node conduction. This later action of verapamil attenuates the increased heart rate from sympathetic tone activation which is seen with nifedipine. In fact, studies show that resting and exercise heart rate may be slower when patients are taking verapamil, as compared to when the patients are taking placebo. Verapamil is particularly useful in controlling the ventricular response of atrial fibrillation. Verapamil, however, should be used cautiously in the elderly because these patients may have occult SA node or AV node disease. Moreover, verapamil depresses gastrointestinal motility which may result in a vexing (especially in the elderly) side effect, namely constipation. Recent data suggest that verapamil taken as secondary prevention improves prognosis in survivors of acute MI at 1-year follow-up.[56] Whether this strategy is better then beta blockade after MI will require further studies.

Diltiazem is an excellent antianginal drug with very few side effects. Diltiazem depresses sinus node activity, AV node conduction, and myocardial contractility, similar to that of verapamil, but it is less potent than verapamil. Nevertheless, it should be used cautiously in the elderly patient who may have sinus node and or AV node disease. Diltiazem is a less potent vasodilator than nifedipine and, for this reason, may be better tolerated in the angina patient, especially the elderly patient. For example, side effects such as syncope and edema are less likely to occur with diltiazem than with nifedipine. Diltiazem is now available in slow release forms which allow once- or twice-a-day dosing regimens.

It should be pointed out that recent studies indicate that chronic diltiazem therapy after MI may worsen prognosis in patients who showed evidence of CHF during their coronary care unit (CCU) stay.

In the Multicenter Ditiazem Post Infarction (MDPT) Study, acute myocardial infarction (AMI) patients with CHF during CCU who were randomized to diltiazem had a higher mortality at 1-year follow-up, compared to patients with CHF who were randomized to placebo.[57] Therefore, we do not recommend that patients with a history of CHF during acute MI routinely receive diltiazem as part of their management of angina pectoris. These patients are best managed by nitrates and or beta blockers. If a calcium channel blocker is needed for angina treatment in these patients, we would recommend a second-generation dihydropyridine, such as amlodipine or felodipine, which does not have negative ionotropic properties. Important recent data from Packer et al[58] has shown that amlodipine is safe in patients with CHF, and its use may even improve prognosis in patients with nonischemic cardiomyopathy.

Bepridil is a new calcium-entry blocker. In addition to its action as a vasodilator and depressor of the SA node and AV node, bepridil has been shown to be a weak sodium channel blocker. This latter property may result in a prolongation of atrial and ventricular refractory periods, which translates to an antiarrhythmic action. However, in some cases, bepridil has been shown to prolong the QT_c interval on the ECG and to cause torsade de pointes. There have been sudden deaths in patients taking bepridil and the mechanism for these deaths has been thought to be due to the proarrhythmic potential of the drug. Accordingly, we do not recommend that bepridil be used as a first-line calcium channel blocker in the treatment of angina. If bepridil is used, we recommend that serial ECGs be performed. If QT_c prolongation is observed during bepridil therapy, we would recommend that bepridil be discontinued and an alternate form of therapy instituted.

Recent disturbing data have called into question the safety of calcium entry blockers in the treatment of various clinical disorders.[55,59-61] The mechanisms for these adverse effects such as increased risk of MI are unclear, but most of the studies show that short-acting nifedipine may be deleterious when used alone in the treatment of angina or hypertension. Accordingly, in most circumstances, until other data are available, we would recommend that dialtiazim or verapamil be preferred over dihydropyridine channel blockers in the treatment of angina and hypertension in the elderly patient.

Management of Angina by Drugs

Single-Drug Therapy

Sublingual nitroglycerin may be the only drug necessary for the treatment of angina in patients with infrequent angina attacks. In patients with frequent angina attacks (i.e., two or more a week), a long-acting antianginal drug should be used for angina prophylaxis. Studies have shown that chronic therapy with either a long-acting nitrate, a beta blocker, or a calcium channel blocker has equal efficacy in angina prevention and improvement in exercise tolerance. Accordingly, the selection of which antianginal drug to use in a given patent must be individualized. For example, in a patient with chronic lung disease and reversible bronchospasm, a long-acting nitrate or calcium blocker should be used for the treatment of angina rather than a beta blocker. Conversely, in patients with a prior MI, a beta blocker, if tolerated, is the ideal antianginal drug because it may improve prognosis, as well as prevent symptoms. A long-acting nitrate is a useful antianginal drug, but it should only be used as monotherapy in patients who do not require 24-hour antianginal prophylaxis. As previously discussed, long-acting nitrate therapy requires a 10- to 14-hour nitrate-free interval to prevent nitrate tolerance. In patients who require 24-hour antianginal prophylaxis, a beta blocker or a calcium channel blocker should be added to the long-acting nitrate drug therapy to ensure this protection.

Combination Drug Therapy

If angina attacks persist despite maximal tolerated doses of either a long-acting nitrate, beta blocker, or calcium-channel blocker, one should consider combination therapy. The combination of a long-acting nitrate with a beta blocker is an excellent rational antianginal drug strategy for the following reasons. Nitrates decrease myocardial oxygen demand by decreasing myocardial wall tension, but they may increase heart rate. Beta blockers decrease heart rate and myocardial contractility. Thus, the combination of a nitrate with a beta blocker decreases all three major determinants of myocardial oxygen demand, wall tension, heart rate, and myocardial contractility. Furthermore, nitrates which relax epicardial coronary arteries and collateral vessels, and improve regional coronary blood flow, may counteract the potential for beta blockers to induce coronary vasospasm. Importantly, controlled clinical studies show that the combination of long-acting nitrates with beta blockers decreases the number of angina attacks and improves exercise tolerance when compared to beta blocker therapy or nitrate therapy alone.[62]

If the patient cannot tolerate a long-acting nitrate, then a combination of a beta blocker with a calcium blocker should be considered. Studies have shown that the combination of a beta blocker with a calcium channel blocker reduces the number of angina attacks and improves exercise capacity when compared to either beta blocker or calcium-channel blocker therapy alone.[63] The choice of which calcium channel blocker should be combined with the beta blocker should be individualized. One should be very cautious of combining a beta blocker with either diltiazem or verapamil, especially in the elderly patient. This combination has the risk of inducing severe bradycardia (i.e., sinus bradycardia and heart block) and provoking CHF. If one chooses this combination, one should use very low doses of each drug and monitor the patient carefully. The combination of a beta blocker and a dihydropyridine calcium channel blocker, especially the second-generation dihydropyridine such as felodipine, does not have the synergistic potential for bradyarrhythmias and worsening of CHF, and should be considered the beta blocker-calcium entry blocker combination of choice in elderly patients at risk for bradyarrhythmias and CHF. However, it should be emphasized that one should initiate this therapy with the lowest possible dose of each drug and titrate slowly upward until clinical efficacy is achieved.

In patients who cannot tolerate a beta blocker, one should consider the combination of a long-acting nitrate with a calcium entry blocker. One should use this drug combination cautiously because both drugs are vasodilators, which increases the risk for hypotension and syncope. To ameliorate the potential for hypotension, we have found it useful not to administer the two drugs together, but to administer them at least 2 hours apart. We have also found that the combination of a long-acting nitrate with the calcium channel blocker, diltiazem, is an effective alternative to the long-acting nitrate and beta blocker combination. Diltiazem tends to slow the heart rate and has a weak, negative ionotropic effect; both of these properties are not clinically present in the dihydropyridine channel blockers.

Triple-drug therapy—a long-acting nitrate, a beta blocker, and a calcium-entry blocker—should be considered in patients who continue to have disabling angina despite double-drug therapy. Notwithstanding, conflicting data on efficacy of head to head comparisons of triple therapy versus double therapy for angina prophylaxis and improvement in exercise tolerance, clinical experience has shown that some patients respond better to triple therapy versus double therapy in the management of their angina.

Unstable Angina

Unstable angina is the most common diagnosis given to patients treated in CCU. The diagnosis of unstable angina is made in patients with new onset angina and in patients with chronic angina, who have an accelerated pattern in their angina, manifested by an increase in frequency, duration, and severity of their angina attacks. Angina at rest is considered the most serious form of unstable angina. ECG changes show that left ventricular ischemia is usually present during these attacks of angina. Braunwald has recently presented a new classification of the various subgroups of unstable angina which should provide uniformity in data analysis for future studies. In Braunwald's classification, type I unstable angina patients include those patients with new onset angina or accelerated angina. These patients do not have rest pain; type II unstable angina patients include those patients with angina at rest within the past month, but not within the preceding 48 hours; and type III unstable angina patients include those patients with rest pain within 48 hours after admission. The patients are further characterized as to the presence or absence of extracardiac conditions that could intensify or provoke myocardial ischemia, and to the presence or absence of a recent MI.[64]

Recent studies have provided insight into the pathogenesis of unstable angina. It is generally believed that the initiating event of unstable angina is the fracturing of the intima of a vulnerable atherosclerotic plaque in an epicardial coronary artery. The mechanism or mechanisms responsible for the plaque fracture is under intense investigation. Some investigators have provided data that suggest that the plaque fractures as a result of hemodynamic factors present within the lumen of the coronary artery. They posit the hypothesis that high shear forces fracture the plaque at the weakest point known as the shoulder region of the plaque.[65,66] Others have provided data supporting the hypothesis that the plaque fractures as a result of an inflammatory reaction within the vulnerable plaque. These investigators suggest that the plaques fracture as a result from the proteolytic action of metaloproteinases, which are released from activated macrophages underlying the fibrous cap of vulnerable atherosclerotic plaque.[67] Whatever the mechanism for the plaque fracture with disruption of the intima, the net result is intraplaque hemorrhage and thrombus overlying the plaque fracture. This results in acute narrowing of the coronary artery, which may compromise coronary blood flow and induce myocardial ischemia. The initial thrombus overlaying the plaque fractures is usually platelet rich, the so-called white thrombus. Later, with the accumulation of fibrin, the thrombus is transformed into a typical fibrin-rich, red thrombus.

During and after the phase of plaque fracture, the affected coronary artery is prone to vasoconstriction. This is the result of localized impaired vasodilatory mechanisms, as well as heightened vasoconstriction activity when the vasoconstrictors serotonin and thromboxane A_2 are released from the platelets within the intracoronary thrombus.[65,66] It is generally accepted that the size of the plaque fracture, the size of the intraplaque hemorrhage, the size of the intracoronary thrombus, the extent of the stenosis of the preexisting atherosclerotic plaque, and the extent of preexisting collateral circulation will determine whether the patient will suffer either unstable angina or an MI. Furthermore, studies indicate that the plaque fracture and associated intraplaque hemorrhage and intracoronary thrombus will resolve over time, usually within 4 to 6 weeks.[67] Accordingly, the fundamental goal in the treatment of patients suspected of having unstable angina is to rapidly stabilize the unstable atherosclerotic plaque.

Unstable angina patients should be admitted to the CCU and monitored for at least 24 hours. Medical therapy includes bed rest, oxygen therapy, antiplatelet therapy, intravenous nitroglycerin, antithrombotic therapy, beta blockers, and, in refractory cases, calcium channel blockers. In addition, extra cardiac factors such as anemia and hyperthyroidism should be ruled out and, if found, should be treated accordingly. Continuous oxygen therapy consists of oxygen at 2 L/min by nasal cannula, if the patient is experiencing pain or if there is any evidence of CHF or other conditions which may induce hypoxemia. Aspirin at a dose of 325 mgm should be chewed and swallowed by the patient on hospital admission to facilitate rapid absorption of the antiplatelet drug. Thereafter, the patient should be treated with enteric-coated aspirin to help prevent gastric toxicity. We recommend that the patient receive an oral dose of 325 mgm of aspirin, daily. It should be emphasized that acute aspirin therapy in the setting of unstable angina and MI reduces death and MI.[24,25,68]

Nitrate therapy should be instituted with intravenous nitroglycerin. We generally start with a dose of 10 μg/min of intravenous nitroglycerin and titrate upward with an incremental dose of 10 μg/min every 2 minutes until chest pain is reduced or, in patients without chest pain, there is a drop in systolic blood pressure of 10 mm Hg or greater, or an increase in heart rate of 10 beats per minute of greater or both. The usual dose of intravenous nitroglycerin is from 10 to 100 μg/min.

Patients should be maintained on intravenous nitroglycerin until they are free of chest pain for at least 24 hours. Thereafter, one may consider discontinuing intravenous nitroglycerin and switching the patient to nitroglycerin patch or an oral nitrate preparation, such as isosorbide dinitrate. Approximately one third of patients will experience a severe nitrate-induced headache, which we have coined the "CCU migraine," during the intravenous nitroglycerin phase of unstable angina treatment. We have used Tylenol and codeine with some success in attenuating this vexing symptom. In patients who cannot tolerate nitrate therapy, beta blockers and nondihydropridine calcium channel blockers should be considered as good antianginal substitutes.

Unstable angina patients, especially those with chest pain and ECG evidence of myocardial ischemia, should be considered for antithrombotic therapy. If there are no contraindications for antithrombotic therapy, the unstable angina patient should receive a 5000 unit bolus of heparin and then the patient should be started on a continuous infusion of heparin at 1000 U/h. The activated partial thromboplastin time (PTT) should be obtained at least every 6 hours and the dose of heparin should be adjusted to maintain the PTT at 55 to 85 seconds. The ideal duration of heparin therapy is unknown, but clinical experience suggests that patients are best treated if the heparin infusion is maintained for at least 48 hours. Moreover, recent studies show that there may indeed be a heparin withdrawal-rebound phenomenon which is manifested clinically as an increased risk for ischemic events to occur shortly after the cessation of heparin therapy.[69,70] Therefore, whenever heparin is discontinued in an unstable angina patient, the patient should be carefully monitored, and if there is an exacerbation of symptoms, heparin should be immediately reinstituted. It has been suggested that aspirin therapy may block the full potential of this clinical phenomenon, thus allowing the discontinuation of heparin to occur without untoward clinical events in the unstable angina patient.

Beta blockers should be started in all unstable angina patients who do not have contraindications for beta blocker therapy. Acute beta blockade has been shown to improve survival in acute MI patients, and it is possible that this benefit is also rendered to unstable angina patients.[71] Very rapid beta blockade can be achieved by giving metoprolol 5 mgm intravenously every 5 minutes for a total dose of 15 mgm. The patient is then started on oral metoprolol therapy. One should only consider intravenous beta blocker therapy in patients with a relative increase in heart rate (heart rate greater then 70 beats per minutes) and a systolic blood pressure greater than 100 mm Hg. It should be pointed out that we have found that the vast majority of unstable angina patients can be managed by an oral beta blocker, such as metaprolol or propranolol alone and, therefore, we rarely resort to intravenous beta blocker therapy. Calcium channel blockers should be given to unstable angina patients who continue to have angina, despite adequate doses of nitrates and beta blockers. It is important to note that nifedipine should not be given alone to an unstable patient without beta blocker therapy. As previously discussed, studies show that treatment of the unstable angina patient with nifedipine alone is correlated with a worse prognosis. The addition of a beta blocker to nifedipine in the unstable angina patient reduces this risk.[55,59-61]

Well over 90% of unstable angina patients can be stabilized with medical therapy within 72 hours after admission. The next decision after the patient is stabilized is whether he or she should undergo coronary angiography, a procedure which should be considered for those patients suspected of having left main CAD and three-vessel CAD with left ventricular disfunction. In both of these conditions, bypass graft surgery had been shown to improve survival.[73-75] Unstable angina patients with a history of PTCA within 6 months of admission should be considered candidates for early angiography because the unstable angina is most likely the consequence of restenosis of the PTCA site. In other patients, decisions for angiography can be made from the results of noninvasive tests, such as low-level exercise stress testing, nuclear studies, or stress echocardiography. In general, if any of these studies show evidence of myocardial ischemia, one should consider performing angiography.[76] In the remaining 10% of unstable angina patients who continue to have ischemia despite medical management, coronary angiography should be performed. Studies show that these are high-risk, unstable angina patients who should be considered for revascularization procedure.[77] Intra-aortic balloon pumping may be useful in these high-risk patients prior to, during, and after coronary angiography.

Recent studies have shown that more potent antithrombotic and antiplatelet therapy may be useful in the unstable angina patient. Studies show that hirudin, a potent antithrombin derived from the leech Hirudo medicinals, dissolves intracoronary thrombi better than heparin.[78] Drugs that block the IIB/IIIA receptor on the platelet result in more platelet dysfunction than that of aspirin. Preliminary studies in unstable angina patients show that these IIB/IIIA blockers improve clinical outcomes compared to placebo.[79] Large controlled clinical trials are now in progress to evaluate these exciting new antithrombin and antiplatelet drugs in patients with unstable angina.

References

1. Wenger WN, Marcus FI, O'Rourke R: Cardiovascular disease in the elderly. *J Am Coll Cardiol* 10:80A-87A, 1987.
2. Elveback L, Lie JT: Continued high incidence of coronary artery disease at autopsy in Olmstead County, Minnesota, 1950 to 1979. *Circulation* 70:345-349, 1984.
3. White NK, Edwards JE, Dry TJ: The relationship of the degree of coronary atherosclerosis with age in men. *Circulation* 1:645-654, 1950.
4. National Center for Health Statistics. *Advance Report of Final Mortality Statistics, 1988 Monthly Vital Statistics Report.* Hyattsville, Maryland: Public Health Service 39(suppl 7):7-1-49, 1990.
5. *National Hospital Discharge Survey.* United States Department of Health and Human Services. Washington, DC: National Center for Health Statistics; 1987.
6. Wei JY: Heart disease in the elderly. *Cardiovasc Med* 9:971-982, 1984.
7. Miller TR, Grossman SI, Schectman KB, et al: Left ventricular diastolic filling in the elderly. *Am J Cardiol* 58:531-535, 1986.
8. Arora RR, Machac J, Goldman MF, et al: Atrial kinetics and left ventricular diastolic filling in the healthy elderly. *J Am Coll Cardiol* 9:1255-1260, 1987.
9. Schulman SP, Weisfeldt ML: Cardiovascular aging and adaptation to disease. In: Schlant RC, Alexander RW (eds). *Hurst's The Heart.* New York: McGraw Hill; 2067-2076, 1994.
10. Aronow WS, Ahn C, Kronzon L, et al: Congestive heart failure, coronary events, and atherothrombotic brain infarction in elderly blacks and whites with systemic hypertension, and with and without echocardiography and electrocardiographic evidence of left ventricular hypertrophy. *Am J Cardiol* 67:295-299, 1991.
11. Applegate WB: Hypertension in elderly patients. *Ann Intern Med* 110:901-915, 1989.
12. Kannel WB, Gordon T, Castell WB, et al: Electrocardiographic left ventricular hypertrophy and risk of coronary heart disease: the Framingham Study. *Ann Intern Med* 72:813-822, 1970.
13. Levy D, Gurrison RJ, Savage DD, et al: Left ventricular mass and incidence of coronary heart disease in an elderly cohort. *Ann Intern Med* 110:101-107, 1989.
14. Aronow WS, Koenigsberg M, Schwartz KS: Usefulness of echocardiographic and electrocardiographic left ventricular hypertrophy in predicting new cardiac events and atherothrombotic brain infarction in elderly patients with systemic hypertension or coronary artery disease. *Am J Noninvas Cardiol* 3:367-373, 1987.
15. Amery A, Birkenhager W, Brixro P, et al: Mortality and morbidity results from the European Working Party on High Blood Pressure in the Elderly Trial. *Lancet* 442:1349-1352, 1985.
16. SHEP Cooperative Research Group: Prevention of stroke by antihypertensive drug treatment in older persons with isolated systolic hypertension: final results of the systolic hypertension in the elderly program (SHEP). *JAMA* 265:3255-3265, 1991 .
17. MRC Working Party: Medical Research Council Trial of Treatment of Hypertension in Older Adults: Principal Results. *Br Med J* 304:405-412, 1992.
18. Jajich CL, Ostfeld AM, Freeman DH: Smoking and coronary heart disease mortality in the elderly. *JAMA* 252:2828-2831, 1984.

19. Blankenhorn DH, Nessim SA, Johnson RL, et al: Beneficial effects of combined colestipol-niacin therapy on coronary atherosclerosis and coronary venous bypass grafts. JAMA 257:3233-3240, 1987.
20. Brown G, Albers JJ, Fisher LD, et al: Regression of coronary artery disease as a result of intensive lipid-lowering therapy in men with high levels of apolipoprotein B. N Engl J Med 323:1289-1298, 1990.
21. The Scandinavian Simvastatin Survival Studs: Randomized trial of cholesterol lowering in 4444 patients with coronary heart disease. Lancet 344:1383-1389, 1994.
22. Adult Treatment Panel II: Detection, evaluation, and treatment of high blood cholesterol in adults. Circulation 89:1329-1445, 1994.
23. Armstrong VW, Cremer P, Eberle P, et al: The association between Lp(a) concentrations and angiography assessed coronary atherosclerosis: dependence on serum LDL levels. Atherosclerosis 62:249-256, 1986.
24. Lewis HD, David JW, Archibald DG, et al: Protective effects of aspirin against acute myocardial infarction and death in men with unstable angina. N Engl J Med 309:396-403, 1983.
25. Cairns JA, Gent M, Singer J, et al: Aspirin sulfinpyrazone, or both in unstable angina: results of a Canadian Multicenter Trial. N Engl J Med 313:1369-1370, 1984.
26. The Writing Group for the PEPI Trial: Effects of estrogen or estrogen/progestin regimens on heart disease risk factors in postmenopausal women: The Postmenopausal Estrogen/Progestin Interventions (PEPI) Trial. JAMA 273:199-208, 1995.
27. Lavie CJ, Milani RV, Littman AB: Benefits of cardiac rehabilitation and exercise training in secondary coronary prevention in the elderly. J Am Coll Cardiol 22:678-683, 1993.
28. Smith SC, Blair SN, Criqui MH, et al: Preventing heart attack and death in patients with coronary disease. Circulation 92:2-4, 1995.
29. Brunton TL: Use of nitrate of amyl in angina pectoris. Lancet 2:97-98, 1867.
30. Ignarro LJ, Lippton H, Edwards JC, et al: Mechanism of vascular smooth muscle relaxation by organic nitrates, nitrites, nitroprusside and nitric oxide: evidence for the involvement of S-nitrosothiols as active intermediates. J Pharmacol Exp Ther 218:739-749, 1981 .
31. Parker JO: Nitrate therapy in stable angina pectoris. N Engl J Med 316:1635-1642, 1987.
32. Flavahan NA: Atherosclerosis of lipoprotein-induced endothelial dysfunction: potential mechanisms underlying reduction in EDRF/nitric oxide activity. Circulation 85:1927-1938, 1992.
33. Ganz P, Abben RP, Barry WH: Dynamic variations in resistance of coronary arterial narrowings in angina pectoris at rest. Am J Cardiol 59:64-74, 1987.
34. Greenberg H, Dwyer EM, Jameson AG, et al: Effects of nitroglycerin on the major determinants of myocardial oxygen consumption: an angiographic and hemodynamic assessment. Am J Cardiol 36:426-432, 1975.
35. Cohen MV, Downey JM, Sonnenblick EH, Kirr ES: The effects of nitroglycerin on coronary collaterals and myocardial contractility. J Clin Inves 52:2836-2846, 1973.
36. Brown BG, Bolson E, Peterson RB, et al: The mechanism of nitroglycerin action: stenosis vasodilation as a major component of drug response. Circulation 64:1089-1097, 1981.
37. Bache RJ, Ball RM, Cobb FR, et al: Effects of nitroglycerin on transmural myocardial blood flow in unanesthetized dog. J Clin Invest 55:1219, 1975.
38. Diodati J, Cannon R0: Effect of nitroglycerin on platelet activation in patients with stable coronary disease. Circulation 84(suppl II):ll-731, 1991.

39. Friesinger GC: Coronary heart disease in the elderly: management considerations. *Am J Geriat Cardiol* 3:42-50, 1994.
40. Olesen J: Hemodynamics. In: Olesen J, Tfelt-Hansen P, Welch KMA (eds). *The Headaches.* New York: Raven Press; 209-222, 1993.
41. Elkayam U: Tolerance to organic nitrates: evidence, mechanisms, clinical relevance and strategies for prevention. *Ann Intern Med* 114:667-677, 1991.
42. Parker J0, Farrell B, Lahey KA, et al: Effect of intervals between doses on the development of tolerance to isosorbide dinitrate. *N Engl J Med* 316:1440-1444, 1987.
43. Demots H, Glasser SP: Intermittent therapy in the treatment of chronic stable angina. *J Am Coll Cardiol* 13:786-793, 1989.
44. Przybojewski JZ, Heyns MH: Acute coronary vasospasm secondary to industrial nitroglycerin withdrawal. *S Afr J* 63:158-162, 1983.
45. Gibson GR, Hunter JB, Raabe DS, et al: Methemoglobinemia produced by high-dose intravenous nitroglycerin. *Ann Intern Med* 96:615, 1982.
46. Danahy DT, Aronow WS: Hemodynamics and antianginal effects of high-dose oral isosorbide dinitrate after chronic use. *Circulation* 56:205-212, 1977.
47. Buck JD, Gross GJ, Warltier DC, et al: Comparative effects of cardioselective versus noncardioselective beta blockade on subendocardial blood flow and contractile function in ischemic myocardium. *Am J Cardiol* 44:657-663, 1979.
48. Schrumpf JD, Sleps DS, Wolfson S, et al: Altered hemoglobin-oxygen affinity with long-term propranolol therapy in patients with coronary artery disease. *Am J Cardiol* 40:76-82, 1977.
49. The Norwegian Multicenter Study Group: Timolol-induced reduction in mortality and reinfarction in patients surviving infarction. *N Engl J Med* 304:801-807, 1981.
50. Aronow WS, Ahn C, Mercando AD, et al: Effect of propranolol versus no antiarrhythmic drug on sudden cardiac death, total cardiac death and total death in patients ≥ 62 years of age with heart disease, complex ventricular arrhythmias, and left ventricular ejection fraction ≥ 40%. *Am J Cardiol* 74:267-270, 1994.
51. Packer M, Bristow MR, Cohn JN: Effect of carvedilol on survival of patients with chronic heart failure. *Circulation* 92:1-142, 1995.
52. Lehtonen A: Effect of beta blockers on blood lipid profile. *Am Heart J* 109:1192-1196, 1985.
53. Miller RR, Olson HG, Amsterdam EA, Mason DT: Propranolol withdrawal rebound phenomenon: exacerbation of coronary events after abrupt cessation of antianginal therapy. *N Engl J Med* 293:416-418, 1975.
54. Agabiti-Rosei E, Muiesan ML, Muiesan G: Regression of structural alterations in hypertension. *Am J Hypertens* 2:705, 1989.
55. Muller J, Morerison J, Stone PH, et al: Nifedipine therapy for patients with threatened and acute myocardial infarction: a randomized, double-blind, placebo-controlled comparison. *Circulation* 69:740-747, 1984.
56. The Danish Study on Verapamil in Myocardial Infarction: The effect of verapamil on mortality and major events after myocardial infarction. The Danish Verapamil Infarction Trial II (DAVIT II). *Am J Cardiol* 66:779-785, 1988.
57. The Multicenter Diltiazem Post Infarction Trial Research Group: The effect of diltiazem on mortality and reinfarction after myocardial infarction. *N Engl J Med* 319:385-392, 1988.
58. Packer, M: The PRAISE Trial (Prospective Randomized Amlodipine Survival Evaluation): Background and Main Results. Presented at the American College of Cardiology Annual Meeting. New Orleans, LA: March, 1995.
59. The Israeli Spring Study Group: Secondary Prevention Reinfarction Israeli Nifedipine Trial (SPRINT): A randomized intervention trial of nifedipine in patients with acute myocardial infarction. *Eur Heart J* 9:351-364, 1988.

60. Yusuf S, Held P, Furberg C: Update of effects of calcium antagonists in myocardial infarction or angina light of the Second Danis Verapamil Infarction Trial (DAVID-II) and other recent studies. *Am J Cardiol* 67:1295-1297, 1991.
61. Psaty BM, Heckbert SR, Koepsell TD, et al: The risk of myocardial infarction associated with antihypertensive drug therapies. *JAMA* 274:620-625, 1995.
62. Bassan MM, Weiler-Ravell D: The additive antianginal action of oral isosorbide dinitrate in patients receiving propranolol: magnitude and duration of effect. *Chest* 83:233-241, 1983.
63. Dargie HJ, Lynch PG, Krikler DM, et al: Nifedipine and propranolol: a beneficial drug interaction. *Am J Med* 71:676-682, 1981.
64. Braunwald E: Unstable angina: a classification. *Circulation* 80:410-414, 1989.
65. Davies MJ, Thomas AC: Plaque fissuring— The cause of acute myocardial infarction, sudden ischaemic death, and crescendo angina. *Br Heart J* 53:363-373, 1985.
66. Davies MJ, Richarson PD, Woolf N, Katz DR, Mann J: Risk of thrombosis in human atherosclerotic plaques: role of extracellular lipid, macrophage, and smooth muscle content. *Br Heart J* 69:377-381, 1993.
67. Kovanen PT, Kaartinen M, Paavonen T: Infiltrates of activated mast cells at the site of coronary atheromatous erosion or rupture in myocardial infarction. *Circulation* 92:1084-1088, 1995.
68. Antiplatelet Trialists' Collaboration: Collaborative overview of randomized trials of antiplatelet therapy— 1: prevention of death, myocardial infarction and stroke by prolonged antiplatelet therapy in various categories of patients.*Br Med J* 308:81-106, 1994.
69. Theroux P, Ouimet H, McCans J, et al: Aspirin, heparin, or both to treat unstable angina. *N Engl J Med* 319:1105-1111, 1988.
70. Theroux P, Waters D, Lam J, Quneau M, McCans J: Reactivation of unstable angina after the discontinuation of heparin. *N Engl J Med* 327:141-145, 1992.
71. ISIS-1 Collaborative Group: A randomized trial of intravenous atenolol among 16,027 cases of suspected acute myocardial infarction. *Lancet* 2:57-66, 1986.
72. Conti CR, Hill JA, Mayfield WR: Unstable angina pectoris: pathogenesis and management. *Curr Prob Cardiol* 14:557-623, 1989.
73. The Veterans Administration Coronary Artery Bypass Surgery Cooperative Study Group: Eleven-year survival in the veterans administration randomized trial of coronary bypass surgery for stable angina. *N Engl J Med* 311:1333-1339, 1984.
74. Luchi RJ, Scott SM, Deupree RH: Comparison of medical and surgical treatment for unstable angina pectoris. *N Engl J Med* 316:977-984, 1987.
75. Parisi AF, Khuris Deupree RH, et al: Medical compared with surgical management of unstable angina: five-year mortality and morbidity in the veterans administration study. *Circulation* 80:1176-1189, 1989.
76. Butman SM, Olson HG, Gardin JM, Piters KM, Hullett M, Butman LR: Submaximal exercise testing after stabilization of unstable angina. *J Am Coll Cardiol* 4:667-673, 1984.
77. Olson HG, Lyons KP, Aronow WS, et al: The high-risk angina patient: identification by clinical features, hospital course, electrocardiography, and Technetium-99m Stannous pyrophosphate scintigraphy. *Circulation* 64:674-684, 1981.
78. Serryus PW, Deckers JW, Close P: A double blind, randomized, heparin controlled trial evaluating acute and long-term efficacy of r-Hirudin in patients undergoing angioplasty. *Circulation* 90:I-394, 1994.
79. Simoons ML, DeBoer MJ, Van Den Brand JBM, the European Cooperative Study Group, et al: Randomized trial of GP IIb/IIIa platelet receptor blocker and refractory unstable angina. *Circulation* 89:596-603, 1994.

Chapter 17

Management of the Acute Myocardial Infarction and the Postmyocardial Infarction Elderly Patient

Robert Forman, MD
Wilbert S. Aronow, MD

Introduction

Although individuals older than 65 years account for only 12% of the population,[1] this age group also accounts for nearly 60% of hospital admissions with acute myocardial infarction (MI), and patients over the age of 75 account for nearly half of these admissions of patients older than 65 years.[2] The in-hospital mortality is higher for this age group; for patients not treated with thrombolytic agents, the mortality rate is approximately 5% in patients less than 65 years of age, 15% in patients 66 to 75 years, and 25% in patients older than 75 years. The postdischarge death rate is particularly high with a 1-year cardiac mortality rate of 12% for patients aged 65 to 75, and 17.6% for patients older than 75 years.[3] About two thirds of these deaths are sudden or related to a new MI.[3] Although ejection fraction is the single most important predictor of 1-year survival in patients post-MI, it was not an important risk factor in mortality in patients ages 65 to 75 years in the Multicenter Investigation of the Limitation of Infarct Size (MILIS) Study[4] or in the group of patients older than 75 years.[3]

Thus, with the high in-hospital and postdischarge mortality, there is a greater potential for improving the survival, and more importantly, the number of lives saved in elderly patients treated with appropriate and optimal therapy. Elderly patients who are free of general, noncardiac debility and who can be expected to live a meaningful life, can

From: Aronow WS, Stemmer EA, Wilson SE (eds). *Vascular Disease in the Elderly.* Armonk, NY: Futura Publishing Company, Inc., © 1997.

and should be offered a comprehensive program to reduce their cardiac morbidity and mortality following an acute MI.

Thrombolytic Agents

It is standard practice to administer thrombolytic agents in younger patients with acute MI, whereas there is a reluctance to use these agents in the elderly because of the generally perceived notion that the complication rate from their use is higher and their effectiveness is inferior in this age group. However, a higher percentage of elderly patients will have contraindications to thrombolytic therapy, including severe hypertension, recent cerebrovascular accident, and bleeding disorder, or arrive too late in the emergency room. Unfortunately, elderly patients had been specifically excluded from many of the earlier randomized trials of thrombolytic agents conducted in the United States, but have been enrolled in the European trials, particularly when streptokinase (SK) has been studied. Elderly patients have since been included in the more recent trials where SK has been compared with tissue plasminogen activator (tPA).

The mortality rates for the major placebo-controlled trials of thrombolytic agents for acute MI have been tabulated according to age (Table 1). Although SK is the only thrombolytic agent that was administered to patients older than age 70 in these trials, we have no reason to believe that these other agents will be less effective in this age group. The Gruppo Italiano per lo Studio della Streptochinasi nell'Infarcto Miocardico (GISSI-1)[5] showed a significant reduction in mortality in patients younger than 66 years treated with SK compared with controls; however, the mortality rate was lower in patient groups older than 65 and 75 who received SK, and the reduction in mortality was not significant. However, the number of lives saved was more than 4 patients per 100 treated in the elderly and only 2 in the younger group. The Intravenous Streptokinase in Acute Myocardial Infarction (ISAM) Trial[6] was the only study in which a greater mortality in the elderly was demonstrated, but the total number of patients in this age group was small and the results were not statistically significant. By far the largest number of elderly patients was randomized to SK or placebo in the Second International Study of Infarct Survival (ISIS-2).[7] In this study, which had four arms (SK, SK with aspirin, and aspirin and placebo), the mortality rate was significantly reduced in the elderly in all three active treatment groups, but particularly when aspirin was combined with SK.

In the Anglo-Scandinavian Study of Early Thrombolysis (ASSET),[8] in which patients were randomized to tPA or placebo and heparin given to both groups, all patients were less than 75 years of age. In this trial, however, the reduction of mortality for patients less than 66 years of age was not significant, but was highly significant for those patients older than 65 years. The results of the APSAC International Mortality Study (AIMS) Trial[9] were similar to those from the ASSET Trial in

Table 1
Effect of Age on Early Mortality Following Thrombolysis

Trial	N	Active/Placebo		Reduction Mortality %	P Value	Lives Saved/1000
Streptokinase						
GISSI-1[5]						
≤75 yrs	10,494	8.7	10.6	18	0.001	19
>75 yrs	1,215	28.9	33.1	13	0.11	42
ISAM[6]						
<70 yrs	1,454	5.1	6.6	23	0.21	15
70–75 yrs	287	13.0	9.6	(35)	0.37	(34)
ISIS-2[7]						
<70 yrs	13,776	7.0	9.6	27	0.001	26
≥70 yrs	3,812	18.2	21.6	16	0.01	34
tPA						
ASSET[8]						
≤65 yrs	3,352	5.4	6.3	14	0.24	11
66–75 yrs	1,679	10.8	16.4	34	0.001	56
APSAC						
AIMS[9]						
<60 yrs	1,257	5.2	8.5	39	0.06	32
60–70 yrs	751	12.2	30.2	60	0.003	180

that the mortality rate was reduced in patients randomized to receive APSAC, but was only significant in the older and not younger patients. In this latter trial, however, all patients were less than 70 years of age and the numbers were relatively small.

A post-hoc subgroup analysis always has the potential danger of producing misleading results and in none of the above studies were patients specifically randomized according to their age. However, the consistent results showing improved short-term mortality in the elderly strongly suggest that this group should not be denied thrombolytic agents because of age alone.

Three large trials have directly compared the outcome of SK with tPA. In the GISSI-2 Trial,[10] 22.5% of the 12,490 patients were older than 70 years, but the results were not separately analyzed according to age. The overall 5-week mortality was not different in the patients receiving either SK or tPA (9.0% and 8.6%, respectively). In the ISIS-3 Trial,[11] 26.1% of the 41,299 patients were 70 years or older and randomized to receive SK, APSAC or duteplase (a double-chain product of tPA). The 5-week mortality was not significantly different (10.6%, 10.5%, and 10.3%, respectively). The results were not separately analyzed according to age. In these two trials, there were additional arms in which the patients did or did not receive subcutaneous heparin. It has been argued that the administration of subcutaneous rather than intravenous heparin might have prejudiced the tPA arm of the trial, but it should be noted that the rate of reinfarction was not higher in the tPA arm.

In the Global Utilization of Streptokinase and Tissue Plasminogen Activator for Occluded Coronary Arteries (GUSTO) Trial,[12] 31,021 patients were randomized into four groups: intravenous heparin with SK; tPA and combination of SK with tPA; and subcutaneous heparin with SK. The tPA was administered in an accelerated and front-loaded protocol over 1.5 hours with two thirds of the dose being given within 30 minutes, instead of the usual total duration of 3 hours. The 30-day mortality in patients less than 75-years-old was significantly reduced in the patients receiving tPA compared with SK (4.4% versus 5.5%, respectively). In this trial, patients older than 75 years of age who constituted 12% of the group, were prospectively randomized and showed no significant difference in mortality (19.3% versus 20.6% for tPA and SK, respectively). The overall benefit in the entire group was significant for those patients who received their tPA within the first 4 hours of the onset of chest pain and for anterior wall MIs.

It may be argued that by administering thrombolytic agents in the elderly one may be necessarily pursuing a more aggressive approach resulting in cardiac catheterization, coronary angioplasty, and bypass surgery. However, in the Thrombolysis in Myocardial Infarction (TIMI-II) Trial,[13] it was shown that these interventions may only be necessary when post-thrombolytic ischemia occurs spontaneously or is provoked. However, even with a conservative approach, one will expect a greater percentage of patients treated with thrombolytic agents to undergo subsequent revascularization procedures.

The fear of causing significant hemorrhage undoubtedly has been a deterrent in the use of thrombolytic treatment in the elderly. Hemorrhagic complications were significantly greater in elderly patients in the TIMI-I and II-A Trials.[14] However, all these patients had invasive procedures within 36 hours of thrombolysis. Probably more relevant was that in the GISSI-1 and ISIS-2 Trials[5,7] in which angiography was not routinely performed, there was a markedly low incidence of major bleeding complications in the elderly.

The most serious hemorrhagic complication following thrombolytic therapy is the occurrence of a cerebral hemorrhage and its dire consequences. The overall incidence of cerebral hemorrhage using conventional doses of thrombolytic agents is reported to be between 0.3% and 0.6%, but is higher in older patients. This rate, however, may be lower than that encountered in the general population receiving thrombolytics because of a more careful selection and exclusion of higher risk patients from the trials. A truer rate of cerebral hemorrhage was reported as 1% in a registry of patients less highly selected than in the randomized trials,[15] and probably more accurately reflects its occurrence.

The rate of strokes complicating three large thrombolytic trials in GISSI-2,[10] ISIS-3,[11] and GUSTO,[12] in which SK was compared with tPA, is shown in Table 2. The stroke rate was significantly higher in all three

Table 2
Stroke and Cerebral Hemorrhage Rate in Patients Receiving Streptokinase and tPA

Trial	Stroke Rate %			Cerebral Hemorrhage Rate %		
	Streptokinase	*tPA*	*P Value*	*Streptokinase*	*tPA*	*P Value*
GISSI-2[10]	0.9	1.1	NS	0.25	0.3	NS
ISIS-3[11]	1.04	1.39	<0.01	0.24	0.66	0.00001
GUSTO[12]						
≤75 years	1.08	1.20	NS	0.42	0.52	NS
>75 years	3.05	3.93	NS	1.23	2.08	<0.05

trials and the cerebral hemorrhage rate was higher in two of these trials in the group of patients receiving tPA. In the first two trials, the results were not separately analyzed according to age, but in the GUSTO Trial a significantly higher stroke and cerebral hemorrhage rate was reported in patients over the age of 75 who received tPA.

Thus, it appears that SK is as effective as tPA in elderly patients and may have an advantage in causing fewer strokes and cerebral hemorrhage in this age group. However, it should be remembered that the stroke rate reported to complicate acute MI in a prethrombolytic era of 1.7% to 2.4% mostly occurred as a result of thromboembolism. The exact role of heparin in the genesis of these hemorrhagic strokes is not clear. However, it can be generally stated that the incidence in thromboembolisms is reduced in patients treated with thrombolysis, aspirin, and subsequent heparin therapy, whereas the incidence of cerebral hemorrhage has increased.

Aspirin

Aspirin diminishes the aggregation of platelets exposed to thrombogenic stimuli by inhibition of the cyclooxygenase enzyme reaction within the platelet, thus blocking the synthesis of thromboxane A2, a powerful stimulus to platelet aggregation and vasoconstriction.[16]

In the ISIS-2 Trial,[7] the use of aspirin was tested for the first time during the acute phase of MI. Administration of 160 mg aspirin daily with initiation of treatment proved highly successful in reducing the early mortality by 21% and, when given together with SK, reduced the mortality a further 25%. The addition of aspirin to SK or placebo in patients 70 years or older resulted in a significant reduction in mortality to 17.6%, compared with 22.3% in the group of patients who did not receive aspirin. Aspirin therapy was also successful in reducing the reinfarction rate from 3.7% in patients receiving SK alone to 1.8% in those patients receiving aspirin and SK.

Immediate administration of 160 to 365 mg of chewable aspirin and its continuation daily thereafter, provided there are no contraindications, is now accepted as standard therapy in the management of acute MI.

A recent very extensive overview of 140 trials has convincingly shown that prolonged administration of aspirin and other antiplatelet drugs significantly reduces the odds ratio of the combined incidence of recurrent MI, stroke, or vascular death in patients following MI by 25%.[17] This analysis reported that patients older than 65 derive as much benefit, if not more than, middle-aged patients. Women also derived similar benefit to men in these studies. Most data pertain to the first year of these studies in which the largest benefit was derived, but an additional benefit was clearly observed in the second year and possibly in the third year of study. However, there is some difficulty in interpreting the data in the later years after randomization before the above conclusions can be accepted.[6]

Although no single trial has shown a statistically significant reduction in mortality alone with the long-term use of aspirin in post-MI patients, a subsequent analysis of the combined results of these randomized trials has shown a significant reduction in cardiovascular mortality by 16%[17] and nonfatal MI by 31%.[18] Although different doses of aspirin have been used, a dose of 75 to 325 mg/d has been shown to provide the maximal benefit.[17]

It is recommended that all patients continue to receive aspirin following MI for an indefinite period, unless there is a specific contraindication to its use.

Heparin

It has become standard practice in North America to administer intravenous heparin with a thrombolytic agent during acute MI. The heparin is usually started as an intravenous bolus of 5,000 units, followed by a maintenance infusion keeping the PTT twice control level and continuing for 3 to 7 days. Heparin has been shown to inhibit the systemic thrombin activity occurring during and following thrombolysis, resulting in a reduced early coronary reocclusion rate.[19] In the ISIS-2 Trial,[7] the early mortality was significantly lower in the group of patients who received intravenous heparin, but the heparin therapy was not randomized in this part of the trial. There was a small increase in bleeding complications in the patients receiving heparin (1.1%), compared with those who did not receive heparin (0.3%). In none of these reports was the effect of age on heparin studied. Although subcutaneous heparin has been used extensively in the European trials, it is not generally recommended for prevention of coronary reocclusion following thrombolysis because it takes 12 to 24 hours for heparin to reach therapeutic levels.

In the Hart Study,[20] heparin (5,000-unit bolus followed by a continuous infusion) appeared to be a more effective antithrombotic agent than low-dose (80 mg) aspirin when they were given in conjunction with tPA for thrombolysis. Angiograms obtained 7 to 24 hours after thrombolysis showed a 82% patency rate in the patients assigned to heparin, compared to 52% in the aspirin group. In contrast, aspirin was at least as effective as heparin in preventing reocclusion between days 1 and 7 post-thrombolysis. Questions have been raised whether an adequate dose of aspirin was used at the onset of the fibrinolytic therapy in this trial.

As stated above, the available evidence strongly supports the use of full-dose aspirin as adjunctive therapy to thrombolysis. However, the routine immediate use of heparin requires testing in randomized trial.[20] The current and ongoing First American Study of Infarct Survival (ASIS-1) Trial[21] will test whether heparin or hirudin will add beneficial effects to aspirin.

Hirudin and hirulog are antithrombin agents which have the advantage over heparin in that they inhibit both free and clot-bound heparin.[22] However, in three recently published trials (GUSTO-IIa,[23] TIMI 9A,[24] and Hirudin for Improvement of Thrombolysis [HIT-III] Study[25]) hirudin was associated with an increase in hemorrhagic stroke and bleeding complications, particularly in the elderly. It was felt that the dose of hirudin used in these trials was excessive. Thus, the results of further investigation will be required before hirudin can be recommended for routine use in acute MI.

All patients, particularly the elderly and those with congestive heart failure (CHF), are at risk for venous thromboembolism, and should be anticoagulated with subcutaneous heparin if they are not fully anticoagulated, and maintained on heparin until the time they are fully mobilized.

Beta-Adrenergic Blockers

During acute MI, excessive reflex activation of the sympathetic nervous system may result in potentially harmful effects of increasing myocardial ischemia, increasing platelet aggregation, and enhancing arrhythmias. The use of beta blockers during and following acute MI has been shown in numerous trials to reverse these potentially harmful effects and improve morbidity and survival.[26] Generally, these studies have excluded patients older than 75 years of age and the effect of age was only considered in post-hoc analysis. The trials have also excluded patients with bradycardia, heart block, severer degrees of CHF, and hypotension. The results of these trials involving early intervention with intravenous beta blockers or the later use of oral beta blocking agents are shown in Table 3.

In the Goteborg Trial, intravenous metoprolol was administered within 48 hours of the onset of acute MI, followed by oral metoprolol for 90 days.[27] There was a significant 36% reduction in mortality of the patients receiving active treatment compared with placebo. When retrospectively analyzed, patients aged 65 to 74 showed a 45% reduction in mortality, and those less than 65 had a 21% nonsignificant

Table 3
Effect of Age on Mortality β-Blocker Therapy for Acute Myocardial Infarction

Trial	N	Follow-Up (Mean)	Active/Placebo %		Reduction in Mortality	P valve
Early Intervention:						
Goteborg[27]						
(Metoprolol)		90d				
<65 years	917		4.5	5.7	21	NS
64–74 years	478		8.1	14.8	45	0.032
MIAMI[29]						
(Metoprolol		15d				
≤60 years	2,965		1.9	1.8	(3)	NS
61–74 years	2,813		6.8	8.2	18	NS
ISIS[30]						
(Atenolol)		7d				
<65 years	10,805		2.5	2.6	4	
≥65 years	5,222		6.8	8.8	33	NS 0.001
Late Intervention:						
Norwegian[3]						
(Timolol)		33(17)				
<65 years	1,152	months	7.7	12.4	38	0.01
65–74 years	732		14.9	21.6	31	0.05
BHAT[35]						
(Propranolol)		36(25)				
<60 years	2,589	months	6.0	7.4	19	NS
60–69 years	1,248		9.8	14.7	33	0.01

reduction in mortality. The difference in mortality was maintained for 2 years, despite the fact that both groups were treated similarly after 3 months,[28] but a subgroup analysis of 2-year survival, according to age, was not included.

A similar regimen of metoprolol administered within 24 hours of acute MI followed by oral treatment was used in the Metoprolol In the Acute Myocardial Infarction (MIAMI) Trial.[29] Administration of metoprolol resulted in a 13% reduction mortality which was not significant (4.9% in placebo versus 3.9% in metoprolol groups). Subsequent subgroup analysis showed that there was an 18% reduction mortality in the elderly patients compared with a 3% increase in mortality in the younger patients, but these results were not statistically significant. The effects of intravenous followed by oral atenolol was studied in the ISIS-1 Trial,[30] where active therapy was commenced within 12 hours of the onset of symptoms. The vascular mortality was reduced by 15% at 7 days and subsequent subgroup analysis of the elderly showed a significant 22.7% reduction in vascular mortality, whereas the mortality was reduced by 4% in the younger patients and this was not significant.

In the TIMI-II Trial,[13] in which the effect of early and delayed coronary angioplasty following thrombolysis was studied, patients were also randomized to receive immediate intravenous followed by oral metoprolol begun on the sixth day after acute MI. The patient group assigned to receive metoprolol therapy had a lower incidence of recurrent ischemia and MI in the first 6 days, but these results were not analyzed according to age of the patients. In the Norwegian Multicenter Study, patients were randomized to receive timolol, a β-blocking agent without intrinsic sympathomimetic activity, or placebo 7 to 28 days following acute MI and followed for 12 to 33 months.[31] In the initial phase of this study, the mortality rate was 17.5% in the placebo group and reduced by 39.4% to 10.6% in the timolol group. The incidence of reinfarction and sudden death were both reduced by 39% in the older patients with a similar rate reduction in the younger patient group.[32,33] After the initial report, patients were treated with an open-labeled drug and followed for a mean of 61 months (50 to 72 months), with 60% of the patients who had originally received timolol and 29% of the placebo group receiving a β-blocking agent during the second phase of the study.[34] The group originally assigned to receive timolol had a significantly lower cumulative mortality rate at 72 months compared with the placebo group (32.3% versus 26.4% in the timolol and placebo groups, respectively). After the first 24 months of the study, the mortality curves of the two groups became parallel and remained so for the duration of the study. The difference in survival in 72 months was significant for patients older than 65 years, but not for those younger.[34]

In the β-Blocker Heart Attack Trial (BHAT), patients were randomized to receive propranolol or placebo 5 to 21 days post-MI and were followed for an average of 25 months.[35] There was an overall reduction in mortality by 26% (9.8% and 7.8% in the placebo and propranolol groups, respectively). A post-hoc subgroup analysis of patients older than 60 years of age revealed a 33% reduction mortality in patients treated with propranolol (14.7% and 9.8% for placebo and propranolol groups, respectively). Reduction in mortality in patients younger than 60 years was 18.9%. The continued benefits in survival up to 3 years of follow-up was due to a reduction in both sudden death and "nonsudden arteriosclerotic heart disease."[36]

Administration of β-blocking agents commenced before discharge from hospital after acute MI and continued thereafter have been shown to be effective in improving the long-term survival. This improved survival can be attributed to reduced sudden death and reinfarction.

The use of β-blocker agents in non-Q wave MI has not been as clearly defined as in Q wave MI, as most of the information relating to the former has been generated from post-hoc subgroup analyses. However, it is concluded from combining information from a meta-analysis of trials that β-blocking agent therapy is likely to reduce the mortality and reinfarction by 25%.[37]

Thus, there is overwhelming evidence that β-blocking agents should be started prior to discharge from hospital after acute MI and continued for at least 3 years in all patients, including the elderly, unless there are specific contraindications to their use. β-blocking agents without intrinsic sympathomimetic activity are currently approved for this use.

Calcium Channel Blocking Agents

Calcium channel blocking agents are known to cause vasodilation, reduction in myocardial oxygen demand, and possible salutary effect on metabolism of ischemic myocytes. It would, thus, have been anticipated that calcium channel blocking agents would be effective in long-term management of patients with MI.

Nifedipine has been used in a number of trials either in-hospital or for short-term, up to 6 weeks, in post-MI patients, and has been shown to have no beneficial and possibly a deleterious effect on these patients.[38]

In the Danish Verapamil Infarction Trial, patients were randomized to receive verapamil or placebo in the second week post-MI and were followed for a mean of 16 months.[39] At the end of 18 months, mortality rates were not significantly different (11.1% and 13.8% in the verapamil and placebo groups, respectively). However, when the patients who did not develop CHF at the time of their MI were separately analyzed, it was shown that there was significant reduction in mortality rate at 18 months in this group of patients from 11.8% in the control group to 7.7% in the verapamil-treated group. In addition, there was a significant reduction in reinfarction rate of 12.7% in the control group to 9.4% in the verapamil group. Although one third of the patients were above the age of 65 years, post-hoc analysis according to age group did not show any significant differences in mortality or morbidity.

In the Multicenter Diltiazem Post Infarction Trial (MDPIT) a total of 2,466 patients 75 years or younger were randomized to either diltiazem or placebo 3 to 15 days following MI and followed for up to 52 months (25 months average).[40] There was a nonsignificant 11% reduction in cardiac events (cardiac death, plus first MI). The cumulative cardiac event rate was significantly increased in those patients randomized to the diltiazem group who showed pulmonary congestion on x-ray at the time of MI and also increased in those patients who had a reduced nuclear ejection fraction. (However, less than half the patients had this study and the increase was not significant.) In contrast, patients without pulmonary congestion (80% of the study population) who received diltiazem had a marginally significant reduction in cardiac event rate compared with their placebo control (11% versus 8% at 1 year in the placebo and diltiazem groups, respectively). Although half the patients in the trial were above the age of 60, the cardiac event rate in those patients older or younger than 60 was not significantly different in their respective diltiazem or placebo groups.

Thus, it is not generally recommended that calcium channel blocking agents be given routinely to post-MI patients. Patients with normal left ventricular systolic function and contraindications to β-blocking agents may benefit from the use of diltiazem or verapamil.

Angiotensin-Converting Enzyme Inhibitors

Angiotensin-converting enzyme (ACE) inhibitors reduce both peripheral vascular resistance and left ventricular filling pressures, and improve ventricular function and exercise capacity in patients with CHF. ACE inhibitors have been shown to be effective in reducing mortality in symptomatic patients with CHF.[41,42] They may also delay the onset of symptoms and the subsequent deterioration in asymptomatic patients with reduced left ventricular systolic function.[43] ACE inhibitors were used in the above studies well after the onset of significant deterioration of left ventricular function. Thus, ACE inhibitors were introduced at the very onset of left ventricular dysfunction at the time of acute MI, and continued for weeks or years in an attempt to reduce the progressive dilation and deterioration in left ventricular function. The results of these studies are shown in Table 4.

In the Survival and Ventricular Enlargement (SAVE) Trial, oral captopril was given to patients 8 to 16 days after they had sustained a large anterior wall MI.[44] These patients had reduced ejection fractions below 40% without overt CHF and were followed for 2 to 4 years. There was a 19% significant reduction in 2-year mortality in those patients receiving captopril (20% versus 25% with the captopril and placebo groups, respectively) and a 36% reduction in CHF in the group treated with captopril. The reduction in mortality was evident as early as 10 months following commencement of therapy. Administration of ACE inhibitors to the older group aged 65 to 70 resulted in a significant, 28% reduction in mortality at 2 years, whereas the reduction in mortality in the younger age group did not reach significance.

The Cooperative New Scandinavian Survival Study (CONSESUS II) differed from other trials in that intravenous ACE inhibitor (enaloprilat) was administered in the first 24 hours after the onset of acute MI and followed by administration of oral enalapril.[45] The patients were followed for only 6 months when the trial was stopped. The mortality rates were slightly, but not significantly higher in the patients receiving enalapril (10.4% versus 9.4% in enalapril and placebo groups, respectively). The difference was more evident in patients older than the age of 70, in whom the mortality was 17 7% higher in those patients receiving enalapril compared with control group, although the difference was not significant.

In the Acute Infarction Ramapril Efficacy (AIRE) Study, the patients were randomized to receive ramapiril 3 to 10 days following acute MI and followed for an average of 15 months.[46] There was a significant, 27% reduction in mortality in the patients who received ACE inhibitors. The mortality was not significantly reduced in those patients under the

Table 4
Effect of Age on Mortality of Angiotensin Converting Enzyme Inhibitor Therapy
Following Myocardial Infarction

Trial	N	Follow-up	Therapy %	Control %	Reduction in Mortality	P Value
SAVE[44]						
(Enalapril)		2–4 years				
<65	1,448		16.6	18.3	5.5	NS
≥65	783		27.9	36.1	22.7	0.02
CONSENSUS II[45]						
(Enalaprilat &						
Enalapril)		6 months				
<70	3,563		5.0	5.6	10.7	NS
≥70	2,540		17.3	14.7	(17.7)	NS
AIRE[46]						
(Ramipril) 2006	Total	15 months	17	23	27	NS
<65			NA	NA	2+	<0.05
≥65			NA	NA	36+	
SMILE[47]		1 year				
(Zofenopril)						
<65	767		5.6	4.0	28.6*	NS
≥65	789		15.4	10.2	33.8*	<0.05
GISSI-3[48]	19,394	6 weeks	6.3	7.1	11	<0.03
(Lisinopril)		(6 months)	NA	NA	—	
>70	5,121		24.8	28.3	12*	NS
						<.004
ISIS-4[49]		5 weeks				
(Captopril)		(12 months)				
<70	42,000		4.3	5.0	14	<0.02
≥70	1,600		14.8	14.7	(1)	NS

* Death or severe heart failure
† Extrapolated from figure
NA = not available
NS = not significant

age of 65 years, whereas it was significantly so in those patients 65 years or older.

In the Survival of Myocardial Infarction Long-Term Evaluation (SMILE) Trial, patients were randomized in the first day of an acute anterior wall MI to either the oral ACE inhibitor zofenopril or placebo and continued treatment for 6 weeks.[47] It is not altogether surprising that the mortality rate was not significantly reduced in this group of patients who were at lesser risk compared with the earlier ACE inhibitor trials described above. However, there was a significant reduction in combined incidents of death and/or severe CHF at 6 weeks (10.6% versus 7.1% for the placebo and zofenopril groups, respectively). At 1 year, there was a significant reduction in mortality in the treatment group compared with the placebo group, despite the discontinuation of study medication (14.1% versus 10.0% in placebo and zofenopril groups, respectively). Again, as in the other trials, the effects of zofenopril were more evident and significant in the older age group and did not reach significance in the younger age group of patients.

Lisinopril was administered within 24 hours of acute MI in the GISSI-3 Trial[48], continued for 6 weeks, and the patient followed for 6 months. The trial did not specifically include patients with large infarctions. There was 11% reduction in mortality at 6 weeks which persisted for 6 months. No reduction in mortality was observed in patients older than 70 years, however there was a 12% reduction in the combined endpoints of death, CHF, and reduction of ejection fraction in these elderly patients.

In the ISIS-4 Trial,[49] oral captopril was given within 24 hours of the onset of acute MI and continued for 1 month. This trial, as in the GISSI-3 Trial, enrolled patients irrespective of infarct size and site. The mortality rate at 5 weeks was significantly reduced from 7.7% to 7.2% in the captopril-treated group and the difference maintained for 1 year. There was no reduction in mortality in patients 70 years and older.

Thus, there is an extensive body of evidence which very strongly suggests that an ACE inhibitor should be prescribed to all patients with large MIs, particularly involving the anterior wall with reduced left ventricular systolic function, and continued with this medication indefinitely in those patients who have reduced ejection fractions. Whether ACE inhibitors have an additional effect on reducing ischemic events, as described in the SAVE Trial, over and above their effect on remodeling, remains to be assessed in prospective trials.

Nitroglycerin

A meta-analysis has reported that administration of nitroglycerin to patients with acute MI results in a favorable outcome.[50] In the two recently published mega trials, no significant beneficial effect was reported. In the GISSI-3 Trial,[48] patients received intravenous nitroglycerin for 24 hours followed by a transdermal patch, and in the ISIS-4 Trial,[49] the patients received 1 month of controlled release isosorbide mononitrate (imdur). In neither of these trials, including the ISIS-4 trial which included a separate analysis according to age, was it shown that nitroglycerin reduced the mortality or infarction rate.

Thus, although it has become standard practice to administer nitroglycerin during acute MI, it has not been shown to significantly reduce mortality and MI rates.

Anticoagulants

The routine use of coumadin following acute MI is controversial. In Chalmers et al's review of more than 30 trials addressing this problem, they indicated that many of these trials that showed significant long-term benefits utilized inadequate controls, while in later trials, small numbers of patients were randomized and the interpretation of the results showed nonsignificant differences were subject to possible beta error.[51] Pooling the data from randomized trials resulted in a small reduction of mortality of 21% in patients receiving oral anticoagulants.[51]

Since this review, three well-controlled trials which have shown a significant reduction in mortality and/or morbidity in patients receiving coumadin or related anticoagulants have been published and the results are shown in Table 5. In the Oslo-based WARIS[52] and the Dutch-based Sixty-Plus Study,[53,54] there was a 43% and 24% reduction in mortality, respectively, whereas in the Anticoagulants in Secondary Prevention of Events in Coronary Thrombosis (ASPECT) Study,[55] also Dutch based, the 10% reduction in mortality was not significant. However, in all these trials there was a significant reduction in reinfarction rate between 33% and 55% and stroke rate of 40% to 55%. All three trials involved elderly patients, but none were analyzed by different age groups.

In the latter three studies, an INR of 2.7 to 4.8 was used to control the anticoagulant therapy. Two recent reviews have suggested that a lower level of anticoagulation could be used with an INR level between 2.0 and 3.0.[56,57]

Systemic embolism has been recorded in approximately 5% of patients who have large anterior and apical Q wave MIs. These patients are generally treated with heparin while in hospital and switched to coumadin before discharge and continued with the anticoagulation for 6 to 12 weeks, whether apical thrombus has been seen on echocardiography or not. There is no reason to believe that an elderly patient should be treated any differently from younger patients in this respect.

Despite these favorable results, it is not as yet standard practice to use anticoagulants in the long-term treatment of uncomplicated MI. Currently, there are two large long-term trials in which patients are being randomized to receive aspirin with or without low-dose coumadin to assess whether the addition of coumadin to aspirin will be superior to aspirin alone.

Dyslipidemia

The relationship between hypercholesterolemia and cardiac mortality has been well established in younger and middle-aged populations,[58,59] but this relationship in the elderly is controversial. It appears that the association between cholesterol level and mortality from coronary heart disease (CHD) weakens with advancing age[60,61]; other studies have reported that hypercholesterolemia remains a significant factor even in the elderly.[62,63] A more recent analysis of the data from the Framingham Study of 1,853 patients aged 65 to 84 years over a period of 7 years showed that hypercholesterolemia remained a significant risk factor for the development of CHD in women, but not in men.[64]

Table 5
Effect of Anticoagulation Therapy on Mortality and Vascular Complications Following Myocardial Infarction

Trial	N	Age	Follow-Up (mean)	Therapy %	Control %	Reduction in Risk	P Value (95% Confidence)
Sixty Plus[53,43]	878	>60	2 years				
Mortality				7.6	13.4	43	0.017
Reinfarction				6.9	15	5	0.005
Stroke				2.7	4.6	41	0.04
WARIS[52]	1214	≤75	63(37) months				
Mortality				15	20	24	0.027
Reinfarction				14	20	34	0.0007
Stroke				3.3	7.2	55	0.0015
ASPECT[55]	3404	all ages	76(37)				
Mortality				10.0	11.1	10	NS
Reinfarction				6.7	14.2	53	(0.38–0.59)
Stroke				2.2	3.6	40	(0.40–0.90)

NS = Not significant

In this study, it was reported that an unfavorable cholesterol/high-density lipoprotein (HDL) cholesterol ratio remained a significant risk factor for both elderly men and women. However, it should be emphasized that although the relative risk of mortality may diminish with advancing age in hypercholesterolemic patients, the absolute difference in mortality, that is the excess number of elderly patients dying with hypercholesterolemia, is larger than in younger patients with elevated cholesterol levels.[63]

The potential for improving mortality and morbidity in patients with preexisting CAD has been well reviewed.[65] In secondary prevention trials, the reinfarction rate is about 6% annually, whereas in primary prevention trials in patients with hypocholesterolemia and at higher risk, the rate is 1% to 2% annually. The 10-year risk of death from cardiovascular disease in patients with preexisting cardiovascular disease was reported to increase from 3.8% to 19.6% with increasing levels of cholesterol, whereas the corresponding risk for patients free of cardiovascular disease had baseline increased from 1.7% to 4.9%.[59]

It has only recently been shown for the first time that overall survival can be improved in the treatment of patients with CAD and cholesterol lowering agents. In the Scandinavian Simvastatin Survival Study (4S) treatment of hypercholesterolemia ranging between 220 to 320 mg in patients, including both males and females, with overt CAD, significantly reduced total mortality and cardiovascular mortality.[66] These patients were followed for a mean of 5.4 years, but a difference in survival was evident at 1 year. Previous studies have shown a significant reduction in cardiac mortality and morbidity in patients treated with lipid-lowering agents, but this is the first time an overall general mortality has shown to be improved with these agents. However, in the 4S Trial, patients over the age of 70 were not enrolled and no prevention (primary or secondary) study has included a significant number or percentage of elderly patients.

It is well established that aggressive treatment of hyperlipemia[66-68] can significantly reduce the size of preexisting plaque and reduce new plaque formation. However, more important in the treatment of patients with preexisting CHD may be the fact that treatment of hyperlipemia can significantly change the composition of the plaque.[69] Thus, softer lipid-laden plaque in areas close to the vascular surface which are more likely to become unstable and rupture are more likely to show a change in lipid composition and regression with lipid-lowering agents.

The standard dietary recommendations in patients with hypercholesterolemia are to reduce total calories derived from fat to 30% and from saturated fat to less than 10%. A recent review of trials employing cholesterol-lowering diets has shown that diet alone can reduce the total cholesterol by at least 10% in seven secondary prevention trials.[70] These trials reported a favorable clinical outcome or prevention of progression of atherosclerotic lesions, but the results were generally not statistically significant and sample sizes were generally small.

It is recommended that elderly patients post-MI who have hyper-cholesterolemia be treated initially with diet and monitoring of their lipid profile, but that lipid-lowering agents be added to their regimen when desired levels of lipids are not achieved.

Hypertension

Respective observational studies have shown that hypertension is a significant factor for the development of MI, stroke, and mortality from cardiovascular disease both in younger and older patients.[71,72] It is, therefore, somewhat surprising that individual randomized trials of treatment of hypertension have not shown a reduction in death or MI. The risk of stroke has been significantly reduced. However, in the Systolic Hypertension in the Elderly Program (SHEP), patients with isolated systolic hypertension older than 60 years of age (72 years average) who were randomized to antihypertensive treatment showed a significant reduction in combined rate of nonfatal MI and CAD death rate of 27%.[73] A meta-analysis of 14 randomized trials showed that the patients who received antihypertensive therapy (which was predominately diuretic or a β-blocking agent), showed a significant reduction in MI by 14% and vascular mortality by 21%.[74] A subsequent analysis of three trials added to the above meta-analysis showed a significant, 17% reduction in the incidence of MI.[75] Pharmacological treatment of hypertension results in a reduction of MI, but only half the expected rate. This smaller than expected reduction has been attributed to possible adverse effects of drug therapy itself.[75,76]

Initial therapy of elderly patients for hypertension in the post-MI period should always include salt and alcohol restriction, weight reduction, and exercise where feasible, before considering pharmacological therapy which should be started with caution and progress slowly in view of the potential downside of treating elderly patients with hypertension.[77]

Smoking

Smoking is reported as a significant risk factor for the development of CAD including patients over the age of 65 years of age. Earlier studies have not always considered smoking as a risk factor in this age group,[72] or have not clearly shown a significant reduction in risk cessation of smoking in the elderly.[78]

In a study of 2,674 patients aged 65 to 75 years of age with more than half being older than 70 years, the risk of smoking increased coronary death rate by 75% or by 52% when multifactorial analysis was carried out taking into account other risk factors. The risk of death after the cessation of smoking reached that of nonsmokers within 1 to 5 years.[79] A more rapid decline in cardiac risk has been described in healthy patients where the risk reaches similar levels to those who never smoked, within 2 to 3 years.

In a prospective survey of three populations greater than 65 years old, the cardiovascular mortality was 100% greater in male smokers (relative risk 2.0) and 60% greater in women smokers (relative risk 1.6).[80] Former smokers had a similar cardiovascular mortality rate as participants who had never smoked. These results were significant for participants above the age of 75 years for men only.

The effect of the cessation of smoking in middle-aged and older patients with known CAD was studied in the CASS registry of patients with known CAD and who did not undergo bypass surgery.[81] It was shown that continued smoking compared with cessation increased the risk of death and nonfatal MI by 1.7 and 1.6, respectively, in patients over the age of 65. The relative risk was similar for patients younger than 65 years of age. However, there were relatively few patients in the study older than 70 years of age.[81]

Ventricular Arrhythmias

It has been well established that the occurrence of ventricular premature depolarizations recorded by Holter monitor the post-MI period is independently associated with a higher risk of mortality following discharge from the hospital.[82] The results of the Cardiac Arrhythmia Suppression Trial (CAST)[83] have significantly influenced our thinking in the use of antiarrhythmic medication in the post-MI for suppression of nonsustained ventricular arrhythmias. In this trial, a significant increase in mortality, including sudden death, was reported in patients who had their arrhythmia successfully suppressed with the anti-arrhythmic agents used in the trial. Subsequent analysis has shown that when these results were analyzed according to age, those patients aged 66 to 79 showed a significantly greater adverse affect and had a higher mortality than in the younger group.[84]

Thus, it has become standard practice to use β-blockers, which are known to have no significant proarrhythmic effects, in the post-MI period to suppress ventricular arrhythmias (see β-blocker section above). Aronow et al[85,86] also reported a prospective study of 245 patients with CHD (64% with prior Q wave MI), complex ventricular arrhythmias, and a left ventricular ejection fraction of 40% or higher in which 123 patients were randomized to propranolol and 122 patients to no anti-arrhythmic drug. At 29-month mean follow-up, compared with no anti-arrhythmic drug, propranolol caused a 47% significant reduction in sudden cardiac death; a 37% significant reduction in mortality caused by propranolol was due to an anti-ischemic effect rather than to an antiarrhythmic effect.[87]

There are conflicting data about the effect of amiodarone on mortality.[85] The use of amiodarone is currently being investigated in the Canadian Amiodarone Myocardial Infarction Arrhythmia Trial and in the European Myocardial Infarct Amiodarone Trial.

Estrogen Replacement

A review of the extensive epidemiological evidence relating to the administration of estrogen on CHD risk in postmenopausal women has shown a significant beneficial effect. Unfortunately, the benefits that are reported have been mostly derived from observational studies rather than prospective trials.[88] Stampfer and Colditz reported in a meta-analysis that estrogen administered in the postmenopausal period resulted in a highly significant reduction in the relative risk of CHD of 0.56. A similar risk reduction of 0.50 was reported when only internally controlled perspective studies were analyzed.[88] However, there is a significant increase in uterine cancer in these patients and probable increase in breast cancer. The increase in uterine cancer can be prevented by administration of progestin for least 10 days each month, but there is little epidemiological evidence for reduction of CHD with utilization of the combination of these hormones. Estrogen therapy has the additional advantage in this age group of reducing osteoporosis and hip fractures.

Estrogen therapy has been shown to reduce the level of low-density lipoprotein (LDL) cholesterol and raise the level of HDL cholesterol while addition of progestin has been reported to attenuate these beneficial effects.[89] An investigational, but nonrandomized, study has reported no deleterious effect of addition of progestin to estrogen on the lipid levels or the risk profile.[90] However, in the recently published Postmenopausal Estrogen/Progestin Intervention (PEPI) Trial in which different progesterone regimens were prospectively randomized, cyclic administration of estrogen with and without micronized progestin had similar beneficial effects on HDL cholesterol and other mix factors.[91] The American College of Physicians has issued guidelines for counseling postmenopausal women[92] and calculated the absolute risk reduction in mortality and morbidity with the use of estrogen with or without progestin.[93]

Thus, the routine prophylactic use of these hormones in the asymptomatic patient is at present considered controversial. However, we are on more certain grounds in recommending their use in patients with significant risk factors or for secondary prevention in patients with known ischemic heart disease and MI.

Conclusion

Elderly patients have a significantly higher mortality and morbidity compared with younger patients in the post-MI period. Results of therapy and reduction of risk factors for CHD are generally equally efficacious, but often superior to the results in younger patients.

References

1. Stenson WB, Sanders CA, Smith HC: Cardiovascular care of the elderly: economic considerations. *J Am Coll Cardiol* 10(suppl a):18a-21a, 1987.

2. Weaver WD, Litwin PE, Martin JS, et al: Effect of age on the use of thrombolytic therapy and mortality in acute myocardial infarction. *J Am Coll Cardiol* 18:657-662, 1991.
3. Smith SC Jr, Gilpin E, Ahnve S, et al: Outlook after acute myocardial infarction in the very elderly compared with that in patients aged 65 to 75 years. *J Am Coll Cardiol* 16:784-792, 1990.
4. Toffler GH, Muller JE, Stone PE, et al: Factors leading to stroke survival after acute myocardial infarction in patients aged 65 to 75 years compared with younger patients. *Am J Cardiol* 62:860-867, 1988.
5. Gruppo Italiano per lo Studio della streptokinasi nell' Infarcto Miocardico (GISSI): Effectiveness of intravenous thrombolytic treatment in acute myocardial infarction. *Lancet* i:397-401, 1986.
6. The ISAM Study Group: A perspective trial of intravenous streptokinase in acute myocardial infarction (ISAM). *N Engl J Med* 314:1465-1471, 1986.
7. ISIS-2 (Second International Study of Infarct Survival) Collaborative Group: Randomized trial of intravenous streptokinase, oral aspirin, both or neither among 17,187 cases of suspected acute myocardial infarction. *Lancet* ii:349-360, 1988.
8. Wilcox RG, Olsson CG, Skene AM, et al: Trial of tissue plasminogen activator for mortality reduction in acute myocardial infarction: Anglo-Scandinavian Study of Early Thrombolysis (ASSET). *Lancet* ii:825-830, 1988.
9. AIMS Trial Study Group: Effect of intravenous APSAC on mortality after acute myocardial infarction: preliminary report of a placebo-controlled clinical trial. *Lancet* i:545-549, 1988.
10. Gruppo Italiano lo Studio Streptokinasi nell' Infarto Miocardico GISSI-2: A factional randomized trial of alteplase versus streptokinase and heparin versus no heparin among 12,490 patients with acute myocardial infarction. *Lancet* 336:65-71, 1990.
11. ISIS-3 (Third International Study of Infarct Survival) Collaborative Group: A randomized comparison of streptokinase versus tissue plasminogen activator versus antistreplase and of aspirin plus heparin versus aspirin alone among 41,299 cases of suspected acute myocardial infarction. *Lancet* 339:753-770, 1992.
12. The GUSTO Investigators: An international randomized trial comparing thrombolytic strategies for acute myocardial infarction. *N Engl J Med* 329:673-682, 1993.
13. The TIMI Study Group: Comparison of invasive and conservative strategies after treatment with intravenous tissue plasminogen activator in acute myocardial infarction: results of the Thrombolysis in Myocardial Infarction (TIMI) Phase II trial. *N Engl J Med* 320:618-627, 1989.
14. Chaitman BR, Thompson B, Wittry MD, et al for the TIMI Investigators: The use of tissue-type plasminogen activator for acute infarction in the elderly: results from Thrombolysis in Myocardial Infarction Phase I Open Label Studies and the Thrombolysis in Myocardial Infarction Phase II Pilot Study. *J Am Coll Cardiol* 14:1159-1165, 1989.
15. DeJaegere PP, Arnold AA, Balk AH, et al: Intracranial hemorrhage in association with thrombolytic therapy: incidence and clinical predictive factors. *J Am Coll Cardiol* 19:289-294, 1992.
16. Patrono C: Aspirin as an antiplatelet drug. *N Engl J Med* 330:1287-1294, 1994.
17. Antiplatelet Trialists' Collaboration: Collaborative overview of randomized trials of antiplatelet therapy—I: prevention of death, myocardial infarction, and stroke by prolonged antiplatelet therapy in various categories of patients. *Br Med J* 308:81-106, 1994.
18. Editorial: Aspirin after myocardial infarction. I:1172-1173, 1980.

19. Hsia J, Hamilton WP, Kleinman N, et al: A comparison between heparin and low-dose aspirin as adjunctive therapy with tissue plasminogen activator for acute myocardial infarction. *N Engl J Med* 323:1433-1437, 1990.

20. Ridker PM, Herbert PR, Fuotes V, et al: Are both aspirin and heparin justified as adjuncts to thrombolytic therapy for acute myocardial infarction. *Lancet* 341:1574-1577, 1993.

21. Ridker PM, O'Donnell CO, Hennekens CH: Direct comparison of aspirin plus hirudin, aspirin plus heparin, and aspirin alone among 12,00 patients with acute myocardial infarction not receiving thrombolysis: rationale and design of First American Study of Infarct Survival (ASIS-1). *J Thrombosis Thrombolysis* 1:119-124, 1995.

22. Huoh J, Fuster V: Guide to anticoagulant therapy, part 1: heparin. *Circulation* 89:1449-1468, 1994.

23. The Global Use of Strategies to Open Occluded Coronary Arteries (GUSTO) IIa Investigators: Randomized trial of intravenous heparin versus recombinant hirudin for acute coronary syndromes. *Circulation* 90:1631-1637, 1994.

24. Antman EM for TIMI 9A Investigators: Hirudin in acute myocardial infarction: safety report from the thrombolysis and thrombin inhibitor in myocardial infarction (TIMI) 9A trial. *Circulation* 90:1624-1630, 1994.

25. Neuhaus KL, Essen R, Tebbe U, et al: Safety observations from the pilot phase of the randomized Hinerdin for Improvement of Thrombolysis (HIT-III) Study. *Circulation* 90:1638-1642, 1994.

26. Yusuf S, Collins R, Lewis J, et al: Beta blockers during and after myocardial infarction: an overview of the randomized trials. *Prog Cardiovasc Dis* 27:335-371, 1985.

27. Hjalmarson A, Herbiz J, Malek J, et al: Effect on mortality of metoprolol in acute myocardial infarction. *Lancet* 2:823-827, 1981.

28. Herlitz J, Elmfeldt D, Holmberg S, et al: Goteborg metoprolol trial: mortality and causes of death. *Am J Cardiol* 53:9D-14D, 1984.

29. MIAMI Trial Research Group: Metoprolol in acute myocardial infarction (MI-AMI): a randomized placebo-controlled international trial. *Eur Heart J* 6:199-226, 1985.

30. ISIS-I (First International Study of Infarct Survival) Collaborative Group: Randomized trial of intravenous atenolol among 16,027 cases of suspected acute myocardial infarction. *Lancet* 2:57-66, 1986.

31. The Norwegian Multicentre Study Group: Timolol-induced reduction in mortality and reinfarction in patients surviving acute myocardial infarction. *N Engl J Med* 304:801-807, 1981.

32. Pedersen TR: The Norwegian Multicentre Study of Timolol after myocardial infarction. *Circulation* 67(suppl I):I49-I52, 1983.

33. Gundersen T, Abrahamsen AM, Kjekshus J, et al: Timolol-related reduction in mortality and reinfarction in patients ages 65-75 years surviving acute myocardial infarction. *Circulation* 66:1179-1184, 1982.

34. Pedersen TR for the Norwegian Multicentre Study Group: Six-year follow-up of the Norwegian Multicentre Study on Timolol after acute myocardial infarction. *N Engl J Med* 313:1055-1058, 1985.

35. β Blocker I Ieart Attack Trial Research Group. A randomized trial of propranolol in patients with acute myocardial infarction. *JAMA* 247:1707-1714, 1982.

36. Hawkins CM, Richardson DW, Vokonas PS: The effect of propranolol in reducing mortality in older myocardial infarction patients: the beta-blocker heart attack trial experience. *Circulation* 67(suppl I):I94-I97, 1983.

37. Yusuf S, Wittes J, Probstfield J: Evaluating effects of treatment subgroups of patients within a clinical trial: the case of non-Q wave myocardial infarction and beta blockers. *Am J Cardiol* 60:220-222, 1990.

38. Roberts MD: Review of calcium antagonists trials in acute myocardial infarction. *Clin Cardiol* 12:III-41-III-42, 1989.
39. The Danish Study Group on Verapamil in Myocardial Infarction: Effect of Vera-pamil on mortality and major events after acute myocardial infarction. *Am J Cardiol* 66:779-785, 1990.
40. The Multicenter Diltiazem Post Infarction Trial Research Group: The effect of diltiazem on mortality and reinfarction after myocardial infarction. *N Engl J Med* 319:383-392, 1988.
41. CONSESUS Trial Study Group: Effects of enalapril on mortality in severe conges-tive heart failure. *N Engl J Med* 316:1429-1435, 1987.
42. The SOLVD Investigators: Effect of enalapril on survival in patients with reduced left ventricular ejection fraction and congestive heart failure. *N Engl J Med* 325:293-302, 1991.
43. The SOLVD Investigators: Effect of enalapril on mortality and development of heart failure in asymptomatic patients with reduced left ventricular ejection fractions. *N Engl J Med* 327:685-691, 1992.
44. Pfeffer MA, Braunwald E, Moye L, et al: Effect of captopril on mortality and morbidity in patients with left ventricular dysfunction after myocardial infarction: results of the survival and ventricular enlargement trial. *N Engl J Med* 327:669-677, 1992.
45. Swedberg K, Held P, Kjekshus J, et al: Effects of early administration of enalapril on mortality in patients with acute myocardial infarction: results of the Coopera-tive New Scandinavian Enalapril Survival Study II (CONSESUS II). *N Engl J Med* 327:678-684, 1992.
46. AIRE Study Investigators: Effect of ramipril on mortality and morbidity of survivors of acute myocardial infarction with clinical evidence of heart failure. *Lancet* 342:821-828, 1993.
47. Ambrosioni E, Borghi C, Magnani B for the Survival of Myocardial Infarction Long-Term Evaluation (SMILE) Study Investigation: The effect of the angiotensin-converting- enzyme inhibitor zofenopril on mortality and morbidity after anterior myocardial infarction. *N Engl J Med* 332:80-85, 1995.
48. Gruppo Italiano per lo Studio della Sopravvivenza nell'infarto Miocardico GISSI-3: Effects of lisinopril and transdermal glyceryl trinitrate singly and together on a 6-week mortality and ventricular function after acute myocardial infarction. *Lancet* 343:1115-1122, 1994.
49. ISIS-4 (Fourth International Study on Infarct Survival) Collaborative Group: A randomized factorial trial assessing early oral captopril, oral mononitrate, and intravenous magnesium sulphate in 58,050 patients with suspected acute myo-cardial infarction. *Lancet* 345:669-685, 1995.
50. Yusuf S, Collins R, McMahon S, et al: Effect of intravenous nitrate on mortality in acute myocardial infarction: an overview of the randomized trials. *Lancet* i:255-259, 1988.
51. Chalmers TC, Matta RJ, Smith H Jr, et al: Evidence favoring the use of anticoagu-lants in the hospital phase of acute myocardial infarction. *N Engl J Med* 297:1091-1096, 1977.
52. Smith P, Arnesen H, Holme I: Effect of warfarin on mortality and reinfarction after myocardial infarction. *N Engl J Med* 323:147-152, 1990.
53. The Sixty Plus Reinfarction Study Group: A double-blind trial to assess long-term oral anticoagulant therapy in elderly patients after myocardial infarction. *Lancet* ii:989-994, 1980.
54. The Sixty Plus Reinfarction Study Research Group: Risks of long-term oral antico-agulant therapy in elderly patients after myocardial infarction. *Lancet* i:64-68, 1982.

55. Anticoagulants in the Secondary Prevention of Events in Coronary Thrombosis (ASPECT) Research Group: Effects of long-term oral anticoagulant treatment or mortality and cardiovascular morbidity after myocardial infarction. *Lancet* 343:499-503, 1994.
56. Hirsh J, Fuster V: Guide to anticoagulant therapy, part 2: oral anticoagulants. *Circulation* 89:1469-1480, 1994.
57. Carins J: Oral anticoagulants or aspirin after myocardial infarction. *Lancet* 343:497-498, 1994.
58. LaRosa JC, Hunninghake D, Bush D, et al: The cholesterol facts: a summary of the evidence relating dietary fats, serum cholesterol, and coronary heart disease: a joint statement by the American Heart Association and the National Heart, Lung and Blood Institute. *Circulation* 81:1721-1733.
59. Pekkanen J, Linn S, Heiss G, et al: Ten-year mortality from cardiovascular disease in relation to cholesterol level among men with and without preexisting cardiovascular disease. *N Engl J Med* 322:1700-1707, 1990.
60. Kannel WB, Castelli WP, Gordon T: Cholesterol in the prediction of atherosclerotic disease. *Ann Intern Med* 90:85-91, 1979.
61. Krumholz HM, Seeman TE, Merrill SS, et al: Lack of association between cholesterol and coronary heart disease mortality and morbidity and all causes of mortality in persons older than 70 years. *JAMA* 272:1335-1340, 1994.
62. Benfante R, Reed W: Is elevated serum cholesterol level a risk factor for coronary heart disease in the elderly? *JAMA* 263:393-396, 1990.
63. Rubin SM, Sidney S, Black DM, et al: High blood cholesterol in elderly men and excess risk for coronary heart disease. *Ann Intern Med* 113:916-920, 1990.
64. Wilson WF, Kannel WB: Hypercholesteremia and coronary risk in the elderly. *Am J Geriatr Cardiol* 3:52-56, 1993.
65. Rossouw JE, Lewis B, Rifkind DM: The value of lowering cholesterol after myocardial infarction. *N Engl J Med* 323:1112-1119, 1990.
66. Scandanavian Simvastatin Survival Study Group: Randomized trial of cholesterol lowering in 4444 patients with coronary heart disease: Scandanavian Simvastatin Survival Study. *Lancet* 344:1383-1389, 1994.
67. Brown G, Albers J, Fisher L: Repression of coronary artery disease as a result of intensive lipid-lowering therapy in men with high levels of apolipoprotein B. *N Engl J Med* 323:1289-1298, 1990.
68. Blankenhorn D, Nessim S, Johnson R, et al: Beneficial effects of combined cholestipol-niacin therapy on coronary atherosclerosis and venous bypass grafts. *JAMA* 257:3233-3240, 1987.
69. Falk E: Why do plaques rupture? *Circulation* 96(suppl III):III-30-III-42, 1992.
70. Denke MA: Cholesterol lowering diets: a review of the evidence. *Arch Intern Med* 155:17-26, 1995.
71. Hypertension Detection and Follow-up Program Cooperative Group: Five-year findings of the Hypertension Detection and Follow-up Program: II. Mortality by race, sex and age. *JAMA* 242:2572-2577, 1979.
72. Stokes J III, Kannel WB, Wolf PA, et al: The relative importance of selected risk factors for various manifestations of cardiovascular disease among men and women from 35-64 years old; 30 years follow-up in the Framingham Study. *Circulation* 75(suppl V):V65-V73, 1987.
73. SHEP Cooperative Research Group: Prevention of strokes by antihypertensive drug treatment in older persons with isolated systolic hypertension: final results of the systolic hypertension in elderly program. *JAMA* 265:4355-4364, 1991.
74. Collins R, Petro R, MacMahon S, et al: Blood pressure, stroke, and coronary artery disease, part 2: short-term predictions in blood pressure: overview of randomized drug trials in their epidemiologic context. *Lancet* 335:827-838, 1990.

75. Manson JE, Toteston H, Ridker PM, et al: The primary prevention of myocardial infarction. *N Engl J Med* 326:1406-1416, 1992.
76. Multiple Risk Factor Intervention Trial Research Group: Multiple risk factor intervention trial risk factor changes and mortality results. *JAMA* 248:1465-1477, 1982.
77. Kaplan NM: The potential downside of treating the elderly with hypertension. *Am J Geriatr Cardiol* Sept/Oct:10-11, 1992.
78. Gordon T, Kannel WB, McGee D, et al: Death and coronary attacks in men after giving up cigarette smoking: a report from the Framingham Study. *Lancet* ii:1345-1348, 1974.
79. Jajich CL, Ostfield AM, Freeman JH: Smoking and coronary heart disease mortality in the elderly. *JAMA* 252:2831-2834, 1984.
80. LaCroix AZ, Lang S, Scherr P, et al: Smoking and mortality among older men and women in three communities. *N Engl J Med* 324:213-217, 1991.
81. Hermanson B, Omen GS, Kronmal RA, et al: Beneficial six-year outcome of smoking cessation in older men and women from coronary artery disease: results from CASS registry. *N Engl J Med* 319:1365-1369, 1988.
82. Ruberman W, Weinblatt E, Goldberg E, et al: Ventricular premature beats and mortality after acute myocardial infarction. *N Engl J Med* 297:750-757, 1977.
83. The Cardiac Arrhythmia Suppression Trial (CAST) Investigators: Preliminary report: effect of encainide and flecainide on mortality in a randomized trial of arrhythmia suppression after myocardial infarction. *N Engl J Med* 321:406-412, 1989.
84. Akiyama T, Pawitan Y, Campbell WB, et al: Effects of advancing age on the efficacy of antiarrhythmic drugs in postmyocardial infarction patients with ventricular arrhythmias. *J Am Geriatr Soc* 40:666-672, 1992.
85. Aronow WS: The management of ventricular arrhythmias in older patients after CAST. *Drugs Aging* 6:112-124, 1995.
86. Aronow WS, Ahn C, Mercando AD, et al: Effect of propranolol versus no antiarrhythmic drug on sudden cardiac death, total cardiac death, and total death in patients 62 years of age with heart disease, complex ventricular arrhythmias, and left ventricular ejection fraction $\geq$ 40%. *Am J Cardiol* 74:267-270, 1994.
87. Aronow WS, Ahn C, Mercando AD, et al: Decrease in mortality by propranolol in patients with heart disease and complex ventricular arrhythmias is more an anti-ischemic than an antiarrhythmic effect. *Am J Cardiol* 74:613-615, 1994.
88. Stampfer MJ, Colditz GA: Estrogen replacement therapy and coronary heart disease: a qualitative assessment of epidemiologic evidence. *Prev Med* 20:47-63, 1991.
89. Martin KA, Freeman MW: Postmenopausal hormone-replacement therapy. *N Engl J Med* 328:1115-1117, 1993.
90. Nabulsi AA, Folsom AR, White A, et al: Association of hormone-replacement therapy with various cardiovascular risk factors in postmenopausal women. *N Engl J Med* 328:1069-1075, 1993.
91. The Writing Group for the PEPI Trial: Effects of estrogen or estrogen/progestin regimens on heart disease risk factors in postmenopausal women. *JAMA* 273:199-208, 1995.
92. American College of Physicians: Guidelines for counseling postmenopausal women about preventive hormone therapy. *Ann Intern Med* 117:1038-1041, 1992.
93. Grady D, Rubin SM, Petitti DB: Hormone therapy to prevent disease and prolong life in postmenopausal women. *Ann Intern Med* 117:1016-1037, 1992.

Chapter 18

Coronary Angioplasty in the Elderly

Randall C. Thompson, MD

There is a large and growing population of elderly patients in our society with symptomatic coronary artery disease (CAD). In the United States 1990 census, there were 31.1 million people, or approximately 12.5% of the population, who were 65 years or older.[1] As the population continues to age, it is estimated that this group will increase by 65% by the year 2020.[2] The incidence of atherosclerosis increases with age, and the number of elderly patients with symptomatic CAD is, therefore, both large and growing. Currently, elderly patients account for most of the hospital admissions for cardiovascular disease, and the majority of patients who undergo coronary artery bypass surgery or ballloon angioplasty are over age 65.[3-6]

Even though the elderly population with symptomatic CAD is large, recent randomized clinical trials of coronary angioplasty versus bypass surgery have not included a large number of elderly subjects, and older randomized trials, such as those of coronary bypass surgery versus medical therapy, have completely excluded older patients. However, from the careful analysis of the expanding and well-described experience of angioplasty and other treatment for CAD in the elderly, clinicians can draw informed conclusions and make rational decisions regarding therapy options.

Percutaneous Transluminal Coronary Angioplasty for Nonemergent Symptomatic Coronary Artery Disease

Older patients, because of factors related to aging and a higher incidence of comorbid medical conditions, have less desirable results compared with younger patients with all therapies for CAD. For exam-

From: Aronow WS, Stemmer EA, Wilson SE (eds). *Vascular Disease in the Elderly.* Armonk, NY: Futura Publishing Company, Inc., © 1997.

ple, older patients do not tolerate medical therapy as well as younger ones, and have a higher incidence of intolerable side effects.[7-9] It is also well established that elderly patients who undergo coronary bypass surgery have increased morbidity and mortality.[5,10-16] There is, thus, a rather obvious attraction for angioplasty as a less invasive alternative for myocardial revascularization. However, it must be accepted that percutaneous transluminal coronary angioplasty (PTCA), like other therapies, will have less desirable results in the elderly than in younger patients.

Characteristics of Elderly Patients Undergoing Percutaneous Transluminal Coronary Angioplasty

The elderly PTCA population has a higher rate of other comorbid medical conditions, and more complex heart disease than younger patients who undergo PTCA. For example, diabetes, hypertension, and previous congestive heart failure (CHF) are significantly more frequent in older patients compared to younger ones.[4,17,18] The National Heart, Lung, and Blood Institute's Coronary Angioplasty Registry from 1985 to 1986 reported that the incidence of previous CHF was 4% in patients under age 65 and 9% in those older than 65 years.[19] Previous CHF is present in 17% to 24% of patients over age 75 undergoing PTCA.[4,19] There is also a greater proportion of women in the elderly PTCA population, and this proportion increases with the age of the patient group.[4,19-21] Nearly 50% of patients over age 75 undergoing PTCA are female.[4,19,21]

As PTCA is utilized with increasing frequency in older patients,[22] the age and complexity of the elderly angioplasty population has steadilty increased.[22,23] For example, an analysis of the Medicare recipient administrative data files of 225,915 patients who underwent PTCA demonstrated that from 1987 to 1990, the mean age increased from 71.2 to 72.0 years, the proportion with a Charlson index score greater than 2 increased from 6.0% to 7.0%, and the number of patients with more than three coded discharge diagnoses increased from 52.2% to 61.6%.[22] Also, the frequency of pulmonary disease, diabetes, and diagnosis of CHF all increased in Medicare patients who underwent PTCA in 1990 versus 1987.[22] In 1990, 9.5% of Medicare PTCA patients over age 65 had a discharge diagnosis of CHF.[22]

Angioplasty Outcome in the Elderly

The technical success rate for angioplasty in the elderly is now very high, essentially equivalent to that achieved in younger patients, and substantially higher than a decade ago.[4,19-40] In more recent reports, the technical success rate has been consistently over 90% in elderly patients. In a Mayo Clinic series of 768 patients 65 years or older who underwent PTCA from 1990 to 1992, the technical success rate was 93.5%.[23] In the subgroup over age 75, the success rate was nearly 92%, substantially better than a similar group undergoing PTCAs at this center from 1980 to 1989,[4,23] or the experience of other centers reporting prior to 1990.[26,33,34,29,41] Despite this high technical success rate, elderly patients have a higher rate of procedural complications, and this is especially true in the very elderly who have a higher rate of procedure related death.[4,19,21,24,27] However, acute PTCA complication rates in the elderly have also improved substantially in recent years. In the Mayo Clinic series of elderly patients undergoing PTCA from 1990 to 1992, the procedure mortality rate was 1.4% versus 3.3% from 1980 to 1989.[23] Although substantially improved compared to just a few years before, the procedure related mortality is still significantly higher in the oldest subgroup of patients. The PTCA related mortality rate in patients over age 75 was 3.3% in this study, down from 6.7% during the 1980s, but the mortality rate was less than .5% for the group of patients ages 65 to 74 years undergoing PTCA from 1990 to 1992.[23] Analysis of the Medicare administrative claims files demonstrated that the overall 30-day mortality of elderly patients undergoing PTCA decreased by 25% between 1987 and 1990, and averaged 3.3%.[22] The Medicare provider data files of over 20,000 octogenarians demonstrated a hospital mortality rate of 7.0%, a 30-day mortality of 7.8%, and a 1-year mortality rate of 17.3%.[22,42] Older series of PTCA in patients over age 80 have reported procedural mortality rates averaging 8% to 10%.[24,26,43-48]

Other complications of PTCA in the elderly have also improved in recent years. In the Mayo Clinic series, the rate of PTCA related myocardial infarction (MI) in patients over the age of 64 fell from 3.9% before 1990 to 2.2% between 1990 and 1992, and the rate of death or MI fell from 6.3% to 3.4%. More strikingly, the rate of emergency coronary artery bypass surgery in patients over age 65 was .65% after 1990 to 1992, versus a more traditionally reported 5.5% during the 1980s.[23]

There have been numerous technical advances which have improved the safety of angioplasty in high-risk patients, such as perfusion balloons for high-risk lesions and abrupt closure,[49-51] long balloons for diffusely diseased segments,[52,53] and more optimal use of anticoagulation, including in-laboratory monitoring of the active clotting time.[53,55] Also, operator experience with PTCA has continued to grow, and the widespread application of intracoronary stents has had a major impact on the rate of emergency bypass surgery. Despite these technical advances, the improved safety of PTCA in the elderly is quite striking. The improved technical success rate does not appear to have resulted in improved long-term event-free survival in elderly patients, perhaps, because the procedure is being appplied to a more complex patient population. [23]

A number of other morbid complications are more common in older patients, especially the very old. Maiello described an approximately 4% rate of requirement for blood transfusion, and 1.1% renal insufficiency in patients over age 70 undergoing PTCA, significantly higher than in younger patients.[39] Very old patients also have longer hospital stays after PTCA.[21] As stents and other percutaneous revascularization devices are used more frequently in the elderly, nonfatal morbid complications such as these will likely increase. Fortunately, the incidence of strokes after PTCA in the elderly is extremely low, even in very old patients, unlike the experience with coronary bypass surgery. This issue is a major factor favoring PTCA versus bypass surgery in older, stroke susceptible patients.

Predictors of Hospital Outcome After Percutaneous Transluminal Coronary Angioplasty

Diffuse CAD, especially multiple diseased coronary segments, has been reported to be the strongest factor predicting hospital death or MI after angioplasty in the elderly.[56] Elderly patients who have multivessel CAD do less well with angioplasty than those with single-vessel disease. For example, Maiello reported a clinical success rate of 100% with PTCA in patients over age 75 with one-vessel CAD, but in patients with three-vessel disease, the PTCA success rate was only 52%, and the hospital mortality rate was 14%.[40] Age appears to be a predictor of procedure related mortality with PTCA in older patients.[4,39] Ischemic complications do not appear to occur more frequently, but the increased procedural mortality appears to be related to lower reserve in older patients, especially very old patients who tolerate these complications more poorly than younger patients, and ischemic complications when they do occur more frequently result in death in the very elderly. Calcified coronary arteries are frequently seen in elderly patients and this factor was found to predict poor outcomes in one study[24] of elderly patients, but was not found to be predictive in another study.[56] Hospitals which perform more PTCAs have lower short-term mortality rates than those which perform fewer procedures,[57] and current guidelines of the American College of Cardiology and American Heart Association recommend that hospitals maintain institutional volume of at least 200 PTCA cases per year.[58]

Intermediate-Term Outcome After Percutaneous Transluminal Coronary Angioplasty in the Elderly

Posthospital survival after PTCA in the elderly, even very elderly patients, is high.[4,20,22-24,28,36,38] In patients over age 75, survival after angioplasty has been reported to be 87% at 3 years,[35] and 83% to 86% at 4 years,[4,24] and overall survival is only slightly less than in patients aged 65 to 74.[4] Event-free survival, however, is not as good as in the younger angioplasty population, and recurrent angina is especially frequent in the oldest patient population.[4,57] Also, although in-hospital success rates have improved in recent years, event-free survival in elderly patients has not improved (Figures 1, 2, and 3).[23] The higher recurrence of angina in elderly postangioplasty patients is in contrast to the coronary bypass surgery experience. Older patients who survive coronary bypass surgery have angina relief and improvement in functional status which is at least as good as younger surgical patients.[10,11,15,60-62] This less durable angina relief with PTCA is at least in part from more extensive CAD and less complete revascularization. The restenosis rate after angioplasty in elderly patients does not appear to be increased when compared with younger patients. Restenosis in older patients has been reported to be between 31% and 44%,[17,25] similar to the restenosis rates in other age groups.[63-70]

Predictors of Posthospital Outcomes

The extensive nature of a patient's CAD is a very important determinate of posthospital survival and event-free survival. Thompson et al used multivariant analysis, and reported that the number of diseased

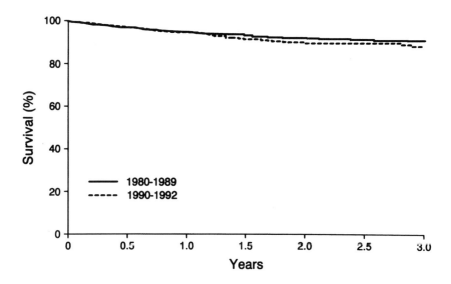

Figure 1. Kaplan-Meier; Curves of survival after hospital dismissal for elderly Mayo Clinic patients undergoing percutaneous transluminal coronary angioplasty (PTCA) between 1980 and 1989, and those undergoing PTCA between 1990 and 1992. (Reproduced with permission from Reference 23.)

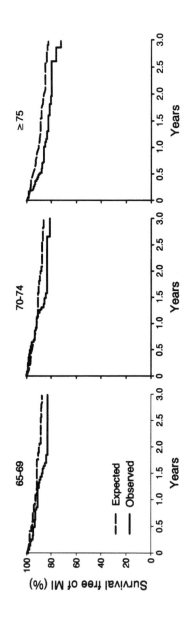

Figure 2. Kaplan-Meier; Curves of survival free of myocardial infarction for three age groups of elderly patients undergoing percutaneous transluminal coronary angioplasty (PTCA) at the Mayo Clinic. The event-free survival curves in patients who underwent PTCA between 1990 and 1992 were not improved compared with risk-adjusted event curves predicted from patients who underwent PTCA between 1980 and 1989. (Reproduced with permission from Reference 23.)

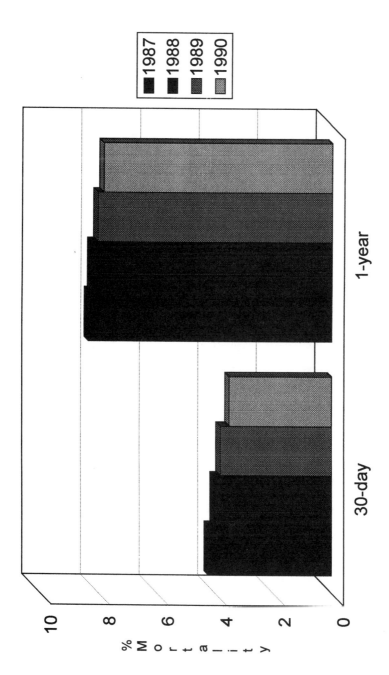

Figure 3. Unadjusted 30-day and 1-year mortality after angioplasty by year of procedure; from the National Medicare Experience (1987 to 1990). (Reproduced with permission form Reference 22.)

coronary segments was the strongest predictor of long-term event-free survival after PTCA in patients over age 65.[56] Likewise, de Jaegere et al reported event-free survival postangioplasty of 81% of patients over age 70 who had single-vessel CAD, but 45% in patients with multivessel disease.[76] Other baseline variables which have been found to be predictors of posthospital event-free survival are measures of left ventricular systolic function, the number of concomitant medical diseases, and the presence of unstable angina.[56,70] High- and low-risk subgroups can be identified, and the heterogeneity of the elderly population should be emphasized. One study used a statistical modeling approach to describe elderly patient groups with potentially low and particulary high rates of event-free survival.[56] For example, an elderly patient with three significant coronary segment stenoses, recent CHF, and two other concomitant medical illnesses would fall into a high-risk category with a 33% rate of major events at 4 years, while an elderly angioplasty patient with a single significant coronary stenosis, no recent CHF, and no other medical illness, would fall in a category with only a 4% event rate of death or MI at 3 years.[70]

Incomplete revascularization has been described as a predictor of late mortality after angioplasty in elderly patients.[70] However, incomplete revascularization is highly correlated with extensive CAD, and completeness of revascularization was not found to be an independent predictor of event-free survival in two other series in which it was analyzed.[36,56]

Completeness of Revascularization With Percutaneous Transluminal Coronary Angioplasty

Approximately 50% of elderly patients having PTCA receive complete revascularization at the time of their procedure.[20-23,40,70,71] In the subgroup of elderly patients with three-vessel CAD, complete revascularization is infrequent, and is obtained in only 16% to 25%.[71,72] Many elderly patients are treated conservatively in an attempt to limit procedure related complications. For example, many frail, elderly patients have limited procedures with the strategy of "culprit vessel angioplasty." Incomplete revascularization after angioplasty has been associated with a high rate of subsequent recurrent angina and bypass surgery.[27,34,71] In addition, the importance of revascularization is well documented in the cardiac surgical population.[73-75] Complete revascularization is desirable and logical when it is feasible. However, it is not clear that more aggressive PTCA procedures would benefit elderly patients. With more extensive angioplasty, the incidence of procedure complications and restenosis is increased, and PTCA, unlike bypass surgery, is easier to repeat.[36,71,76] Elderly patients also have a higher incidence of silent ischemia, and there are more cardiac events in elderly patients who have silent ischemia.[77] However, it is not known whether angioplasty in these patients would alter the outcome. One logical approach would seem to be to dilate all functionally significant coronary stenoses in elderly patients when feasible. Patient selection and individualization of therapy are key.

Percutaneous Transluminal Coronary Angioplasty for Acute Myocardial Infarction in the Elderly

Direct PTCA is an attractive therapy for treatment of acute MI in elderly patients. The mortality rate of elderly patients treated with conventional therapy is quite high. In patients over age 80, mortality for an acute MI is typically over 30%.[78-80] For example, Naylor et al reported a mortality rate of 35.9% in 3,406 octogenarians in Ontario who had an MI between 1981 and 1991.[80] Thrombolytic therapy has been shown to benefit older patients, but a minority of elderly patients, especially the very elderly, are actually treated with thrombolytic drugs, and the risk of major hemorrhage including hemorrhagic stroke is increased in the aged.[81-83] Also, although there is a mortality benefit, very elderly patients treated with thrombolytic therapy have a high mortality rate, nonetheless.[81] For example, in the subgroup of patients over age 75 in the Global Utilization of Streptrokinase and Tissue Plasminogen Activator for Occluded Coronary Artery (GUSTO) Study, the mortality rate of those treated with tissue plasminogen activator was 19.3%. There was also a 3.9% rate of stroke in this patient group.[81] PTCA has been shown to result in higher infarct-related artery patency, fewer recurrent ischemic events, lower in-hospital mortality, and a lower instance of stroke compared with thrombolytic treatment.[84-89] The experience of direct PTCA for acute MI in the elderly is not large, but the reported results appear encouraging and compare favorably to historical descriptions of other therapies (Table).[88-91] For example, in the Primary Angioplasty in Myocardial Infarction (PAMI) trial, the subgroup of patients over age 65 treated with PTCA had a marked reduction of combined end point of death or reinfarction as compared with patients treated with thrombolytic therapy (8.6% versus 20%).[91]

Laster et al described the experience with direct angioplasty for acute MI in octogenarians at the Mid America Heart Institute. Thirty-day mortality was 16%, but was only 10% in patients who were hemodynamically stable and not in cardiogenic shock at the time of presentation.[88] In the study by Laster and another one from the same institution,[89] there were no strokes in elderly patients treated with direct PTCA, but Stuckey et al reported a stroke rate of 5.3% in 75 patients over age 75 who had primary PTCA for acute MI.[90] For the very elderly patients who present in cardiogenic shock with an acute MI, there is a very high mortality rate regardless of therapy. In Laster's study, the survival rate was only 33% in octogenarians presenting with cardiogenic shock.[88] Treatment of MI with cardiogenic shock in the very elderly with direct PTCA remains controversial because of the poor prognosis. Thus, most reports of primary

Table 1
Change in Hospital Outcome of Angioplasty in the Elderly

	1981–1989				1990–1992			
	65–69 years	70–74 years	>75 years	p	65–69 years	70–74 years	>75 years	p
Number of patients	400	300	282		257	241	270	
Men %	67.5	58.7	56.4	0.006	72	75.5	60.4	<0.001
Success rate per segment	84.6	86.5	88.8	0.16	93.7	91.5	90.8	0.31
Success rate per patient	87.3	88	89.4	0.7	95.7	93	91.9	0.18
Death % (n)	1.5 (6)	2.3 (7)	6.7 (19)	<.001	.8 (2)	0 (0)	3.3 (9)	0.01
CABG within 24 hrs. % (n)	7.7 (31)	6.3 (19)	1.4 (4)	0.001	1.2 (3)	.8 (2)	0 (0)	0.01
Myocardial infarction % (n)	3.3 (13)	5.0 (15)	7.1 (20)	0.07	2.3 (6)	3.7 (9)	5.2 (14)	0.23
Death or MI % (n)	4.5 (18)	6.7 (20)	12.1 (14)	0.001	2.7 (7)	3.7 (9)	8.2 (22)	0.01

(Reproduced with permission from *J Am Col Cardiol* 27:8–14, 1996.)

Table 2
Direct PTCA for Acute MI in the Elderly

STUDY *(Ref)*	*Treatment*	*n*	*Age Group*	*Mortality (%)*
PAMI (89)	t-PA	75	>65	15.0
PAMI (89)	PTCA	75	>65	5.7
Lee (87)	PTCA	105	>70	18.0
Laster (86)	PTCA	55	>80	16.0

PTCA in elderly patients have been encouraging, but further study is warranted at this stage.

Application of Intracoronary Stents in the Elderly

Numerous new intracoronary devices have extended or improved the application of PTCA. Balloon expandable intracoronary stents, in particular, are being utilized with growing enthusiasm. Stents have been shown to be an effective treatment for abrupt or threatened closure during PTCA, and there is a reduced rate of restenosis with primary stenting compared with PTCA.[92-94] In older patients, intracoronary stents can be used effectively, but one should expect less desirable results than in younger patients. Early reports of elective placements of the Palmaz-Schatz intracoronary stent suggest a lower clinical success rate in very elderly patients. For example, Yokoi et al reported a technical success rate of 95% in patients 65- to 74-years-old, but only 68% in patients over 75.[95] The hospital mortality rate was 1.2% in patients 65- to 74-years-old versus 4.1% in the group over age 75. Very elderly patients have a higher incidence of calcified coronary lesions, and this factor could contribute to a lower success rate. However, as experience with the Palmaz-Schatz intracoronary stent grows and the technology is improving, the technical success rate is also improving.

In the initial group of patients who underwent intracoronary stenting with the Cook stent for abrupt or threatened closure during PTCA at the Mayo Clinic, there were 113 patients over age 65. The technical success rate was 89.4% versus 93.2% in younger patients.[96] The rate of emergency bypass surgery in these patients (who had for the most part failed PTCA) was less than 3% for both groups.[96]

Intracoronary stents are a significant advance for PTCA in both elderly and younger patients because of the reduced need for emergency bypass surgery and reduction in the rate of restenosis for de novo lesions. As experience with intracoronary stents grows, the relative limits and benefits in elderly patients should become more apparent.

Percutaneous Transluminal Coronary Angioplasty Versus Bypass Surgery in the Elderly

Trials of bypass surgery versus multivessel coronary angioplasty have not included large enough numbers of elderly patients to allow subanalysis in older patients. However, there is a large reported clinical experience with revascularization in older patients, and certain conclusions can be drawn. For example, in the Emory Angioplasty Surgery Trial (EAST), in which the average age was 61.6 years, there was no difference between the angioplasty and surgical groups for the primary end points of composite death, Q-wave MI, or large reversible thallium defect at 3 years.[97] The hospital mortality rate was 1% for both PTCA and surgical patients at the end of 3 years. Overall survival was excellent, over 93% in both groups. Repeat coronary revascularization was more frequent in the angioplasty group. Similar randomized trials of angioplasty and surgery have shown similar outcomes to the EAST study for patients who can be treated with either PTCA or bypass surgery.[98-100]

Although direct comparisons of PTCA and bypass surgery in the elderly are not available, indirect comparisons have been made. For example, O'Keefe et al performed a nonrandomized retrospective comparison of angioplasty versus bypass surgery in patients over age 70.[70] This study found that the short-term mortality was lower in patients receiving PTCA, but at 1 year, the mortality rate was about the same for the two therapies, and mortality curves were quite similar between the fourth and fifth years. As with the randomized trials in younger patients, O'Keefe's study showed that more postangioplasty patients required additional revascularization procedures.[70]

The operative mortality rates in the elderly surgical patient population is generally higher than the mortality rate in the elderly angioplasty population.[45,47,48,101-103] The mortality rate increases with advancing age with coronary bypass surgery, and is 10% to 12% in octogenarians.[22,104] However, very elderly patients who survive coronary surgery have very good angina relief.[58,105] Recurrent angina appears to be more frequent in very elderly patients who undergo angioplasty, perhaps because of the difficulrty in achieving full revascularization in many of the oldest patients.[4,59] In elderly patients, especially very elderly patients, coronary bypass surgery can be considered more durable and definitive but riskier than PTCA.

Costs

In the EAST study, total costs were slightly lower at 3 years for patients who underwent PTCA versus the bypass surgical group ($23,734.00 versus $25,310.00).[105] However, there were more hospitalizations and more anginal medications given to patients in the angioplasty group which would further reduce the small difference in cost.[105] In the elderly, the length of hospital stay is understandably longer, especially in those patients having bypass surgery.[66,106] The cumulative cost of both angioplasty and bypass surgery is greater in the elderly than in younger patients.

Stroke and Cognitive Dysfunction

Stroke after coronary bypass surgery increases in frequency with advancing age. In patients over age 65, the stroke rate is approximately 2.5% versus 1% or less in younger patients.[10] The rate of stroke is extremely low in even very elderly patients undergoing PTCA. Also unlike PTCA, postoperative cognitive dysfunction commonly occurs in older bypass patients.[60,105] Reversible confusional states are common in the elderly, and neuropsychological testing indicates that up to 60% of patients undergoing cardiac surgery have subclinical neuropsychological disturbances. Cognitive dysfunction is symptomatic in about 10% of the total surgical population.[108,109] Elderly patients are even more likely to develop these neuropsychological deficits.[110]

Predicting Success With Coronary Bypass Surgery

A number of factors have been shown to predict poor outcomes after coronary bypass surgery in elderly patients. Depressed left ventricular systolic function, emergency surgery, class IV anginal symptoms, unstable angina, previous MI, hypertension, smoking, prior coronary bypass surgery, cachexia, female sex, and emergency surgery have all been described as predictors of poor outcome.[10-12,14,110-117] The patient characteristics which are predictors of outcome with surgery are not necessarily the same as the ones which predict angioplasty success. For example, cachexia, previous MI, and emergency procedure have *not* been shown to be important for PTCA procedural success. Measures of left ventricular systolic function predict event-free survival for elderly angioplasty and surgical groups, as well as most other populations of patients with CAD. Left ventricular systolic function appears to be relatively less important for immediate success with PTCA.[10,12,56] Concomitant medical ilness is also a factor which predicts long-term survival in the elderly angioplasty and surgical populations.[10,56,117]

Recommending Coronary Surgery Rather than Percutaneous Transluminal Coronary Angioplasty in the Elderly

Many elderly patients with symptomatic CAD are not technically suited for PTCA, but are acceptable candidates for coronary bypass surgery, and surgery is, therefore, the appropriate therapy. Also, coronary bypass surgery has been shown to improve survival in elderly patients with left main coronary stenosis, as well as those with three-vessel CAD and poor left ventricular systolic function.[13,117-119] Coronary bypass surgery appears to give better results than PTCA in elderly patients with decreased left ventricular contractile dysfunction and multivessel CAD.[120,121] In elderly patients who have multivessel CAD and poor left ventricular systolic function, bypass surgery is frequently more appropriate than angioplasty, especially if surgery can more easily obtain complete revascularization.

Elderly patients in whom the risk of morbid complications with coronary bypass surgery is increased may be more appropriate for balloon angioplasty. Also, for patients who are frail and have multiple medical probelms, the risk of surgery is higher. In particular, patients who are at increased risk of stroke because of diffuse aortic atherosclerotic disease or preexisting cerebrovascular disease should be considered for PTCA.

Approach to the Elderly Patient Who Needs Revascularization

Careful patient selection is the key to optimal outcome in the treatment of the elderly. The elderly are a heterogeneous group, and appropriate treatment strategies and goals of therapy vary, especially between the "young-old" and "old-old." In younger patients, the goals of therapy are improvement in long-term survival, maintenance of an active lifestyle, and symptom relief. However, in very elderly patients, the focus is different. In them, maintenance of independence and relief of disabling symptoms are the primary goals of therapy. Given the increased risk of intervention, it is particularly important that elderly patients play an important role in the treatment decision. PTCA, when technically feasible, is an appropriate therapy for many elderly patients.

References

1. Tauber C: Sixty-five plus in America. *Current Population Reports Series* P-23, No. 178. Washington, DC: US Government Printing Office, 1992.
2. US Bureau of the Census: Projections of the population of the United States by age, sex, and race—1988 to 2080. *Current Population Reports Series* P-25, No. 1018. Washington, DC: US Government Printing Office.
3. National Center for Health Statistics: Current estimates from the National Health Interview Survey, United States, 1989. *Vital and Health Statistics Series* 10, No. 176. Rockville, MD: US Department of Health, Education, and Welfare, 1990.
4. Thompson RC, Holmes DR Jr, Gersh BJ, Mock MD, Bailey KR: Percutaneous transluminal coronary angioplasty in the elderly: early and long-term results. *J Am Coll Cardio* 17:1245-1250, 1991.
5. Findleib M, Havlik R, Gillum RF, Pokras R, McCarthy E, Morine M: Coronary heart disease in related procedures: National Hospital Discharge Survey Data. *Circulation* (suppl)79:113-118, 1989.

6. Ltyle BW, Cosgrove D, Loop FD: Future implications of current trends in bypass surgery. *Cardiovasc Clin* 21:265-268, 1991.
7. Backes RJ, Gersh BJ: The treatment of coronary artery disease in the elderly. *Cardiovasc Drugs Ther* 5:449-455, 1991.
8. Nolan L, O'Malley K: Prescribing for the elderly. Part I. Sensitivity of the elderly to adverse drug reactions. *J Am Geriatr Soc* 36:142-149, 1988.
9. Gurwitz JH, Col NF, Avorn J: The exclusion of the elderly and women from clinical trials in acute myocardial infarction. *JAMA* 2687:1417-1422, 1992.
10. Loop FD, Lytle BW, Cosgrove DW, Goormastic M, Taylor PC, Golding LAR: Coronary artery bypass graft surgery in the elderly: indications and outcome. *Cleve Clin J Med* 55:23-34, 1988.
11. Horvath KA, DiSesa VJ, Peigh PS, Couper GS, Collins JJ Jr, Cohn LH: Favorable results of coronary artery bypass grafting in patients older than 75 years. *J Thorac Cardiovasc Surg* 99:92-96, 1993.
12. Mullany CJ, Darling GE, Pluth JR, Orszulak TA, Schaff HB, Ilstrup GM: Early and late results after isolated coronary bypass surgery in 159 patients aged 80 years and older. *Circulation* 82 (suppl 4):IV-29-IV-36, 1990.
13. Horneffer PJ, Gardner TJ, Manolio TA, et al: The effects of age on outcome after coronary bypass surgery. *Circulation* 76 (suppl 5):VI-XII, 1987.
14. Weintraub WS, Craver JM, Guyton RA: Influence of age on results of coronary artery surgery. *Circulation* 84 (suppl) III-226-III-235, 1991.
15. Salamon NW, Page US, Biegelo JC, Krause AH, Okies JE, Metzdorff MT: Coronary artery bypass grafting in elderly patients: comparative results in a consecutive series of 469 patients older than 75 years. *J Thorac Cardiovasc Surg* 101:209-218, 1991.
16. Kahn SS, Kupfer JM, Matloff JM, Tsai TP, Nessim S: Interaction of age and preoperative risk factors in predicting operative mortality for coronary bypass surgery. *Circulation* 86 (suppl 2): II-186-II190, 1992.
17. Macaya C, Alfonso F, Iniguez A, Zarco P: Long-term clinical and angiographic follow-up of percutaneous transluminal coronary angioplasty in patients ≥65 years of age. *Am J Cardiol* 66:1513-1515, 1990.
18. Mock MB, Holmes DR Jr, Vliestra RE, Gersh BJ, Detre KM, Kelsey SF, et al: Percutaneous transluminal coronary angioplasty (PTCA) in the elderly patient: experience in the National Heart, Lung and Blood Institute PTCA registered approved. *Am J Cardiol* 53:89C-91C, 1984.
19. Kelsey SF, Miller DP, Holubkov R, Lu AS, Cowley MJ, Faxon DP, et al: Investigators from the NHLBI PTCA Registry: results of percutaneous transluminal coronary angioplasty in patients ≥65 years of age. *Am J Cardiol* 66:1033-1038, 1990.
20. Voudris V, Antonellis J, Salcahis A, et al: Coronary angioplasty in the elderly: immediate and long-term results. *Angiology* 44:933-937, 1993.
21. Forman DE, Berman AD, McCabe CH, Balm DS, Wei JY: The "young-old" versus the "old-old." *J Am Geriatr Soc* 40:19-22, 1992.
22. Peterson ED, Jollis JG, Bebchuk, et al: Changes in mortality after myocardial revascularization in the elderly: the National Medicare Experience. *Ann Intern Med* 121:919-927, 1994.
23. Thompson RC, Holmes DR Jr, Grill DE, Bailey KR: Changing outcome of angioplasty in the elderly. *J Am Coll Cardiol* 27:8-14, 1996.
24. Buffet P, Danchin N, Julliere Y, Feldman L, Marie PY, Selton-Suty C, et al: Percutaneous transluminal coronary angioplasty in patients more than 75 years old: early and long-term results. *Int J Cardiol* 37:33-39, 1992.
25. Jackman JD Jr, Navetta FI, Smith JE, Techen JE, Davidson CJ, Phillips HR, et al: Percutaneous transluminal coronary angioplasty in octogenarians as an effective therapy for angina pectoris. *Am J Cardiol* 68:116-119, 1991.

26. Rizo-Patron C, Hamad N, Paulus R, Garcia J, Beard E: Percutaneous transluminal coronary angioplasty in octogenarians with unstable coronary syndromes. *Am J Cardiol* 66:857-858, 1990.
27. O'Keefe JH Jr, Rutherford BD, McConahay DR, Johnson WL Jr, Giorgi LV, Ligon RW, et al: Multivessel coronary angioplasty from 1980 to 1989: procedural results and long-term outcome. *J Am Coll Cardiol* 16:1097-1102, 1990.
28. Ellis SG, Cowley MJ, DeSciascio G, Deligonul U, Topol EJ, Bulle TM, Vandormael MG, The Multivessel Angioplasty Prognosis Study Group: Determinants of 2-year outcome after coronary angioplasty in patients with multivessel disease on the basis of comprehensive preprocedural evaluation: implications for patient selection. *Circulation* 83:1905-1914, 1991.
29. Vandormael M,, Deligonul U, Taussig S, Kern MJ: Predictors of long-term cardiac survival in patients with multivessel coronary artery disease undergoing percutaneous transluminal coronary angioplasty. *Am J Cardiol* 67:1-6, 1991.
30. Rich JJ, Crispino CM, Saporito JJ, Domat I, Cooper WM: Percutaneous transluminal coronary angioplasty in patients 80 years of age and older. *Am J Cardiol* 65:675-676, 1990.
31. Dorros G, Janke L: Percutaneous transluminal coronary angioplasty in patients over the age of 70 years. *Cathet Cardiovasc Diagn* 12:223-229, 1986.
32. Mills TJ, Smith HC, Vliestra RE: PTCA in the elderly: results and expectation. *Geriatrics* 44:71-79, 1989.
33. Holt GW, Sugrue DD, Bresnahan JF, Vliestra RE, Bresnahan DR, Reeder GS, et al: Results of percutaneous transluminal coronary angioplasty for unstable agina pectoris in patients 70 years of age and older. *Am J Cardiol* 61:994-997, 1988.
34. Bedotto JB, Rutherford BD, McConahay DR, Johnson WL Jr, Giorgi LV, Shimshak TM, et al: Results of multivessel percutaneous transluminal coronary angioplasty in persons age 65 years and older. *Am J Cardiol* 67:1051-1055, 1991.
35. Simfendorfer C, Raymond R, Schrader J, Badhwar K, Dorosti K, Franko I, et al: Early and long-term results of percutaneous transluminal coronary angioplasty in patients 70 years of age and older with angina pectoris. *Am J Cardiol* 62:959-961, 1988.
36. de Jaegere P, de Feyter P, van Domburg R, Suryapranata H, van den Brand M, Serruys PW: Immediate and long-term results of percutaneous coronary angioplasty in patients aged 70 and over. *Br Heart J* 67:138-143, 1992.
37. Lindsay J Jr, Reddy VM, Pinnow EE, Little T, Pichard AD: Morbidity and mortality rates in elderly patients undergoing percutaneous coronary transluminal angioplasty. *Am Heart J* 128:697-702, 1994.
38. Reynen K, Kunkel B, Bachmann K, Gansser R, Maratus P: PTCA in elderly patients: acute results and long-term follow-up. *Eur Heart J* 14:1661-1668, 1993.
39. Maiello L, Colombo A, Gianrossi R, Thomas J, Feinci L: Percutaneous transluminal coronary angioplasty in patients aged 70 years and older: immediate and long-term results. *Int J Cardiol* 36:1-8, 1992.
40. Maiello L, Columbo A, Gianrossi R, Thomas J, Feinci L: Results of coronary angioplasty in patients aged 75 years and older. *Chest* 102:375-379, 1992.
41. ten Berg JM, Ball ET, Tjon Joe Gin RM, Ernst JNPG, Nast EG, Ascoop CAPL, et al: Initial and long-term results of percutaneous transluminal coronary angioplasty in patients 75 years of age and older. *Cath Cardiovasc Diagn* 26:165-170, 1992.
42. Jollis JG, Peterson ED, Bebchuck JD, DeLong ER, Humphreys JO, Muhlbaier LH, et al: Coronary angioplasty in 20,006 patients over age 80 in the United Sates (abstr). *J Am Coll Cardiol* (suppl)1:47A, 1995.
43. Kern, MJ, Deligonul U, Galan K, Zelman R, Gabliani G, Bell ST, et al: Percutaneous transluminal coronary angioplasty in octogenarians. *Am J Cardiol* 61:457-458, 1988.

44. Jeroudi MO, Kleinman NS, Minor ST, Hess KR, Lewis JM, Winters WL Jr, et al: Percutaneous transluminal coronary angioplasty in octogenarians. *Ann Intern Med* 113:423-428, 1990.
45. Myler RK, Webb JG, Nguyen K, et al: Coronary angioplasty in octogenarians: comparison to coronary bypass surgery. *Cathet Cardiovasc Diagn* 23:3-9, 1991.
46. Santana JO, Haft JI, LaMarche NS, Goldstein JE: Coronary angioplasty in patients 80 years of age or older. *Am Heart J* 124:13-18, 1992.
47. Weyrens FJ, Goldenberg I, Mooney JF, et al: Percutaneous transluminal coronary angioplasty in patients aged ≥90 years. *Am J Cardio* 74:397-398, 1994.
48. Mick MJ, Sinpfendarfer C, Arnold AZ, Piedmonte M, Lytle BW: Early and late results of coronary angioplasty and bypass in octogenarians. *Am J Cardiol* 68:1316-1320, 1991.
49. Quigley PJ, Hinohara T, Phillips HR, et al: Myocardial protection during coronary angioplasty with an autoperfusion balloon catheter in humans. *Circulation* 78:1128-1134, 1988.
50. Turi CG, Campbell CA, Gottimukkala MV, Kloner RA: Preservation of distal coronary perfusion during prolonged balloon inflation with an autoperfusion angioplasty catheter. *Circulation* 75:1273-1280, 1987.
51. Leitschuh ML, Mills RM Jr, Jacobs AK, Ruocco NA Jr, LaRosa D, Faxon DP: Outcome after major dissection during coronary angioplasty using the perfusion balloon catheter. *Am J Cardiol* 67:1056-1060, 1991.
52. Tenaglia AN, Zidar JP, Jackman JD Jr, et al: Treatment of long coronary artery narrowings with long angioplasty balloon catheters. *Am J Cardiol* 71:1274-1277, 1993.
53. Brymer JF, Khaja F, Kratt PL: Angioplasty of long or tandem coronary artery lesions using a new longer balloon dilation catheter: a comparative study. *Cathet Cardiovasc Diagn* 23:84-88, 1991.
54. Rath B, Bennett DH: Monitoring the effect of heparin by measurement of activated clotting time during and after percutaneous transluminal coronary angioplasty. *Br Heart J* 63:18-21, 1990.
55. Ogilvy JD, Kopelman HA, Klein LW, Agarwal JB: Adequate heparinization during PTCA: assessment using activating clotting times. *Cathet Cardiovasc Diagn* 18:206-209, 1989.
56. Thompson RC, Holmes DR Jr, Gersh BJ, Bailey KR: Predicting early and intermediate-term outcome of coronary angioplasty in the elderly. *Circulation* 88:1579-1587, 1993.
57. Jollis JG, Peterson ED, DeLong ER, et al: The relationship between the volume of coronary angioplasty procedures at hospitals treating Medicare beneficiaris and short-term mortality. *N Engl J Med* 331:1625-1629, 1994.
58. Ryan TJ, Bauman WB, Kennedy JW, et al: Guidelines for percutaneous transluminal coronary angioplasty. *Circulation* 88:2987-3007, 1993.
59. Imburgia M, King TR, Soffer AD, Rich MW, Krone RJ, Salimi A: Early results and long-term outcome of percutaneous transluminal coronary angioplasty in patients age 75 years or older. *Am J Cardiol* 63:1127-1129, 1989.
60. Guadagnoli E, Ayanian JZ, Cleary PD: Comparison of patient reported outcomes after elective coronary artery bypass grafting in patients aged ≤ and ≥ 65 years. *Am J Cardiol* 70:60-64, 1992.
61. Kowalchuk GJ, Siu SC, Lewis SM: Coronary artery disease in the octogenarian: angiographic spectrum and suitability for revascularization. *Am J Cardiol* 66:1319-1323, 1990.
62. Knapp WS, Douglas JS Jr, Quaver JM, Jones EL, King SB III, Bone BK, et al: Efficacy of coronary artery bypass grafting in elderly patients with coronary artery disease. *Am J Cariol* 47:923-930, 1981.

63. McBride W, Lange RA, Hillis LD: Restenosis after successful coronary angioplasty: pathophysiology and prevention. N Engl J Med 318:1734-1737, 1988.
64. Leimgruber PP, Roubin Gs, Hollman J, Cotsonis GA, Meier B, Douglas JS, et al: Restenosis after successful coronary angioplasty in patients with single-vessel disease. Circulation 73:710-717, 1986.
65. Holmes DR Jr, Vlietstra RE, Smith HC, Vetrovec GW, Kent KM, Cowley NJ, et al: Restenosis after percutaneous transluminal coronary angioplasty (PTCA): a report from the PTCA Registry of the National Heart, Lung and Blood Institute. Am J Cardiol 53:77C-81C, 1984.
66. Bourassa MG, Lesperance J, Eastwood C, Schwartz L, Cote G, Kazim F, et al: Clinical, physiologic, anatomic, and procedural factors predictive of restenosis after percutaneous transluminal coronary angioplasty. J Am Coll Cardiol 18:386-376, 1991.
67. Hirshfeld JW Jr, Schwartz JS, Jugo R, MacDonald RG, Goldberg S, Savage MP (the M-Heart Invertigators), et al: Restenosis after coronary angioplasty: a multivariant statistical model to relate lesion and procedure variables to restenosis. J Am Coll Cardiol 18:647-656, 1991.
68. Serruys PW, Luitjan HE, Beatt KJ, et al: Incidence of restenosis after successful coronary angioplasty: a time related phenomenon. A quantitative angiographic study in 342 consecutive patients at one, two, three, and four months. Circulation 77:361-366, 1988.
69. Leimgruber PP, Roubin GS, Hollman J, et al: Restenosis after successful coronary angioplasty in patients with single-vessel disease. Circulation 73:710-713, 1986.
70. O'Keefe JH Jr, Sutton MB, McAllister BB, et al: Coronary angioplasty versus bypass surgery in patients ≥ 70 years old matched for ventricular function. J Am Coll Cardiol 24:425-430, 1994.
71. Bell MR, Bailey KR, Reeder GS, Lapeyre AC III, Holmes DR Jr: Percutaneous transluminal angioplasty in patients with multivessel coronary disease: how important is complete revascularization for cardiac event-free survival? J Am Coll Cardiol 16:553-562, 1990.
72. Reeder GS, Holmes DR Jr, Detr K, Costigan T, Kelsey SF: Degree of revascularization in patients with multivessel coronary disease: a report from the National Heart, Lung and Blood Institute Percutaneous Transluminal Coronary Angioplasty Registry. Circulation 77:638-644, 1988.
73. Lawrie GM, Morris GC, Silvers A, et al: The influence of residual disease after coronary artery bypass on the 5-year survival rate of 1274 men with coronary artery disease. Circulation 66:717-723, 1982.
74. Jones EL, Craver JM, Guyton RA, Bone DK, Hatcher CR Jr, Riechwald N: Importance of complete revascularization in performance of the coronary bypass operation. Am J Cardiol 51:7-12, 1983.
75. Bell MR, Gersh BJ, Schaff HV, Holmes DR Jr, Fisher LD, Alderman EL, Investigators of the Coronary Artery Surgery Study: Effect of completeness of revascularization on long-term outcome of patients with three-vessel disease undergoing coronary artery bypass surgery: a Report from the Coronary Artery Surgery Study (CASS) Registry. Circulation 86:446-457, 1992.
76. Bourassa MG, Holubkov R, Yeh W, Detre KM: Strategy of complete revascularization in patients with multivessel coronary artery disease: a report from the 1985-1986 National Heart, Lung and Blood Institute Percutaneous Transluminal Coronary Angioplasty Registry. Am J Cardiol 70:174-178, 1992.
77. Aronow WS, Mercando AD, Epstein S: Prevalence of silent myocardial ischemia detected by 24-hour ambulatory electrocardiography, and its association with new coronary events at 40-month follow-up in elderly diabetic and nondiabetic patients with coronary artery disease. Am J Cardiol 69:555-556, 1992.

78. Goldberg RJ, Gore JM, Gurwitz JH, Alpert JS, Brady P, Strohsnitter W, et al: The impact of age on the incidence and prognosis of initial acute myocardial infarction: the Worcescer Heart Attack Study. *Am Heart J* 117:543-549, 1989.
79. Latting CA, Thorberman ME: Acute myocardial infarction in hospitalized patients over age 70. *Am Heart J* 100:311-318, 1980.
80. Naylor CD, Chen F: Population mortality trends among patients hospitalized for acute myocardial infarction: the Ontario Experience, 1981-1991. *J Am Coll Cardiol* 24:1431-1438, 1994.
81. The GUSTO Investigators: An international randomized trial comparing four thrombolytic strategies for acute myocardial infarction. *N Engl J Med* 329:673-682, 1993.
82. Lew As, Hanoch H, Cercek B, Shah PK, Ganz W: Mortality and morbidity rates of patients older and younger than 75 years with acute myocardial infarction treated with intravenous Streptokinase. *Am J Cardiol* 59:1-5, 1987.
83. TIMI Study Group: Comparison of invasive and conservative strategies after treatment with intravenous tissue plasminogen activator in acute myocardial infarction. *N Engl J Med* 320:618-627, 1989.
84. Grines CL, Browne KF, Marco J, et al: A comparison of immediate angioplasty with thrombolytic therapy for acute myocardial infarction. *N Engl J Med* 328:673-679, 1993.
85. Zijlstra F, Jan deBoer M, Hoorntje JCA, Reiffers S, Rerber JHC, Surgapranata H: A comparison of immediate coronary angioplasty with intravenous Streptokinase in acute myocardial infarction. *N Engl J Med* 328:680-684, 1993.
86. Gibbons RJ, Holmes DR Jr, Reeder GS, Bailey KR, Hopfenspringer MR, Gersh BJ: For the Mayo Coronary Care Unit and Catheterization Laboratory Groups. Immediate angioplasty compared with the administration of a thrombolitic agent followed by conservative treatment of myocardial infarction. *N Engl J Med* 328:685-691, 1993.
87. DeBoer MJ, Ghoontje JC, Ottervanger JP, Reitters S, Suryapranata H, Zijlftro F: Immediate coronary angioplasty versus intravenous Streptokinase in acute myocardial infarction: left ventricular ejection fration, hospital mortality, and reinfarction. *J Am Coll Cardiol* 23:1004-1008, 1994.
88. Laster SB, Rutherford BD, Giorgi LV, et al: Results of direct percutaneous transluminal coronary angioplasty in octogenarians. *Am J Cardiol* 77:10-13, 1996.
89. Lee TC, Laramee A, Rutherford BD, McConahay DR, Johnson WL Jr, Giorgi LV, et al: Emergency percutaneous transluminal coronary angioplasty for acute myocardial infarction in patients 70 years of age and older. *Am J Cardiol* 66:663-667, 1990.
90. Stuckey T, Bradie B, Hamsen C, Muncy D, Weintraub R, Kelly T, et al: Primary angioplasty for acute myocardial infarction in elderly thrombolytic candidates: is it the best option? (abstr). *J Am Coll Cardiol* (suppl)1:47A, 1995.
91. Stone GW, Grines CL, Browne KF, et al: Predictors of in-hospital and six-month outcome after acute myocardial infarction in the reperfusion era: the Primary Angioplasty and Myocardial Infarction (PAMI) Trial. *J Am Cardiol* 25:370-377, 1995.
92. Swigart W, Urban P, Golf S, Kaufman U, Imbent C, Fischer A, et al: Emergency stenting for acute occlusion after coronary balloon angioplasty. *Circulation* 78:1121-1127, 1988.
93. Serruys PW, de Jaegere P, Kicmene JF, et al: A comparison of balloon expandable-stent implantation with balloon angioplasty in patients with coronary artery disease. *N Engl J Med* 331:489-494, 1994.
94. Fischman DL, Leon MB, Bam DS, et al: A randomized comparison of coronary-stent placement and balloon angioplasty in the treatment of coronary artery disease. *N Engl J Med* 331:496-501, 1994.

95. Yokoi H, Kimaura T, Sawada Y, Nosaka H, Nouyoshi M: Efficacy of safety of Palmaz-Schatz stent in elderly (≤75 years old) patients: early and follow-up results (abstr). *J Am Coll Cardiol* (suppl) 1:47A, 1995.

96. Thompson RC, Holmes DR Jr, Garrett KN: Use of intracoronary stents in the elderly: early and intermediate-term results. *J Inv Cardiol* 53C, 1995.

97. King SB, Lembo NJ, Weintraub WS, et al: A randomized trial comparing coronary angioplasty with coronary bypass surgery. *N Engl J Med* 331:1044-1050, 1994.

98. Hamm CW, Reimers J, Ischinger T, Rupprecht HJ, Berger J, Bleifeld W: A randomized study of coronary angioplasty compared with bypass surgery in patients with symptomatic multivessel coronary disease. *N Engl J Med* 331:1037-1043, 1994.

99. BARI Investigators: Protocol for the bypass angioplasty revascularization investigation. *Circulation* 84(suppl)V:V1-V27, 1991.

100. Hampton JR, Henderson RA, Jullian DG, et al: Coronary angioplsty versus coronary artery bypass surgery: the randomized intervention treatment of angina (RITA) trial. *Lancet* 331:573-580, 1993.

101. Iniguez A, Macaya C, Alfonso F, et al: Percutaneous transluminal coronary angioplasty for postinfarction and angina in elderly patients. *Age Aging* 22:31-36, 1993.

102. Rich MW, KellerAJ, Schechtman KB, Marshall G, Kouchoukos NT: Morbidity and mortality of coronary bypass surgery in patients 75 years or older. *Ann Thorac Surg* 46:630-634, 1988.

103. Ko W, Krieger KH, Lazenby WD, et al: Isolated coronary artery bypass grafting in 100 consecutive octigenarian patients: a multivariant analysis. *J Thorac Cardiovasc Surg* 102:532-538, 1992.

104. Peterson ED, Coupers PA, Jollis JG, et al: Outcomes of coronary artery bypass graft surgery in 24,461 patients aged 80 years or older. *Circulation* 92 (suppl 95):II85-II91, 1995.

105. Carey JS, Cunningham RA, Singer LKM: Quality of life after myocardial revascularization: effect of increasing age. *J Thorac Cardiovasc Surg* 103:108-115, 1992.

106. Stason WB, Sanders CA, Smith AC: Cardiovascular care of the elderly: economic considerations. *J Am Coll Cardiol* 10 (suppl A):182A-121A, 1987.

107. Lipowski ZJ: Delirium in the elderly patient. *N Engl J Med* 320:578-582, 1989.

108. Sotaniemi KA, Mononen H, Hokkanen TE: Long-term cerebral outcome after open-heart surgery: a five-year neuropsychological follow-up study. *Stroke* 17:410-416, 1986.

109. Townes BD, Bashein G, Hornbein TF, et al: Neurobehavioral outcomes in cardiac operations: a prospective controlled study. *J Thorac Cardiovasc Surg* 98:774-782, 1989.

110. Slogoff S, Girgis KZ, Keats AS: Etiologic factors in neuropsychiatric complications associated with cardiopulmonary bypass. *Anesth Analg* 61:903-911, 1982.

111. Acinapra AJ, Rose DM, Cunningham JN Jr, Jacobowitz IJ, Kramer MD, Zisbrod Z: Coronary artery bypass in septuagenarian: analysis of mortality and morbidity. *Circulation* 78 (suppl)1:I-=179-I-184, 1988.

112. Faro RS, Golden MD, Javid H, Serry C, DeLaria GA, Monson D, et al: Coronary revascularization in septuagenarians. *J Thorac Cardiovasc Surg* 86:616-620, 1983.

113. Tsa TP, Matloff JM, Gray RJ, Chaux A, Kass RM, Lee ME, et al: Cardiac surgery in the octogenarian. *J Thorac Cardiovasc Surg* 91:924-928, 1986.

114. Rich MW, Keller AJ, Schechtman KB, Marshall WB Jr, Kouchoukos NT: Morbidity and mortality of coronary bypass surgery in patients 75 years of age or older. *Ann Thorac Surg* 46:638-644, 1988.

115. Dorros G, Lewin F, Daley P, Assa J: Coronary artery bypass surgery in patients over age 70: report from the Milwaukee Cardiovascular Data Registry. *Clin Cardiol* 10:377-382, 1987.

116. Lahey SJ, Borlase BC, Lavin PT, Levitsky S: Preoperative risk factors that predict hospital length of stay in coronary artery bypass patients >60 years. *Circulation* 86 (suppl)2:II-181-II185, 1992.

117. Gersch BJ, Kromal RA, Schaff HB, et al: Comparison of coronary artery bypass surgery and medical therapy in patients 65 years of age or older: a nonrandomized study from the Coronary Artery Surgery Study (CASS) Registry. *N Engl J Med* 313:217-224, 1985.

118. Jeffery DL, Vijayanagar RR, Bognollo DA, Eckstein PF, Kerpchar JB, Natarajian P, et al: Coronary bypass for left main disease in patients over 70 years of age. *J Cardiovasc Surg* 26:212-216, 1985.

119. Chaitman BR, Davis KB, Kaiser GC, Mud G, Weins RD, Ng GS, participating CASS Hospitals, et al: The role of coronary bypass surgery for "left main equivalent" coronary disease: the Coronary Arteries Surgery Study Registry. *Circulation* 74 (suppl)3:III-17-III-25, 1986.

120. O'Keefe JH Jr, Allen JJ, McAllister BB, et al: Angioplasty versus bypass surgery for multivessel coronary artery disease with ventricular ejection fraction ≤40%. *Am J Cardiol* 71:897-901, 1993.

121. Munger TM, McGregor CGA, Bailey KR, Danielson GK, Holmes DR Jr: Long-term retrospective follow-up for outcome of percutaneous transluminal coronary angioplasty versus coronary artery bypass surgery in patients with severely depressed left ventricular function. *JACC* 17:63A, 1991.

Chapter 19

Surgical Management of Coronary Artery Disease in the Elderly

Stewart M. Scott, MD
Edward A. Stemmer, MD

A major share of physicians' time and the nation's resources are being directed toward decreasing the prevalence of ischemic heart disease and preventing its morbidity and mortality. Reduction in the number of deaths from coronary arterial disease (CAD) has been identified by the Public Health Service as 1 of 22 priority areas for health improvement in the United States by the year 2000.[1]

William Harvey, in the mid 1600s, appreciated the nutritive function of the coronary arteries. Heberden, in the late 1700s, introduced the term *angina pectoris*. Although the condition was generally associated then and for many years thereafter with sudden death, Heberden did not make the connection between this "painful and most disagreeable sensation in the breast" and CAD. It was almost 150 years later, in 1912, that Herrick established that acute occlusion of the coronary arteries could produce myocardial infarction (MI) without resulting in immediate death. Less than 5 years after Herrick published his work and before acute MI was recognized as a common occurrence, surgeons were attempting to relieve the symptoms of coronary heart disease. Over the next 50 years, numerous procedures to treat the consequences of CAD were devised and performed, often with questionable results.

After the multiple randomized studies conducted in the 1970s had demonstrated that certain subsets of patients benefited from coronary arterial bypass grafting (CABG), the procedure began to be performed in older groups of patients. By 1990, approximately 300,000 CABGs were being performed annually, in addition to 310,000 percutaneous angioplastic procedures (PTCA).

In recent years, the performance of coronary arterial revascularization in a growing number of elderly patients with limited potential for survival has raised questions not only about the effectiveness of CABG

From: Aronow WS, Stemmer EA, Wilson SE (eds). *Vascular Disease in the Elderly*. Armonk, NY: Futura Publishing Company, Inc., © 1997.

in the elderly, but about the justification for expending resources for this purpose. This chapter is intended to provide objective data by which the value of CABG in the elderly can be judged.

If the risks and benefits of cardiac surgery in the elderly are to be properly assessed, however, it is important to first provide an overview of the nature and prevalence of CAD in the general population and an understanding of the historical backgrounds for both medical and surgical treatment.

Prevalence of Coronary Artery Disease

Clinically apparent heart disease affected 19,307,000 people of all ages in the United States in 1990 for a prevalence rate of 80.7 per thousand civilian, noninstitutionalized individuals. Ischemic disease is the major component of these heart conditions, with rheumatic heart disease, hypertensive heart disease, and all other types of heart disease making up the remainder. Not unexpectedly, the prevalence of clinically established heart disease in a noninstitutionalized population increases with age. Under age 45 years, the prevalence in men in 1990 was 27.3 per 1000 persons rising to 404.8 per 1000 at ages 75 years or older. Prevalence in females was lower at all ages above 45 years (Table 1).[2] An estimated 6.2 million Americans have significant CAD.[3] The true incidence of CAD in the United States, however, is largely unknown, since many patients have "silent" disease in that they are either asymptomatic or do not recognize the significance of their symptoms. This population remains untreated until the onset of angina pectoris, MI, congestive heart failure (CHF), arrhythmias, or sudden death. Nevertheless, an approximation of the true incidence of CAD can be obtained from both autopsy studies and epidemiological studies in asymptomatic individuals.

Autopsy Studies

In a 1950 autopsy study, White et al[4] and Ackerman et al[5] examined 100 hearts in each of 6 decades from the fourth through the ninth. The

Table 1
Prevalence of Heart Conditions (All Forms)
United States by Age and by Gender per 1000 Persons, 1990 (Civilian, noninstitutionalized)

Age Group	Men	Women
Under 45 yrs	27.3	34.2
45 to 64	137.4	101.5
65 to 74	275.2	242.5
75 and over	404.8	292.3

prevalence of significant CAD (stenosis ≥60% of at least one coronary artery) ranged from 7.2% in women during the fourth decade of life to 75.1% in men during the sixth decade of life (Table 2).[4,5] Fleg et al, in reviewing this series, pointed out that the prevalence of CAD peaked 2 decades later in women than it did in men, but that the prevalence of the disease was nearly identical in both sexes over the age of 70.[6] In 1953, Enos et al reported on an autopsy study of 300 United States soldiers killed in action in Korea.[7] Seventy-seven percent of these individuals, with an average age of 22 years, had evidence of CAD. Fifteen percent had noteworthy obstruction, while 10% had total or near total occlusion of a major coronary vessel.[7] In 1971, McNamara et al[8] reported on a study of United States soldiers killed in Vietnam. Forty-five percent of those individuals had coronary atherosclerosis that was thought to be minimal, but 5% were found to have severe occlusive disease.[8]

Epidemiological Studies

Harris,[9] in 1970, described a 1964 National Center for Health Statistics study in which the prevalence of definite and suspected heart disease was analyzed in the United States population aged 18 to 79 years. Definite heart disease was present in 13.2% of the group, while suspected heart disease was present in another 11.7%. In the 75- to 79-year age group, 42.3% had definite heart disease, while an additional 25.2% had suspected heart disease, percentages very close to those found by Ackerman and White in their autopsy studies.[9] In 1976, Froelicher found that 21.7% of asymptomatic airman with abnormal treadmill stress tests had significant CAD.[10] In 1980, Gerstenblith et al demonstrated that the prevalence of CAD when assessed by resting criteria (history of angina pectoris or MI on a resting electrocardiogram) was less than half that when resting criteria were supplemented by stress electrocardiography or thallium testing (Table 3).[11] In 1983, Hertzer et al,[12] reviewing 1000 coronary arteriograms performed in patients with peripheral vascular disease, found that 37% of patients without clinical

Table 2
Prevalence of Coronary Artery Disease
Autopsy Series: Percentage of Hearts with Stenosis Greater Than 60% in at Least One Coronary Artery

Decade of Life	Men	Women
Fourth	13.6	7.2
Fifth	36.7	12.8
Sixth	75.1	22.3
Seventh	70.2	30.3
Eighth	67.1	59.1
Ninth	65.4	59.1

Table 3
Comparison of the Frequency of Coronary Arterial Disease Detected by Clinical
(Resting) Information and Clinical Information Supplemented by Stress Testing

Age Group	Number of Individuals Studied	Percent Meeting Criteria Resting	Resting Plus Stress
50 to 59 years old	70	13	24
60 to 69	73	15	37
70 to 79	36	22	56
80 to 89	10	20	50

Resting criteria = classical angina, myocardial infarction, MI by EKG
Stress criteria = stress EKG and Thallium scan at maximal exercise

indications of CAD had greater than 70% stenosis of one or more coronary arteries. The age range of their patients was 29 to 95 years with a mean of 64 years.[12] In 1991, Gould commented that up to 13% of middle-aged men in the general population have coronary atherosclerosis, most of it clinically silent. Further, he noted that coronary arteriography revealed disease in 15% to 35% of asymptomatic men between 40 to 55 years old. Of those shown to have CAD, 7% to 35% were found to have anatomically severe disease.[13]

It is apparent that CAD in the United States is a much greater problem than would be suspected from the overt manifestations of the disease.

Manifestations of Coronary Arterial Disease
Mortality

In 1990, there were 489,200 deaths from ischemic heart disease, giving a crude death rate of 196.7 per 100,000 residents in the United States.[14] Approximately one third of all deaths from ischemic heart disease occur in individuals with no prior history of CAD. Approximately one half of all deaths from ischemic heart disease are sudden.[15] Approximately 300,000 of those dying from CAD will never reach a hospital alive. More than 156,000 deaths per year from cardiovascular disease occur before the age of 65. More than half of those dying from cardiovascular disease will be women.[3]

Deaths from heart disease of all types escalate rapidly after the age of 35. In 1990, men between the ages of 45 and 54 had a rate of death from ischemic heart disease of 123.8 per 100,000 population. Between the ages of 75 and 84, the death rate was 2,953.7 per 100,000 individuals. Women had lower death rates in all age intervals above the age of 25 (Table 4).[16]

Table 4
Death Rates from Ischemic Heart Disease by Age and by Gender per 100,000
Persons, 1990 (Residents, United States)

Age Group	Men	Women
45 to 54	123.8	33.6
55 to 64	375.4	135.4
65 to 74	898.5	415.2
75 to 84	2129.6	1287.6
85 and over	5120.7	4257.8

Sudden Death

Sudden death from ischemic heart disease is a persistent and serious problem not only because of its unpredictable nature, but because it is the mode of death in a large number of patients with CAD. Kannel and Thomas,[15] reviewing the results of the Framingham Study, noted that at least half of all deaths from CAD in patients aged 45 to 74 are "sudden" in that they occur within 1 hour of the onset of symptoms. Almost two thirds of coronary fatalities occur outside the hospital. Both transient attacks of myocardial ischemia and clinically evident MI can trigger sudden death, although the relative role of each in sudden death is unclear. Ventricular fibrillation is the usual mechanism causing death.[15] Half of those who present with sudden death have no prior history of CAD. Conversely, in the Framingham Study, 17% of men and 13% of women who did suffer a known coronary attack presented with sudden death as their first and last symptom. Even more disturbing are the observations of Kannel and Thomas[15] and others that it is unusual for patients with known CAD to develop or report specific prodromata that would provide a warning of impending death. The incidence of sudden death increases steadily with increasing age in both men and women, although compared with men, women do not reach the same incidence of sudden death until 20 years later in life.[15,17,18]

Kannel and Thomas[15] observed that death from CAD is as likely as not to be sudden, unexpected, and unheralded by known prior CAD or its symptoms. Treatment of these patients is likely to be unsuccessful and prevention difficult in the absence of known disease. It is true, however, that a high-risk group can be identified by retrospective studies. The individuals suffering sudden death are predominantly male, overweight, hypertensive, and cigarette smokers. Most have a type A personality. A significant number have engaged in moderate or strenuous activity shortly before collapsing.[15] Other authors have commented that only 2% to 5% of sudden deaths attributable to coronary atherosclerosis will occur during physical exertion, only 8% to 12% at work, and 4% while driving. The vast majority occur at home in bed.[19]

The reported incidence of coronary arterial thrombosis in patients dying suddenly varies considerably. Kannel and Thomas commented that antemortem thrombosis could be incriminated in no more than 5% to 10% of instances of sudden death.[15] Autopsy studies by Spain and Baroldi found coronary thrombosis in fewer than 20% of patients dying within the first hour of the onset of ischemic symptoms.[20] The frequency with which coronary thrombosis was found after sudden death appeared to increase with longer survival after the acute episode. Other studies have found recent coronary thrombi in from 74% to 91% of sudden death patients.[20,21]

Acute Myocardial Infarction

In 1988, CAD was the underlying cause of 1.5 million MIs in the United States.[13] In 1990, approximately 675,000 individuals were discharged from the hospital with a diagnosis of acute MI.[3] Acute MI is the initial presentation of CAD in 20% of women and 40% of men (Table 5).[18] Of those who survive their initial MI, 20% of men and 40% of women can be expected to die within the first year. High-risk groups have as high as a 50% risk of death within the first year. In subsequent years, the average mortality per year in patients who have suffered an MI is about 5%, a frequency that is three to four times that of the general population.[22] In patients surviving an acute MI, 86% were found to have total occlusion of a coronary artery when studied during the first 6 hours after the event. When patients were studied between 6 and 24 hours after the acute episode, 67% were found to have total occlusion of a coronary vessel.[20]

Of those who survive an acute MI, 40% will have persistent angina pectoris, CHF, or arrhythmias; 25% of the presumably asymptomatic

---

Table 5

Distribution and Frequency of Initial Clinical Manifestations of Coronary Heart Disease in 427 Patients from the Framingham Study

| Category or Manifestation | Percentage of Individuals in Whom Event was the Initial Manifestation of Coronary Heart Disease | | |
	Men	Women	Both Sexes
Angina pectoris	36.6	66.7	46.1
Coronary insufficiency	7.9	9.6	8.4
Myocardial infarction	40.8	17.8	33.5
Death	14.7	5.9	12.0
Total	100.0	100.0	100.0
Number of Patients	**Distribution of Patients**		
Total patients	2336	2873	5209
Number developing CHD	292	135	427

patients will have a positive treadmill test, and 20% to 30% of the entire group will have silent ischemic episodes.[23,24]

Angina Pectoris

Angina pectoris and MI are the cardiac equivalents of intermittent claudication and gangrene that occurs in the extremities with one major exception. In 1990, peripheral vascular disease was directly responsible for only about 1% of deaths from major cardiovascular disease. Ischemic heart disease was responsible for over 50% of deaths due to major cardiovascular disease.[25] The prevalence of angina pectoris in the general population is approximately 1.6%. In the population of 6.2 million with significant coronary heart disease, the prevalence of angina pectoris is approximately 60%.[3,23] Angina pectoris is the initial presentation of CAD in two thirds of women and one third of men (Table 5).[18] Angina pectoris as a symptom of CAD varies from one population group to another, and tends to be lower in older individuals and in diabetics. In a review of patients over the age of 65, only 19% presented with angina prior to an acute MI.[26]

Although significant CAD can be present without angina pectoris, the presence of angina pectoris is associated with an 89% to 90% likelihood of significant stenosis in one or more of the major coronary arteries.[27]

Silent Ischemia

Silent ischemia occurs when there is an imbalance between myocardial oxygen demand and supply without recognizable symptoms, such as dyspnea on exertion, angina pectoris, or MI. It can be present in patients who have never experienced any cardiac symptoms, as well as in those who have had an MI, but are currently asymptomatic. Episodes of silent myocardial ischemia can also occur in the presence of established angina pectoris.

The true incidence of silent ischemia in a general population is, of course, unknown. Moreover, CAD can exist in the absence of either silent or symptomatic ischemia. Silent myocardial ischemia without symptomatic ischemia can be documented by treadmill testing in approximately 12% of patients surviving an acute MI. About 75% of the four million patients in the United States being treated for angina pectoris will also have episodes of silent ischemia.[23] Droste[24] commented that two thirds of all spontaneous ischemic episodes are silent. Two percent to 4% of all healthy men ages 40 to 60 have episodes of silent ischemia. Instances of silent ischemia occur in 20% to 30% of all patients following MI. In symptomatic patients with CAD, 60% to 90% have episodes of silent ischemia in addition to their manifest symptoms.[24]

Silent ischemia is a prominent characteristic of coronary heart disease in the elderly. Aronow et al,[25] conducting a study of 1489 elderly diabetic and nondiabetic patients with a mean age of 80 years, was able to document CAD in 599 (40.2%). Silent myocardial ischemia was found in 34.2% of this group. Typical angina pectoris was present in only 19 of the 599 patients. While diabetics had a significantly higher prevalence of CAD, there was no difference in the prevalence of silent ischemia between diabetics and nondiabetics.[28] Gerstenblith et al,[11] employing noninvasive techniques, found that the prevalence of silent ischemia in patients known to have coronary heart disease progressed from 11% in patients 50- to 59-years-old to 30% in those 80- to 89-years-old (Table 3).[11]

Silent ischemia is not a benign event. Weiner et al[29] compared the outcomes in three groups of patients with known coronary heart disease. One group had silent ischemia, the second had symptomatic ischemia, while the third group had CAD without ischemic events. The two groups with ischemia had almost identical survivals at 7 years (60% and 55%), while the group without ischemic events had a 73% survival.[29] Patients with silent ischemia soon after an acute MI have a higher mortality at 1 year than do those without silent ischemia (27% versus 2%).[23]

Historical Perspectives

Evolution of the current medical and surgical treatment of CAD can be divided into three periods: 1) recognition of the disease; 2) development of basic diagnostic tools; and 3) implementation of accurate diagnosis and surgical treatment. The significant events took place over a period of 200 years. During the eighteenth century, angina pectoris was recognized as a common and lethal illness that frequently attacked without warning and was associated with sudden death. Its relationship to arterial disease was recognized. During the nineteenth century, the basic instruments necessary for detecting CAD were developed, as were the basic medications for treating its symptoms. MI was recognized as a pathological entity. The early and mid-portion of the twentieth century saw the development of sophisticated diagnostic techniques that made modern treatment of CAD and its complications a reality during the last half of the twentieth century.

Recognition of the Disease

Appreciation and understanding of the role of the coronary arteries in the production of cardiac disease did not begin to develop until the late eighteenth century when Heberden introduced the term *angina pectoris* (Greek for strangling or choking, breastbone or breast) during a lecture before the Royal College of Physicians of London in July, 1768. He described symptoms he had observed in "at least twenty men almost all above 50-years-old, most with a short neck, and inclining to be fat." Heberden commented that angina pectoris was "not extremely rare," that it was associated with walking, particularly after eating, and that the uneasiness vanished the moment the patient stood still. He noted that the symptoms worsened with time and could occur while lying down. He reported that although the natural tendency of the illness was to kill the patient suddenly, the disorder could last "near twenty years." Because the patient's pulse was not usually disturbed by the pain, Heberden concluded that "the heart is not disturbed by it." He ascribed the illness to "a strong spasm sometimes accompanied by an ulcer," but commented that he had never had it in his power to "see anyone opened who had died of it." Heberden published his report in 1772.[30-32]

In 1775, Edward Jenner helped his close friend, John Hunter, perform an autopsy on one of Heberden's patients who died suddenly following an anginal attack associated with a sense of impending death. Ossified coronary vessels were found, but the arteries were not carefully examined. In 1785, Jenner made the connection between angina pectoris and CAD, but did not publish his conclusions until 1799 (in a letter to Parry who included it in his text *Syncope Anginosa*). John Hunter, who had initially developed angina pectoris in 1773, finally died of the disease in 1793 at age 65 years. His death occurred suddenly during a dispute with the board of St. George's Hospital. Jenner's delay in reporting his conclusions about the basis of angina pectoris until after Hunter's death has been attributed to his desire not to alarm his life-long friend.[33-35]

Developing the Tools

Although the frightening and disabling nature of angina pectoris was clearly recognized as a major clinical problem during the nineteenth century, little that was new was added to the basic understanding of CAD. Burns, in Scotland, in his 1809 textbook on diseases of the heart, attributed angina pectoris to myocardial ischemia. Laennec introduced the stethoscope in 1819. In 1840, Williams, in Edinburgh, suggested that an obstructed coronary artery was the cause of the pallid, yellowish appearance of a segment of myocardium discovered at autopsy. The term *myocardial infarction* was not then in use (as late as 1884, what is now known as an MI was referred to as "fibrinoid degeneration"). In 1867, Brunton, in England, introduced amyl nitrite for the treatment of angina pectoris. Nitroglycerin, the mainstay of the treatment of angina pectoris even today, was introduced by Murrell in England in 1879. Riva-Rocci, in Italy, developed the first practical sphygmomanometer in 1891. The year following the serendipitous discovery of x-rays by Roentgen in 1895, Roentgen studies of the heart were being performed by Williams in the United States. That same year, Marie, in France, writing his thesis on complications of cardiac disease used the term MI. Dock, in 1896, was the first physician in the United States to make a diagnosis of coronary thrombosis during life.[33,36,37]

Diagnosis

Widespread appreciation of the relationship between CAD, angina pectoris, and MI did not occur until the second quarter of the twentieth century. Sir Clifford Allbutt, in 1900, attributed angina pectoris to disease of the aorta, an understandable conclusion in view of the likelihood of coronary ostial occlusion secondary to the syphilitic aortitis that was so common at the time.[37] A major contribution to establishing the pathophysiology of CAD was made by Einthoven in Holland in 1903 when he developed a practical method for performing electrocardiography. Sir William Osler commented in 1910 that he had not seen a case of coronary thrombosis until he became a Fellow of the Royal College of Physicians.[38] CAD remained virtually unrecognized as a cause of death until 1912 when Herrick in Chicago described (in six patients) the clinical features of sudden obstruction of the coronary arteries, including the gross changes that occurred in the myocardium in the region of the infarct. He noted that prior attacks of angina had generally been experienced, but that the fatal thrombosis might be the first evidence of coronary disease.[39] In 1918, he republished his data and reported electrocardiographic studies conducted in patients with coronary artery thrombosis.[40] Paul Dudley White commented that in the mid 1920s, in Massachusetts General Hospital, a diagnosis of coronary artery thrombosis and of MI was rare among the autopsies performed.[32] He himself, "that doyen of cardiologists," stated that he did not see his first patient with an MI until he was in his second year of practice in 1921. Wearn, in 1923, wrote that "coronary thrombosis with infarction of the heart as a clinical entity is a condition which is generally classed among the rarities of medicine."[38] In the United States, the most famous instance of failure to recognize the signs and symptoms of fatal CAD occurred in San Francisco on August 2, 1923 when Warren Harding, the 29th president of the United States, died following an acute MI. His death was attributed to acute indigestion or (by *The New York Times*) to a "stroke of apoplexy." By the late 1920s, however, coronary thrombosis, alias MI, was a well-established diagnosis.

In 1929, a German intern, Werner Forssmann,[41] having heard of an experiment by Claude Bernard, threaded a catheter through his antecubital vein into his right atrium. His goal was to devise a technique to speed delivery of drugs to a patient and to understand the "mysteries of the heart" and circulatory system.[41,42] Discouraged from pursuing his experiments by Sauerbruch, the professor of surgery, Forssmann became a urologic specialist. Cournand and Ranges, in New York, became aware of Forssmann's work, and by 1941 had developed the technique for catheterizing the right heart in humans.[43] Zimmerman, in 1950, and Seldinger, in 1953, developed the techniques of left heart catheterization. In 1958, in Cleveland, Ohio, F. Mason Sones, Jr. accidentally injected the right coronary artery with contrast material producing the first selective coronary angiogram. Louis Pasteur is credited with the statement "chance favors the prepared mind." Sones et al[44] not only recognized the potential value of his serendipitous observation, but pursued the development of the technique of selective coronary arteriography making it a practical diagnostic procedure. The presentation of his results during the 1959 meeting of the American Heart Association introduced the modern era of medical and surgical treatment of CAD.[44]

Surgical Treatment

At about the time of Herrick's report that sudden occlusion of a major coronary artery was not "almost universally fatal," surgeons began their attempts to relieve the pain of angina pectoris. Francois Franck, in 1899, proposed removal of the cervical and first thoracic ganglia. His intent was to accomplish a "complete cure of certain cases of Grave's disease, which were complicated by aortitis and angina."[45] Bilateral extirpation of the cervical sympathetic chain, together with removal of both thoracic ganglia, was first performed by a Bucharest surgeon, Jonnesco in 1916 (for the treatment of angina pectoris).[46]

From 1916 through 1982, no less than 59 different variations of surgical procedures had been performed for the treatment of CAD. The procedures ranged from those designed to interrupt the afferent nerve pathways from the heart to those developed to replace the heart. The surgical approaches to CAD can be divided into four broad categories: extrapericardial procedures; techniques for indirect myocardial revascularization; direct revascularization of the coronary arteries; and cardiac replacement (Table 6).[42,47-49] A few of these procedures were performed only in experimental animals, some represented variations of a more basic concept, many were devised by more than one individual, and most were performed in humans at one time or another often over a period of many years. Eventually, all but a few were found to be ineffective or minimally effective.

A major share of the credit for the development of modern coronary arterial surgery belongs to Claude Beck of Western Reserve University and to his persistent efforts to prevent sudden death in patients with a heart "too good to die." Beginning in 1935, he devised and applied numerous variations of his Beck I and Beck II operations. He noted that increases of arterial flow of as little as 5 mL/min into anoxic areas of the myocardium could relieve the pain of angina pectoris and could afford protection against a fatal heart attack.[50,51] About 10 years later, Arthur Vineberg of McGill University began advocating implantation of systemic arteries into the myocardium, thus beginning the era of indirect myocardial revascularization.[52] Widespread application of the current techniques of direct myocardial revascularization began with the reports of Favoloro, Johnson et al, Urschel et al, and Kerth in 1969.[53-56] The first transplantation of a human heart was performed by Christiaan Barnard in 1967 in South Africa.[57] By the mid 1970s, 70,000

Table 6
Classification of Surgical Procedures Designed to Treat Coronary Arterial Disease

Extrapericardial Procedures
    A. Denervation procedures
    B. Procedures to decrease metabolic demand of myocardium
    C. Procedures to redirect blood flow to coronary arteries

Indirect Myocardial Revascularization Procedures
    A. Cardio-pericardiopexy procedures
    B. Epicardial grafting procedures
    C. Procedures to increase retrograde flow into native vessels
    D. Procedures to increase oxygen extraction
    E. Procedures to stimulate collateral development
    F. Myocardial channelization procedures
    G. Myocardial implant procedures

Procedures for Direct Revascularization of the Coronary Arterie
    A. Angioplastic (endarterectomy) procedures
    B. Replacement grafting
    C. Bypass grafting

Cardiac Replacement
    A. Transplantation
    B. Mechanical heart

CABGs were being performed annually in the United States.[54] By 1990, the number had grown to 300,000 per year.

As early as 1971, however, there were those who questioned the efficacy of aortocoronary bypass grafting and the justification for its widespread application. The objections and criticisms were based in part on the long history of failures and marginal results of surgical procedures intended to treat CAD; they were also based in part on what were considered to be the high risks inherent in coronary arterial surgery, and in part on the availability of techniques of medical management that presumably could yield results comparable or superior to those achieved by operation. These concerns led to the performance of numerous controlled studies that compared the outcomes of medical and surgical therapy. Before summaries of the major, pertinent studies are presented, however, the natural history of angina pectoris needs to be addressed since it is, of necessity, the background against which any medical or surgical treatment of CAD must be evaluated. Curiously, it was not until attempts at surgical management of coronary disease were well under way that substantial efforts to determine the natural history of angina pectoris were attempted.

The Natural History of Angina Pectoris

Once the significance of angina pectoris was understood, its natural history and prognosis became a major concern. Early studies by Herrick

(1918) and by White (1926, 1931, 1943) were handicapped by the inability to determine the extent of the disease in the coronary arteries during life.[40,58-60] In addition, patients with angina pectoris who also had associated diseases such as hypertension, valvular disease, previous MI, and congestive failure were often lumped together. In these early series, the annual mortality for patients with angina pectoris ranged from 2.5% to 9.0%.[61] Later studies were difficult to analyze because of surgical intervention. As a result of the constraints described above, a study that would accurately determine the true natural history of angina pectoris would have had to have been conducted after the common techniques of diagnosis were available (including coronary arteriography), but before modern medical and surgical treatment was in widespread use; that is, between the years 1960 and 1970, a narrow window. Interestingly, there have been several studies that come close to meeting these criteria.

Oberman et al[62] analyzed the course of 246 patients who underwent coronary arteriography for chest pain between 1965 and 1970, a time period prior to the advent of aortocoronary bypass grafting in their institution. At 22 months, there were no deaths in patients with one-vessel disease and small hearts, or in those with one-vessel disease and no electrocardiographic evidence of an old transmural infarction. In contrast, the annual mortality rate was 35% in those patients with two-vessel disease and a history of CHF. Patients with angina complicated by associated cardiovascular disease or by serious noncardiovascular diseases were excluded from the study. The annual mortality for all patients with one-vessel disease was 2.0%. The annual mortality for all patients with two-vessel disease was 13.0% and for three-vessel disease, 15.0%. The presence of an old MI, a history of CHF, or an enlarged heart markedly increased the annual mortality in patients with angina pectoris.[62] Oberman identified seven independent predictors of increased annual mortality in patients with angina pectoris: cardiomegaly; stenosis of the left anterior descending artery; dyspnea on effort with either paroxysmal nocturnal dyspnea or orthopnea; tachycardia; stenosis of the left main coronary artery; stenosis of the left circumflex artery; and stenosis of the right coronary artery.[62]

Reeves et al[61] combined the results of five studies of patients with angina pectoris. Each of the studies had been conducted prior to 1970. Average follow-up ranged from 15 to 84 months. There were a total of 265 patients with one-vessel disease, 220 with two-vessel disease, and 220 with three-vessel disease. Separate analyses for risk factors other than angina pectoris and the number of vessels diseased were not conducted. In this pooled group, the average annual mortality rate was 2.2% for patients with one-vessel disease, 6.8% for those with two-vessel disease, and 11.4% for those with three-vessel disease.[62]

Thus, angina pectoris taken by itself is a poor predictor of survival. Individuals with single-vessel disease and angina pectoris uncomplicated by a history of transmural MI, CHF, cardiomegaly, associated cardiovascular disease, or serious noncardiovascular disease appear to have an annual mortality rate of 1% to 2%. Support for this point of view came from a study conducted by Russek[63] in the late 1960s. He identified a "good risk" group of patients with severe and refractory angina pectoris. All were placed on maximal medical management and followed. The probability of death over a period of 5 years was 6% or 1.2% per year.[63] The use of subsets in evaluating clinical outcomes in patients with angina pectoris was to assume even greater importance as aortocoronary bypass grafting and the analysis of its results became commonplace.

Randomized Studies

Since 1972, five large randomized studies have compared the results of CABG, plus medical therapy with medical therapy of angina pectoris. Stable angina pectoris was the subject of three studies; unstable angina was the subject of two studies. While various criticisms can be made of the design and conduct of the studies, the conclusions drawn from them have shaped the practice of CABG around the world. The effect of age on outcome was evaluated in these studies but patients over 65 years of age were either excluded from entry or were present in small numbers. Even so, the results of the randomized studies became guidelines for the performance of CABG in the elderly.

Early Veterans Administration Studies

In the mid 1960s, cardiologists and thoracic surgeons in the Veterans Administration (VA) became interested in evaluating current surgical procedures to revascularize the ischemic heart. Before CABGs were being widely performed, two operations were studied employing randomization techniques: the Beck "poudrage" procedure and the Vineberg implant procedure. Analyses of the Beck procedures did not reach the literature. A total of 146 patients (75 medical and 71 surgical) were entered into the internal mammary implant study between 1966 and 1972. Thirty-day operative mortality was 12.3%. Visualization of the implant 1 year after operation was accomplished in half of the eligible patients. There was a 50% patency rate in the single implant group and 69% in the double implant group. At 12 years, 41% of the medical group and 42% of the surgical group were alive. Eighty-one percent of the deaths in both the medical and surgical groups were due to cardiac disease. The study ended partly because of these findings and partly because of the shift to direct revascularization of the coronary arteries.[64]

Veterans Administration Stable Angina Study

Six hundred eighty-six patients were entered into the stable angina study between 1972 and 1974. Three hundred fifty-four individuals were randomized to medical therapy; 332 were randomized to medical plus surgical therapy. Ninety-one patients had greater than 50% stenosis of the left main coronary artery (43 medical, 48 surgical). Five hundred ninety-five patients were "non-left main" (311 medical and 284 surgical). All patients were men. The ages of those in the study ranged from 27 to 68 years, with a mean age of 50.5 years. Patients with all degrees of angina were accepted. No minimum for ejection fraction was set. During 11 years of follow-up, 38% of the 354 patients assigned to medical treatment underwent bypass surgery. Twenty-two of those crossing over had left main CAD.

At 11 years, survival for patients without significant left main disease was 58% in both treatment groups. Survival between treatment groups of patients with one-vessel or three-vessel disease was not significantly different at either 7 or 11 years. At 11 years, survival for patients with two-vessel disease treated surgically was marginally worse than for their counterparts treated medically (55% versus 69%, p = 0.045). Patients treated surgically for left main disease clearly did better than those treated medically (88% versus 65%, p = 0.016). Patients who were categorized as high risk by angiographic criteria, clinical criteria, or by a combination of both had significantly better survival with surgical treatment. Patients were classified as angiographically high risk if they had three-vessel disease and impaired left ventricular function. They were classified as clinically high risk if they had at least two of the following: resting ST depression, a history of MI, or a history of hypertension. Survival at 11 years in the high clinical risk group was 49% for the surgical group and 36% for the medical group (p = 0.015). In the low clinical risk group, survival at 11 years was 63% for the surgical group and 73% for the medical group (p = 0.066). In the angiographically high-risk group, survival at 11 years was 50% for surgical patients and 38% for medical patients (p = 0.026). In the angiographically low-risk group, the corresponding survival data were 61% and 68% (p = 0.105). In the combined angiographically and clinically high-risk group, survival at 11 years was 54% in the surgical group and 24% in the medical group (p = 0.005). Corresponding survivals in the combined angiographically and clinically low-risk group were 66% and 76% (p = 0.092). During the first 7 years of the study, the average annual mortality for all surgical patients without left main disease was 3.3%; for medical patients without left main disease annual mortality was 4.0%. During the next 4 years, the corresponding annual mortality rates were 4.8% and 3.5%. Thus, in terms of survival, three groups of patients benefited from surgical treatment: those with significant left main disease; those with extensive CAD associated with reduced ventricular function; and those who fell into clinically or angiographically high-risk categories.

Quality of life was better in those patients treated surgically. At 5 years, 41% of surgical patients and 17% of medical patients reported marked improvement in symptoms. Twenty percent of the surgical patients and 42% of the medical patients described worsening symptoms. Over the 5-year period, the benefits of surgery decreased, but even at 5 years were still significantly better (p = 0.0014). The incidence of nonfatal MI was not significantly different between the two treatment groups. At 5-year follow-up, left ventricular function remained unchanged in both treatment groups.[65-68]

Veterans Administration Unstable Angina Study

Four hundred sixty-eight patients were entered into the unstable angina study between 1976 and 1982 (237 medical, 231 medical plus surgical). Three hundred seventy-four patients were identified as type I (accelerated angina, rest angina, and recent onset angina); 94 were identified as type II (prolonged angina unrelieved by nitrates and accompanied by ST segment changes on electrocardiogram). All patients were men. The age range in the study was 32 to 73 years with a mean age of 56 years. Patients with all degrees of angina were accepted. Patients with ejection fractions below 30% and those with left main lesions greater than 50%, recent MI, or prior coronary artery surgery were excluded. At the end of 10 years, 50% of patients randomized to medical treatment had crossed over to surgery.

At 10 years, survival was 61% for surgical patients and 62% for medical patients. At 5 years and 8 years, there was significantly better survival for patients with three-vessel disease treated surgically (89% versus 77% and 77% versus 65%, respectively). At 10 years, however, the surgical advantage was no longer significant (63% versus 57%, p = 0.190). At 8 years, survival of patients with three-vessel disease and an ejection fraction of 58% or less was significantly better in the surgical group (79.5% versus 57.1%, p = 0.018). In contrast, survival at 8 years in those with one or two-vessel disease and an ejection fraction greater than 58% was significantly better with medical treatment (83.2% versus 67.8%, p = 0.022).

A major finding in this study was the effect of surgical treatment on survival of patients with an ejection fraction between 30% and 58% if crossovers from medicine to surgery are censored (counted as lost to follow-up at the time of crossover). When this was done, there was a strong advantage to surgical treatment throughout the 10 years of follow-up (59% versus 43%, p = 0.007).[69]

Continued smoking was an independent predictor of death in the surgical group at 2, 5, and 10 years. At 10 years, New York Heart Association (NYHA) Class III or IV, age, and diabetes mellitus were additional independent predictors of mortality in the surgical group. In the medically treated group, decreased ejection fraction and the number of vessels diseased were consistent, independent predictors of mortality.

As in the stable angina study, quality of life was better in the surgically treated group with superior pain control, reduced medication requirements, and significantly fewer new cardiovascular hospitalizations over the 10-year observation period (p = 0.0001). At the end of 10 years, the number of nonfatal MIs were not significantly different between the treatment groups.[70-72]

European Coronary Surgery Study Group

Seven hundred sixty-eight patients were entered into the study between 1973 and 1976 (373 medical, 395 surgical). One patient was lost to follow-up before operation leaving 394 surgical patients. All were men under the age of 65 years (mean age 50 years). Those with severe angina pectoris, as well as those with ejection fractions below 50% or single-vessel disease were excluded from the study. Patients with left main lesions of 50% or more were included on a discretionary basis (31 medical, 28 surgical). Patients assigned to medical treatment could cross over to the surgical group if they had unacceptable symptoms despite adequate medical therapy (24% did cross over within 5 years). All patients were followed for 5 years: 60% for 6 years; 25% for 7 years; and 10% for 8 years.

At 5 years, 92.4% of the surgical patients and 83.6% of the medical patients were alive (p = 0.00025). In those patients with left main disease, there was a markedly increased 5-year survival with operation, but because of the small numbers, the difference was not significant (81.7% versus 67.9%, p = 0.11). Survival was markedly improved in the surgical group with three-vessel disease and also in the group with two- or three-vessel disease when it was associated with stenosis of 50% or greater in the proximal left interior descending artery. An abnormal electrocardiogram, ST segment depression of 1.5 mm or more during exercise, and the presence of peripheral vascular disease, were each independent predictors of better survival with operation. Survival at 10 years in patients over the age of 53 was significantly better in the surgical group (72% versus 57%, p = 0.007). Below age 53 years, age was not a significant factor affecting outcome between the two treatment groups. A conclusion drawn from the study was that the greatest benefits of surgery occurred in the high-risk groups of patients. Surgery was unlikely to improve 5-year survivals in patients with good left ventricular function, ST segment depression less than 1.5 mm on exercise, a normal resting electrocardiogram, and absence of peripheral vascular disease. These conclusions closely resemble those reached in both the stable and unstable VA randomized studies.[73-76]

Operation markedly improved the quality of life as measured by the percentage of patients free of angina or by increased exercise tolerance. As in other studies, these effects diminished with time although the advantage over medical treatment remained statistically significant at 4 years for exercise performance (p = 0.001) and throughout the study for angina relief (p = 0.001).[74]

Coronary Artery Surgery Study

Randomized Study

In 1973 the National Heart, Lung and Blood Institute organized a patient registry and a randomized trial, the Coronary Artery Surgery Study (CASS), designed to compare results of medical and surgical therapy in patients with CAD. The goal of the randomized trial was to test the hypothesis that CABG significantly reduced the mortality rate and the incidence of MI in patients with mild angina, or in those who were asymptomatic after an MI (but who had CAD documented by angiography).[76,77]

Between 1975 and 1979, 780 patients were entered into the study (390 medical, 390 surgical). Ninety percent of the patients were men. All enrollees were 65 years of age or less; the mean age was 51.2 years. Patients with angina more severe than Canadian Class II were excluded as were those with unstable angina, progressive angina, CHF, previous CABG, or serious coexisting illness. Patients with an ejection fraction less than 35% and those with left main lesions greater than 70% were also excluded. Patients with a well-documented MI more than 3 weeks before randomization were accepted into the study. Analyses were performed on the basis of treatment assigned.[73,77]

At 8 years, 87% of the surgical patients and 84% of the medical patients were alive (p = 0.14). However, in the subset of patients with ejection fractions below 50%, 84% of the surgical patients and 70% of the medical patients were alive at 7 years (p = 0.012). When this subset of patients was analyzed by the number of vessels diseased, a significant difference in survival was found only in those patients with three-vessel disease (88% in the surgical group, 65% in the medical group, p = 0.0094). At 5 years, there was no significant difference between treatment groups in the occurrence of nonfatal MI. At 5 years, the crossover rate from medicine to surgery was 24%.[76]

At 5 years, the surgical group had significantly less chest pain (p < 0.0001), had fewer activity limitations (p < 0.0001), and required less beta blockade (p < 0.0001). In the surgical group, treadmill exercise tests documented less exercise-induced angina, less ST segment depression, and longer treadmill times.[78]

National Cooperative Study Group

Unstable Angina

Under the auspices of the National Heart, Lung and Blood Institute, a prospective, randomized study was initiated comparing intensive medical therapy with urgent CABG for the management of patients with unstable angina. Between 1972 and 1976, 288 patients were entered into the study (147 medical, 141 surgical). Eighty-two percent were men. All enrollees were under the age of 70 years. The patients had to have angina associated with transient ST segment or T wave changes on electrocardiogram. Ninety percent of the patients had rest pain while in the hospital. To be eligible, the patients had to have greater than 70% occlusion of at least one coronary artery. Seventy-six percent of the patients had multivessel CAD; 30% of individuals in the study had proximal left anterior descending arterial disease. Thus, the group corresponded to patients with type II symptoms in the VA unstable angina study. An ejection fraction of 30% or less and greater than 50% narrowing of the left main coronary artery were reasons for exclusion, as were an MI within 3 months, or serious illness other than CAD.

At 65 months, there was no significant difference in survival between surgical and medical patients (85% surgery versus 84% medical). Forty-three percent of patients crossed over from medicine to surgery (34% of NYHA Classes I and II, 60% of NYHA classes III and IV). Crossover occurred sooner in patients with more severe angina.[79]

At the end of the first year, severe angina was significantly more common in medically treated patients with one-vessel ($p < 0.05$), two-vessel ($p < 0.01$), and three-vessel ($p < 0.01$) disease. There was no significant difference in the incidence of nonfatal MI between the two treatment groups.[80]

Overview

While the general goal of all of the randomized trials summarized above was to compare the results of medical and surgical treatment of CAD, it is clear that the individual studies differed substantially in mortality data, study design, patient selection, and patient recruitment. It is nevertheless striking that there are a number of major conclusions for which there is substantial agreement among the studies:

1. Angina pectoris is, of itself, not an indication for surgery.
2. Surgery does not increase survival over that obtained by medical therapy for one- or two-vessel disease, unless the patients fall into a high-risk category.
3. Surgery has a clear advantage in the treatment of significant left main disease.
4. Surgery results in a significantly increased survival percentage in patients with three-vessel disease and abnormal left ventricular function.
5. Surgical treatment results in better survival in patients who are high risk by clinical or angiographic criteria, or a combination of both.
6. Quality of life is uniformly better in the group surgically treated. Exercise tolerance and freedom from angina are better in the surgical group. Requirements for medication and new hospitalizations for cardiovascular events are less in the surgical group.
7. In those groups that benefited from operation, the benefits, particularly as they concerned quality of life, tend to decrease

with time. Even so, the advantages of surgical treatment continue for 5 to 10 years.

It is of interest that a small randomized study of CABG, begun in 1971 by two of the editors,[81,82] reached many of the same conclusions as those reported from the much larger trials. This study found that: 1) overall survival in the medical and surgical groups was not significantly different; 2) the incidence of nonfatal MI was the same in both treatment groups; 3) there was no improvement in ejection fraction as a result of surgery; 4) freedom from angina was more frequent in the surgical group; 5) surgically treated patients required less medication than medically treated patients; 6) surgical patients had better exercise performance than did medically treated patients; and 7) the benefits of surgical treatment decreased with time. Because of the small size of the study, outcome in what might have been critical subgroups could not be determined.[81,82]

The primary issues addressed by the studies cited above were operative mortality and survival. Measurements of the quality of life were secondary endpoints. In some circumstances, however, quality of life is of more concern to the patient than is quantity of life.

Outcome of Coronary Arterial Surgery in the Older Patient

Whenever containment of costs or the issue of unnecessary surgery is raised in the scientific or lay literature, two topics will almost certainly be prominent parts of the presentation: the volume of cardiac surgery being performed in the United States, and the costs of providing medical care for the elderly. How then do we evaluate, in a factual manner, the benefits of CABGs in the elderly? Is such surgery justified? If so, on what basis? Comparative data that is so easily obtained for younger patients may not be applicable to older patients and can be difficult if not impossible to find.

It is important to understand at the outset that the goals of health care in the older patient are different than those in the young and middle-aged population. In the younger patient, the primary goal is to reduce the chance of dying from specific diseases. As Hippocrates observed almost 2,500 years ago, older patients frequently have multiple chronic diseases that are not curable and will result in death or disability, or both. Rather than cure, the goals of health care in these patients are independence, relief of symptoms, preservation of function, and the extension of useful and active life. Clearly, survival is a necessary consideration, but from the patient's point of view, quality of life may be more important.

In this scenario, the questions that surround cardiac surgery and coronary bypass in particular have high visibility. Do the conclusions reached in the randomized studies of younger patients apply to older groups of patients? Are the procedures technically feasible in the elderly, or is the CAD too extensive? Can the operation be performed with an acceptable mortality? What are the consequences of performing the operation electively or of waiting until it is urgent or emergent? How serious is the morbidity of the procedure in the short-term or the long-term? Does the patient live long enough to reap the benefits of the treatment? To what degree, and for how long, are the symptoms relieved? Are future adverse events prevented? Can alternative procedures be as effective as CABG? In short, do the improvements in the length of life and its quality justify the risks, discomforts, complications, and expense of CABG? There are no large, randomized studies available to compare the results of medical and surgical treatment of CAD in the elderly. However, there are data from several large nonrandomized studies that can provide many of the answers to the questions posed above.

Frequency of Inoperable Coronary Arterial Disease

In 1984, Hertzer et al reported a series of 1,000 coronary angiograms performed in patients with stable peripheral vascular disease.[12] Six hundred eighty-five of the patients were men; 315 were women. Three hundred ninety-nine were 60- to 69-years-old, 245 were 70- to 79-years-old, and 33 were over 80 years of age. The age range was 29 through 95 years, with a mean of 64 years. The patients were divided into five groups on the basis of angiographic findings: normal coronary arteries; mild to moderate CAD; advanced, but compensated CAD; severe, correctable CAD; and severe, inoperable CAD. Severe, inoperable CAD was defined as greater than 70% stenosis of multiple coronary arteries and the lack of adequate targets for grafts because of diffuse distal disease or generalized ventricular impairment. The patients were analyzed as a group and by whether or not CAD was suspected prior to angiography.

Severe, inoperable CAD was found in 5.8% of the entire group. It was more common in those who were suspected of having CAD on clinical grounds than in those who had no clinical indications of CAD (9.7% versus 0.9%). In the group as a whole, the prevalence of both severe, inoperable CAD and severe, correctable CAD increased with increasing age. The frequency of severe, correctable CAD among those suspected of having CAD, however, remained approximately the same across all age groups. The frequency of severe, correctable CAD was significantly greater in men than in women (29% versus 17%, p = 0.001), but there was little difference between the sexes in the frequency of severe, inoperable CAD (6.0% versus 5.4%)(Table 7). Severe, inoperable CAD was found in 15% of those who had angina, but only 7.2% of those who did not (p < 0.001).

While severe, inoperable CAD did increase with age in patients with suspected CAD, severe, correctable CAD occurred with about the same frequency in all age groups with suspected CAD. The presence of selected risk factors markedly increased the frequency of both severe, correctable and severe, inoperable disease (Tables 7 and 8).[12]

Table 7

Comparison of the Frequency of Severe, Correctable and Severe, Inoperable CAD Between Patients Suspected of Having CAD and Those Without Clinical Evidence of CAD (in percentages)

Age Group (number patients)	All Patients		Suspect CAD		No Clin CAD	
	Correct	Inop	Correct	Inop	Correct	Inop
Less than 50 years (71)	21	1	31	3	14	0
50 to 59 (252)	22	2	36	4	10	1
60 to 69 (399)	24	6	34	7	13	0
70 and over (278)	30	11	35	16	21	3
All Patients (1000)	25	6	34	10	14	1

CAD = coronary arterial disease; correct = severe, correctable coronary arterial disease; Inop = severe,inoperable coronary arterial disease.

Table 8

Correlation of Selected Risk Factors with Frequency of Severe, Correctable or Severe, Inoperable Coronary Disease
1000 Patients with Stable Peripheral Vascular Disease
Mean Age 64 Years

Risk Factor	Percentage Occurrence	
	Severe, Correctable CAD	Severe, Inoperable CAD
All 1000 patients	25	6.0
Presence of angina		
Yes	51	15.0
No	19	3.5
History of Infarct		
Yes	32	14.0
No	23	3.3
EKG Finding		
Normal	19	2.2
Myocard infarct	32	12.0
ST, T wave abnor	33	7.5
Hypertension	26	7.0
Diabetes Mellitus	22	12.0
Hyperten Plus Diab	24	11.0

Medicare Data

Peterson et al analyzed the outcomes of CABG in 24,161 Medicare patients 80 years of age or older who had been operated upon between 1987 and 1990. Patients with end stage renal disease, failed coronary angioplasty, or combined open-heart procedures were excluded from the original group of 202,488, as were those who had been operated upon in health maintenance organizations, non-US hospitals or federal hospitals. Eighty-three percent of the patients were 80- to 85-years-old, 13% were 86- to 90-years-old, and 1% was 90-years-old or older. Men constituted 57.4% of the group. Outcome data in this group were compared with similar data in 147,822 Medicare patients who had undergone CABG between the ages of 65 and 70 years. Octogenarians were significantly more likely than those in the younger group to be women, to have been admitted for an acute MI before bypass, to have CHF, or to have cerebrovascular disease. The octogenarians were less likely to have pulmonary disease or diabetes mellitus. The rate of CABGs performed in octogenarians is rising. In the 65- to 70-year-old group, it rose from 38.1 per 10,000 in 1987 to 42.1 per 10,000 in 1990. Corresponding figures for the octogenarians are 7.2 and 12.0.

Independent predictors of increased 30-day mortality in the octogenarians were increasing age, female gender, and evidence of impaired MI (acute MI or CHF before bypass). The presence of comorbid conditions (cerebrovascular disease, peripheral arterial disease, or chronic renal disease) also predicted a higher 30-day mortality. Independent predictors of mortality at 3 years included all of the 30-day predictors, plus diabetes mellitus and pulmonary disease.[83]

The effects of increasing age, female gender, and the presence of myocardial impairment were reported by Peterson et al in another article in which he reviewed outcomes following CABG in 357,885 Medicare patients over the age of 65.

In the 65- to 69-year-old group, 30-day mortality was 4.3% while mortality at 1 year was 8.0%. Corresponding figures for the 70- to 74-year-old group were 5.7% and 10.9%, for the 75- to 79-year-old cohort, 7.4% and 14.2%, and for those aged 80 or more, 10.6% and 19.5%. In spite of the higher mortalities in the octogenarians, however, their survival at 3 years was essentially the same as that of octogenarians in the general population in the United States (71.2% versus 73.4%).[83,84]

In the 65-year-old and older group, women suffered a higher 30-day mortality than men (7.3% versus 5.1%). Survival at 1-year post-CABG was essentially the same for women and men (87.6% versus 89.7%).[84]

Thirty-day mortality was higher for those who underwent CABGs during an admission for acute MI than it was for those who had not been admitted for an acute MI, but underwent CABG (9.6% versus 5.2%). Survival of the MI group at 1 year was poorer than that of the CABG only groups (84.7% versus 89.7%).[84]

Peterson's study also compared charges and costs for bypass surgery in the 65- to 70-year-old group with those in the 80-year-old and older group. Mean costs for the younger group were $21,700, with a range of $14,000 to $23,000. Mean costs for the octogenarians were $27,000, with a range of $17,000 to $30,000. Costs were standardized to 1990 dollars. Median values for hospital stay, charges, and costs were 38%, 22%, and 21% higher in octogenarians than in those 65-to 70-years-old.[83]

It is clear from this study that elderly patients can undergo coronary arterial revascularization with an increased, but still relatively low operative mortality, with the result that their survival at 3 years closely approximates that of the general population of the United States in the same age ranges. Evaluation of cardiac risk factors and comorbid disease is essential. Delay in operation until the patient has a complication of CAD, specifically an acute MI, has a markedly adverse effect on outcome in both the short-term and the long-term.

Coronary Artery Surgery Study

Registry Data

In 1985, Gersh et al reported on a series of 1491 nonrandomized patients 65 years of age or older. There were 630 patients in the medical treatment group and 861 in the surgical treatment group. One thousand eighty-four were 65- to 69-years-old, 329 were 70- to 74-years-old, and 78 were 75-years-old or older. The patients ranged in age from 65 to 82 years. Four hundred thirty-four in the medical group were men; 635 in the surgical group were men. The group treated medically included more women, more patients with left ventricular dysfunction, and more patients with associated medical diseases. Surgically treated patients had a higher incidence of severe angina and more frequent three-vessel disease. There were no significant differences between the treatment groups in terms of age distribution or other major risk factors. In an effort to compensate for the nonrandomized nature of the data, the series was analyzed by establishing a "lower risk" subset of medical and surgical patients and, in addition, dividing the entire group into quartiles based on a prognostic index. The lower risk subset was defined by excluding patients with moderate or marked functional impairment of the left ventricle, as well as those with acute coronary insufficiency and those with critical left main stenosis. The quartiles were based on the sum of weighted risk factors identified as independent predictors of survival.

Cumulative 6-year survivals of the two treatment groups without risk adjustment for prognostic factors were 80% in the surgical group and 63% in the medical group (p < 0.0001). Survival following surgical treatment was significantly better in all age groups until age 75 years. Even in patients 75-years-old or older, the 6-year survival in the surgical group was better than in the medical group, but the difference did not reach significance because of the small number of patients (75% versus 56%, p < 0.14). When survival curves were adjusted for major prognostic variables, the surgical advantage persisted (79% versus 64%, p < 0.0001). Survival at 6 years was also a function of the number of vessels diseased, the functional status of the left ventricle, and the risk quartile into which the patients fell. Patients with two-vessel disease, three-vessel disease, and those in the higher risk category fared better in terms of survival with operation. Those who fell in the lower risk subset (125 medical, 109 surgical) had essentially equal survivals between treatment groups (83% surgical versus 82% medical, p = 0.9650). In the lower risk subset, the number of vessels diseased were not factors in survival between the two treatment groups. Survival in patients with normal left ventricular wall motion (NLVWM) was not significantly different between treatment groups. In the highest risk quartile, survival at 6 years was 62% in the surgical group and 33% in the medical group (p < 0.0001) (Table 9).[85]

While survival at 6 years in either treatment group was good to excellent considering the age of the patients, it is illuminating to review the causes of death in the 293 patients who died during the study. Noncardiac causes were responsible for death in 45% of the surgical patients, but only 13% of the medical patients (p < 0.0001). Clearly, coronary revascularization cannot protect against death from associated diseases, but it did protect the patients treated surgically against death from cardiac causes.[85]

Table 9
Comparison of Survivals Following Coronary Arterial Bypass Surgery and Medical Therapy in Patients 65-Years-Old or Older
1,491 Nonrandomized Patients from CASS Registry

Category or Manifestation	Percentage Survival at 6 Years		P Values
	Surgery	Medicine	
Entire series	80	63	<0.001
Series adj for risk	79	64	<0.0001
65 to 69 year olds	81	67	<0.0001
70 to 74	77	51	<0.0001
75 years old and older	75	56	<0.14
One vessel disease	82	81	<0.64
Two vessel disease	89	70	<0.0002
Three vessel disease	75	47	<0.0001
Norm left ventr motion	87	83	<0.13
"Lower risk" category	83	82	0.9650
Risk quartile one	92	84	0.0203
Risk quartile two	86	81	0.4845
Risk quartile three	76	66	0.0322
Risk quartile four (highest risk)	62	33	<0.0001

In terms of quality of life, at 1 year, 71% of the surgical patients were free of chest pain in contrast to 25% of medical patients. At 5 years, 62% of the surgical patients and 29% of the medical patients were free of chest pain (p < 0.00001).[85]

In summary, Gersh's study demonstrated that 65-year-old or older patients in the high-risk categories and those with two- or three-vessel disease, but not in the "lower risk" group, benefited from surgical treatment with 6-year survivals ranging from 62% to 92%. In addition, patients treated surgically received substantial protection from death due to cardiac causes. Sixty-two percent of patients undergoing CABG were free of chest pain at 5 years. Six-year medical survival in this group of patients ranged from 33% to 84%.

Risks Versus Benefits

Oliver Wendall Holmes Jr., justice of the United States Supreme Court until he was 91 years old, commented in 1900 that, "Life is an end in itself, and the only question is whether there is enough of it."[86] His statement describes succinctly the concerns of this section.

Risks

It is clear that the elderly are exposed to greater risks of both death and complications following CABG than are their younger counterparts. Although increasing age is an independent predictor of death in both the short-term and the long-term following CABG, it is uncommon for age to be the only risk factor present in the elderly. Older patients who undergo CABG have more extensive CAD, are more likely to have left main CAD, have more severe symptomatology, and are more likely to have had CHF. They are more likely to have major noncardiac associated diseases at the time of operation. When the elderly undergo operation, the procedure is more likely to be performed urgently or emergently.

In large studies of patients undergoing CABG, three-vessel disease was present in 50% to 90% of those over the age of 70 and in 30% to 70% of those younger than 60-years-old. Significant left main disease was present two to three times more often in those over the age of 70, than in those less than 50 years of age. Almost 85% of preoperative patients over the age of 80 were in NYHA Classes III or IV, in contrast to 60% of those less than 60-years-old. Two thirds of those over the age of 70 had unstable angina prior to operation, in contrast to less than half of those under the age of 70. Moderate to severe impairment of left ventricular function was found almost twice as often in those over age 70, than in those under age 70 years. A history of CHF was present in 10% of those over the age of 80, but in less than 3% of those younger than 50 years of age. Coronary arterial revascularization was performed as an emergency procedure in over 20% of patients over the age of 80, but in only 10% of patients less than 80-years-old.[87-89]

Patients over the age of 50 were more likely to be hypertensive, than those less than 50-years-old. The prevalence of diabetes mellitus increased steadily until the eighth decade, then decreased. Coexistent peripheral vascular disease and cerebrovascular disease were two to three times more common in those over the age of 70 than in those under the age of 70. Interestingly, pulmonary disease was less frequent above the age of 80, than it was in those in the 65- to 70-year age group.[83,87,90]

Operative mortality following CABG in the elderly has varied widely, largely as a result of differences in baseline characteristics of the study population, and differences in the prevalence of associated diseases. Of special note is the effect on operative mortality of performing urgent or emergent procedures in the elderly. In Weintraub et al's study[87] of 13,625 patients, CABGs were performed as emergencies in 9% of those between the ages of 50 and 70, in 10.4% of those 70- to 79-years-old, and in 23.3% of those over the age of 80. Hospital mortality in the three groups was 5.0%, 11.4%, and 8.8%, respectively.[87] Kaul et al reported a 2.2% hospital mortality in octogenarians undergoing elective CABG, 5.94% in those undergoing urgent operation, and 28.6% in those undergoing emergency operation.[91] Peterson et al, in a study of 357,885 Medicare patients undergoing CABG, found a 4.3% 30-day mortality for patients 65- to 69-years-old, 5.7% for patients aged 70 to 74 years, 7.4% for those aged 75 to 79 years, and 10.6% for those 80 years old or older.[84] Kennedy et al[92] reported that hospital mortality increased steadily with increasing age following revascularization within 30 days of an acute MI. For those less than 60 years of age, mortality was 2.5%; for those 60- to 69-years-old, it was 4.8%; for those aged 70 to 79 years, operative mortality was 13.2%; and in those 80-years-old or older, the mortality was 20.0%.[92]

Peterson et al[83] measured the relative effect of selected baseline characteristics on 30-day operative mortality following CABG in 24,461 octogenarians. The factors measured and their respective odds ratios were as follows:

Age	1.37	Cerebrovascular disease	2.22
Female gender	1.19	Peripheral vascular disease	1.42
Nonwhite race	1.02	Acute myocardial infarction	1.73
Pulmonary disease	0.96	Congestive heart failure	1.77
Diabetes mellitus	0.93	Chronic renal disease	2.42

They noted that it was not always possible to determine whether the condition occurred preoperatively or postoperatively. They also cautioned that because of limitations in the coding of diagnoses, the effect of some factors could have been overestimated.[83]

Evaluation of the risks of CABG in the elderly should not overlook the risks of cardiac catheterization. Ko et al reported a 6.2% mortality following cardiac catheterization in the elderly, compared with a rate of 1% or less in the general population.[93]

Elderly patients also suffer more complications after CABG. Overall major and minor morbidity following CABG is approximately 55% in octogenarians, 28% in those 70- to 79-years-old, and 16% in those less than 70-years-old.[91] The incidence of major complications in patients 70-years-old or older is approximately 20%.[90] Approximately 45% of octogenarians develop arrhythmias, primarily atrial fibrillation and bradycardia, following coronary arterial revascularization. Respiratory problems, primarily pneumonias, develop in about 20% of patients. Nonfatal wound infections occur in approximately 1% of those less than 50 years old and 4% of those 80-years-old or older. Nonfatal neurological events, primarily strokes, occur in less than 1% of those under 60 years of age, and in 2% to 3% of those over the age of 70. Acute renal failure is about three times more frequent in patients over the age of 70. Perioperative MI occurs in about 2% of patients undergoing CABG, but are not significantly more frequent in the older patients.[87,88,90,91,94]

Benefits

Because survival is clearly the most certain criterion by which the effectiveness of different modalities of treatment can be evaluated, it is invariably employed in the evaluation of surgical procedures sometimes to the exclusion of other measurements. Establishing the proper role for CABG in the elderly, however, requires that other outcomes be assessed in as measureable a form as possible. Of major importance are factors such as the degree of relief from angina, the frequency of return of angina, the prevention of further myocardial injury, the frequency with which reintervention is necessary, and the effect of noncardiac causes of death on survival. Less easily quantified, but also important, are additional quality of life measurements such as ability to perform activities of daily living, degree of independence, functional status, employability, and patient perception of health.

To place survival data following CABG in the elderly in perspective, it is helpful to consider the likelihood of survival of comparable segments of the general population in the United States over similar periods of time. The data that follow are from 1989: 5-year survival at age 60 years, 93% of individuals; at age 65, 90%; at age 70, 85%; at age 75, 78%. At age 80 years, 68% of individuals can expect to live another 5 years. For octogenarians specifically, 81% can expect to live another 3 years; 75%, 4 years; 68%, 5 years; and 60%, 6 years.

Tsai et al[95] reported that, in a group of 303 octogenarians undergoing CABG, 82% lived 1 year; 72%, 3 years; and 62%, 5 years. Corresponding values for the 70- to 79-year-old group were 90% at 1 year and 76% at 5 years.[95] Peterson et al, reviewing post-CABG survivals in 147,822 patients aged 65 to 70 years, found that 92.9% survived 1 year; 89.7%, 2 years; and 86.9%, 3 years. In a post-CABG group of 24,461 octogenarians, corresponding survivals were 80.8%, 76.3%, and 71.2%.[83] Acinapura et al reported that 94% of 3,142 CABG patients under the age of

70 years and 85% of 685 CABG patients over the age of 70 years survived 6 years.[88] Thus, survival of elderly patients following CABG closely approaches the survival of the general population of like age. The differences in survival are small and approximate the operative mortalities observed within the corresponding age groups.[83,93]

The obvious question is: what would the survivals have been without CABG? The natural history of CAD in the elderly is simply unknown. Neither are there randomized studies from which to draw conclusions. Nevertheless, the data that are available clearly suggest that the survival of elderly patients following CABG is better than that following other treatment modalities, particularly in a high-risk subset of elderly patients. Krumholz et al, describing a small, nonrandomized study of 93 octogenarians treated by CABG, PTCA, or medical management, following an acute MI, noted that 80% of the surgical patients, 70% of the PTCA patients, and 44% of the medical patients were alive at 46 months.[96] Ko et al reported that 77.4% of octogenarians treated surgically survived 3 years compared with 55.2% of patients treated medically.[93] Cumulative 6-year survivals of 1491 nonrandomized CASS patients aged 65 years or older were 80% in the surgical group and 63% in the medical group.[85]

What then about the quality of life following CABG in the elderly? Vogt et al,[97] reviewing 98 patients aged 70 years or older, compared outcomes between patients treated by either medical management, PTCA, or CABG. Six to 12 months following treatment, 80% of those treated surgically were free of angina, compared with 43% of those treated by PTCA, and 25% of those treated medically.[97] Hochberg et al reported that 91% of 67 CABG patients less than 70 years of age and 94% of 64 CABG patients 70 years of age or older were free of angina at 22 months. The same authors found a decrease in NYHA score from 3.0 to 1.3 in the CABG group younger than age 70, and from 3.3 to 1.4 in the CABG group older than 70 years.[98] Acinapura reported similar results.[88] Ko et al, comparing results in medically and surgically treated patients, found that at 26 months the surgical patients had improved from an average NYHA class of 3.4 at baseline to 1.2 while the medically treated patients had remained essentially unchanged (2.8 to 2.5).[93]

Krumholz et al, following a group of 93 octogenarians who had been treated by CABG, PTCA, or medical therapy, reported that at 1 year, none of the CABG patients had suffered a recurrent MI, while 6% of the PTCA patients and 28% of the medically treated patients had reinfarcted.[96]

In two series, one by Gersh et al, the other by Ko et al, cardiac events as a cause of late mortality in elderly patients were less common in patients treated surgically for CAD than in those treated medically.[85,93] Gersh et al found that late deaths (within 6 years) were due to cardiac causes in 87% of medical patients, but only 55% of surgically treated patients (p < 0.0001). Thus, CABG appears to not only extend elderly patients' lives, but protect them from cardiac deaths in the long-term.

Other measurements of the quality of life also give the advantage to surgical treatment of CAD in the elderly. In a group of patients 70-years-old or older, Vogt found that at 6 to 12 months, shortness of breath was relieved in 66% of those treated by CABG, but in only 10% of those treated by PTCA. The frequency with which shortness of breath was reported by medical patients post-treatment actually increased (p = 0.001). Patients managed by CABG scored significantly better than their PTCA or medically managed counterparts in basic and intermediate activities of daily living, as measured by Jette et al's Functional Status Questionnaire (p = 0.030, p = 0.026).[99] The surgical patients, in contrast to the PTCA and medically managed groups, reported better improvement in their general well-being, as well as in their satisfaction with their health (79.2%, 55.2%, 44.2%, p = 0.022).[97] In Krumholz et al's series[96] of 93 octogenarians, patients who had undergone CABG or PTCA were more likely to be able to care for themselves and live independently, than those who had been managed medically (89%, 89%, 52%). Similarly, those who had undergone revascularization procedures (either CABG or PTCA) were more likely to consider the quality of their lives to be good or excellent (89%, 86%, 44%).[96] Unlike survival statistics, long-term data on the quality of life in elderly patients are difficult to find. Thus, the question of the durability of these results remains unanswered. In the final chapter of this text, Tresch addresses in some detail the subject of quality of life following CABG, as well as other forms of vascular therapy.

Summary and Comment

Despite the lack of controlled, randomized studies, it is still possible to draw valid conclusions about the use of CABG in the elderly. First, the long-term survival of older patients following CABG approximates that of the general population of comparable age. Second, following CABG, the elderly experience excellent relief of symptoms. Third, their quality of life is significantly enhanced, particularly when it is compared to that following medical management. Fourth, in general, the indications for CABG in the elderly are the same as those developed from the randomized studies of younger patients.

In almost every series, operative and in-hospital mortality for CABG is higher for patients over the age of 70. For octogenarians, in-hospital mortalities of 8% to 10% are commonly cited. On the other hand, several authors report mortalities in the range of 2% to 3% for elective procedures performed in 70- and 80-year-old patients.[89,91,93] It is clearly evident that urgent or emergent operation in these patients is associated with a substantial increase in operative mortality. It is also apparent that there is a general reluctance to operate on elderly patients, particularly those over the age of 80, until they develop an urgent or emergent problem (Weintraub reported that 23.3% of 146 patients over the age of 80 were operated upon as emergencies). The result, of course, is a higher overall operative mortality than would have been the case if a more aggressive approach had been taken in the treatment of the elderly patient. Jones,[100] in an article entitled "In search of the optimal surgical mortality," cited data on 5,809 patients from the Duke Cardiovascular Databank. He pointed out that while less severe CAD was associated with a lower operative mortality, it was also associated with a lower absolute benefit from operation. Conversely, although increasing severity of CAD was associated with increasing operative mortality, it was associated with increased absolute benefits from operation. He concluded that within the limits of the data, there was no level at which the cardiac disease was so severe that the magnitude of operative risk canceled all potential benefits of operation. Similar conclusions were reached in the VA Unstable Angina Study, when patients with low ejection fractions were randomized to medical or surgical treatment.[69-72,100]

The increased life expectancy of older patients undergoing CABG is not insignificant. A 60-year-old individual in the United States has a life expectancy of 21.1 years; at age 70, life expectancy is 14.2 years; and at age 80, life expectancy is 8.5 years.[101] From the information given in this chapter and in the final chapter of this text, it is clear that these extra years are active and of good quality, at least from the perspective of the patient.

From the data that have been presented, the indications outlined by Aronow for performance of CABG in the elderly seem appropriate.[102] They are:

1. Significant left main CAD.
2. Significant three-vessel disease, especially in the presence of a decreased left ventricular ejection fraction and ischemia.
3. Significant two-vessel disease, decreased left ventricular ejection fraction, and proximal left anterior descending CAD.
4. Clinical evidence of CHF during ischemic episodes with ischemic, but viable myocardium.
5. Unacceptable symptoms, despite optimal medical management.

In addition, the increased frequency and significance of silent myocardial ischemic disease in the elderly needs to be recognized and considered in the identification of patients who would benefit from coronary revascularization.

References

1. Healthy People 2000: *National Health Promotion and Disease Prevention Objectives.* Washington, DC. US Government Printing Office; 391-413, 1991.
2. US Bureau of the Census: *Statistical Abstract of the United States.* 113th Ed. Washington, DC: US Government Printing Office; Table 206, 135, 1993.
3. Community approach to ECC: prevention and the chain of survival. In: Cummins RO (ed). *Advanced Cardiac Life Support.* Dallas: Scientific Publishing, American Heart Association; (16)1, 1994.
4. White NK, Edwards JE, Dry TJ: The relationship of the degree of coronary atherosclerosis with age. *Circulation* 1:645-654, 1950.

5. Ackerman RF, Dry TJ, Edwards JE: Relationship of various factors to the degree of coronary atherosclerosis in women. *Circulation* 1:1345-1354, 1950.
6. Fleg JL, Gerstenblith G, Lakatta EG: Pathophysiology of the aging heart and circulation. In: Messerli FH (ed). *Cardiovascular Disease in the Elderly.* Boston: Martinus Nijhoff; 11-34, 1984.
7. Enos WF, Holmes RH, Beyer J: Coronary disease among United States soldiers killed in action in Korea: preliminary report. *JAMA* 152:1090-1094, 1953.
8. McNamara JJ, Molot MA, Stremple JF, et al: Coronary artery disease in combat casualties in Vietnam. *JAMA* 216:1185-1188, 1971.
9. Harris R: Aging and the cardiovascular system. In: Harris R (ed). *The Management of Geriatric Cardiovascular Disease.* Philadelphia: JB Lippincott, Co.; 3-16, 1970.
10. Froelicher VF, Yanowitz FG, Thompson AJ Jr, et al: The correlation of coronary angiography and the electrocardiographic response to maximal treadmill testing in 76 asymptomatic men. *Circulation* 48:597-604, 1973.
11. Gerstenblith G, Fleg JL, Vantosh A, et al: Stress testing redefines the prevalence of coronary artery disease in epidemiologic studies (abstr). *Circulation* 62:III-308, 1980.
12. Hertzer NR, Beven EG, Young JR, et al: Coronary artery disease in peripheral vascular patients: a classification of 1000 coronary angiograms and results of surgical management. *Ann Surg* 199:223-233, 1984.
13. Gould KL: Physiology of coronary circulation. In: Gould KL (ed). *Coronary Artery Stenosis.* New York: Elsevier Science Publishing, Co., Inc.; 1, 1991.
14. US Bureau of the Census: *Statistical Abstract of the United States.* 113th Ed. Washington, DC: US Government Printing Office; Table 126, 91, 1993.
15. Kannel WB, Thomas HE Jr: Sudden coronary death: The Framingham Study. In: Greenberg HM, Dwyer EM Jr (eds). *Sudden Coronary Death.* New York: The New York Academy of Sciences; 3-21, 1982.
16. US Bureau of the Census: *Statistical Abstract of the United States.* 113th Ed. Washington, DC: US Government Printing Office; Table 132, 96, 1993.
17. Goldstein S: *Sudden Death and Coronary Heart Disease.* Mt. Kisco, NY: Futura Publishing Co., Inc.; 1-22, 1974.
18. Gordon T, Kannel WB: Premature mortality from coronary heart disease: The Framingham Study. *JAMA* 215:1617-1625, 1971.
19. Davies MJ, Robertson WB: Diseases of the coronary arteries. In: Pomerance A, Davies MJ (eds). *The Pathology of the Heart.* Oxford, England: Blackwell Scientific Publications; 106, 1975.
20. Lew WYW, LeWinter MM: Acute myocardial infarction: pathophysiology. In: Chatterjee K, Karliner J, Rapaport E, et al (eds). *Cardiology: An Illustrated Text/ Reference. Vol. 2. Cardiovascular Disease.* New York: Gower Medical Publishing; 7.112-7.133, 1991.
21. Hudson REB: Necropsy studies. In: Hudson REB (ed). *Cardiovascular Pathology.* Vol. 3. London, England: Edward Arnold, Ltd.; S.405-S.408, 1970.
22. Kannel WB: An overview of the risk factors for cardiovascular disease. In: Kaplan NM, Stamler J (eds). *Prevention of Coronary Heart Disease: Practical Management of the Risk Factors.* Philadelphia: WB Saunders, Co.; 1-19, 1983.
23. Parmley WW: Silent ischemia. In: Chatterjee K, Karliner J, Rapaport E, et al (eds). *Cardiology: An Illustrated Text/Reference. Vol. 2. Cardiovascular Disease.* New York: Gower Medical Publishing; 7.91-7.99, 1991.
24. Droste C: Silent myocardial ischemia. *Am Heart J* 118:1087-1092, 1989.
25. US Bureau of the Census: *Statistical Abstract of the United States.* 113th Ed. Washington, DC: Government Printing Office; Table 125, 90, 1993.
26. Hudson REB: Coronary artery disease in the elderly. In: Hudson REB (ed). *Cardiovascular Pathology.* Vol 3. London, England: Edward Arnold, Ltd.; S.415, 1970.

27. Hudson REB: Coronary arteriography. In: Hudson REB (ed). *Cardiovascular Pathology.* Vol. 3. London, England: Edward Arnold, Ltd.; S.402-S.405, 1970.
28. Aronow WS, Mercando AD, Epstein S: Prevalence of silent myocardial ischemia detected by 24-hour ambulatory electrocardiography, and its association with new coronary events at 40-month follow-up in elderly diabetic and nondiabetic patients with coronary artery disease. *Am J Cardiol* 69:555-556, 1992.
29. Weiner DA, Ryan TJ, McCabe CH, et al: The role of exercise-induced silent myocardial ischemia in patients with abnormal left ventricular function: a report from the Coronary Artery Surgery Study (CASS) registry. *Am Heart J* 118:649-654, 1989.
30. Heberden W: Some account of a disorder of the breast. *Medical Transcripts of the Royal College of Physicians* 2:58, 1772.
31. Roth N: William Heberden (1710-1801). *Medtronic News* 15(2):27-29, 1985.
32. White PD: Coronary heart disease, angina pectoris, coronary thrombosis, and myocardial infarction. In: White PD (ed). *Heart Disease.* 4th Ed. New York: The Macmillan Co.; 517-577, 1951.
33. White PD: The evolution of our knowledge of the heart and its diseases. In: White PD (ed). *Heart Disease.* 4th Ed. New York: The Macmillan Co.; 1-24, 1951.
34. Kittle CF: John Hunter, 1728-1793, the architect of modern surgery. *Bull Am Coll Surg* 61(1):7-11, 1976.
35. Bloch H: John Hunter, Esq, FRCS (1728-1793). *Am J Surg* 151:640-642, 1986.
36. Schmidt JE: *Medical Discoveries.* Springfield, IL: Charles C. Thomas; 126-128, 1959.
37. Hudson REB: Ischemic heart disease and myocardial infarction. In: Hudson REB (ed). *Cardiovascular Pathology.* Vol. 3. London, England: Edward Arnold, Ltd.; S.410-S.415, 1970.
38. Davies MJ, Robertson WB: Diseases of the coronary arteries. In: Pomerance A, Davies MJ (eds). *The Pathology of the Heart.* London, England: Blackwell Scientific Publications; 89, 1975.
39. Herrick JB: Clinical features of sudden obstruction of the coronary arteries. *JAMA* 59:2015-2018, 1912.
40. Herrick JB, Nuzum FR: Angina pectoris: clinical experience with 200 cases. *JAMA* 70:67-70, 1918.
41. Forssmann W: Die sondierung des rechten Hertzens. *Klin Wchnschr* 8:2085-2087, 1929.
42. Hall RJ: Myocardial revascularization: historical considerations. *Tex Heart Inst J* 21(4):280-287, 1994.
43. Cournand A, Ranges HA: Catheterization of the right auricle in man. *Proc Soc Exp Biol Med* 46:462-466, 1941.
44. Sones FM JR, Shirey EK, Proudfit WL, et al: Cine-coronary arteriography (abstr). *Circulation* 20:773-774, 1959.
45. Franck F: Signification physiologique de la resection du sympathique dans la maladie de Basedow, l'epillepsie, l'idiotie et le glaucome. *Bull de l'Acad de Med* 41:594, 1899.
46. Jonnesco T: Traiment chirurgical de l'angine de poitrine par la resection du sympathique cervico-thoracique. *Bull de l'Acad de Med* 84:93, 1920.
47. Lindskog GE, Liebow AA, Glenn WWL: Coronary heart disease. In: Lindskog GE, Liebow AA, Glenn WWL (eds). *Thoracic and Cardiovascular Surgery with Related Pathology.* New York: Appelton-Century Crofts; 871-879, 1962.
48. Urschel HC Jr, Razzuk MA: Surgery for coronary artery disease. In: Norman JC (ed). *Cardiac Surgery.* 2nd Ed. New York: Appelton-Century Croft; 447-472, 1972.

49. Cutler EC: The surgery of the heart and pericardium. In: Walters W (ed). *Lewis' Practice of Surgery.* Hagerstown, MD: WF Prior, Co., Inc.; 46-59, 1948.
50. Beck CS: The development of a new blood supply to the heart by operation. *Ann Surg* 102:801, 1935.
51. Beck CS, Leighninger DS: Coronary heart disease treated by operation. *Arch Surg* 85:383-389, 1962.
52. Vineberg AM: Development of anastomosis between coronary vessels and transplanted internal mammary artery. *Can Med Assoc J* 55:117, 1946.
53. Portrait: Rene Favaloro: Pan-American pioneer of bypass. *Cardiology* 2(5)46-47, 1985.
54. Johnson WB, Flemma RJ, Lepley D Jr, et al: Extended treatment of severe coronary artery disease: a total surgical approach. *Ann Surg* 170:460-468, 1969.
55. Urschel HC Jr, Miller ER, Razzuk MA, et al: Aorta-to-coronary artery vein bypass graft for coronary artery occlusive disease. *Ann Thorac Surg* 8:114-120, 1969.
56. Kerth WJ: Aorta-coronary bypass grafts. *J Thorac Cardiovasc Surg* 57:487, 1969.
57. Matthews FP: Medicine. In: Paradise J, Waxman ML, Shores L (eds). 1968 Yearbook. New York: *Crowell-Collier Educational Corp.;* 350-354, 1968.
58. White PD: The prognosis of angina pectoris and of coronary thrombosis. *JAMA* 87:1525-1530, 1926.
59. White PD, Bland EF: A further report on the prognosis of angina pectoris and of coronary thrombosis: a study of five hundred cases of the former condition and of 200 cases of the latter. *Am Heart J* 7:1-14, 1931.
60. White PD, Bland EF, Miskall EW: The prognosis of angina pectoris: a longtime follow-up of 497 cases, including a note on 75 additional cases of angina pectoris decubitus. *JAMA* 123:801-804, 1943.
61. Reeves TJ, Oberman A, Jones WB, et al: Natural history of angina pectoris. *Am J Cardiol* 33:423-430, 1974.
62. Oberman A, Jones WB, Riley CP, et al: Natural history of coronary artery disease. *Bull NY Acad Med* 48:1109-1125, 1972.
63. Russek HI: "Natural" history of severe angina pectoris with intensive medical therapy alone. In: Norman JC, Lawrence EP (eds). *Coronary Artery Medicine and Surgery: Concepts and Controversies.* New York: Appelton-Century Crofts; 23-31, 1975.
64. Bhayana JN, Gage AA, Takaaro T: Long-term results of internal mammary artery implantation for coronary artery disease: a controlled trial. *Ann Thorac Surg* 29:234, 1980.
65. The Veterans Administration Coronary Artery Bypass Surgery Cooperative Study Group: Eleven-year survival in the Veterans Administration randomized trial of coronary bypass surgery for stable angina. *N Engl J Med* 311:1333-1339, 1984.
66. Takaro T, Pifarre R, Fish R: Left main coronary artery disease. In: Hultgren H (ed). Veterans Administration Cooperative Study of Medical Versus Surgical Treatment for Stable Angina: Progress Report. *Prog Cardiovasc Dis* 28(3):229-234, 1985.
67. Detre K, Peduzzi P, Scott SM, et al: Long-term survival results in medically and surgically randomized patients. In: Hultgren H (ed). Veterans Administration Cooperative Study of Medical Versus Surgical Treatment for Stable Angina: Progress Report. *Prog Cardiovasc Dis* 28(3):235-243, 1985.
68. Hultgren H, Takaro T, Kroncke G, et al: Summary and clinical applications. In: Hultgren H (ed). Veterans Administration Cooperative Study of Medical Versus Surgical Treatment for Stable Angina: Progress Report. *Prog Cardiovasc Dis* 28(5):397-401, 1986.
69. Scott SM, Deupree RH, Sharma GVRK, et al: VA study of unstable angina: ten-year results show duration of surgical advantage for patients with impaired ejection fraction. *Circulation* 90(5):II-120-II-123, 1994.

70. Luchi RJ, Scott SM, Deupree RH, et al: Comparison of medical and surgical treatment for unstable angina pectoris: results of a Veterans Administration Cooperative Study. *N Engl J Med* 316:977, 1987.
71. Booth DC, Deupree RH, Hultgren HN, et al: Quality of life after bypass surgery for unstable agina: 5-year follow-up results of a Veterans Affairs Cooperative Study. *Circulation* 83:87-95, 1991.
72. Scott SM, Luchi RJ, Deupree RH: VA Cooperative Study comparing medical and surgical therapy for unstable angina. In: Morrison DA, Serruys P (eds). *Medically Refractory Rest Angina*. New York: 121-143, 1992.
73. Takaro R, Bhayana J, Dean D: Historic perspective. In: Hultgren H (ed). Veterans Administration Cooperative Study of Medical Versus Surgical Treatment for Stable Angina: Progress Report. *Prog Cardiovasc Dis* 28(3):213-218, 1985.
74. European Coronary Surgery Study Group: Long-term results of prospective randomized study of coronary artery bypass surgery in stable angina pectoris. *Lancet ii:* 1173-1180, 1982.
75. Varnauskas E, The European Coronary Surgery Study Group: Twelve-year follow-up of survival in the randomized European coronary surgery study. *N Engl J Med* 319:332-337, 1988.
76. Karliner JS: Coronary artery bypass surgery. In: Chatterjee K, Karliner J, Rapaport E, et al (eds). *Cardiology: An Illustrated Text/Reference. Vol. 2. Cardiovascular Disease.* New York: Gower Medical Publishing; 7.249-7.261, 1991.
77. CASS Principal Investigators and Their Associates, Coronary Artery Surgery Study (CASS): A randomized trial of coronary artery bypass surgery: survival data. *Circulation* 68:939-950, 1983.
78. CASS Principal Investigators and Their Associates, Coronary artery surgery study (CASS): A randomized trial of coronary artery bypass surgery: quality of life in patients randomly assigned to treatment groups. *Circulation* 68:951-960, 1983.
79. Conti CR, Becker LC, Biddle TL, et al: Unstable angina: NHLBI cooperative study group to compare medical and surgical therapy: long-term morbidity and mortality (abstr). *Am J Cardiol* 49:1007, 1982.
80. Russell RO Jr, Moraski RE, Kouchoukos N, et al: Unstable angina pectoris: national cooperative study group to compare surgical and medical therapy. II. In-hospital experience and initial follow-up results in patients with one, two, and three vessel disease. *Am J Cardiol* 42:839-848, 1978.
81. Aronow WS, Stemmer EA: Bypass graft surgery versus medical therapy of angina pectoris. *Am J Cardiol* 33:415-420, 1974.
82. Aronow WS, Stemmer EA: Two-year follow-up of angina pectoris: medical or surgical therapy. *Ann Intern Med* 82:208-212, 1975.
83. Peterson ED, Cowper PA, Jollis JG, et al: Outcomes of coronary artery bypass graft surgery in 24,461 patients aged 80 years or older. *Circulation* 92(suppl II):II-85-II-91, 1995.
84. Peterson ED, Jollis JG, Bebchuk JD, et al: Changes in mortality after myocardial revascularization in the elderly: the national medicare experience. *Ann Intern Med* 121:919-927, 1994.
85. Gersh BJ, Kronmal RA, Schaff HV, et al: Comparison of coronary artery bypass surgery and medical therapy in patients 65 years of age or older: a nonrandomized study from the Coronary Artery Surgery Study (CASS) registry. *N Engl J Med* 313:217-224, 1985.
86. Bartlett J: *Familiar Quotations.* Boston: Little, Brown and Co.; 644, 1980.
87. Weintraub WS, Craver JM, Cohen CL, et al: Influence of age on results of coronary artery surgery. *Circulation* 84(suppl III):III-226-III-235, 1991.
88. Acinapura AJ, Rose DM, Cunningham JN Jr, et al: Coronary artery bypass in septuagenarians: analysis of mortality and morbidity. *Circulation* 78(suppl I):1-179-I-184, 1988.

89. Curtis JJ, Walls JT, Boley TM, et al: Coronary revascularization in the elderly: determinants of operative mortality. *Ann Thorac Surg* 58:1069-1072, 1994.
90. Gehlot AS, Santamaria JD, White AL, et al: Current status of coronary artery bypass grafting in patients 70 years of age and older. *Aust N Z J Surg* 65:177-181, 1995.
91. Kaul TK, Fields BL, Wyatt DA, et al: Angioplasty versus coronary artery bypass in octogenarians. *Ann Thorac Surg* 58:1419-1426, 1994.
92. Kennedy JW, Ivey TD, Misbach G, et al: Coronary artery bypass graft surgery early after acute myocardial infarction. *Circulation* 79(suppl I):I-73-I-78, 1989.
93. Ko W, Gold JP, Lazzaro R, et al: Survival analysis of octogenarian patients with coronary artery disease managed by elective coronary bypass surgery versus conventional medical management. *Circulation* 86(suppl II):II-191-II-197, 1992.
94. He GW, Acuff TE, Ryan WH, et al: Risk factors for operative mortality in elderly patients undergoing internal mammary artery grafting. *Ann Thorac Surg* 57:1453-1461, 1994.
95. Tsai TP, Chaux A, Matloff JM, et al: Ten-year experience of cardiac surgery in patients aged 80 years and over. *Ann Thorac Surg* 58:445-451, 1994.
96. Krumholz HM, Forman DE, Kuntz RE, et al: Coronary revascularization after myocardial infarction in the very elderly: outcomes and long-term follow-up. *Ann Intern Med* 119:1084-1090, 1993.
97. Vogt AR, Funk M, Remetz M: Comparison of symptoms, functional ability, and health perception of elderly patients with coronary artery disease managed with three different treatment modalities. *Cardiovasc Nursing* 30:33-38, 1994.
98. Hochberg MS, Levine FH, Daggett WM: Isolated coronary artery bypass grafting in patients 70 years of age and older: early and late results. *J Thorac Cardiovasc Surg* 84:219-223, 1982.
99. Jette AM, Davies AR, Cleary PD, et al: The functional status questionnaire: reliability and validity when used in primary care. *J Gen Intern Med* 1(3):143-149, 1986.
100. Jones RH: Comment: in search of the optimal surgical mortality. *Circulation* 79(suppl I):I-132-I-136, 1989.
101. US Bureau of the Census: *Statistical Abstract of the United States.* 115th Ed. Washington, DC: US Government Printing Office; Table 116, 87, 1995.
102. Aronow WS: Appropriate use of coronary artery bypass graft surgery and percutaneous transluminal coronary angioplasty in older patients. *Clin Ger* 4(2):15-22, 1996.

Chapter 20

Occlusive Disease of the Aorta

Luis A. Sanchez, MD
William D. Suggs, MD
Frank J. Veith, MD

Introduction

Severe aortoiliac occlusive disease can manifest as incapacitating claudication or limb-threatening ischemia of the lower extremities. Male cigarette smokers under the age of 65 have been considered in the past as the group with the highest prevalence of the disease. Over the past 20 years, it has been noted that there are increasing numbers of women affected with occlusive disease of the aortoiliac segment.[1] In addition, with the graying of the population and the increased life expectancy of individuals, the number of elderly patients presenting with significant aortoiliac occlusive disease is continuously increasing and becoming a significant and growing percentage of the patients that require intervention for this disease.[2] Over the past 10 years, the average age of patients requiring aortoiliac reconstructions at our institution has increased from 63 to 68 years.

The options for the treatment of aortoiliac occlusive disease have evolved over the past 40 years, since the initial aortoiliac reconstructions were performed in the 1950s using an arterial prosthesis. Multiple options for arterial reconstructions have been developed to accommodate varied patient arterial anatomy and risks of intervention. Advances in catheter-based techniques, vascular imaging, and other noninvasive tests have paralleled the development of new surgical techniques and procedures. Further advances in the treatment of aortoiliac occlusive disease are based on the combination of percutaneous techniques and surgical skills used to develop and perform endoluminal bypasses.

Patient Assessment

The initial evaluation of elderly patients with aortoiliac occlusive disease is critical. Atherosclerotic disease of the aortoiliac segment is

From: Aronow WS, Stemmer EA, Wilson SE (eds). *Vascular Disease in the Elderly.* Armonk, NY: Futura Publishing Company, Inc., © 1997.

often asymptomatic in many elderly patients, secondary to their sedentary lifestyle. Few elderly patients present with lower extremity or buttock claudication. Instead, they more commonly present with limb-threatening lower extremity ischemia (rest pain, ischemic ulceration, or gangrene) secondary to multilevel arterial occlusive disease. The combined aortoiliac and infrainguinal arterial occlusive disease can be more difficult to assess and treat in this patient population. After a complete physical examination that includes a careful pulse examination, noninvasive studies are used to better evaluate the patients' arterial disease. The vascular laboratory may aid in the evaluation and selection of patients with single or multilevel revascularization.[3] If an intervention is indicated, further necessary invasive studies are performed to define the best intervention for each individual patient.

Ankle-Brachial Indices, Segmental Pressures, and Pulse Volume Recordings

The ankle-brachial index (ABI) is determined by dividing the ankle pressure on each lower limb by the higher of the two brachial pressures. Patients with normal circulation have ABIs from 1.0 to 1.2, those with claudication have ABIs from 0.40 to 0.95, and those with limb-threatening ischemia have ABIs from 0 to 0.5. A very important limitation of the measurement of lower extremity pressures occurs in patients with heavily calcified vessels, mostly diabetics and patients with end stage renal disease. In these patients, the ABIs are falsely elevated due to the higher pressure required to occlude calcified vessels and, in some cases, will not occlude with pressures higher than 300 mm Hg. Gradients of more than 20 mm Hg between measuring sites are diagnostic of occlusive disease in the intervening segment.

Pulse volume recordings (PVRs) are obtained using a calibrated airplethysmograph. A PVR waveform is generated for different levels of the lower extremity using standard blood pressure cuffs. The increase in pressure within the cuff resulting from the volume increase during systole is recorded as a pulse wave. The tracings are characterized as normal when there is a brisk rise during systole and a dicrotic notch, moderately abnormal when there is loss of the notch and a more prolonged downslope, and severely abnormal when there is a flattened wave. The absolute amplitudes are not comparable from patient to patient, but serial PVRs have been shown to be very reproducible making them very useful to follow the course of patients with severe peripheral vascular disease.[4] ABIs and PVRs cannot differentiate proximal femoral disease from iliac occlusive disease.

Duplex Scanning

Duplex scanning can be a useful noninvasive way to assess the aortoiliac system. A variety of studies have recently evaluated the ability of this technique to predict iliac artery stenoses. Kohler et al initially suggested that duplex scanning had excellent sensitivity (89%) and specificity (90%) when used to predict a 50% or more iliac stenosis.[5] Three subsequent studies by Langsfeld et al,[6] Moneta et al,[7] and Legemate et al[8] have corroborated these findings with sensitivities ranging from 81% to 89% and specificities ranging from 88% to 99%. These noninvasive evaluations may be useful to better evaluate the elderly prior to invasive procedures such as angiography.

Spiral CT Scanning and Magnetic Resonance Angiography

Conventional CT scanning has limited use in the evaluation of aortoiliac occlusive disease, but can be helpful to identify severely calcified arteries or lesions that may alter treatment plans. In addition, faster, new spiral CT scanners that have the capability of three-dimensional reconstructions may provide better images, but these studies are not routinely used for the evaluation of patients with aortoiliac occlusive disease.

Magnetic resonance angiography (MRA) is noninvasive, does not require contrast agents, and may allow for good arterial imaging. Studies by Owens et al[9] and Carpenter et al[10] have shown that MRA may be more sensitive than arteriography when imaging distal lower extremity runoff vessels. Carpenter[11] also reported that MRA had a 100% positive predicted value and a 98.6% negative predicted value when compared to contrast angiography in the evaluation of patients with aortoiliac occlusive disease. These findings have not been widely reproduced, but this noninvasive modality has the potential to replace contrast arteriography in the evaluation of these patients. Current images are generally inadequate for therapeutic planning in most centers, but as the associated hardware and software improve, the role of MRA in the assessment of occlusive disease of the aortoiliac segments will increase.[12]

Angiography

Intra-arterial contrast angiography is considered the gold standard for the evaluation of patients with aortoiliac occlusive disease. This modality provides essential diagnostic information necessary to appropriately plan the treatment of most vascular patients with arterial occlusive disease. A complete evaluation of the existing arterial disease from the aorta to the pedal vessels is necessary for most elderly patients, since they commonly have concomitant infrainguinal arterial occlusive disease. The addition of intra-arterial pressure measurements at the time of arteriography improves the accuracy for detecting clinically significant disease. Resting pressure gradients greater than 5 mm Hg during angiographic pull-back pressure measurements in the aortoiliac system are abnormal and indicate a hemodynamically significant stenosis. In addition, pressure measurements after intra-arterial injection of a vasodilatory drug like papaverine are used to evaluate the significance of aortoiliac stenoses under conditions of stress that require increased blood flow through these vessels. A systolic pressure gradient across the lesion of more than 15 mm Hg is considered hemodynamically significant.[13]

The complication rate of arteriography in the general population is only 1.7% to 3.3%.[14] Elderly patients with severe aortoiliac disease have to be carefully evaluated before the procedure, since local and systemic complications are more likely than in the general population. The transfemoral approach is the safest, but other options like the translumbar, transbrachial, or transaxillary approach may have to be used for patients with weak or nonpalpable femoral pulses. These alternative approaches have higher local complication rates. These include hematomas, pseudoaneurysms, dissections, thrombosis, and embolization.

Renal insufficiency is an important complication of angiography. Renal impairment associated with contrast agents occurs in 6.5% to 8.2% of patients who undergo arteriography.[15,16] Patients with preexisting azotemia and a baseline creatinine greater than 2.0 are at the highest risk for renal complications after angiography. Elderly patients have lower creatinine clearances for a given serum creatinine level, so they should always be considered at a higher risk for nephrotoxicity. All possible precautions should be taken to limit the renal insult. The use of low osmolar contrast agents has been shown by some authors to decrease the incidence of renal impairment,[17,18] but these findings are not universal.[19] Adequate hydration prior to arteriography is a very effective maneuver to diminish the risk of contrast nephropathy. Mannitol is used for its osmotic diuretic effect to help prevent contrast toxicity. Vasodilators like dopamine have also been used because the nephrotoxic effect of contrast agents is considered to be partly due to intrarenal vasoconstriction. Dopamine has been shown to be better than mannitol at preventing contrast-related renal insufficiency.[20] Unfortunately, many elderly patients have moderate to severe cardiac disease and aggressive hydration may lead to congestive heart failure, cardiac ischemia, and arrhythmias. In addition, the use of dopamine may also lead to cardiac complications. Careful hydration and judicious use of mannitol, dopamine, and contrast agents can decrease the incidence of renal impairment associated with arteriography.

Intravascular Ultrasound

Intravascular ultrasound (IVUS) is a new method of evaluating arterial stenoses from within the blood vessel. It allows accurate calculation of the degree of stenosis, but at this time, it is only an adjunct to arteriography. It may become very useful to evaluate specific arterial lesions before interventions and to better assess the immediate results after angioplasty or stent placement procedures. The catheters used are costly, and their role in the evaluation and treatment of arterial disease is still under evaluation.

Therapeutic Options

Elderly patients with mainly aortoiliac occlusive disease rarely require an intervention. Patients with claudication should be treated initially by maximizing the management of known risk factors for the development of atherosclerosis, an exercise or walking program, and the use of potentially helpful oral agents like pentoxifylline. The small group of patients with severe, debilitating claudication that has failed the initial treatment protocol will generally request an intervention. In addition, the patients that present with limb-threatening ischemia secondary to multilevel occlusive disease should be considered for intervention.

Percutaneous Transluminal Angioplasty and Stents

The use of percutaneous balloon angioplasty for the treatment of aortoiliac occlusive disease, with or without the use of intravascular stents, flourished over the past decade. It is crucial that these new technologies are used under optimal circumstances to obtain good long-term results. Only patients with significant symptomatic disease should be considered for treatment by a technique with demonstrable benefit to the patients relative to the risks involved.

The location of the lesion has to be considered before therapy is determined. Isolated aortic stenoses are uncommon. A variety of small series of aortic angioplasty for stenotic disease have been published. The initial success ranges from 90% to 100%,[21-24] with 5-year patency rates of 70%.[21,23] Stents have been used infrequently alone or as attachment devices for endovascular grafts for the treatment of aortic lesions to date.[25]

Stenotic lesions of the iliac arteries have been successfully treated with balloon angioplasty. The 5-year patency rate of iliac angioplasty in a large literature review by Becker et al was 72%.[26] Multiple series in the literature have described a variety of factors that can affect the long term results of iliac angioplasty. Predictors of a long-term successful outcome after balloon angioplasty include the location of the lesion (common iliac lesions respond better than external iliac artery lesions), the indication for therapy (patients with claudication respond better than those with limb-threatening ischemia), the severity of the lesion (arterial stenoses respond better than arterial occlusions), and the arterial runoff distal to the lesion (lesions with good runoff respond better than those with poor runoff). Johnston et al reported a 60% 5-year patency rate for common iliac artery angioplasty, as compared to a 48% 5-year patency rate for external iliac artery lesions.[21] Series containing predominantly claudicants have 5-year secondary patency rates of up to 83%.[27] An early series by Spence et al reported 2-year patency rates of 79% for patients with claudication and 50% for those treated for limb salvage.[28] A more recent study on diabetics reported 5-year patency rates of 70% for claudicants and only 29% for patients with limb-threatening ischemia.[29] Johnston found that common iliac artery stenoses with good runoff had a 65% 5-year patency rate versus 52% for arteries with poor runoff.[21] In diabetics, the 5-year patency rate for lesions with good runoff has been reported at 76%, while it was only 20% for those lesions with poor runoff.[29]

In 1990, Palmaz et al reported on 171 procedures in 154 patients in which stents were placed in the iliac arteries to treat occlusive disease.[30] The indications at that time were for unsatisfactory angioplasty, restenosis of previous angioplasty, or complete occlusion. At the average of 6 months of follow-up 113 of 154 patients remained asymptomatic. A randomized German trial of iliac stent placement versus angioplasty alone implied that stenting was superior to angioplasty. The 5-year patency for stenting was 92% versus 64% for angioplasty.[31] Other studies have supported the use of stents in the iliac arteries particularly for total occlusions, dissection, and restenosis (Figure 1).[32-35] Vorwerk and Gunther reported a 90% initial success rate in their last series of 50 patients with total occlusions.[36] The use of stents for the treatment of angioplasty failures, dissections, or more complex lesions has improved the results of iliac artery interventions, but the long-term durability of the treatment of complex lesions has yet to be confirmed.

Aortofemoral Bypass

Aortofemoral bypass remains the standard to which other procedures must be compared to in the treatment of aortoiliac occlusive disease. Operative morbidity and mortality are low with 5-year patency rates of 80% to 90%.[37-40] Ten-year patency rates of 70% to 80% have been achieved in patients who have ceased smoking after operation (Figure 2).[37,38] A significant portion of patients requiring iliac reconstruction will also have significant femoropopliteal disease. The majority of patients are best served by correction of their inflow disease prior to infrainguinal reconstruction. Patients with severe rest pain or those with gangrene or nonhealing ulcerations may need simultaneous aortoiliac and infrainguinal bypasses to achieve limb salvage.

Femoral to Femoral Bypass

Crossover bypass for unilateral iliac artery occlusion has been traditionally reserved for high-risk patients, but have been used more recently in good risk patients. This procedure can easily be performed under regional or local anesthetic if required. Patency rates have ranged from 60% to 90% at 5 years.[39-43] When concurrently performed fem-fem bypasses were compared to aortobifemoral bypasses in low-risk patients, fem-fem bypasses were inferior in terms of patency and hemodynamic performance to aortobifemoral bypasses (primary patency 61% versus 87% at 3 years). Interestingly, in this series, limb salvage rates were similar for both procedures in patients initially admitted with limb-threatening ischemia.[40] Femoral to femoral graft is also useful to treat a unilateral occlusion of a limb of a bifurcated aortic graft.[44]

Direct iliofemoral bypass is another option for unilateral iliac artery occlusion. In a randomized study in France, aortofemoral and iliofemoral bypasses were compared with femorofemoral or iliofemoral crossover bypass. Primary patency rates for direct reconstruction were better at 4 years (89%) than for crossover grafts (52%) with no difference in morbidity.[41] Five-year secondary patency rates for iliofemoral versus femorofemoral bypass were 69% versus 65%, respectively, in a report by Harrington.[42]

Axillofemoral Bypass

Traditionally, high-risk patients with aortoiliac occlusive disease have been treated with axillofemoral bypasses. Axillofemoral grafts were considered inferior to aortobifemoral grafts in terms of long-term patency. However, after the introduction of externally supported prostheses by Kenney,[45] patency rates of axillofemoral grafts dramatically improved. Recent papers have demonstrated patency rates for axillary grafts that approach those from historic series for aortobifemoral grafts.[46,47] Passman et al[40] found that axillofemoral grafts compared favorably to aortic grafts in terms of limb salvage. In their comparative series of concurrently performed procedures, the aortic grafts had better long-term patency, but equivalent results in terms of limb salvage. In this report, the group of patients undergoing axillary to femoral artery bypasses were an older and sicker group of patients with a significantly decreased survival when compared to the patients undergoing aortic procedures. Therefore, one can conclude that patients with limited life expectancy can achieve results from axillary bypasses which should be equivalent to those of aortic reconstruction, but should continue to use direct aortic reconstruction for the younger, better risk patients.[48]

Endoluminal Grafts

An alternative method for treating long segment aortoiliac disease uses endovascular stented grafts placed across the area of occlusion or stenoses. These devices may be inserted under local or regional anesthesia, require less operative dissection, and can be done with minimal blood loss. They can be applied to long or multiple lesions for which balloon angioplasty and stents have not been proven to be durable.[47-49] Prelimi-

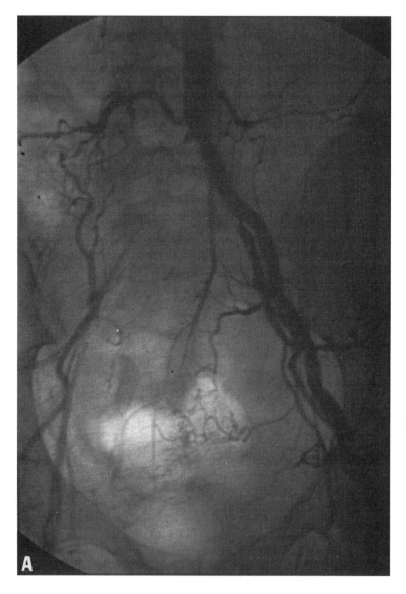

Figure 1A. Sixty-five-year-old female admitted with one half block right leg claudication with a history of two failed femoral-femoral artery bypasses. Pelvic angiogram shows total occlusion of the right common iliac artery.

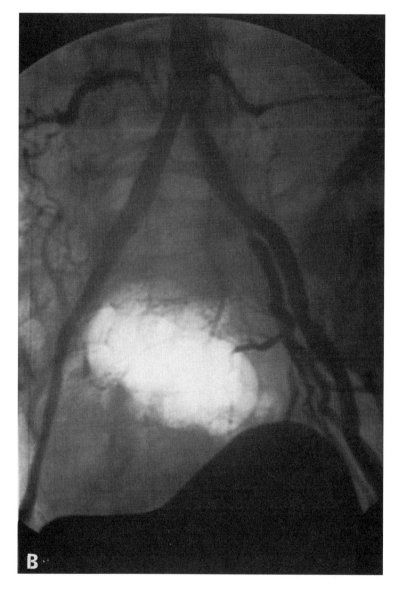

Figure 1B. Sixty-five-year-old female admitted with one half block right leg claudication with a history of two failed femoral-femoral artery bypasses. The iliac artery occlusion was corrected by balloon angioplasty and wall stent placement.

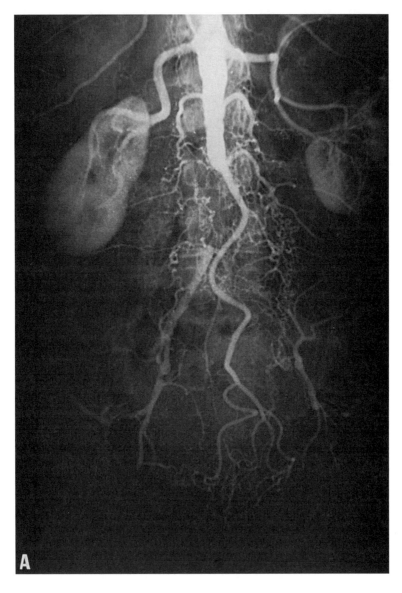

Figure 2A. This is an aortogram of a 72-year-old female with a total occlusion of the distal aorta.

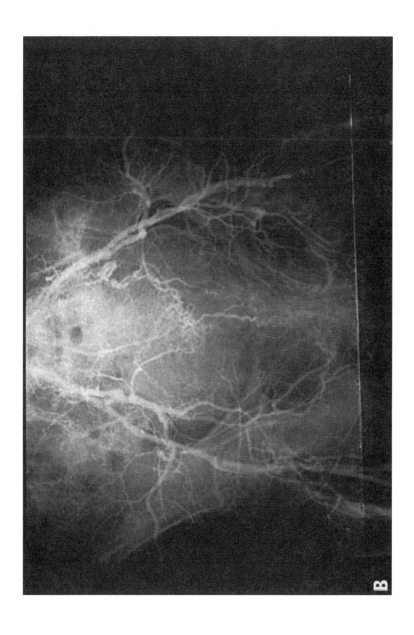

Figure 2B. This angiogram shows reconstitution of the femoral arteries bilaterally; this patient underwent a successful aortobifemoral bypass.

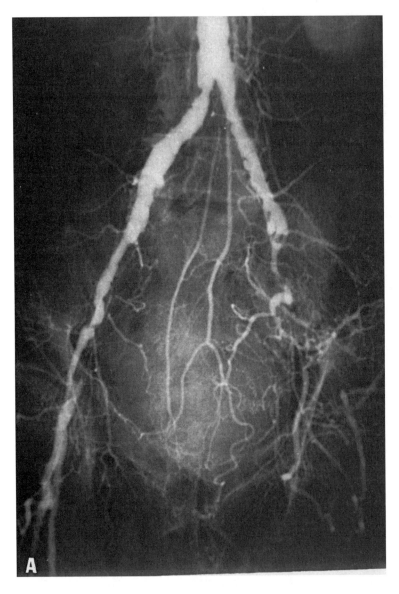

Figure 3A. Sixty-two-year-old woman admitted with limb-threatening ischemia of the left lower extremity. Pelvic arteriogram shows diffuse iliac disease on both sides with a left external iliac artery occlusion.

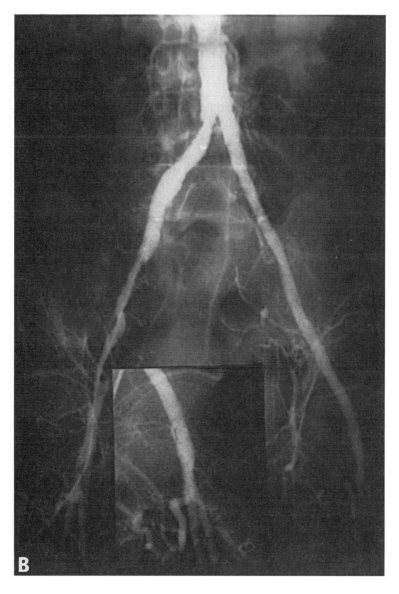

Figure 3B. Sixty-two-year-old woman admitted with limb-threatening ischemia of the left lower extremity. The iliac artery occlusion was corrected by use of an endovascular stented graft from the proximal common iliac artery to the femoral artery, which was extended to the popliteal artery in a standard fashion.

nary reports of aortoiliac reconstruction utilizing stented grafts in 43 high-risk patients demonstrated primary and secondary patency rates at 18 months of 77% and 95%, respectively.[25] In addition, these endoluminal grafts can be combined with conventional infrainguinal bypass techniques to achieve limb salvage. Seventeen such cases have been successfully performed with a 1-year patency rate of 94% and a limb salvage rate of 93% (Figure 3).[50-52] These methods will undoubtedly have an increased application in the management of multilevel aortoiliac and infrainguinal occlusive disease as technology improves.

Conclusions

With the increasing age of our population, the number of elderly individuals that will present with significant aortoiliac occlusive disease will continue to increase. The types of interventions used to treat these elderly patients' disease processes should be tailored to their ages and associated medical conditions. The increasing utilization of interventional techniques, such as angioplasty with stents and endoluminal stented grafts, should allow for the treatment of elderly patients with diminishing morbibity and mortality rates.

References

1. Cronenwett JL, Davis JR Jr, Gooch JB, et al: Aortoiliac occlusive disease in women. *Surgery* 88:775-784, 1980.
2. Veith FJ, Gupta SK, Wengerter KR, et al: Changing atherosclerotic disease patterns and management strategies in lower-limb threatening ischemia. *Ann Surg* 212:402-414, 1990.
3. Moneta GL, Yeager RA, Taylor LM Jr, et al: Hemodynamic assessment of combined aortoiliac/femoropopliteal occlusive disease and selection of single or multilevel revascularization. *Semin Vasc Surg* 7:3-10, 1994.
4. Baker JD, Dix D: Variability of Doppler ankle pressures with arterial occlusive disease: an evaluation of ankle index and brachial-ankle pressure gradient. *Surgery* 79:134-137, 1976.
5. Kohler TR, Nance DR, Cramer MM, et al: Duplex scanning for diagnosis of aortoiliac and femoropopliteal disease-a prospective study. *Circulation* 76:1074-1080, 1987.
6. Langsfeld M, Nupute J, Hershey FB, et al: The use of deep duplex scanning to predict hemodynamically significant aortoiliac stenoses. *J Vasc Surg* 7:395-399, 1988.
7. Moneta GL, Yeager RA, Antonovic R, et al: Accuracy of lower extremity arterial duplex mapping. *J Vasc Surg* 15:275-284, 1992.
8. Legemate DA, Teeuwen C, Hoenveld H, et al: Value of duplex scanning compared with angiography and pressure measurement in the assessment of aortiliac lesions. *Br J Surg* 78:1003-1008, 1991.
9. Owens RS, Carpenter JP, Baum RA, et al: Magnetic resonance imaging of angiographically occult runoff vessels in peripheral arterial occlusive disease. *N Engl J Med* 326:1577-1581, 1992.
10. Carpenter JP, Owen RS, Baum RA, et al: Magnetic resonance angiography of peripheral runoff vessels. *J Vasc Surg* 16:807-815, 1992.

11. Carpenter JP, Owen RS, Holland GA, et al: Magnetic resonance angiography of the aorta, iliac, and femoral arteries. *Surgery* 116:17-23, 1994.
12. Arlart IP, Guhl L, Edleman RR: Magnetic resonance angiography of the abdominal aorta. *Cardiovasc Intervent Radiol* 15:43, 1992.
13. Brewster DC, Waltman AC, O'Hara PJ, et al: Femoral artery pressure measurement during aortography. *Circulation* 60:120-124, 1979.
14. Hessel SJ, Adams DF, Abrams HL: Complications of angiography. *Radiology* 138:273-281, 1981.
15. Gomes AS, Baker JD, Martin-Paredero V, et al: Acute renal dysfunction after major arteriography. *AJR* 145:1249-1253, 1985.
16. Martin-Paredero V, Dixon SM, Baker JD, et al: Risk of renal failure after major angiography. *Arch Surg* 118:1417-1420, 1983.
17. Nikonoff T, Skau T, Berglund J, et al: Effects of femoral arteriography and low osmolar contrast agents on renal function. *Acta Radiol* 34:88-91, 1993.
18. Katholi RE, Taylor GJ, Woods WT, et al: Nephrotoxicity of nonionic low-osmolality versus ionic high osmolality contrast media: a prospective double-blind randomized comparison in human beings. *Radiology* 186:183-187, 1993.
19. Lautin EM, Freeman NJ, Schoenfeld AH, et al: Radiocontrast-associated renal dysfunction: a comparison of lower-osmolality and conventional high-osmolality contrast media. *Am J Roentgenol* 157:59-65, 1991.
20. Hall KA, Wong RW, Hunger GC, et al: Contrast-induced nephrotoxicity: the effects of vasodilator therapy. *J Surg Res* 53:317-320, 1992.
21. Johnston KW, Rae M, Hogg-Johnston SA, et al: 5-Year results of a prospective study of percutaneous transluminal angioplasty. *Ann Surg* 206:403, 1987.
22. Ravimandalam K, Rao VRK, Kumar S, et al: Obstruction of the infrarenal portion of the abdominal aorta: results of treatment with balloon angioplasty. *Am J Roentgenol* 156:1257-1262, 1991.
23. Odunry A, Colapinto RF, Sniderman KW, et al: Percutaneous transluminal angioplasty of abdominal aortic stenoses. *Cardiovasc Intervent Radiol* 12:1-6, 1989.
24. Yakes WF, Kumpe DA, Brown SB, et al: Percutaneous transluminal aortic angioplasty: techniques and results. *Radiology* 172:965-970, 1989.
25. Marin ML, Veith FJ, Cynamon J, et al: Transfemoral endovascular stented graft treatment of aortoiliac and femoropopliteal occlusive disease for limb salvage. *Am J Surg* 168:156-162, 1994.
26. Becker GJ, Katzen BT, Dake MD: Noncoronary angioplasty. *Radiology* 170:403-412, 1989.
27. Gallino A, Mahler F, Probst P, et al: Percutaneous transluminal angioplasty of the arteries of the lower limbs: a 5-year follow-up. *Circulation* 70:619-623, 1984.
28. Spence RK, Freiman DB, Gatenby R, et al: Long-term results of transluminal angioplasty of the iliac and femoral arteries. *Arch Surg* 116:1377-1386, 1981.
29. Stokes KR, Strunk HM, Campbell DR, et al: Five-year results of iliac and femoropopliteal angioplasty in diabetic patients. *Radiology* 174:977-982, 1990.
30. Palmaz JC, Garcia OJ, Schatz RA, et al: Placement of balloon-expandable intraluminal stents in iliac arteries: first 171 procedures. *Radiology* 174:969-975, 1990.
31. Richter GM, Roeren I, Brado M, et al: Further update of the randomized trial: iliac stent placement versus PTA-morphology, clinical success rates, and failure analysis. *JVIR* 4:30, 1993.
32. Liermann D, Strecker EP, Peters J: The Strecker stent: indications and results in iliac and femoropopliteal arteries. *Cardiovasc Intervent Radiol* 15:298, 1992.
33. Palmaz JC, Laborde JC, Rivera FJ, et al: Stenting of the iliac arteries with the Palmaz stent: experience from a multicenter trial. *Cardiovasc Intervent Radiol* 15:291-297, 1992.

34. Hausegger KA, Cragg AH, Lammer J, et al: Iliac artery stent placement: clinical experience with a Nitinol stent. *Radiology* 190:199-202, 1994.
35. Vorwerk D, Gunther RW: Stent placement in iliac arterial lesions: three years of clinical experience with the Wallstent. *Cardiovasc Intervent Radiol* 15:285-290, 1992.
36. Vorwerk D, Gunther RW: Chronic iliac artery occlusion. Presented at the International Congress, University of Heidelberg, Zermatt, April, 1993.
37. Brewster DC, Darling RC: Optimal methods of aortoiliac reconstruction. *Surgery* 84:739-748, 1978.
38. Piotrowski JJ, Pearce WH, Jones DN, et al: Aortobifemoral bypass: the operation of choice for unilateral iliac occlusion? *J Vasc Surg* 8:211-218, 1988.
39. Schneider JR, Besso SR, Walsh DB, et al: Femorofemoral versus aortobifemoral bypass: outcome and hemodynamic results. *J Vasc Surg* 19:43-57, 1994.
40. Passman MA, Taylor LM Jr, Moneta GL, et al: Comparison of axillofemoral and aortofemoral bypass for aortoiliac occlusive disease. *J Vasc Surg* 23:263-271, 1996.
41. Hanafy M, McLoughlin GA: Comparison of iliofemoral and femorofemoral crossover bypass in the treatment of unilateral iliac arterial occlusive disease. *Br J Surg* 78:1001-1002, 1991.
42. Harrington ME, Harrington EB, Haimov M, et al: Iliofemoral versus femorofemoral bypass: the case for an individualized approach. *J Vasc Surg* 16:841-842, 1992.
43. Farber MA, Hollier LH, Eubanks R, et al: Femorofemoral bypass: a profile of graft failure. *South Med J* 83:1437-1443, 1990.
44. Nolan KD, Benjamin ME, Murphy TJ, et al: Femorofemoral bypass for aortofemoral graft limb occlusion: a ten-year experience. *J Vasc Surg* 19:851-857, 1994.
45. Kenney DA, Sauvage LR, Wood SJ, et al: Comparison of noncrimped, externally supported (EXS) and crimped, nonsupported Dacron prostheses for axillofemoral and above-knee femoropopliteal bypass. *Surgery* 92:931-946, 1982.
46. El-Massry S, Saad E, Sauvage LR, et al: Axillofemoral bypass with externally supported, knitted Dacron grafts: a follow-up through 12 years. *J Vasc Surg* 17:107-115, 1993.
47. Taylor LM Jr, Moneta GL, McConnell DB, et al: Axillofemoral grafting with externally supported polytetrafluoroethylene. *Arch Surg* 129:588-595, 1994.
48. Harrington ME, Harrington EB, Haimov M, et al: Axillofemoral bypass: compromised bypass for compromised patients. *J Vasc Surg* 20:195-201, 1994.
49. Martin EC: Percutaneous therapy in the management of aortoiliac disease. *Semin Vasc Surg* 7:17, 1994.
50. Tegtmeyer CJ, Hartwell GD, Selby JB, et al: Results and complications of angioplasty in aortoiliac disease. *Circulation* 83(suppl 1):I-53-I-60, 1991.
51. Johnston KW: Iliac arteries: reanalysis of results of balloon angioplasty. *Radiology* 186:207-212, 1993.
52. Marin ML, Veith FJ, Sanchez LA, et al: Endovascular aortoiliac grafts in combination with standard infrainguinal arterial bypasses in the management of limb-threatening ischemia: preliminary report. *J Vasc Surg* 22:316-325, 1995.

Chapter 21

Infrainguinal Arterial Occlusive Disease in the Elderly

Ian L. Gordon, MD, PhD

Introduction

Modern efforts to ameliorate arterial occlusive disease have yielded amazing advances in the diagnosis and treatment of disease in many territories including the lower extremity. All the technical innovations applied in other territories have been translated into the leg, sometimes with greater success, as the leg seems to tolerate ischemia better than the brain or heart, and the consequences tend not to be as mortal. Amputation, a procedure that is rarely practical in other territories, is commonly employed as a form of management for severe manifestations of lower extremity ischemia, adding additional complexity to the decision making surrounding clinical problems. As the number of therapeutic options expands, the choices are increasingly difficult. Controversy surrounds many common clinical practices or attitudes, and more than a few important issues are disputed. Partly this is due to both vascular surgery and endoluminal therapy being new and rapidly evolving clinical enterprises. Partly this is due to a lack of definitive knowledge regarding the long-term consequences of particular interventions.

The author hopes that this chapter will serve as an exposition of the basic facts and practices that underlie current surgical management of atherosclerotic disease below the inguinal ligament. In many of the cases where controversies or differences in viewpoints exist, an effort has been made to put forward both sides (or more) of the argument. The author's own experiences as a vascular surgeon have undoubtedly colored the presentation of the virtues and risks of various therapies, and the need to be concise has required oversimplification and condensation of material that deserved more careful discussion. For these faults the author begs forgiveness, hoping that readers will appreciate the difficulties of exposing the underlying patterns in the large amount of information relevant to this broad topic.

From: Aronow WS, Stemmer EA, Wilson SE (eds). *Vascular Disease in the Elderly.* Armonk, NY: Futura Publishing Company, Inc., © 1997.

Of historical interest, the Roman Emperor Claudius (Tiberius Claudius Drusus Nero Germanicus; 10 B.C. to 54 A.D.) "had a certain majesty and dignity of presence, which showed to best advantage when he happened to be standing or seated—and especially when he was in repose. This was because, though tall and well built, with a handsome face, a fine head of white hair and a firm neck, he stumbled as he walked owing to weakness of his knees . . . ."[1]

Although the emperor's limp was congenital rather than due to vascular insufficiency, the association of his name with lower extremity disease is apt, as his family name, *Claudius,* is cognate with *claudicare* (to limp), thus sharing with claudication the same Latin root. It is as if a President of the United States was named Stumbler, and he was unsteady on his feet.

Definitions

We shall use the acronym PAOD (peripheral arterial occlusive disease) to refer to atherosclerosis affecting the large arteries below the inguinal ligament, recognizing the many other terms such as arterial insufficiency, peripheral vascular disease (PVD), and arteriosclerosis obliterans in common use. Chronic critical limb ischemia (chronic CLI) was defined by the Second European Consensus Document on Chronic Critical Leg Ischemia by either of two criteria:

> *. . . persistently recurring ischemic rest pain requiring analgesics lasting more than 2 weeks, with ankle systolic pressures of ≤ 50 mm Hg and/or a toe systolic pressure of ≤ 30 mm Hg; or ulceration or gangrene of the foot or toes, with an ankle systolic pressures of ≤ 50 mm Hg or a toe systolic pressure of ≤ 30 mm Hg.*[2]

Fontaine classes 1 and 2 correspond to moderate and severe intermittent claudication, and Fontaine classes 3 and 4 (rest pain and tissue loss) correspond to chronic CLI.

Natural History

Several sites in the lower extremity vasculature (Figure 1) are particularly susceptible to narrowing or occlusion from atherosclerosis. The distal segment of the superficial artery as it passes through the Hunter's canal to merge into the popliteal artery is the most common site of involvement. The common femoral artery, the midportion of the popliteal artery, and the origins of the tibial arteries are other sites with high predilections for atherosclerotic plaque formation. Often the distribution of lesions in one lower extremity is strikingly similar to that found in the other.

Arterial insufficiency in the lower extremity usually presents as a slowly progressing chronic problem, with symptoms and signs related to the degree of blood flow restriction. The severity of ischemia is influenced by the number of diseased arterial segments, the degree of

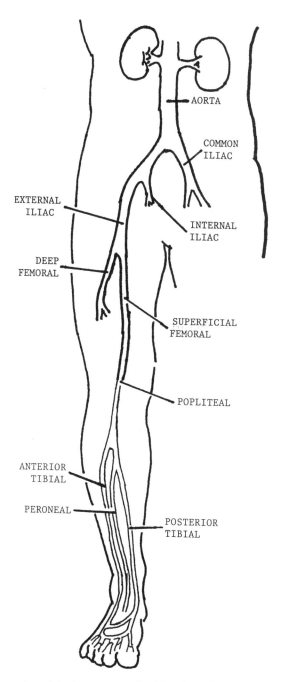

Figure 1. *Major arteries of the lower extremity.* Note how the anterior and posterior tibial arteries communicate directly with the pedal arteries.

narrowing in each segment, the adequacy of collateral flow around areas of occlusion, and the physiological demands placed upon the circulation. Other conditions which may mimic the symptoms of PAOD include arthritis and neurological syndromes, such as spinal stenosis or nerve root radiculopathy from disk herniation.

With acute occlusions such as those resulting from vascular graft occlusions, or embolism to the native arteries of the lower limb, flow through collateral channels may be inadequate to preserve limb viability. Embolism, thrombosis, and trauma are the major causes of acute occlusions. The overall incidence of acute occlusions is high, perhaps 10% to 20% of all admissions to hospital for PAOD are secondary to acute occlusions rather than for chronic ischemia. About half of all emboli lodge in either the superficial femoral or popliteal arteries, one third lodge in the aorta or iliac vessels, and the remainder occlude vessels below the knee. The heart is the most common source of emboli, which also originate from plaques and aneurysms in the thoracic and abdominal aorta. Bilateral extremity involvement is common when the origin is proximal; unilateral involvement is the rule with embolism from the iliac or more distal vessels. Arterial thrombi may form in the lower extremity from a variety of causes besides atherosclerosis, including arterial injury, collagen vascular disorders, myeloproliferative diseases, and dysproteinemias. The distinction between acute thrombosis and embolism may be difficult even with angiography, and the exact cause of arterial obstructions is not always determined.

Acute arterial occlusion leads to a sudden onset of symptoms. On examination, pulses are absent, the limb is cool and pale, and neurological symptoms suggestive of nerve ischemia are present—weakness, paralysis, or paresthesia. Five Ps connote acute arterial occlusion—pain, pallor, pulselessness, paralysis, and poikilothermia (for coolness). The long nerves of the lower extremity are the tissues most sensitive to ischemia, and the urgency of intervention correlates with the degree of diminished sensation and power in the limb. In the absence of good collateral flow, acute occlusion causes dramatically progressive symptoms. Initial numbness developing in the first hour can be followed by ischemic muscle contracture, subcutaneous hemorrhage, focal gangrene, and fixed skin staining. Irrevocable tissue and/or limb loss may occur in as little as 6 hours. Often, even when the foot is cool and rest pain is present, collateral flow is sufficient to preserve the limb for a short period, allowing diagnostic studies to precede operative intervention. If complete paralysis, muscle tenderness or rigidity, or thrombosis of superficial cutaneous vessels is present, the probability of limb loss is high, even with successful revascularization.

Emergent intervention is less often indicated with presentations of chronic symptoms, even if tissue necrosis is already present. The indolent pace of chronic disease reflects the tendency for slowly progressive arterial obstruction to be opposed, with varying success, by collateral formation. Detailed history taking and thorough physical examination of arterial pulses, neurological function, and the skin help to determine the chronicity and severity of PAOD. Evaluation of capillary and vein refill times, skin temperature and staining, blistering, cyanosis, collapse of superficial veins, and calf tenderness or rigidity help to decide the pace with which revascularization needs to be pursued. Rubor, hair loss, and normal neurological findings suggest chronic rather than acute ischemia, allowing more deliberation and less haste for diagnosis and therapy.

With chronic arterial insufficiency, mild to moderate impairment of arterial flow leads to muscle pain when walking or exercising, commonly referred to as intermittent claudication. The ischemic muscle pain induced by exercise is generally experienced as a painful cramp localized to a specific muscle group. The most common site affected is the calf, but the thigh, foot, and buttocks may also be affected. Some patients will describe a premonition that the leg can go no further, or tightness, tingling, or burning rather than cramping as the predominant symptom. The hallmark of intermittent claudication is close association of symptoms with walking and rapid resolution with rest.

Claudication represents an imbalance between the increased demand of exercising muscle for nutrient oxygen and glucose and the limited ability of the diseased arterial system to meet the increased demand. Thus, claudication represents a *functional* impairment in blood flow. With more severe arterial occlusion, the limitation of flow is inadequate to meet the requirements of resting metabolism, causing CLI.

CLI may manifest as either constant pain at rest or as tissue loss. Rest pain is generally experienced in the foot, usually in the toes or over the metatarsal heads. Early on, the patient may experience painful paresthesias with the leg elevated that are relieved by dependency. As the disease progresses, pain may be constant, particularly at night. Patients often report that they dangle their legs over the side of the bed or even stand up to walk so as to relieve symptoms. Rest pain at night should be distinguished from nocturnal calf cramps (which develop during sleep, are relieved by massage, respond to quinine, and are not due to CLI). Without intervention, the limb afflicted with rest pain from critical ischemia generally goes on to develop some form of tissue loss, either in the form of skin ulceration or gangrene.

Ulcers resulting from arterial insufficiency develop in the ankle, leg, or foot, often after minor trauma that otherwise would heal. The heel and malleoli are common sites, but any site in the distal limb may ulcerate. Arterial ulcers tend to be bland without intense inflammation or infection. Fibrinopurulent exudate or necrotic tissue forms the base (Figure 2). The ulcers may be painful, but not necessarily, particularly in diabetics with neuropathy. Arterial ulcers need to be distinguished from pure neuropathic ulcers secondary to diabetes or other neurological conditions, and also from venous ulcers. Neuropathic ulcers tend to form over plantar pressure points, such as the heel and metatarsal heads, and result when reflex mechanisms protecting the skin from pressure fail due to diminished sensation and/or bony deformity. Neuropathic ulcers may result in infection of underlying bone (osteomyeli-

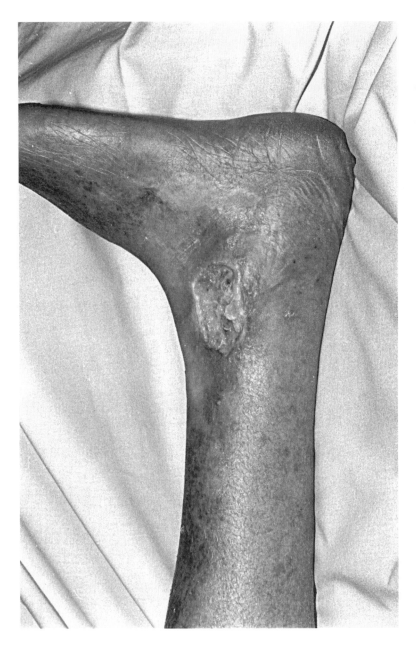

Figure 2. *Arterial ulcer.* The **base** of the ulcer is fibrinopurulent exudative tissue. Little surrounding inflammation is evident.

tis). Venous ulcers tend to be confined to the anterior and medial surface of the leg, with characteristic surrounding brawny skin hyperpigmentation. Although venous ulcers usually can be distinguished from arterial ulcers without difficulty, occasionally both venous disease and arterial insufficiency are present, such that the routine local care that usually heals venous ulcers fails. When a venous ulcer fails to respond to conventional therapy (e.g., Unna boots), PAOD may be present.

Gangrene represents death of tissues from ischemia. The damage to the tissues is analogous to a stroke causing cerebral infarction. The infarcted tissue may become mummified and appear as a dry, black spot or toe, or present as a bland crust on the skin overlying an area of devitalized soft tissue (Figure 3). In severe cases, the entire foot or lower portion of the limb may become necrotic from gangrene. Initially, the infarcted tissue is dry ("dry gangrene"), but with time, supervening bacterial infection leads to suppuration ("wet gangrene") with the serious consequences of systemic infection and sepsis. In some cases, CLI presents as a cellulitis of the foot or leg without ulceration or gangrene. Left untreated, the limb may be lost, but optimal medical therapy centered around antibiotics may salvage the limb temporarily. Unless the arterial supply is improved, major amputation is usually required to control infection and achieve wound healing (Figures 4 and 5).

Once tissue loss is present, conventional surgical wisdom is that intervention is mandated for limb salvage or amputation will be inevitable. Sometimes, particularly after an acute thrombotic event such as a bypass graft closure, sufficient collaterals will develop for rest pain and ulceration to resolve after weeks or months, but this is generally believed to be rare. In fact, recent studies suggest that small ischemic ulcers do frequently heal spontaneously, perhaps as much as 40% of the time, with conservative measures.[3] As with claudication, objective hemodynamic measurements predict the risk of disease progression to amputation better than clinical assessments of pain or ulceration. The absence of detectable Doppler flow signals (see below) is particularly ominous, indicating a high risk of limb loss if restoration of blood flow is not accomplished.

Epidemiology of Peripheral Arterial Occlusive Disease

One factor confounding attempts to accurately estimate the incidence of PAOD is the dissociation between the anatomical severity of lesions causing arterial occlusion and the severity of symptoms elicited. Epidemiological surveys based on the gold standard of angiography overestimate the incidence of symptomatic patients, as over half of subjects with documented large vessel arterial obstruction on angiogram will not report symptoms.[4] Many subjects with complete occlusions of a major lower limb artery (e.g., the superficial femoral) are more limited by weakness or shortness of breath secondary to cardiopulmonary dis-

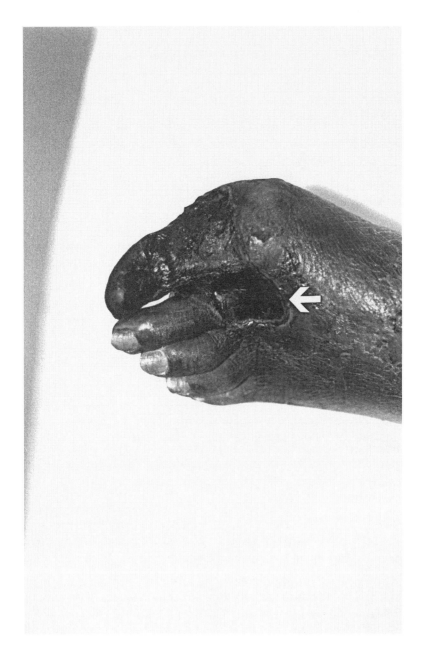

Figure 3. *Ischemic gangrene.* The great toe is mummified, and skin infarction is seen extending over the interspace between the first and second toes **(arrow)**.

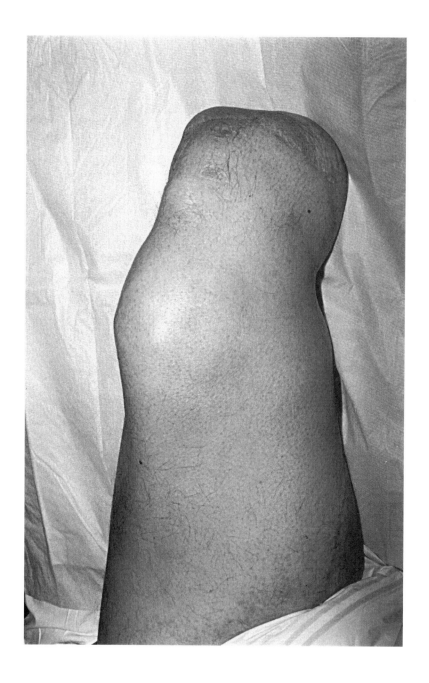

Figure 4. Below knee amputation (BKA).

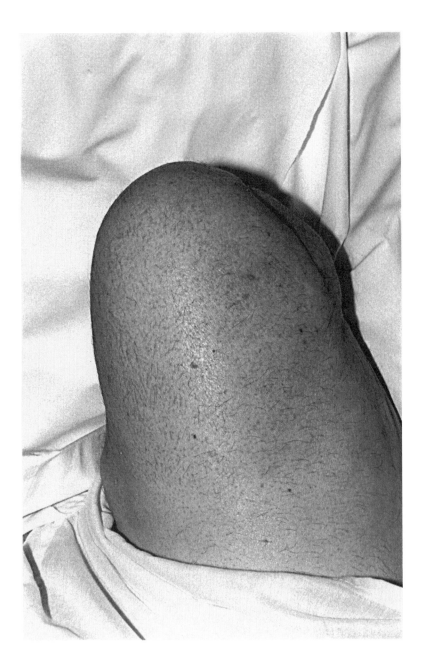

Figure 5. Above knee amputation (AKA).

ease, and do not walk far enough to develop claudication symptoms. Elderly subjects appear to often accept decreased mobility, whether due to arthritis, neurological disease, or PAOD, as a natural consequence of aging, and will avoid the subject or deny the significance during health assessments.

As a consequence of this symptom, anatomical lesion dissociation, it should be appreciated that rates of detection for PAOD depend on the diagnostic criterion employed. Angiograms will detect more cases than noninvasive ultrasound or symptom questionnaires. With increasingly stringent definitions of ischemia, the prevalence of PAOD will be measurably less, as subjects with functional ischemia greatly outnumber those with CLI.

Estimates of the prevalence of PAOD show variation with age, sex, and geographic location. Reported prevalence figures range from a low value of 0.4% in Danish men aged 40 to 59[5] to 14% in American men and women over the age of 65.[6] Figure 6 is a representative demonstration of the relation between PAOD prevalence and age derived from surveys in Scotland. Note the higher prevalence in men compared to women, with the gap narrowing with advancing age. Also, note the steep increase in prevalence starting at age 50, with men under 50 having less than 1% prevalence, compared to men older than 60, who have a fivefold increased prevalence.[7] This age dependence was confirmed in a Swiss study, based on careful physical examination as well as symptoms, in

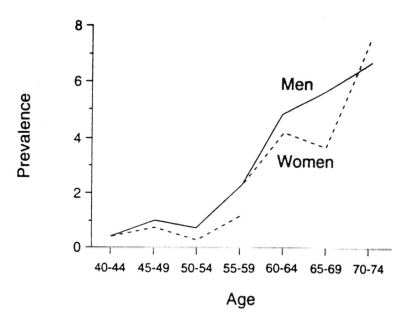

Figure 6. Prevalence of peripheral arterial occlusive disease (PAOD) in men and women. (Reproduced with permission from Reference 7.)

which the prevalence of PAOD between the ages of 35 and 44 was 0.6% compared to 7.5% for those 60- to 64-years-old.[4]

The Framingham Study measured the incidence of intermittent claudication in rates per 10,000 person-years and demonstrated the effect of aging on the tendency to develop PAOD. Young men (ages 30 to 34) had only one tenth the incidence rate: 6 per 10,000 person-years, versus 61 per 10,000 person-years in men older than 65. Woman had half the incidence rate of men until reaching 65, at which point the incidence of claudication in women was only slightly lower than men: 54 versus 61 per 10,000 person-years.[8,9]

A low ankle/brachial pressure index ([ABPI]; see section on noninvasive testing) found on noninvasive testing is probably a better marker of PAOD than either angiography or symptoms, as it reflects more accurately the physiological restriction in blood flow. Based on noninvasive testing, approximately 15% to 25% of Europeans or Americans over age 60 have PAOD when an ABPI of less than 0.9 is used as a criterion.[10,11] Based on noninvasive testing, over 30% of Italians 80 years and older had PAOD, which is one of the highest prevalence rates reported.[12]

In 1960, before the modern era of vascular surgery, Boyd[13] reported the outcomes in 1440 patients with claudication followed for 10 years. Only 12% ultimately required amputation. Progressive deterioration of functional ischemia to chronic CLI occurs in only a minority. In the Framingham Study, after an 8-year follow-up, only 1.6% of claudicants had required amputation. When noninvasive tests are used to objectively define PAOD and rule out other diagnoses, higher progression rates for functional to critical ischemia are evident, with as many as 20% to 40% of claudicants progressing to rest pain or tissue loss within 5 years.[14,15] A consensus view is that somewhere between 15% to 20% of functional ischemia patients will progress to CLI.[16] Based on extrapolation from incidence and prevalence measurements overall, 1% of men over the age of 55 in the industrialized West develop critical ischemia.

Based on the available incidence and prevalence data, it appears that 20% of patients with PAOD will develop CLI, of whom about one quarter will ultimately require amputation. The estimated crude rate for lower limb amputations resulting from PAOD in the United States is 280 per million population per year,[17] suggesting a crude incidence for CLI of 500 to 1000 per million per year. This is comparable to another estimate that 150,000 patients per year in the United States develop limb-threatening ischemia from infrainguinal atherosclerosis.[18]

Risk Factors

Smoking, diabetes, hyperlipidemia, and hypertension are all important risk factors that both heighten the risk of developing PAOD and increase the likelihood that functional PAOD will progress to CLI. Not surprisingly, these are the same factors most strongly associated with atherosclerosis in other territories. Tobacco use is the most important risk factor for claudication. In the Framingham Study, heavy smokers were twice as likely as nonsmokers, with otherwise identical risk profiles, to develop claudication, and overall 80% of claudicants have a smoking history.[9] Smokers are nine times more likely to develop PAOD than nonsmokers.[19] Continued tobacco consumption once claudication develops worsens the prognosis. In one study from the Mayo Clinic,[20] 11% of claudicants who continued smoking required amputation within 5 years, compared to no amputations in those who did not. Similarly, patency in lower extremity bypass grafts is worse in smokers than nonsmokers.[21] Interestingly, despite the well-known appreciation in the general public for the association of smoking with heart disease, most patients are ignorant of the association of smoking with PAOD.[22]

Diabetes is another important independent factor related both to the development of PAOD and to the risk of progression to CLI. The incidence of type II diabetes rises with age. In Europeans, the prevalence of diabetes at age 50 is about 3%, rising to 6% at the age of 70.[2,23] Ethnic and geographic factors lead to even higher rates. Eleven percent of Germans aged 60 and older have been estimated to have diabetes.[24] Diabetics have at least a fivefold increased risk of CLI compared to nondiabetics. Ulcers and gangrene will occur in 10% of elderly diabetics, and over a 5-year period in the Swiss study, 6.8% of diabetics underwent lower extremity amputations compared to 0.6% of nondiabetics.[2,16] Approximately 20% of diabetics with claudication progress to amputation within 5 years, compared to about 3% of nondiabetics.[19,25] Diabetics who continue to smoke have the worst prognosis for progression to amputation.

The Framingham Study found hypertension to be associated with an approximate threefold increased incidence of claudication.[9] Whether treatment of hypertension influences the progression of claudication is unknown, but it is reasonable to surmise that it should.

Control of hyperlipidemia with diet and medications that reduce low-density lipoproteins (LDL) and raise high-density lipoprotein levels (HDL) has been shown to reduce the incidence of cardiovascular events in many studies. Blankenhorn and Hadis showed, using angiographic methods, that regression of plaque could be induced in the femoral artery with aggressive medical management of serum cholesterol.[26] In diabetics, tight control of hyperglycemia and reduction in serum triglyceride levels are associated with decreased manifestations of PAOD.[27] The net import of these and many similar studies is that optimal medical management of the risk factors for atherosclerosis diminishes the incidence of PAOD and slows the progression of functional ischemia to CLI.

Location of disease and the number of levels affected by atherosclerosis correlates with age and also the risk of functional ischemia progressing to CLI. Isolated aortoiliac involvement is regarded as a favorable pattern, with disease below the inguinal ligament associated with worse outcomes.[15,20] Infrainguinal disease is found in 65% of patients over age 40 compared to only 25% in younger patients, who are more likely to have aortoiliac disease. Multiple segment involvement, rather than single segment disease, is more common in the elderly.[16,28] When multiple segments are involved, the chance of claudication progressing to CLI within 5 years is 25%, compared to 15% when only single level disease is present.[29] Multiple segment involvement is also associated with decreased survival and increased coronary artery disease (CAD)(see *Association of Peripheral Arterial Occlusive Disease With Atherosclerosis in Other Territories*).

The severity of initial claudication has an association with the risk of amputation that parallels the association between number of segments involved and risk of progression to CLI. Patients who present with moderate claudication have less than a 3% risk of amputation at 2.5 years, compared to 15% amputations in severe claudicants.[30] Decreasing ABPI with serial follow-up is another poor prognostic sign.[14,15,31]

Based on recent series following the fate of claudicants, it can be shown that the risk of progression of claudication within 5 years to limb threat or tissue loss is 27% and the risk of amputation within 5 years is 4%. About 69% of claudicants will continue to have claudication or die within a 5-year interval, and one third will deteriorate, but not develop critical ischemia. Estimates of survival vary, but an average of multiple series puts 5-year survival for claudicators at about 70%, which is significantly diminished compared to age matched controls without PAOD.[16]

Diagnostic Methods in Peripheral Arterial Occlusive Disease

Two modes of diagnostic testing dominate current evaluation of PAOD: noninvasive ultrasound tests and contrast arteriography. The tests are complementary, with noninvasive ultrasound better at assessing the severity of ischemia, but lacking the precision of arteriography. Arteriography provides detailed and accurate information regarding the localization and morphology of arterial lesions, but does not reliably depict the physiological impact of restricted blood flow.

Doppler ultrasound instruments detect flowing blood in vessels based on the frequency shift induced in a beam of ultrasound after reflection of moving red blood cells. Accurate measurement of blood pressures at various levels in the lower extremity can be achieved using tourniquets and Doppler stethoscopes in a manner similar to determination of arm (brachial artery) blood pressure with a cuff, manometer, and stethoscope. The ankle/brachial pressure index (ABPI) is particularly helpful in assessing lower extremity ischemia. Normally the ABPI is 1.0 to 1.2, with any values below 1.0 suggesting arterial occlusive disease. The lower the ABPI, the more severe the restriction of blood flow (Table 1), and the more serious the ischemia. Not only is the ratio of ankle to arm pressures important, but the actual systolic pressure at the ankle has prognostic significance, with pressures below 50 mm Hg

Table 1
Correlation Between ABPI and Severity of Symptoms in PAOD

Severity of PAOD	Ankle/Brachial Pressure Index
Normal	1.0–1.2
Mild claudication	.8–.5
Moderate—severe claudication	.5–.8
Severe claudication—rest pain. Possible tissue loss	.3–.5
Limb threat	<0.3

ABPI = ankle brachial pressure index

PAOD = peripheral arterial occlusive disease

The table represents for each range of ABPI the symptoms likely to be present. In the absence of diabetes, tissue loss or gangrene is uncommon with ABPI > 0.5, but may be present in diabetic patients.

in the pedal arteries accepted as a reliable determinant of CLI. The determination of pressures at different levels by placing cuffs at different positions—high thigh, above knee, below knee, and calf—allows the level of obstruction to be identified when a clear gradient in pressure is demonstrated. One technical problem with segmental pressure measurements is that occasionally the tibial arteries are not compressible, due to calcification from renal failure or diabetes. Such noncompressible arteries yield falsely elevated ABPI values.

Ultrasound methods measure blood flow velocity based on the Doppler frequency shift in ultrasound reflected off moving red blood cells. This allows a flow velocity versus time waveform to be constructed (Figure 7), depicting the phasic flow of blood through the cardiac cycle. Normally, the waveform is triphasic, with reversal of flow in diastole at the level of the common femoral artery, and may be biphasic or triphasic in the pedal arteries. Biphasic or monophasic flow in the femoral artery, or monophasic flow at the ankle, represents significant occlusion proximal to the measurement. Analysis of Doppler velocity waveforms allows inferences to be drawn regarding arterial obstruction, even when ABPI measurements are falsely elevated from calcification.[32]

Duplex ultrasound is the most powerful method of noninvasive vascular diagnosis. It combines Doppler frequency measurements with two-dimensional images of blood vessels (Figure 8). Duplex ultrasound allows sophisticated hemodynamic analyses based on velocity power spectra, velocity waveforms, and ratios of systolic and diastolic flows. The severity of flow restriction induced by a stenosis can, thus, be accurately assessed and disturbed flow reliably detected.[33]

Noninvasive ultrasound studies help determine whether invasive investigations such as arteriography are necessary. Measurements of skin perfusion performed by laser Doppler techniques or Clark electrode determination of partial skin oxygen pressure ($tcPO_2$) and assessment

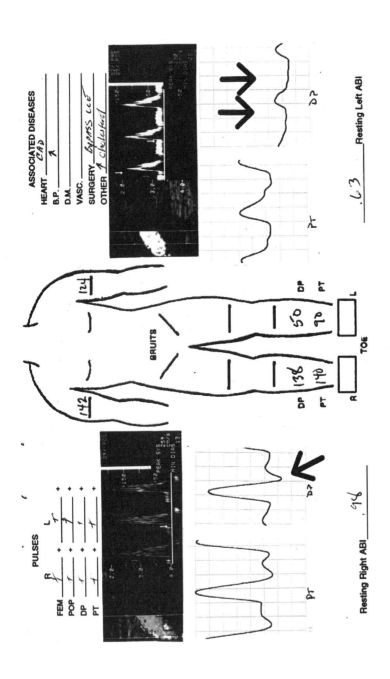

Figure 7. *Noninvasive ultrasound laboratory report.* The patient's right leg has normal ankle/brachial pressure index (ABPI) and velocity waveforms. The **single arrow** points to reversed flow during diastole which represents the normal flow pattern. The left leg has reduced ABPI, and the waveform is blunted and lacks reversed flow (**double arrows**).

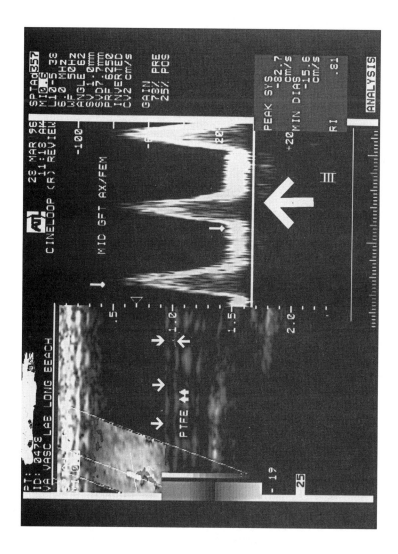

Figure 8. *Duplex ultrasound of polytetrafluoroethylene (PTFE) graft.* The figure displays the velocity versus time power spectrum obtained from insonating the midportion of a graft. Note the narrow dispersion of velocities during systole, characteristic of laminar flow **(single arrow).** The wall of the graft can be discerned in the two-dimensional image on the figure right **(multiple arrows).**

of walking distance on a low speed (2 mph) treadmill are other helpful tests. The vascular laboratory is particularly good in documenting hemodynamic responses to interventions aimed at improving the circulation. After arterial reconstruction, increased ABPI pressures or improvements in the blood velocity waveform reliably indicate improved blood flow. Bypass grafts are easily assessed via ultrasound for patency and the presence of significant stenosis. Figure 9 is an example of a study obtained on a femoropopliteal bypass. The information provided by ultrasound regarding flow of blood and vessel patency or occlusion allows critical management decisions to be taken, without depending on arteriography. These features make the vascular noninvasive laboratory an indispensable element of the medical resources required to treat vascular disease.

Arteriography (angiography) is a diagnostic procedure generally performed by specialists such as cardiologists and radiologists; vascular surgeons also perform angiographic procedures inside the operating room as an adjunct to operative reconstructions. Arteriography entails placing a catheter in the arterial system via an arterial puncture. The femoral artery is most commonly employed, with the axillary or brachial arteries being other common sites for access. Precise localization of the tip is controlled by passing it over a guidewire.[34] Once the catheter is positioned, contrast material is injected and radiographic images made as the contrast flows through the blood vessels. Video and digital subtraction technologies are increasingly employed to enhance the images obtained with fluoroscopy, as the amount of contrast and the time required for examinations are reduced. The excellent anatomical detail provided by contrast angiography makes it the continuing gold standard for diagnostic evaluation of arterial disease in the lower extremity. Figure 9 shows a normal angiogram with the pedal arches receiving their predominate inflow from the posterior tibial artery.

The costs and risks of contrast angiography limit its use. In 1996, the typical lower extremity arteriogram might cost between $3,000 to $4,000, independent of any therapeutic maneuvers employed. Because the procedure requires prolonged immobilization and the contrast injection is painful, intravenous sedatives and narcotics are usually employed, mandating close monitoring. Although usually performed on an outpatient basis, patients on anticoagulants or with renal failure may require hospitalization for angiography. Renal damage may occur from the contrast agents employed. To prevent this, close attention to administered fluids is required: dehydration increases the risk of renal damage while overhydration may induce congestive heart failure (CHF). Diabetics with preexisting renal disease have the highest risk for contrast-induced nephropathy.[35] Although rarely serious, bleeding and hematoma formation are frequent complications. Axillary puncture may cause nerve damage or lead to hematomas that require emergency decompression. Retroperitoneal hemorrhage, after femoral puncture for diagnostic or therapeutic procedures, can be fatal.[36-38]

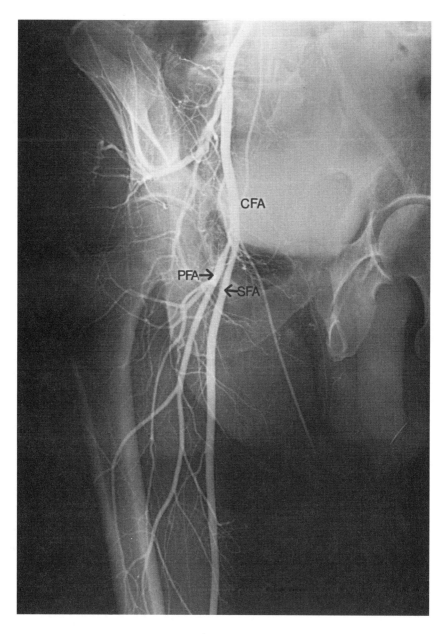

Figure 9A.

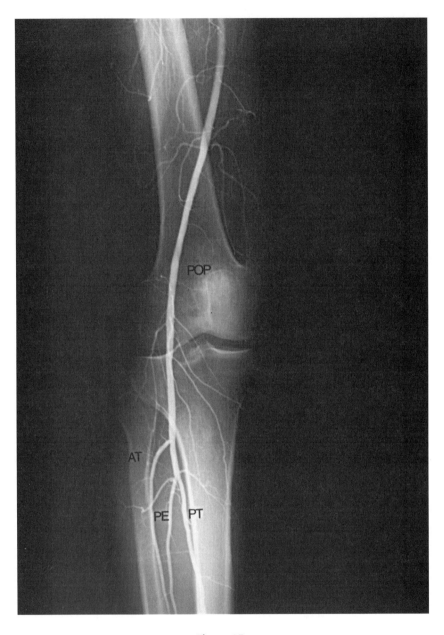

Figure 9B.

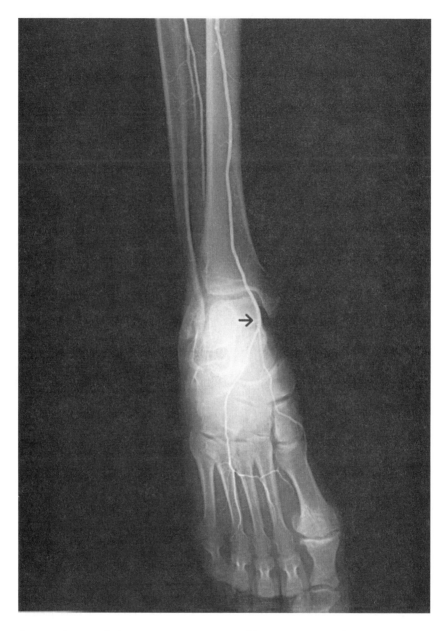

Figures 9A, B, and C. *Contrast arteriogram of lower extremity.* The normal arterial supply is shown, except the pedal arch is predominantly fed by the posterior tibial artery **(arrow)**. CFA=common femoral artery; SFA=superficial femoral artery; PFA= profunda femoris artery; POP=popliteal artery; AT=anterior tibial artery; PE=peroneal artery; PT=posterior tibial artery.

A new imaging method using catheters bearing rotating ultrasound transducers at their tip allows images of the blood vessel wall from inside to be constructed during radiological procedures. Intravascular ultrasound (IVUS) is more accurate than contrast angiography in assessing stenosis severity, as the latter technique routinely underestimates stenosis dimensions because of several technical limitations. IVUS may help after balloon angioplasty to check for residual stenosis or intimal flaps that require correction.

New imaging modalities, such as helical computed tomography ("spiral CT") and magnetic resonance imaging (MRI), provide images similar to contrast angiograms, although not yet as precise. Because these techniques are less invasive, they will be increasingly employed in the future in lieu of arteriography, especially as their resolution improves with advances in technique. MRI and CT angiography will probably never replace contrast fluoroscopy, since the stunning advances in catheter-based therapy will continue in the foreseeable future to make the interventional radiologist a critical and necessary component of the medical team treating vascular disease.

Pathophysiology of Peripheral Arterial Occlusive Disease

Although much of the pathophysiology of PAOD remains obscure, certain concepts that reconcile epidemiological findings with clinical and laboratory investigations have gained widespread acceptance. One concept is that reduced tissue perfusion is partially a consequence of inappropriate activation of local inflammatory responses in the microcirculation. Stenosis or obstruction of large vessels causes reduced perfusion of distal microcirculatory beds. Occasionally, other disease processes also contribute, such as diabetic small vessel disease or Buerger's disease (thromboarteritis obliterans). CLI develops when compensatory mechanisms such as collateral supply are inadequate to maintain the nutrition of the peripheral tissues, and is more common in multisegmental disease. Concomitant venous disease may also contribute to CLI, as well as decreased cardiac output from arrhythmia, myocardial ischemia, and possibly certain drugs (e.g., beta blockers).[2,39-41]

It has been proposed that progression of ischemia in the diseased limb is enhanced by activation of platelets and leukocytes, either by passage over ulcerated plaques or through poststenotic turbulent vortices. After activation, these cells stimulate local microthrombosis in the distal microvascular beds. Alternatively, defective prostanoid synthesis or fibrinolysis in diseased plaque tissue may promote local microthrombosis.[42]

The skin microcirculation (arterioles, capillaries, and postcapillary venules) can be divided into thermoregulatory and nutritional vessels. Nutritional capillaries normally carry less than 15% of total blood flow to the foot, with regulation of flow between thermoregulatory and nutritional vessels the result of a complex interplay between autonomic nervous system activity, local intrinsic mediators, and circulating humoral factors. Healthy nutritional capillaries are regularly perfused with a rhythmic distribution of flow (vasomotion) resulting from a periodic relaxation and contraction of arteriolar sphincters; the pattern of local smooth muscle sphincter tone can accommodate to decreased perfusion pressure and maintain tissue perfusion in a process known as autoregulation. Endothelial cells influence autoregulation of flow via vasodilatory mediators (prostacyclin and nitric oxide [NO]) and contractile mediators such as endothelin.[2]

Endothelial cells play an important role in controlling local hemostasis and thrombosis via regulation of thrombin activity (thrombomodulin, Protein C, Protein S) and modulation of the antithrombin III system with glycosaminoglycans. Endothelium also affects fibrinolysis through release of tissue plasminogen activator (tPA) and plasminogen inhibitors. Other properties of the endothelium such as surface charge, expression of cell adhesion molecules (CAM), and elaboration of NO influence the interaction of the vessel wall with leukocytes and platelets. Normally, blood-borne cells provide appropriate reactions to injury and inflammation without compromising nutritional capillary flow.

Arteriolar vasodilation, mediated through local vasoactive substances, acts to maintain nutritional capillary flow despite large vessel occlusion. In some patients, paradoxically increased skin flow (presumably from maximum local vasodilation) can be demonstrated next to areas of severe ischemia, suggesting that both maldistribution of flow and absolute reduction in flow account for critical ischemia in PAOD. In CLI, laboratory findings in the area of ischemia include tissue edema which may cause collapsed capillaries, pericapillary hemorrhage, reduced numbers of perfused capillaries, delayed perfusion of open capillaries based on fluorescence videomicroscopy, and inhomogeneous distribution of flow to the skin microcirculation. All of these factors are associated with reduced $tcPO_2$ and metabolic activity. Occlusion of the microcirculation from aggregates of ischemia activated leukocytes and platelets is one of several potentially important mechanisms for tissue damage that is currently under investigation.[2,43,44]

CLI may also adversely influence the role of vasomotion in maintaining skin flow. The frequency of vasomotion cycles is sensitive to oxygen tension, and abnormal vasomotion is evidenced by capillary microscopy in CLI. Chronic vasodilation in one area may preclude normal vasomotion activity in nearby tissues, causing reduction or maldistribution of nutritional capillary flow. The influence of ischemia on platelets, leukocytes, erythrocytes, endothelium, and the clotting system may influence vasomotion. Erythrocytes and leukocytes deform easily to pass through the smallest capillaries under normal perfusion pressures and shear rate. These cells may become relatively less deformable under the influence of decreased perfusion and shear. This effect is probably more important for leukocytes which are inherently less deformable than red cells; even the red cells have been found to be less deformable in CLI because of increased fibrinogen and local abnormalities in pH and osmolarity.[2,45]

Another key influence on the natural history of PAOD is the response of the arterial wall to iatrogenic trauma, such as surgery or balloon angioplasty. With either intervention, some portions of the arterial wall are traumatized. The response of the injured arterial wall is to elaborate new tissue in a process called myointimal hyperplasia. Smooth muscle cells, partially under the influence of platelet-derived growth factors (PDGF) elaborated at the site of injury, migrate from the media into the intima and transform into unique myointimal cells, which proliferate and lay down fibrous tissue. The resulting lesion is histologically distinct from atherosclerotic plaque, but has many of the same consequences including reduction in blood flow and promotion of thrombosis.[46,47] The proliferative response of the arterial wall after catheter interventions for stenosis may lead to delayed complete occlusions, and every vascular surgeon has had the experience of seeing a technically perfect bypass graft fail after only a few months due to myointimal hyperplasia occluding an anastomosis.

Peripheral Arterial Occlusive Disease and Diabetes

Diabetic patients have an increased risk for PAOD and have worse outcomes. Probably the mechanisms that underlie the microcirculatory disturbances in CLI are exaggerated in diabetes. Several other factors unique to diabetes aggravate the effects of large vessel occlusion. These include neuropathy, diabetic angiopathy, and enhanced susceptibility to infection.

Peripheral neuropathy is frequently found with diabetes. The most common form, distal symmetric polyneuropathy, involves sensory, autonomic, and motor fibers. Affected diabetics do not perceive the noxious stimuli that result from temperature extremes, foreign bodies, and poorly fitted shoes. This leads to increased tissue trauma, calluses, and ulceration. Muscle weakness due to motor fiber damage and limited proprioception secondary to neuropathy may lead to foot deformity and abnormal distribution of pressures on the plantar surface. Abnormal autonomic innervation may cause loss of sweating and dry, fissured skin. Increased arteriovenous shunting at the expense of nutritional capillary flow may also be a consequence of the autonomic dysfunction. Even without ischemia, the net effect of these factors may cause ulcers of the foot, particularly over bony prominences, known as neuropathic ulcers.

Diabetic angiopathy is another factor contributing to the increased incidence of CLI in diabetics. Electron microscopy is required to demonstrate the characteristic thickening of capillary basement membranes and microaneurysms in patients with diabetic angiopathy. These ultrastructural changes are present in 88% of diabetics compared to 23% of normals.[48] In addition to large artery atherosclerosis and microvascular angiopathy, diabetics tend to have more severe involvement of the tibial arteries (often with sparing of the peroneal artery) than nondiabetics as part of a pattern of diffuse, multisegmental distribution of lesions both above and below the inguinal ligament. All the ravages of atherosclerosis tend to occur at a younger age than in nondiabetics.

The chronic hyperglycemic state is known to inhibit leukocyte immune function and phagocytosis, aggravating infection in the wounds induced by CLI. Loss of autonomic fibers may impair postural vasoconstriction responses and responses to vasodilatory influences. Together, these deficits in blood flow, neurological function, and immune function, greatly increase the risk in diabetes for PAOD, CLI, sepsis, and amputation.

Sometimes, neuropathic ulcers are difficult to distinguish from neuroischemic ulcers in which PAOD is a contributing factor. Neuroischemic ulcers raise particularly difficult problems in clinical management. The fundamental problem is that ulcers with only a moderate ischemic component that normally heal, cause limb loss in diabetes. Aggressive application of diagnostic tests and early vascular intervention is warranted in diabetics, particularly in older patients, given their increased risk of amputation. Compared to nondiabetics they tend to have a faster rate of atherosclerotic progression, and the presence of neuropathy may prevent recognition of CLI before severe tissue loss occurs. Noninvasive tests of arterial supply should be performed in all diabetics with ulcers. Arteriography should be considered at an early stage, even when the patient is thought to have neuropathic ulcer, if the ulcer does not heal or there is doubt regarding the arterial circulation. The investigation of neuroischemic ulcers in diabetes should be the same as for nondiabetic patients.[2]

Association of Peripheral Arterial Occlusive Disease With Atherosclerosis in Other Territories

Patients with PAOD are at increased risk for atherosclerosis in other territories. Independent of the common risk factors (smoking, hyperlipidemia, diabetes, hypertension), PAOD correlates with an increased risk of CAD. This heightened association is a consequence of the tendency for atherosclerosis to involve arteries systemically rather than being restricted to just one organ. The most important consequence of this systemic pattern is decreased survival in PAOD. Claudicants have 72% 5-year and 50% 10-year survival rates, compared to 90% 5-year and 75% 10-year survival rates in age matched controls.[39] When matched to patients with identical risk factors except for the presence of PAOD, claudicators have a three- to sixfold higher risk of cardiovascular mortality.[49]

The increased risk of death correlates with whether single or multiple levels of disease in the lower limb are present. As shown in Figures 10 and 11, when multisegment disease is present, overall survival decreases and cardiac deaths increase. These findings are corroborated by another study which found that claudicators undergoing bypass had 55% survival at 5 years compared to CLI patients who had 35% survival.[50] Over 80% of deaths in patients with PAOD are due to myocardial infarction (MI)(60%), stroke (12%), and other vascular catastrophes (10%) such as ruptured aneurysm and mesenteric ischemia.[39] As might be expected based on this natural history, a high incidence of diseased coronary and carotid arteries is found when PAOD patients are studied. Significant carotid occlusive disease was found by duplex ultrasound

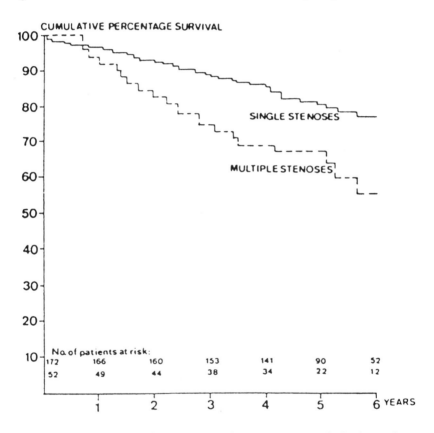

Figure 10. *Impact of multiple segment involvement on survival.* The figure depicts the relative cumulative survival for peripheral arterial occlusive disease (PAOD) patients with either single or multiple arterial segmental disease in the lower extremity. The numbers of patients refer to the **upper** and **lower curves**, respectively. The survivorship curves are significantly different (*P*<0.002), even after adjusting for slight differences in age and the presence of coronary heart disease (CHD). (Reproduced with permission from Reference 182.)

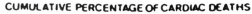

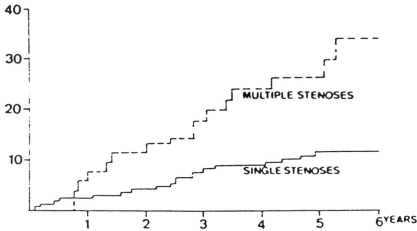

Figure 11. *Cumulative percentage of cardiac deaths.* A higher rate of death from cardiac causes was evident in the multiple stenosis group compared to the single stenosis subjects (*P*<0.001) even after adjustment for age and coronary heart disease (CHD). (Reproduced with permission from Reference 182.)

scanning in over 50% of claudicants in one study,[51] and the incidence of severe stenosis (>60%) may be as high as 10%.[52] Hertzer et al[53] studied CAD via angiography in 1000 peripheral vascular patients being prepared for surgery. Over 90% had detectable CAD, with 31% having severe enough disease that coronary intervention was a consideration. In 27% of the patients with PAOD and severe CAD, the presence of significant coronary stenosis was not suspected based on clinical findings or ECG.[53]

The associations between PAOD and atherosclerosis in other territories can be summarized as: 1) they are frequently found together; 2) significant CAD may be missed, because PAOD can prevent exercise-induced angina from being elicited; 3) patients with PAOD have increased death rates from atherosclerotic complications in other territories, particularly stroke and MI; and 4) more severe PAOD correlates with more severe manifestations of atherosclerosis in other territories.

Treadmill ECG, a relatively inexpensive and reliable screening modality, usually is not practical for evaluation of PAOD patients because of their limited ambulation. Increasingly complicated and costly screening algorithms to detect CAD in PAOD patients using noninvasive methods, such as radionuclide cardiac imaging or echocardiography, have been advocated, with proponents of these methods arguing that they allow a cost-effective identification of those warranting cardiac catheterization.[54,55]

What is very difficult to address, as there is virtually no relevant clinical data,[56] is how helpful extensive cardiac assessment is when a patient with PAOD requires surgery. On the surface, it would seem beneficial to detect occult life-threatening CAD before subjecting PAOD patients to stressful procedures. What is not clear, is how much effort to detect such lesions is optimal, and when coronary lesions detected by a diligent search require intervention. It is generally accepted that if conventional indications for coronary intervention based on symptoms (e.g., angina) or morphological features of a coronary angiogram (e.g., severe diffuse three-vessel disease) are present, coronary revascularization should precede peripheral arterial intervention. What is very unclear is how often "prophylactic" coronary revascularization is beneficial. In prophylactic coronary revascularizations, the indication is essentially that noncardiac surgery is required and that there is CAD amenable to intervention. Virtually no studies have adequately addressed the risk/benefit issues raised. It is expected that survivors of prior coronary interventions will probably have improved mortality when undergoing second procedures such as lower extremity bypass. The important question is whether overall survivorship is improved with aggressive treatment of silent CAD.

To answer this question, a study has to be performed in which patients with PAOD requiring surgery are divided into two groups treated with different strategies. In the first group, every patient would undergo extensive cardiac testing, and significant coronary lesions, when detected, would be treated by angioplasty or coronary bypass surgery. In the other group, less extensive cardiac evaluation would be performed, and the indicated lower extremity surgery would be performed with a much lower rate of prior coronary interventions. The second group should have higher rates of perioperative cardiac complications including MI and death. On the other hand, the first group of patients will probably have a higher rate of coronary interventions and suffer complications from these procedures. Would the overall survival of the patients undergoing two procedures be better than those only undergoing one? This is the type of study that needs to be applied to the questions surrounding the role of cardiac diagnosis and therapy in patients with severe PAOD. Until such data is available, the most helpful point of view is the recommendation of the European Consensus Group:

> Before major peripheral arterial surgery is performed, the possibility of the patient first requiring coronary revascularization or carotid endarterectomy should be considered. Patients with objective evidence of severe myocardial ischemia or symptomatic carotid stenoses should be referred for a specialist's opinion. In practice, coronary revascularization or carotid endarterectomy is rarely indicated before the interventional management of critical limb ischemia.[2]

As lower extremity ischemia is rarely the only problem of an older patient, its management is perceived by most clinicians as palliative. The underlying disease is not curable, and long-term survival is poor. The best result often achieved is for the patient to die of a stroke or heart attack before progressing to the point where lower extremity amputation is necessary. Each patient's symptoms has to be evaluated in the light of the risks created by disease in other organs and the impact success or failure of a vascular intervention will have on the overall quality of life. Patients with equivalent angiographic findings may require completely different management strategies because of psychological, social, and medical factors not directly related to the arterial lesion. The claudicator who cannot work as a mailman requires a different approach than the golfer who is unhappy about having to use an electric cart at the golf course or the comatose patient with gangrene of the foot. The frequent association of PAOD with atherosclerotic degeneration of other organs poses particularly difficult challenges. Often the risk/benefit ratio for limb salvage is prohibitive due to CAD, and the agonizing decision to amputate rather than attempt arterial reconstruction has to be made.

Therapy of Peripheral Arterial Occlusive Disease

Current therapies and interventions for PAOD include medical management, interventional radiology methods such as thrombolysis and balloon angioplasty, conventional surgical reconstruction of arteries via bypass or endarterectomy, and, finally, amputation. The next four sections present an overview of these therapies, concentrating on their distinguishing features.

Medical Management

The most important aspect of managing lower extremity ischemia is distinguishing between limb-threatening CLI and the functional ischemia of claudication. This distinction is generally easy except when neuropathy is present, as the patient may not experience the rest pain associated with inadequate tissue perfusion. Detailed noninvasive studies and even angiography are warranted whenever doubt exists as to the severity of ischemia, particularly in diabetes. The remainder of medical management revolves around reducing risk factors for atherosclerosis in the hopes of slowing disease progression, teaching proper local care of the foot, encouragement of exercise, and providing drug therapy when appropriate.

Given that continued tobacco consumption gravely affects the likelihood of disease progression, it is most helpful if a physician can influence the patient to cease smoking. Approaches combining techniques such as a written contract between patient and physician, counseling, group therapy, biofeedback, and nicotine patch appear to increase abstinence. Even when tissue loss is already present, it is not too late to see tobacco cessation lead to healing and limb salvage. Control of cholesterol, hyperglycemia, and hypertension with diet and medication also help arrest the progression of disease. Both dietary modifications and drug therapy may be warranted to minimize the impact of metabolic abnormalities.

Exercise is very effective in management of claudication. Most patients can double their walking distance within 3 months with a daily exercise routine, leading to improved joint mobility, better neuromuscular function, and a lower incidence of cardiovascular events.[57] These beneficial effects probably are achieved by promoting the formation of arterial collateral vessels, inducing changes in mitochondria and oxidative enzymes in the muscle cell, and, possibly, improved cardiac performance. With advancing age, ambulation consumes a greater proportion of the total possible energy expenditure an individual is capable of. As a consequence, most of the benefits of strenous exercise in the young are achieved in the aged by simple walking.[58] The usual prescription is for the patient to walk at 2 mph for 30 to 60 minutes daily outside or on a treadmill. Increasing the pace to 3 mph or raising the treadmill to a mild incline are useful training modifications.[59] Stationary bicycles and other exercise machines are helpful, but probably are not as effective as treadmills for increasing walking ability. It is important to frequently stress to PAOD patients the benefits of exercise as, with moderation and common sense, they can only help themselves.

In many cases, avoidable trauma to the foot or leg leads to ischemic wounds and ultimate amputation. Patients must be careful to wear properly fitted, sturdy shoes and avoid walking barefoot. Small objects such as a key inside the shoe may cause serious wounding. Careless nail clipping or stepping on sharp objects when walking barefoot equally may be the prologue to a catastrophe. One marker of the pervasiveness of this problem is that many of the patients seen by podiatrists and chiropodists are elderly with circulatory problems. Feet should be bathed daily and the skin kept moist with topical ointments to prevent cracking, which can be a portal of entry for bacterial infections. Similarly, fungal infections should be treated aggressively. Socks should be made of wool or other thick fabrics, and as necessary, cotton waste or lamb's wool should be placed between toes to prevent pressure sores. Diabetics with bony deformity and neuropathy require special efforts to prevent pressure ulceration using measures such as prosthetic boots and orthotic inserts. Diabetic pressure ulcers are more difficult to treat than to prevent.

A few medications have a proven role in the management of chronic lower extremity ischemia. These include anticoagulant and antiplatelet drugs, and the putative rheological agent pentoxifylline. Several experimental agents also seem to have sufficient promise that they warrant mention, despite incomplete clinical evaluation.

Medications which interfere with platelet aggregation, degranulation, and binding to endothelium are of proven efficacy in treating several manifestations of vascular disease. Saphenous vein graft patency is improved by chronic aspirin therapy, as is the incidence of MI.[60] The need for peripheral arterial surgery was reduced in men receiving daily low-dose therapy of 325 mg aspirin.[61] Aspirin inhibits platelet cyclooxygenase, thus inhibiting arachidonic acid synthesis and platelet prostaglandin levels—in particular thromboxane, which promotes platelet aggregation. Another antiplatelet drug, ticlopidine, inhibits platelet aggregation by antagonizing ADP-dependent activation of platelet membrane glycoprotein II_b/III_a receptors. Ticlopidine has a modest effect on claudication in placebo-controlled trials[62] and has effects similar to aspirin on the incidence of MI and stroke.

Anticoagulants other than aspirin are often employed in the management of PAOD. In acute ischemic episodes, heparin therapy is standard, often stabilizing or improving severe ischemia, allowing more time to optimally prepare the patient for surgical intervention. It should be remembered that clotting is the result of fibrin monomer production from fibrinogen cleaved by thrombin. Plasminogen binds to the clot as it forms, and under certain circumstances will be activated to the proteolytic enzyme, plasmin, which divides fibrin into small fragments and causes clot lysis. Heparin inhibits thrombin and platelet aggregation, and shifts the equilibrium between clotting and lysis toward the unopposed action of plasmin, thus favoring clot lysis. After heparin has been employed in the immediate management of managing a thrombotic episode, anticoagulation is maintained for a prolonged period with oral coumadin. A typical scenario is the patient who suffers an acute occlusion of arterial bypass graft. After a successful thrombectomy, it would be common to place such a patient on lifelong anticoagulation with coumadin or coumadin and aspirin. The latter combination with its increased risk of hemorrhage tends to be reserved for patients who clot while on coumadin alone. Current conventional wisdom is that all PAOD patients, with or without grafts, warrant chronic antiplatelet therapy.[2] The optimal roles of aspirin, ticlopidine, warfarin, and various anticoagulant combinations in managing PAOD have not yet been adequately elucidated by prospective clinical trials.

Pentoxifylline is widely used to treat moderate claudication, despite a limited understanding of its mode of action or actual effectiveness. It may significantly improve microcirculatory blood flow by increasing the deformability of the erythrocyte membrane and lowering fibrinogen levels. Alternatively, its effects may be more anti-inflammatory, via an effect on macrophage production of inflammatory mediators or leukocyte adherence to the endothelium.[63,64] Treadmill walking is increased 45% in claudicators on pentoxifylline compared to 23% in placebo controls.[65] The author's impression is that it helps about one third of those receiving it, generally those with the least severe symptoms; an occasional patient reports dramatic or complete resolution of his symptoms with pentoxifylline therapy. As a consequence, it is appropriate to place many claudicants on a short trial, discontinuing the drug if no benefit is apparent at 1 to 3 months.

Prostaglandin E_1 (PGE_1) is a very potent arterial vasodilator. Several analogues, e.g., iloprost, have shown moderate efficacy in promoting ischemic ulcer healing.[66,67] Prostaglandins have short circulating half-lives, as they are readily taken up in the pulmonary circulation; lipid emulsions have been employed to stabilize the drug for intravenous use. Despite difficulties in formulating long-acting compounds, several formulations are continuing to be evaluated in clinical trials.

Arterial Reconstruction

Infrainguinal Bypass

Only a few reconstructive procedures have earned a lasting place in the armamentarium of the vascular surgeon treating PAOD. These include arterial bypass, profundaplasty, endarterectomy, thrombectomy, and sympathectomy. Most reconstructions affecting the lower limb are classified as either *inflow* or *outflow* procedures, depending on whether the immediate effect is increased inflow into the femoral bifurcation or increased flow from the bifurcation distally. Bypasses in which the femoral or a more distal artery is the donor vessel are classified as *outflow* procedures. In contrast, aortofemoral bypass to improve flow into the femoral bifurcation is classified as an *inflow* procedure.

Below the inguinal ligament, bypass surgery is the most common arterial reconstruction, and its results are the standard to which other interventions are compared. It is important to understand the endpoints typically employed to measure bypass success: patency; secondary patency; limb salvage; and patient survival. *Patency* refers to the percentage of bypass grafts that are found to have blood flow at the end of a specified period by life-table analysis. A graft is considered to have *primary patency* if it has had uninterrupted blood flow without any procedures performed to restore flow. A graft is considered to have *secondary patency* if flow is present at the end of the time period under consideration, but has required one or more corrective procedures to restore flow such as thrombectomy and/or revision. In some instances, a graft is recognized to be failing due to progressive intimal hyperplasia or atherosclerosis or some technical defect, and a corrective procedure is carried out to prevent graft thrombosis. Grafts managed in such a manner are deemed to have *assisted primary patency*.

Limb salvage rates and survival rates are also determined by life-table analysis, with limb salvage considered to be achieved if no major amputation has been performed and minor procedures, if necessary, were necessitated by irreversible tissue loss present prior to revascularization. A patient undergoing femoropopliteal bypass whose wounds healed after a subsequent transmetatarsal amputation would be considered a case of successful limb salvage if forefoot gangrene had been present prior to the bypass.

Kunlin first reported the successful use of autologous saphenous vein for infrainguinal bypass in the femoropopliteal position in 1949.[68] Since then, a variety of materials employed as conduits for blood flow have been implanted, and the anatomical variations on infrainguinal bypass have increased. The graft materials most frequently employed today are autologous saphenous vein (in either the reversed or in situ configuration) and expanded polytetrafluoroethylene (PTFE).[69] Other conduits that have been employed with variable degrees of success include Dacron cloth grafts,[70] autologous veins from the arm,[71] human umbilical vein (HUV) heterografts fixed with glutaraldehyde,[72] and glutaraldehyde-fixed carotid arteries from sheep and cows.[73] It is generally agreed that autologous vein conduits yield the best long-term patency rates, particularly with bypass below the knee, and prosthetic materials and heterografts are avoided in distal bypass situations. The success of vein conduits appears to result, at least in part, from decreased anastomotic intimal hyperplasia when vein intima is sewn directly to artery intima; consequently, vein patches at the anastomoses of PTFE grafts have become popular, as this technique improves graft patency.[74]

There are four main classes of bypass below the inguinal ligament, defined by the position of the distal anastomosis. These are *above knee femoropopliteal bypass*, *below knee femoropopliteal bypass*, *tibial bypass*, and *pedal bypass*. Figures 12 and 13 depict femoropopliteal and popliteal-tibial grafts. Depending on whether the popliteal artery is used above or below the knee, a procedure is also labeled as either *suprageniculate* or *infrageniculate*. Tibial bypass encompasses reconstructions where the distal bypass anastomosis employs either the tibioperoneal trunk (the segment distal to the popliteal artery beyond the origin of the anterior tibial artery) or a tibial artery above the ankle. Bypass to the tibial arteries at the level of the ankle or below is occasionally referred to as *paramalleolar* or *inframalleolar bypass*; we employ *pedal bypass* to refer to both. *Infracrural* refers to bypass to distal arteries beyond the popliteal.

Conventionally, bypasses are named by the position of the proximal and distal anastomoses. The most common donor artery is the common femoral, so bypasses based upon this segment are known as *femoropopliteal*, *femorotibial*, or *femoropedal*. The profunda femoris artery may serve as the origin in some circumstances; bypass between the deep femoral and popliteal arteries would be appropriately referred to as a *profundapopliteal graft*. Similarly, a graft based on the popliteal artery and connected to the anterior tibial artery would be properly described as a *popliteal-anterior tibial bypass*. Occasionally, *sequential* grafts are constructed in which two distal anastomoses are created, increasing the runoff of blood flow into the distal circulation. Sequential grafts may employ either side-to-side or end-to-side anastomoses, and are thought to possibly improve long-term patency in cases where high peripheral resistance due to diffuse disease is a problem.[75]

The literature reporting on the results of vascular interventions employs graphic representations of life-table analyses to demonstrate cumulative limb salvage, patency, and survival. Figure 14 shows the relations between these endpoints that have been discerned from the many studies following the fate of patients undergoing bypass surgery.[76-78] Several trends or relations are represented in the figure. First, secondary

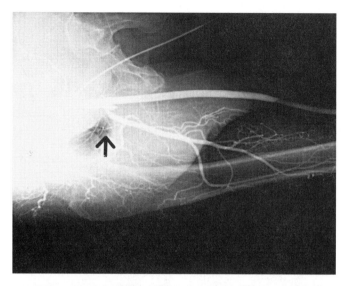

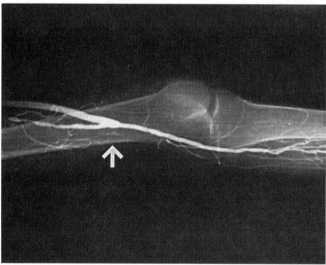

Figures 12A and B. *Contrast arteriogram of patent femoropopliteal bypass graft.* The radiograph shows the origin of the polytetrafluoroethylene (PTFE) graft just proximal to the origin of the deep femoral artery at the bifurcation of the common femoral artery **(black arrow).** The distal anastomosis with the above knee popliteal artery is also shown **(white arrow).**

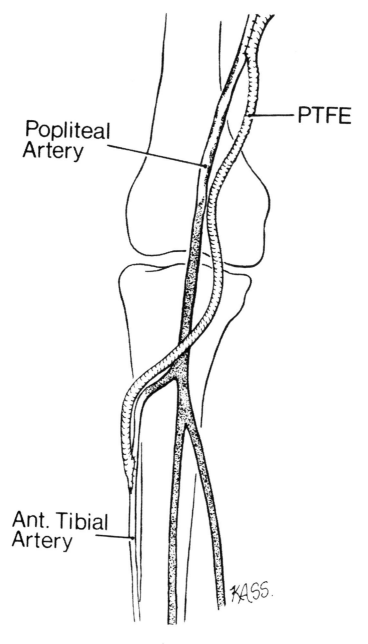

Figure 13. *Popliteal-anterior tibial bypass.* An externally supported ringed polytetra-fluoroethylene (PTFE) graft connecting the proximal popliteal artery to the anterior tibial artery is depicted. (Reproduced with permission from Reference 179.)

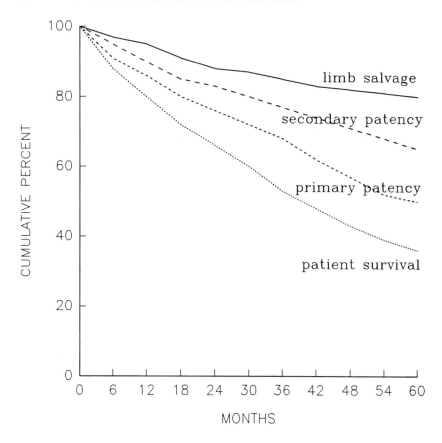

Figure 14. *Life-table analysis of results from infrainguinal bypass.* The idealized relation between limb salvage, graft patency, and patient survival is shown. The relations shown could be for any particular bypass, such as above-knee saphenous vein femoropopliteal bypass. If a more distal anastomosis had been employed, overall rates of salvage, patency, and survival would be shifted downward, but the relative positions of the curves would remain unchanged.

patency of grafts is always better than primary patency, as it represents both grafts that were reopened after occlusion and grafts which never closed. Second, limb salvage rates exceed graft patency rates. In part, this is a result of some bypasses being performed for rest pain or claudication, so failure of the graft does not necessarily mandate amputation. More important is the understanding that when a limb threatened by critical ischemia is salvaged by bypass, the graft often slowly fails with time from progressive atherosclerosis or intimal hyperplasia. When a failing graft finally thromboses, sufficient collaterals often have developed to allow continued limb survival. In this setting, bypass has acted as a bridge allowing the limb to survive until sufficient collaterals have developed. The other important feature depicted in Figure 14 is the tendency for patient survival to be worse than either graft patency or limb salvage. Patients with PAOD, as noted earlier, have accelerated mortality from CAD and cerebrovascular disease, and tend to die after successful limb salvage before critical ischemia leads to amputation.

Several factors influence the expected rates of patency, limb salvage, and survival after infrainguinal bypass. The most important determinants are severity of the ischemia leading to operation, level of the distal anastomosis, quality of runoff arteries below the distal anastomosis (distal resistance), and the type of conduit employed.[79] When the indication for operation is claudication, overall patency rates, limb salvage rates, and patient survival are better than when critical ischemia is the indication. This relation is shown in Figure 15, which depicts survivorship after bypass. Survival is highest in claudicators, intermediate in rest pain, and lowest when tissue loss was the indication for intervention. The correlation of operative indications with mortality is a consequence of more diffuse disease in the leg correlating with more severe manifestations of atherosclerosis in other territories, such as the coronary circulation. If limb salvage had been chosen as the endpoint, the relations depicted in Figure 15 would still hold, as symptom intensity roughly correlates with the degree of atherosclerotic occlusion in the leg. Compared to claudication, more of the tibial vasculature tends to be compromised when rest pain is present. Tibial occlusion correlates with higher resistance in the runoff flow from proximal bypasses, and correlates with decreased graft patency and limb salvage. Similarly, with tissue loss as the indication for bypass, increased limb atherosclerosis tends to result in higher rates of graft failure and amputation. One of the main lessons to be drawn is that the more severe PAOD is at the time of presentation, the more imminent are limb loss and death, even with successful arterial reconstruction.

Figure 16 shows the influence of both conduit employed and the level of bypass. The figure compares limb salvage rates obtained with autologous vein and PTFE grafts. Saphenous vein grafts to the popliteal artery provide the best results, and PTFE grafts to distal tibial vessels the worst. Intermediate rates of limb salvage are achieved with proximal PTFE grafts and distal vein grafts. Knowledge regarding the relative success of these different procedures influences surgical judgment. Most surgeons employ saphenous vein whenever possible for distal bypass because of the poor results obtained when PTFE is used below the knee. Below knee bypass is more technically difficult than above knee femoropopliteal bypass; tibial and pedal bypasses are more challenging yet. Because of these difficulties, and decreased patency and limb salvage rates, distal bypasses are reserved for limb threat and avoided for claudication.

The patency of the tibial arteries is another factor correlating with outcomes. For either above or below knee femoropopliteal bypass, the more tibial vessels are open, the better the results in terms of patency, limb salvage, and survival, with three patent tibial vessels free of disease correlating with much better results than single-vessel tibial runoff.[77,80,81]

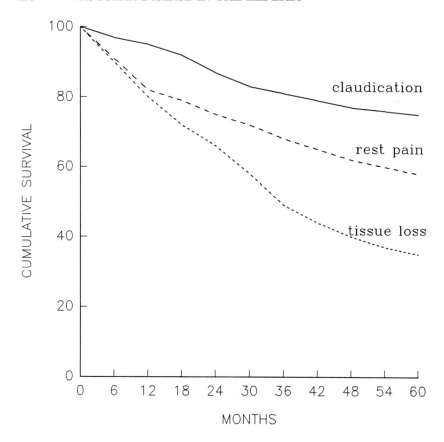

Figure 15. *Survival versus indication for bypass.* The idealized relation between cumulative survival and indication for revascularization is shown. For the same operation (e.g., above knee femoropopliteal bypass), claudicators will have higher long-term survival than those with rest pain or tissue loss. If survival after femorotibial bypass were plotted based on indication, the curves would be shifted downward (as more distal disease correlates with increased vascular death), but the relative positions would be unchanged. Similarly, if limb salvage after above knee vein bypass were plotted, the curves would be shifted up, and the relative positions would remain unchanged.

Two methods are commonly employed when autologous vein is used as the bypass conduit. *Reversed vein* techniques are similar to those used in cardiac bypass: the vein is completely mobilized, checked for leaks or other technical flaws, and anastomosed to the recipient arteries in a reversed configuration relative to the proximal and distal ends. The initial proximal vein end is sewn to the distal artery and the initial distal vein end is sewn to the proximal artery. In the reversed configuration, the valves in the vein offer no resistance to flow.

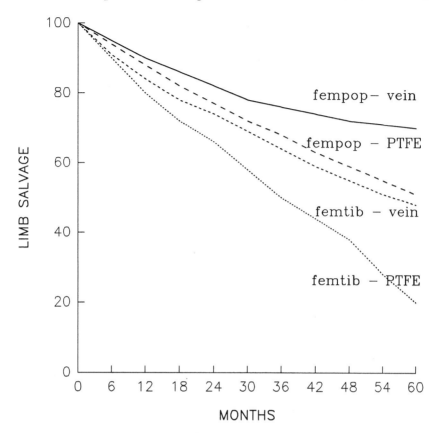

Figure 16. *Limb salvage after different bypass procedures.* The idealized relation between type of bypass and cumulative limb salvage is depicted. The influence of graft material is evident, as for both proximal and distal bypass, saphenous vein grafts yield better limb salvage results than polytetrafluoroethylene (PTFE). With the same graft material, bypass to more distal sites correlates with lower limb salvage rates, as atherosclerosis is more advanced and grafts tend to fail sooner when distal bypass is required.

The in situ method entails passing valvulotomes through the vein to cut the valve cusps and allow retrograde blood flow (Figures 17 and 18). With this method, the vein is not mobilized from its bed. The method was introduced by Hall[82] and subsequently popularized by others.[63,83] The advantages claimed for the in situ technique are: 1) fewer incisions on the leg; 2) improved match between the caliber of the distal vein and artery; and 3) shorter operating time. Proponents of reversed vein technique point out the increased risk of technical problems such as arteriovenous fistula and retained valves with the in situ method, and are concerned that the passage of valvulotomes may damage some veins.

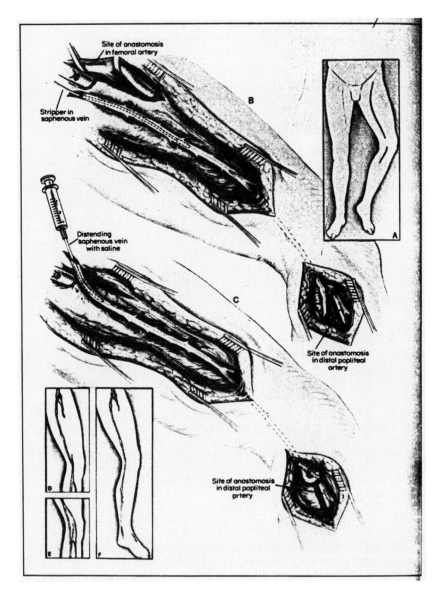

Figure 17. *Method of in situ bypass.* The figure shows the incisions and operative exposure employed to use the saphenous vein without removing it from its bed. (Reproduced with permission from Reference 63.)

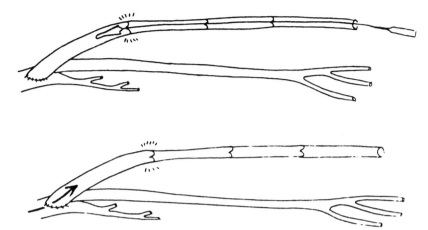

Figure 18. Retrograde valvulotome employed to cut valves with in situ technique. The figure depicts a retrograde valvulotome being passed through the saphenous vein at operation to cut valves and allow reversal of flow through the vein. Many types of valvulotomes are employed for in situ bypass grafting. (Reproduced with permission from Reference 63.)

Randomized prospective studies have not shown any significant advantage of one technique over the other,[84,85] although with either method, small saphenous vein diameter is associated with decreased patency (Figure 19). Good results also have been reported using arm veins[71] and composite grafts made from prosthetic materials and vein segments.[86,87]

Prosthetic cloth grafts (most commonly PTFE) have worse patency and limb salvage rates than autologous vein. The discrepancy is less marked with above knee bypass, where 5-year patency is approximately 50% for PTFE compared to about 70% for vein.[79] With distal bypass, the difference between PTFE and vein are magnified, with primary patency rates of about 50% for vein compared to approximately 20% for PTFE when tibial and pedal bypasses are performed.[86,87] The results of above knee bypass with HUV and Dacron are about the same as with PTFE, although a significant percentage of HUV bypasses undergo significant aneurysmal degeneration within 5 years.[88-90]

It is generally conceded that, compared to patients managed with saphenous vein bypass in the lower limb, PTFE grafts have about a 30% or higher risk of subsequent interventions to maintain patency. Long-term survival of bypass patients is thought not to be sensitive to the choice of graft materials; however, the increased risk of secondary revascularization and amputation procedures appears to make them more expensive in the long-term than vein grafts.[159]

The results achieved with prosthetic grafts like PTFE in the above knee position support their use in patients who can tolerate only short operations (emergency bypass or high-risk patient), or in whom the need

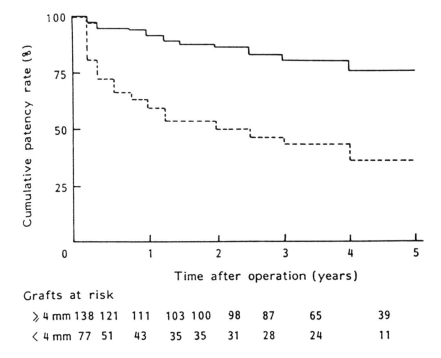

Figure 19. *Influence of vein diameter on saphenous vein graft patency.* The figure shows the results of life-table analysis for vein graft patency. The **top curve** and **row of numbers** represent cumulative patency for veins with a minimum diameter of 4 mm or larger. The **bottom curve** and **row of numbers** represents the patency for veins with minimum diameters less than 4 mm. Highly significantly different patencies are evident (*P*<0.02). (Reproduced with permission from Reference 173.)

to preserve the saphenous vein for possible future coronary bypass is a consideration. Unfortunately, given the association between PAOD and CAD, many patients are high risk, and preservation of the saphenous vein is always a consideration. Although with prosthetic grafts like PTFE the need for secondary procedures is higher due to poorer graft patency, the shortened life expectancy of PAOD patients means that many will die prior to prosthetic graft failure. Given these factors, the indications for use of autologous vein versus prosthetic materials is very controversial. Some argue that because of poor patency, prosthetic grafts should never be employed except when veins are not available. Others argue that the saphenous veins should be preserved for possible coronary bypass, and that prosthetic grafts, particularly for proximal bypass, yield limb salvage rates sufficiently greater than survival to justify their use. This controversy will not subside in the near future. Nested within the vein versus prosthetic graft debate is a nearly as convoluted argument over the proper configuration (reversed or in situ) that is optimal for vein. Potential future improvements in prosthetic graft engineering, such as seeding with endothelial cells[91] or impregnation of the cloth with medications that inhibit intimal hyperplasia, may someday provide better alternatives to autologous vein. Until then, the results achieved with autologous vein, which have been confirmed in numerous studies from multiple centers, will continue to be the gold standard by which all interventions, either surgical or by radiology methods, are judged.

The complications of standard bypass are equally well known. These include perioperative death, early graft failure, wound complications such as lymphorrhea and infection, and leg edema. As shown in Table 2, the overall incidence of death within 30 days of bypass is 2% to 5%, and is predominantly due to MI from CAD.[76,77,79,92] (Also shown in Table 2 are mortality rates associated with older versus younger patients.) Early graft thrombosis is reported to occur in as many as 20% of difficult distal bypasses[93] and may be higher overall in the community. Early graft thrombosis tends to be a consequence of undetected or unavoidable technical flaws at surgery, such as intimal flap, stenosis of an anastomosis, small vein caliber, arteriovenous fistula, and often can be corrected with immediate reoperation. Other factors associated with early graft failure include poor runoff, hypercoaguable states, and systemic hypotension.[94] Wound complications occur in 8% to 19% of reported series of infrainguinal bypass, and include the relatively minor complications of superficial necrosis of skin with delayed healing, and the more significant problems of wound fluid collections and lymphorrhea. The most dreaded complication is deep infection involving the graft. Infected cloth grafts generally require excision of the infected portions of the graft and complex revascularization procedures; prosthetic graft infections are associated with high rates of limb loss. Fortunately, the overall risk of graft sepsis with the modern use of perioperative antibiotics is on the order of 1% to 2%, even when established infection is present in the limb prior to surgery.[95]

Table 2
Mortality of Lower Extremity Bypass

Author (Year)	Number of Patients	Mean Age	30-Day Mortality
Rosenblatt[73] (1990)	171	64	0
Vieth[156] (1990)	857	—	3.1
Taylor[76] (1992)	484	68	2.3
Moody[173] (1992)	226	68	1.8
Whittemore[79] (1995)	3005	—	2.0
Plecha[174] (1985)	2377	<75	2.2
	571	>75	6.7
Gregg[139] (1985)	186	<70	3.5*
	89	>70	15.6*
Bunt[140] (1994)	183	<70	2.2

* hospital mortality

Thrombectomy

Patients who present with a sudden onset of acute limb threat often have embolized clots from a cardiac or peripheral source into the infrainguinal arteries. In many instances, the thrombosis of a previously patent bypass graft creates an identical clinical picture. Surgical management entails operative exposure of one or more of the vessels occluded, fashioning an incision (arteriotomy) into the artery, and extraction of the offending thrombus via the arteriotomy. Embolectomy catheters specifically designed for these procedures are passed via the arteriotomy into the proximal and distal arterial segments. A tip mounted balloon is inflated and traps the thrombus, leading to its extraction as the catheter is gently removed out of the artery. Repeated passes of the thrombectomy catheter will usually result in satisfactory removal of clot and restoration of blood flow.

Adjunctive therapy in patients requiring urgent thrombectomy includes the use of systemic heparin, and other anticoagulants such as aspirin. Diagnostic angiography before surgery is helpful in planning the operation, and intraoperative contrast angiography can be used to position thrombectomy catheters over guidewires and to confirm the restoration of blood flow. Thrombolytic drugs may be administered as part of the operation to dissolve clots either that are incompletely removed by embolectomy catheters or that are lodged in tibial or pedal vessels beyond their reach. The combination of fluoroscopic guidance of embolectomy catheters and the use of intraoperative thrombolytic drugs both improves the overall success of operative interventions and allows distal thrombi to be adequately managed via femoral and popliteal incisions.[96,97] The use of proximal incisions is an advantage, as they avoid arteriotomies of more distal vessels with the risk of intimal hyperplasia and late thrombosis. An additional concern is that incisions below the knee may compromise amputation stump healing if revascularization is unsuccessful.

The overall immediate success rate with surgical thrombectomy and embolectomy for limb salvage in the face of acute occlusion is good, on the order of 70% to 90%. Overall patient mortality, however, is strikingly high; compared to elective limb bypass surgery, the reported mortality ranges from 4% to 39%, with an average rate of about 20% in recent series.[98] Some of the factors responsible for high mortality are metabolic disturbances which accompany acute arterial occlusion of the lower extremity including hyperkalemia, acidosis, and renal failure secondary to rhabdomyolysis. Some of these disturbances are a consequence of cellular necrosis due to ischemia, and may be exacerbated by the reperfusion injury that often attends successful revascularization after severe ischemia. Delay in operative treatment of limb-threatening ischemia correlates with poor outcomes. In one series, treatment instituted within 12 hours of symptom onset led to a limb salvage rate of 93% and 12% mortality. After 12 hours, limb salvage fell to 78% and mortality increased to 31%.[99]

Another factor in the high mortality of embolism is the overlay of severe cardiac disease that is often found, and the frequency of other comorbid diagnoses including advanced malignancy. Increased mortality is associated with advanced age; in one series, those less than 70-years old were found to have 7% mortality compared to 22% for those older than 70.[100]

Occluded bypass grafts are often treated by thrombectomy using techniques similar to those employed with primary thromboembolism. Balloon catheter methods are usually sufficient to allow restoration of flow, and results are good if attendant technical defects restricting flow (most commonly stricture of the distal anastomosis or stenosis in the native artery just beyond) are also corrected. Saphenous vein grafts are more difficult to salvage with thrombectomy than prosthetic grafts. Often in graft thrombosis, clot propagates into the arteries beyond the distal anastomosis (e.g., the tibial origins may be occluded after a femoropopliteal graft clots), and successful thrombectomy requires supplemental removal of thrombus in these distal segments.

Endarterectomy

In 1944, Dos Santos reported on the use of operative thromboendarterectomy[101] in the management of short atherosclerotic occlusions. Modifications of the technique using open and semi-open methods employing special extraction loops and even CO_2 gas dissection methods soon followed.[102,103] In the late 1950s and 1960s, long continuous endarterectomy reconstructions of the femoral and popliteal arteries were widely performed. As long-term follow-up became available, the patency of long endarterectomies of the superficial femoral and popliteal arteries at 5 years (30% to 35%) was significantly worse than femoropopliteal bypass with autogenous vein (>70%). This discrepancy contributed to the general recognition in the 1970s that bypass was the preferred method for long occlusions.[104] Short segment endarterectomy remains reasonable as an alternative method of arterial reconstruction in certain circumstances, and continues to be an adjunct to bypass surgery, when endarterectomy at or near the site of an anastomosis is necessary.

The method of long endarterectomy of the superficial femoral artery (SFA) entails exposure of the vessel throughout the area of significant stenosis and occlusion, making 1 to 3 arteriotomies, and extraction of the plaque via the arteriotomies with careful attention to creating a smooth tapering endpoint at the junction of the endarterectomized and native segments of the artery. The arterial wall is frequently patched with prosthetic graft or autogenous vein.

Endarterectomy of the common femoral artery, distal SFA near the adductor hiatus, and the popliteal artery is still performed for short occlusions isolated to a single arterial segment. The results are good with the larger, proximal arteries (5-year patencies of 94% and 66%

for common femoral artery (CFA) and SFA endarterectomy), but decreased in more distal segments (44% 5-year patency in the popliteal artery).[104]

Profundaplasty

The profunda femoris artery (PFA or deep femoral artery) is the major source of collateral blood flow to the popliteal artery when the SFA is occluded. Distal branches of the PFA form a series of arcades that anastomose with the geniculate branches of the popliteal artery above the knee. The proximal PFA is a common site for atherosclerotic plaque development, with the plaque usually confined to the first 2 to 3 cm of the artery at its origin.

In some circumstances, patients with PAOD who have occlusion of the SFA gain significant benefit from operative reconstruction of the origin of the PFA (*profundaplasty*), allowing increased flow of external iliac blood into the PFA and ultimately the popliteal artery via collaterals. Reconstruction of the PFA aims to improve inflow of blood into the lower limb at the level of the femoral bifurcation and, thus, is classified as an inflow procedure. Profundaplasty is most commonly performed during aortoiliac reconstructions such as aortofemoral and femorofemoral bypass when the SFA is occluded and the origin of the PFA is stenosed. The operative technique employed is to extend the common femoral incision through the origin of the PFA and, using endarterectomy techniques, the atherosclerotic plaque is removed and an adequate arterial lumen constructed. The inflow graft is then tailored and sutured as a tongue to close the profunda arteriotomy in a patch-like manner.

Profundaplasty can also be performed alone. The common femoral, superficial femoral, and profunda arteries are dissected, with the exposure of the distal arteries carried out for several centimeters beyond their origins. An arteriotomy from the common into the deep femoral artery is made and plaque removed. A patch of either prosthetic graft, autologous vein, or frequently, the wall of the adjacent occluded SFA is used to close the incision. The most appropriate use of profundaplasty as a sole intervention is when the origin of PFA is stenosed greater than 50%, the SFA is occluded, and diffuse disease makes bypass to more distal vessels problematic. The 5-year limb salvage rate for profundaplasty alone is about 35% compared to 80% when it is combined with an inflow procedure (Figure 20). As is the case for other infrainguinal reconstructions, isolated profundaplasty has better long-term patency when performed for claudication (>80%) as opposed to limb salvage (<20%).[105,106]

Sympathectomy

Sympathetic denervation of the lower extremity was a widespread practice in the early and middle parts of this century, prior to the

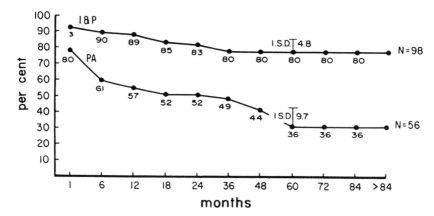

Figure 20. *Cumulative patency after profundaplasty.* Patency after performance of profundaplasty as part of an inflow procedure (e.g., aortofemoral bypass) is shown in the **top curve**, and patency with profundaplasty performed as an isolated procedure is shown in the **bottom curve**. (Reproduced with permission from Reference 106.)

development of direct arterial reconstruction methods. The underlying rationale for sympathectomy is that arterioles and precapillary sphincters are chronically constricted due to nerve impulses conveyed over sympathetic nerve fibers, and that improved blood flow results from removing the vasoconstriction induced by the sympathetic nervous system. The operative technique entails exposure of the sympathetic ganglia of the lumbar vertebra via a small flank incision, and excision of two or more ganglia in continuity. Good results after sympathectomy are particularly likely in patients with causalgia and vasospasm, but the results with PAOD are mixed, and the operation has fallen out of favor.[107] It is now reserved for PAOD patients who are otherwise deemed inoperable and have physiological features suggesting that they may respond to sympathectomy. Potential complications of sympathectomy include injury to the ureter and genitofemoral nerve, retrograde ejaculation, and other sexual disturbances in men, and usually transient postsympathectomy neuralgias.[108]

The immediate effect of sympathectomy in the absence of PAOD is to increase total limb blood flow and skin blood flow in particular.[109] The microcirculation of skeletal muscle is mostly under the control of local vasogenic mediators and insensitive to sympathetic nervous influences. In contrast, the skin has a rich network of arteriovenous anastomotic channels which normally are closed to blood flow because of tonic vasoconstriction mediated by sympathetic fibers. After sympathectomy, increased blood flow is predominantly directed into these skin arteriovenous communications rather than nutritive capillaries supplying skin or muscle. Although skin temperature often prominently increases immediately after sympathectomy, the effect is usually transient as vasomotor tone returns to baseline levels. The limited period of efficacy is due partly to denervated smooth muscle developing increased sensitivity to circulating norepinephrine.[110] In animal models of limb ischemia, sympathectomy does not induce significant improvement in muscle blood flow, and in patients undergoing sympathectomy skin perfusion is similarly unaffected.[111,112]

Despite the laboratory data, in some clinical studies, sympathectomy appears to ameliorate rest pain and improve ulcer healing.[113] The effect on rest pain may be due more to an alteration in the nerve pathways for noxious stimuli rather than improved tissue perfusion, but the wound healing effects observed in a minority of patients indicate that improved skin perfusion might be achieved in some cases. The argument that sympathectomy may improve graft patency by decreasing peripheral resistance and increasing graft blood flow has been put forward, but convincing evidence for this interesting hypothesis is lacking. Current recommendations are that sympathectomy be reserved for inoperable critical ischemia in patients with an intact sympathetic nervous system (diabetics with neuropathy often do not) who have a good response to test injections of local anaesthetic into the sympathetic chain. As an ABPI less than 0.3 prognosticates failure of sympathectomy, the procedure should be restricted to patients with ABPI ≥ 0.3.[114]

Endovascular Interventions

Percutaneous Balloon Angioplasty

The practicality of treating arterial lesions via percutaneous dilation was established by Dotter and Judkins in 1964.[115] The development by Gruntzig in the 1970s of balloon catheters steerable over a guidewire for percutaneous angioplasty has revolutionized the management of atherosclerotic occlusive disease in virtually all territories.[116] Interventionalists trained in radiology, cardiology, or surgery are capable of dilating lesions without surgical exposure of the diseased vessel. Balloon angioplasty is frequently performed as the sole therapy of occlusive lesions during diagnostic angiography and as an adjunctive measure during open-surgical procedures. Studies have shown that when lower extremity stenotic arterial lesions are amenable to either balloon angioplasty or standard surgical therapy, such as patch angioplasty or endarterectomy, interventional techniques provide equivalent outcomes.[117] Long-term follow-up data for the most widely employed intervention, percutaneous balloon angioplasty (PBA), is now available, making an informed discussion of the merits of PBA compared to surgery feasible.

Several factors help predict success or failure of PBA in the management of PAOD including: 1) whether the lesion being treated is a stenosis or a complete occlusion; 2) lesion length; 3) the severity of symptoms, i.e., claudication or limb threat; 4) the anatomical position of the lesion, i.e, femoral, popliteal, or tibial; and 5) the quality of the tibial runoff vessels—how many of the three vessels are patent and relatively disease free. Although femoropopliteal lesions are more frequently encountered than iliac lesions, iliac lesions are technically easier to treat. Much of what has been learned regarding the results of PBA (and other catheter-directed therapies) in PAOD has been derived from iliac artery studies, but the basic influence of the factors enumerated above appear to translate to more distal arterial segments.

The best results with PBA tend to be achieved with short (<5 cm) focal lesions. A good example of the results that can be achieved is demonstrated in Figure 21, showing the effect of a balloon dilatation of a focal popliteal stenosis. Complete occlusions tend to be longer than stenotic lesions, with 94% of iliac stenoses and 79% of femoropopliteal stenoses being 5 cm or less, compared to 30% of iliac occlusions and 9% of femoropopliteal occlusions.[118] The overall 5-year patency rate for all iliac lesions treated with PBA is 70% compared to 52% for all femoropopliteal lesions, which may, in part, reflect the influence of the longer average length of femoropopliteal lesions.[119] Five-year patency after iliac PBA has been reported as 63% in patients with good SFA runoff compared to 51% with occluded SFAs.[120] A comparable study in diabetics found 1-year patency to be 95% with good SFA runoff versus 76% with poor SFA runoff. When follow-up was extended to 5 years, iliac patency after PBA was 77% with good runoff compared to 20% with poor runoff.[121]

Whether the lesion is an occlusion or stenosis is significant in predicting success. In the femoropopliteal position, PBA of stenotic lesions has been reported to achieve a 5-year patency of 77% with good tibial runoff (two or three vessels patent) compared to 59% with poor runoff (zero or one patent vessels).[122] With femoropopliteal occlusions and good tibial runoff, PBA yields a 5-year patency of 34% compared to only 20% when the tibial runoff is poor.[120] The results of PBA in claudicators with long SFA occlusions (mean length = 18 cm) were examined in one study. Seventy-eight percent of all patients with occluded SFAs had immediately successful guidewire recanalization of the occlusion. Balloon angioplasty led to an overall 1-year patency of 40%. Short lesions (≤ 5 cm) had a 62% 1-year patency after PBA compared to 31% with lesions longer than 25 cm.[123]

In most centers, the typical femoropopliteal lesions treated with PBA are short rather than long, and more likely to be stenoses than complete occlusions. Like bypass, the success of PBA appears to be related to the severity of symptoms warranting intervention, with better results found in claudicators than critical ischemia, reflecting the influence of lesion severity and multiple level involvement. With claudication as the indication for femoropopliteal PBA, 62% patency at 3 years has been reported compared to 43% patency in limb-threat patients. Most failures after PBA appear to occur within the first 2 years, with decreasing rates of failure thereafter.[124]

PBA of tibial artery lesions is feasible, and is being performed on an increasingly frequent basis, but often not as the sole intervention performed. Reports on the patency at 2 to 3 years have varied from 75%

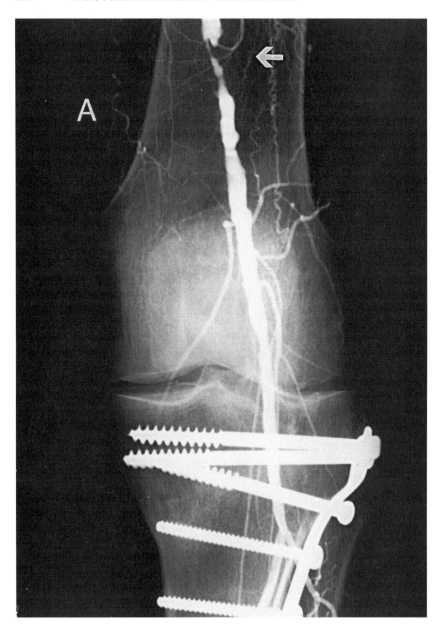

Figure 21A and B. *Percutaneous balloon angioplasty (PBA) of a high-grade popliteal artery stenosis.* **A** and **B** are before and after contrast arteriograms of a popliteal stenosis **(arrows)** treated with balloon angioplasty. The patient's symptoms of claudication ceased after the procedure and the ankle/brachial pressure index (ABPI) increased from 0.62 to 0.84.

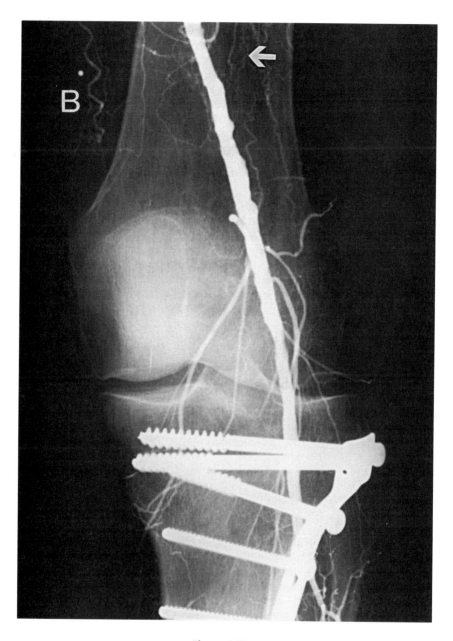

Figure 21B.

to 33%, without obvious reasons for the discrepancy; it is still too early to adequately assess tibial balloon angioplasty.[125,126]

Several factors act in concert to limit the success of balloon angioplasty. First, an angioplasty catheter cannot always be placed in the proper position, even if a wire has been passed. This may be a problem with complete occlusions, or when stenoses are very tight or multiple lesions are present. Second, there is a tendency of atherosclerotic plaque to recoil back into the lumen after balloon dilation. As the offending plaque material is not physically removed during angioplasty, effective displacement out of the lumen implies a contained rupture or dissection of the vessel wall. Third, the vessel wall damaged by mechanical trauma (such as PBA) often responds with a proliferative response known as myointimal hyperplasia, setting the stage for delayed restenosis.

PBA has become an accepted and important part of the management of PAOD. It should be appreciated, however, that this mode of therapy has its own risks, including embolization of clot into distal vessels (which may precipitate limb-threat crises or worsen ischemia), bleeding including retroperitoneal hemorrhage, arteriovenous fistula, and hematoma at the puncture site. All of these risks are greater than those encountered with pure diagnostic angiography, as larger catheters tend to be employed and the length and complexity of the angiographic procedures are increased.

Stents

Stents are metal coils that can be deployed with catheter techniques and expanded at the site of balloon dilations. The inflated stent prevents elastic recoil of atheroma into the lumen, thus preventing immediate restenosis and thrombosis, and represent a major improvement in the endoluminal management of PAOD. A variety of balloon expandable and self-expanding stents are currently in use in Europe or undergoing clinical trials, but the Palmaz stent is the only device currently approved for intravascular use in the United States. The largest experience with stents in PAOD has been in the management of iliac lesions, where at 36-months patency has been found to be 26% better for stented arteries compared to PBA alone.[127,128]

So far, the experience with stents below the inguinal ligament is limited. Our center has one of the largest experiences with stenting of infrainguinal occlusions, having treated over 50 limbs since 1994 with wire recanalization, balloon angioplasty, and deployment of stents to open chronic occlusions of the SFA. Compared to historical controls treated with PBA alone, stented arteries have a 1-year patency rate of over 70% compared to 40% for PBA alone.[129] These findings suggest that stenting below the inguinal ligament, particularly for occlusions, may be a signal improvement in the capability of endoluminal methods to manage PAOD.

Stents do not prevent tissue growth through the interstices. We have seen significant intimal hyperplasia leading to restenosis in about half of our patients with SFA occlusions (Figure 22). Repeat PBA of the hyperplastic tissue is feasible and often is effective, but tissue ingrowth may represent an important inherent limitation on stent therapy, particularly in arteries of small caliber. The vascular community is waiting with great interest the introduction of stents coated with prosthetic materials like PTFE and Dacron, as such devices may, except at the end points, be relatively impervious to restenosis from myointimal hyperplasia.

Lasers and Atherectomy Catheters

The use of laser energy to remove atherosclerotic plaque and penetrate complete obstructions was the subject of intense clinical investigation during the late 1980s. Despite great promise, results were disappointing, as the lased arterial surface often was thrombogenic and led to unwanted clotting, and arterial perforation was a frequent complication. Patency rates for arterial occlusions treated by various laser devices have not been significantly better than those achieved by cold guidewire penetration of occlusions and PBA.[130] At this writing, enthusiasm has waned, and the centers that purchased laser devices rarely use them now.

Atherectomy catheters represent another approach toward endoluminal management of atherosclerotic lesions. These are devices passed over a wire which have a cutting element at the tip to remove plaque. Three catheters have been employed in the United States in recent clinical trials, and represent the spectrum of devices likely to be available in the near future. The Auth Rotablator has a high-speed, diamond-studded burr at its tip. This creates the ability to both drill a channel through complete obstructions and remove plaque. It produces a slurry of small particles, and is claimed to selectively destroy only calcified or fibrous tissue, leaving elastic soft tissue, like the arterial media, uninjured.[131] The Simpson AtheroCath is another device whose cutting element is a spins inside a metal housing at the tip of a flexible catheter. Plaque is forced through a slot toward the cutting element by inflation of a balloon on the opposite side of the catheter tip, giving the operator some directional control. The cut pieces of plaque are trapped inside the metal housing.[132] The Transluminal Endarterectomy Catheter (TEC) is another wire-directed catheter with a screw-like cutting element rotating rapidly inside a metal housing at the tip.[133] Vacuum suction bottles are connected to recover particles and prevent embolization.

Several problems and limitations hamper the current applications of these devices. First, all of them create a potential risk of embolization, which may create significant obstruction, particularly in the tibial circulation. Proponents of the Rotablator claim that the small size of the particles produced by this device avoids this problem; they claim that the tiny particles produced lodge in the microcirculation, avoiding obstruction of larger vessels. Second, the degree of plaque actually removed by these devices may not be sufficient to warrant their applica-

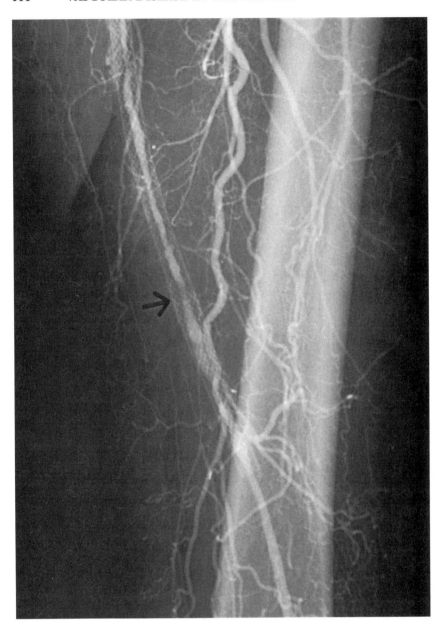

Figure 22. *Contrast arteriogram of stent in superficial femoral artery 1 year later.* One year previous to the arteriogram, the patient had undergone recanalization of a complete occlusion of the supeficial femoral artery with balloon angioplasty and deployment of a Schneider Wallstent. The lumen is now restricted along the length of the stent, presumably due to ingrowth of intimal tissue, since immediately after the angioplasty no stenosis was evident.

tion. Inability to reduce stenoses to less than 50% was a problem in early studies of the Rotablator. Similarly, IVUS studies of TEC atherectomy in our institution indicated that only a small proportion of the total plaque was removed from complete obstructions.[134] A final problem is that the application of these mechanical devices may lead to restenosis from myointimal hyperplasia as a result of arterial wall trauma, overwhelming the short-term benefits. Most studies of the efficacy of these catheters have reported only brief follow-up, and longer periods of observation are required to establish their efficacy.

Catheter-Directed Thrombolysis

Most occlusions in arteries represent a focal area of severe stenosis harboring a blood clot occluding the lumen. With time, the thrombus may propagate and occlude a longer segment of the artery. If fibroblasts invade the clot, tissue is laid down and replaces the thrombus in a process known as organization. The clots in arteries are amenable to dissolution with thrombolytic drugs, particularly within the first month before organization has progressed, but often even after 6 months or longer. Clots within prosthetic bypass grafts may be susceptible to thrombolysis longer, as tissue ingrowth appears to be retarded by the prosthetic cloth. The drugs commonly employed are streptokinase, urokinase, and tPA. All the drugs have a common mechanism, as they activate plasminogen into plasmin, which cleaves polymerized fibrin into small fragments, thus destroying the clot. Although similar efficacy and complications are found with all three drugs, urokinase currently has achieved a position of dominance (at least in North America) for therapy of peripheral arteries because of its better cost:risk:efficacy profile compared to the other drugs. All the thrombolytic drugs carry a significant risk of inducing hemorrhage at remote locations, such as the brain (the risk of stroke due to intracerebral hemorrhage is about 1% to 2%) or the arterial puncture site.[135,136]

Thrombolytic drugs delivered systemically by intravenous infusions have been shown to modestly improve the outcome after acute coronary artery thrombosis in large international trials employing thousands of patients at multiple sites. The standard practice in peripheral arterial surgery, however, is to place catheters directly into the artery for delivery of urokinase into the clot. When the catheter can be optimally positioned, local arterial therapy is more reliable and successful than systemic therapy. Skilled interventional radiologists can tell with fair accuracy when they pass a guidewire through an obstruction whether it is a clot and whether it is likely to be lysed.

During the last 10 years, thrombolytic drugs have become integrated into the clinical armamentarium for vascular disease, leading to a paradigm shift in the management strategy for thrombotic arterial occlusions. Based on randomized prospective trials, it seems that if an arterial occlusion is amenable to either surgery or thrombolysis, similar outcomes are achieved when either therapy is employed as the first step. Both the immediate and long-term (1 year) limb salvage and mortality rates are comparable when either surgery or thrombolysis is the first step.[137] The results with either therapy are very similar when clotted bypass grafts are treated, and the efficacy of thrombolysis as a first step is marginally diminished compared to surgery when long native arterial segments are involved.

Thrombolysis and surgery are best regarded as complementary therapeutic options rather than equivalent approaches. The patient who fails one intervention may be successfully managed by the other, and thrombolysis is a useful adjunct to operative procedures such as balloon thrombectomy. A key concept is that when thrombolysis has been successful in the initial management of an acute lower extremity thrombosis, subsequent surgery or intervention is still usually required to correct the underlying derangement in arterial anatomy. After thrombolysis, precise depiction of the offending lesion by contrast arteriography often allows a less invasive intervention to be performed than otherwise would be needed. For example, after thrombolysis of an acute SFA occlusion, balloon angioplasty of a stenosis may be performed as the definitive intervention in lieu of bypass.

In the acute setting, choosing thrombolysis as the initial therapeutic intervention for limb threat is an accepted and often optimal decision. Although the patient is exposed to the bleeding risks of thrombolysis, including stroke, this appears to be an acceptable trade-off as it decreases the scope of operative procedures, and allows for better preoperative planning.

Amputation

Frequently in PAOD, a decision has to be made whether to pursue vascular reconstruction for limb salvage or to perform amputation. Current practice, when limb salvage is attempted, is to pursue revascularization first, hoping to salvage as much of the limb as possible, and to defer amputation until the maximum benefit of arterial reconstruction has been achieved. In some cases, primary amputation is performed in lieu of revascularization for patients with rest pain or advanced gangrene. There are three major considerations which favor amputation over arterial reconstruction: 1) tissue loss has progressed beyond the point of salvage, even with revascularization; 2) the patient has such severe concomitant medical problems that make vascular surgery too risky, and amputation is perceived as a safer alternative; and 3) limitations in life expectancy or functional ability make limb salvage benefits outweighed by the potential risks and costs.

In most cases, amputation for PAOD is undertaken for gangrene or severe rest pain. It should be emphasized that revascularization and amputation are not mutually exclusive, and although usually performed separately, limited debridement or toe amputation is occasionally performed concomitantly with vascular procedures.

Several principles guide the management of the patient with CLI once the decision to amputate is reached. The amputation ideally will remove all necrotic, painful, or infected tissue. The blood supply to the amputation stump should be sufficient to allow primary healing. The amputated limb should be suitable for fitting to a prosthesis to allow rehabilitation. Finally, as the functional capability of the amputated limb is highly dependent on length, when the patient is a candidate for rehabilitation, as distal a level as possible should be selected for the amputation.

Amputations can be considered as *major* or *minor*, depending on the level selected. Minor amputations such as amputation of one or more toes (toe or ray) or amputation of the distal forefoot (transmetatarsal), provide a foot suitable for walking without a prosthesis; in some cases, depending on the number of digits lost and the level, special shoes or inserts are required. Disarticulation at the level of the tarsal bones is generally unsatisfactory, unless the ankle is fused, as the result is unstable for weight bearing. More proximal amputations at the ankle or higher have increased costs and time required for rehabilitation, and decreased probability of successful restoration of independent ambulation. Transmalleolar (Symes), below knee (BKA), through knee (TKA), and above knee (AKA) amputations are the major amputations usually performed for vascular disease, with BKA and AKA the most common (Figures 23 to 25).

Vascular amputation has a high associated morbidity and mortality, including the need for surgical revision of nonhealing stumps, contralateral limb amputation, and early death.

Hospital stays associated with amputation generally are long and expensive. Long hospitalization may be attributable in part to complications like wound necrosis, stump revision, flexion contractures, and decubitus ulcer formation.

In-hospital death (Table 3) after lower extremity amputation due to PAOD ranges from 5% to 17% within 30 days in modern series, being higher with sepsis and AKA, and lower when sepsis is absent and with distal amputations. Thirty-day mortality figures do not adequately reflect the serious nature of amputation, as within 30 to 60 days after amputation, an equivalent number of patients die as within the first 30 days.[138,139] Survivors of amputation have reduced longevity compared to age matched controls. Long-term survival rates for vascular amputees have varied in reported series (Table 4). Five-year survival for major amputations is approximately 50% to 60%, but significantly poorer survival appears to result from AKA compared to BKA, and advanced age correlates with diminished survival. Bunt and Malone reported only 50% 1-year survival after amputation in patients older than 70, compared to 84% in younger patients.[140] This corresponds to Couch et al's finding that 5-year survival was three times higher in patients under 60 compared to those older than 60 (75% versus 24%).[141]

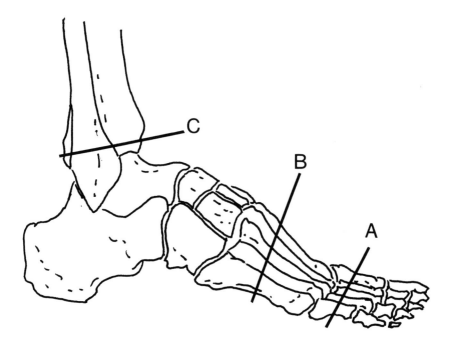

Figure 23. *Levels of foot amputation:* **A.** Level for toe or ray amputation; **B.** Level of transmetatarsal amputation; and **C.** Level of Symes (ankle) amputation.

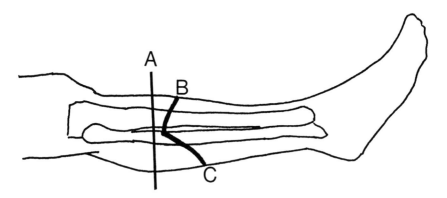

Figure 24. *Below knee amputation (BKA):* **A.** Level of bone division; and **B and C.** skin incision.

As noted earlier, diabetic patients have a four- to tenfold increased risk of ever requiring a major amputation for PAOD. Twenty percent of diabetic admissions to hospital are the result of infections of lower extremity, half of which involve the foot. About half of the foot infections will lead to amputation. The estimated incidence of lower extrem-

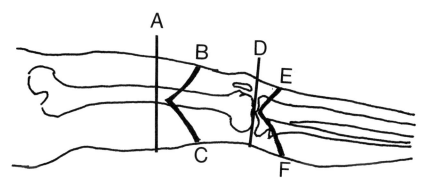

Figure 25. *Through knee and above knee amputations.* **A.** Level of bone division for above-knee amputation (AKA); **BC.** Skin flaps; **D.** Level of disarticulation for through knee amputation (TKA); and **EF.** TKA skin incision.

Table 3
Mortality of Lower Extremity Amputation

Author (Year)	Number of Patients		Mean Age	Mortality
Huston[175] (1980)	AKA	100	65	15
Gregg[139] (1985)	BKA	62	—	8*
	AKA	43	—	23*
Rush[176] (1981)	BKA	110	64	7
	AKA	146	67	16
Couch[141] (1977)		242	60	13
Houghton[151] (1992)		440	72	17*
Plecha[174] (1985)		783	<75	9.8
			>75	14.7
Bunt[140] (1994)		212	<70	1.5
		253	>70	8.0

* hospital mortality

ity amputation in high-risk diabetics is 6% to 12% per year. After amputation, diabetics have an increased risk for contralateral amputation (40% within 3 years) compared to nondiabetic patients. The overall risk of contralateral amputation within 5 years is estimated as 20% to 40% for nondiabetics, and may be as high as 50% within 5 years for diabetics who have already had a major amputation. In one study, diabetics had a 39% 5-year survival after amputation compared to a 75% 5-year survival in nondiabetic amputees, and an 85% 5-year survival in age matched controls.[142-144]

Table 4
Long-Term Survival After Amputation or Revascularization for Critical Ischemia

Author (Year)	Procedure	Mean Number	Age	Survival
Huston[175] (1980)	AKA	100	65	56% at 2 years
Couch[141] (1977)	BKA + AKA	32	<60	75% at 5 years
		141	>60	24% at 5 years
Rush[176] (1981)	BKA	121	64	63% at 5 years
	AKA	146	67	51% at 5 years
Bunt[140] (1994)	BKA + AKA	212	<70	84% at 1 year
	BKA + AKA	253	>70	50% at 1 year
Whittemore[79] (1995)	bypass	230	65	60% at 5 years
Vieth[179] (1981)	bypass	522	—	48% at 5 years
Taylor[76] (1990)	bypass	498	68	38% at 5 years
Hobson[178] (1985)	BKA	172	67	58% at 5 years
	bypass	375	66	59% at 5 years
Ouriel[177] (1988)	BKA + AKA	158	70	54% at 3 years
	bypass	204	68	80% at 3 years

Approximately 20% of BKA and 10% of AKA fail to heal primarily, leading to prolonged hospitalization, repeated surgery, and extended convalescence.[144,145] Early complications in stump healing are usually a consequence of inadequate arterial inflow, and the main factors determining the level of amputation, other than the extent of necrosis and infection present, are preoperative and intraoperative assessments of blood flow. To a large degree, the two main goals of amputation surgery, fashioning a stump which heals primarily and preservation of limb length, are in conflict. The higher the level chosen, the more likely healing is to be successful, but at the expense of functional performance. Alternatively, lower levels of amputation increase the risk of wound complications. Techniques used to assess blood flow include noninvasive ultrasound measurements of ABPI and velocity waveforms, $tcPO_2$,[146,147] and in some centers, measurements of skin or limb perfusion via laser Doppler techniques, calorimetry, or dye or isotope clearance. Whatever method of blood flow assessment is employed, the goal is to accurately choose the lowest level of amputation that is likely to heal.

It is important to understand the physiological impact of amputation on the elderly patient's functional ability and quality of life. Several factors play a role. First, ambulation with a prosthesis requires more energy expenditure than ambulation on an intact limb. The higher the level of amputation, the more energy is demanded for ambulation. Table 5 uses oxygen consumption as a marker of energy expenditure, and shows the expected increased total energy requirement for ambulation with a prosthesis after amputation. Ambulation by a unilateral BK amputee requires 33% more energy expenditure, 87% more in the unilat-

Table 5
Energy Expenditure with Ambulation in Vascular Amputees*

Amputation Increase	Oxygen Cost (mL O₂/kg-meter)**	%
Normals	0.15	—
Unilateral		
Symes	0.17	13
Unilateral BKA	0.20	33
Unilateral AKA	0.28	87
Bilateral BKA	0.31	106

** Determined by oxygen consumption measurements during walking on a level surface at a comfortable walking speed.
(Reproduced with permission from Reference 149.)

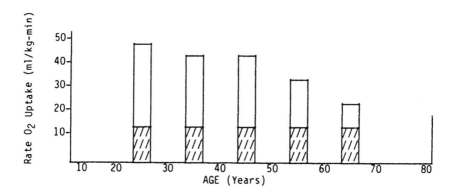

Figure 26. *Relation between age, ambulation, and maximal aerobic capacity.* The **height of each bar** corresponds to the maximal sustained O₂ consumption possible at each age. **Hatched areas** represent the rate of energy expenditure with ambulation. With increasing age, the energy required for ambulation represents an increasing percentage of maximal energy expenditure. (Reproduced with permission from Reference 183.)

eral AK amputee, and over 100% more in the bilateral BK amputee. Secondly, as shown in Figure 26, although the energy of ambulation, measured as oxygen uptake (mL 0₂ /kg per min) remains fairly constant with age, with increasing age, the overall ability to expend energy decreases. As a consequence, the percentage of total energy output devoted to normal ambulation increases from about 30% at age 25 to 55% at age 65.[148] It can be readily discerned, based on the data shown in Table 5 and Figure 26, that many geriatric amputees will be incapable of meeting the physiological demands of prosthetic ambulation with even a BKA, and that a unilateral AKA should make ambulation impossible for most older patients.

Because elderly patients do not have the cardiovascular reserve for ambulation with a prosthesis, they are much less likely to be rehabilitated than younger patients. This is despite advances in prosthetic design and the introduction of improved rehabilitation methods, such as early postoperative ambulation on prostheses. In one series, only 30% of geriatric amputees with AKAs were ambulatory with a prosthesis compared to 70% of BKA patients.[141] A recent study limited to just reasonable candidates found that less than two thirds of patients were, in fact, significantly rehabilitated after BKA.[149] Every series has shown that with AKA or bilateral amputation, the prospects of rehabilitation are worse than those found with BKA. A particularly important point to emphasize is that with advanced age, the average level required for amputation rises. In one study, patients less than age 55 required AKA 12.5% of the time, those between ages 55 and 74 required AKA about 50% of the time, and patients 75 and older required AKA 68% of the time.[139] Not only do older patients have decreased energy reserves for rehabilitation, they generally require higher levels of amputation.

Some caution is warranted when assessing claims for successful rehabilitation. Published reports asserting excellent rehabilitation rates usually come from special centers with a high mix of young trauma patients. An additional problem is the loose manner in which successful rehabilitation is defined in the literature. Some authors have considered the ability to wear a prosthesis as evidence of rehabilitation, without measuring functional aspects of ambulation and mobility.

A grim perspective on the potential for rehabilitation is offered by a recent British survey of vascular amputees. Four hundred forty patients (median age 72) at eight different centers underwent amputation between 1986 and 1988 (193 unilateral AKAs, 193 unilateral BKAs, 54 others). Seventy-five patients died in hospital, 113 were deemed unsuitable, and the remaining 252 patients (57%) were actually referred for prosthesis fitting. Of the survivors referred for prosthesis rehabilitation, only 12% achieved mobility independent of a wheelchair; another 29% were able to achieve limited mobility around their homes with the prosthesis. Nearly half the amputees actually fitted never wore their prostheses. Using the entire population of 440 amputees, only 5% ultimately achieved independent ambulation and another 12% achieved partial rehabilitation. Rates of rehabilitation were approximately twice as high with BKA as with AKA.[150]

Similar findings were reported from the American community experience.[139] With patients below the age of 75, 40% with AKA and 80% with BKA actually wore a prosthesis. In contrast, with patients 75 and older, only 5% of AKA and 40% of BKA patients were subsequently found to be actually wearing a prosthesis. These results are discouraging. The low likelihood of achieving rehabilitation of geriatric amputees remains a tremendous problem, and is the major impetus for the development of revascularization methods.

Strategies in Choosing Therapy for
Peripheral Arterial Occlusive Disease

The goal of vascular surgeons and other specialists treating patients with PAOD is to assess the severity of symptoms and risk of limb loss, and apply therapy which appropriately matches, in terms of potential benefit and risk, the needs of the individual patient. Table 6 shows the potential interventions appropriate for each level of ischemia, and reflects the prevailing practice patterns in the United States in 1996. The table lists options—not every therapy is meant to be applied to a patient. Symptoms are difficult to quantitate, and do not correlate precisely with objective measurements of ischemia such as ABPI. As a consequence, the therapy chosen for one patient may be quite different than that chosen for another, although clinical findings are equivalent.

It also should be remembered that standard surgical and endoluminal interventions carry some risks of either failing to provide benefit or worsening a patient's symptoms; as a consequence, particularly for patients with moderate claudication, there may be no compelling reason to pursue any therapy other than medical management with an emphasis on exercise therapy. A group at Oxford conducted a particularly interesting study which examined the outcome when claudicators were assigned to either exercise rehabilitation or balloon angioplasty. The two groups had equal disease based on initial walking distance and ABPI. Immediately after balloon angioplasty, patients had significant elevations in ABPIs. At the end of 1 year, however, there was no significant difference in ABPI between the two groups, and the claudicators assigned exercise training were walking three times further than their baseline.[151] This result supports reserving surgical or endovascular ther-

Table 6	
Indications for Therapy in PAOD	
Symptoms	*Interventions*
mild to moderate claudication	medical management of risk factors
	adjust beta and calcium channel blockers
	diabetic foot education
	graded walking program
	± pentoxifylline
severe/incapacitating claudication	medical management (see above)
	angiography ± endoluminal therapy
	± arterial surgery
critical limb ischemia (rest pain or gangrene)	angiography
	arterial surgery
	± endoluminal therapy
	± amputation

PAOD = peripheral arterial occlusive disease

apy, in the absence of limb-threatening ischemia, for patients temperamentally incapable of entering into a graded exercise program.

There is a case for performing angiography and potentially intervening with endoluminal techniques when claudication is very severe or disabling. As balloon angioplasty is in fact relatively safer than surgery, it seems appropriate to offer this form of therapy for patients whose quality of life is severely diminished, even though the long-term risk of limb loss is moderate, and the progression from functional to critical ischemia is usually sufficiently slow to allow timely surgical intervention for limb salvage. It is important to remember, however, that there is no evidence that either surgical or endoluminal interventions are more effective than medical management in preventing limb loss or improving quality of life. Endoluminal and surgical procedures carry risks of thrombosis, embolism, and bleeding that occasionally precipitate limb-threatening emergencies and even, rarely, limb loss or death. These catastrophes instill in the conscientious practitioner a healthy regard for the principle that every therapeutic intervention has an equal and opposite potential complication.

Despite these widely appreciated concerns, it is increasingly common to perform contrast angiography to diagnose PAOD, hoping to find lesions amenable to endoluminal therapy in patients who would not necessarily be considered surgical candidates. Many centers perform angiography with the understanding that during the procedure, arterial lesions amenable to catheter-directed therapy will be treated. Claudicators are advised that surgery is unlikely to be recommended, unless a lesion which is particularly favorable to surgical reconstruction, e.g., a common femoral obstruction which can be treated with endarterectomy, is found. With diabetic patients, the standards for intervention perhaps should be relaxed, because they do not experience the same symptoms that nondiabetics do. A more aggressive approach to revascularization seems appropriate in order to reduce the risk of limb loss, when clinical findings of marked ischemia, corroborated by noninvasive testing, are present.

With critical ischemia, the decision to intervene is much easier, as the limb is threatened and amputation may be required if revascularization is deferred or unsuccessful. The issue is not whether to treat, but which therapy, surgical reconstruction, endoluminal therapy, or amputation should be chosen. Two decisions need to be made, first whether to pursue revascularization or amputation (see below), and if revascularization is elected, whether to attempt endoluminal or conventional surgical therapy.

Once the decision is made to pursue revascularization and an angiogram is obtained, two new issues arise. First, is an inflow procedure (a suprainguinal bypass or femoral reconstruction) required, or an outflow procedure (infrainguinal reconstruction), or both? Second, the issue is raised whether strictly endoluminal methods such as balloon angioplasty should be employed, or standard arterial reconstructive surgery, or a combination of both. In some cases, both inflow and outflow procedures are required, and endoluminal techniques are used to reconstruct one segment and surgical techniques the other. An example would be a patient with iliac stenosis and occlusion of the SFA. Limb salvage might entail balloon angioplasty of the iliac lesion as an inflow procedure, and a femoropopliteal bypass as an outflow procedure.

In determining whether endoluminal methods are to be employed, the most important concern is whether the identified lesions are practically amenable to endoluminal methods. A guidewire must be capable of being passed through the lesion in most instances to make endoluminal therapy possible. Another concern is the length of the lesion. Short stenoses and obstructions (<5 cm) may be reasonably managed with balloon angioplasty and possibly stent deployment. For long lesions above the knee, or short occlusions below the knee, endoluminal methods yield less satisfactory outcomes, and bypass is the conventional first choice when limb threat is present. In CLI, when a clot amenable to catheter-directed thrombolysis is found during angiography, the available data suggests that comparable results (amputation-free survival) are achieved with either initial thrombolysis or initial surgery; increasingly, thrombolysis is elected.

Although there are no hard and fast rules for when to use endoluminal versus surgical methods, several general principles have evolved from the continuous evolution in clinical judgment that is emerging from fruitful (albeit at times adversarial) interplay between interventional radiologists and vascular surgeons. In the absence of limb threat, endoluminal methods are generally preferable and, as if feasible, such procedures appear to expose the patient to lower risks and costs, without usually increasing the risk of progression on to limb threat. When limb-threatening ischemia is present, and only a single level of occlusion is found, and the lesion is short, endoluminal methods are favored. If the responsible lesion is long or multiple segments are involved, surgical reconstruction, usually bypass, is more often preferable.

Endoluminal interventions are increasingly employed as the first step in the management of severe PAOD, as endoluminal interventions are both cheaper than surgical arterial reconstruction and require shorter hospital stays.[152] It also appears that when restenosis or occlusion occurs after initially successful angioplasty, second or even third endoluminal interventions are feasible, without creating undue hazards for the patient.[153,154]

The data in Table 7 is drawn from one center with a reputation for aggressive limb salvage efforts.[155] It illustrates the role that balloon angioplasty (and increasingly endovascular stents) has, along with other procedures, undertaken for limb salvage. Taken from a time before stents were generally employed, this data illustrates in practice how endoluminal and surgical methods are married. Several important features are demonstrated including: 1) a low incidence of primary amputation; 2) most limbs required more than one procedure (the average number per limb being 1.67); 3) 24.5% of limbs required only inflow procedures, 62.5% only outflow procedures, and 13% both types of procedures; and

Table 7
Distribution of Procedures Performed in 393 Threatened Limbs*

Type of Procedure	Number	(% limbs)
all	658	(100)
all amputations	56	(14.2)
primary amputation	21	(5.3)
secondary amputation	35	(8.9)
total inflow	190	(48.3)
balloon angioplasty	95	(24.2)
bypass graft	95	(24.2)
total outflow	447	(113.7)
balloon angioplasty	88	(26.2)
bypass graft	344	(87.5)
suprainguinal only	96	(24.5)
infrainguinal only	246	(62.5)
suprainguinal + infrainguinal	51	(13.0)

The table shows the distribution of procedures reportedly performed to manage the limb threatening ischemia over a 2-year period (1988–1989) at one institution. The raw numbers of each type of procedure are shown, as well as the percentage of limbs requiring each type. The total number of procedures, 658, represents an average of 1.67 procedures being performed for each limb.

(Reproduced with permission from Reference 156.)

4) half of the inflow procedures were performed with balloon angioplasty compared to 23% of the outflow procedures. Some conclusions that could be drawn from this data are: 1) primary amputation can be avoided with aggressive revascularization with therapy of multiple levels; 2) outflow procedures are more likely to be needed than inflow procedures with limb threat; 3) although an important option in managing infrainguinal disease, angioplasty is more likely to be helpful with aortoiliac rather than distal disease; and 4) most salvaged limbs require infrainguinal bypass as part of the overall revascularization.

Does Revascularization Lead to Lower Amputation Rates?

It should be appreciated that the frequency with which PBA has been applied to patients with PAOD has dramatically increased over the last 20 years. Between 1979 and 1989, the rate of angioplasty in the state of Maryland increased from 1 to 24 per 100,000 (excluding those under 25 years old); during the same interval, bypass surgery rates increased from 32 to 65 per 100,000, and amputation rates remained stable at 30 per 100,000 (Figure 27).[156] At face value, this observation has the disturbing implication that PBA does nothing to prevent the need for bypass or amputation, and it even has been taken to indicate

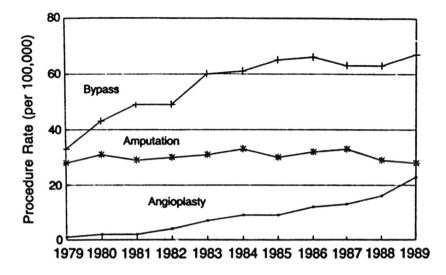

Figure 27. *Utilization of angioplasty, bypass, and amputation over a 10-year period.* The figure shows crude rates of procedure employment (ignoring subjects younger than 25 years of age) from 1979 through 1989. A marked increase in the use of angioplasty was evident during this period, along with an increase in bypass utilization. Crude amputation rates remained stable. The data is drawn from all nonfederal hospitals in Maryland. (Reproduced with permission from Reference 157.)

that revascularization is ineffective, given the stability of amputation rates over a period of time where the rate of revascularizations increased. Such an interpretation fails to consider the tendency to use PBA more for claudication than limb threat, or if used in critical ischemia, to be used in conjunction with infrainguinal bypass. Given the overall low chance of claudication to lead to limb threat, it is not surprising that balloon angioplasty has not a had a major impact on the utilization of bypass or amputation.

The data from Maryland is too crude to justify any inferences regarding the efficacy of revascularization in diminishing amputation. First, the data for amputations does not distinguish between minor and major amputations, and does not distinguish between BKA and AKA. Did the average level of amputation decline over the decade of study? A trend over 10 years for more lower levels of amputation to be employed would indicate that attempts at limb salvage were at least partially successful. More detailed information regarding the type of amputations performed is required. A second problem with interpreting this data is the failure to use age-adjusted rates for amputation and revascularization. Later data from Maryland by the same group show how procedure rates vary with age, with amputation more frequently applied to older patients (Figure 28). Given the aging that occurred in the Maryland population over the study interval, the observation that overall amputa-

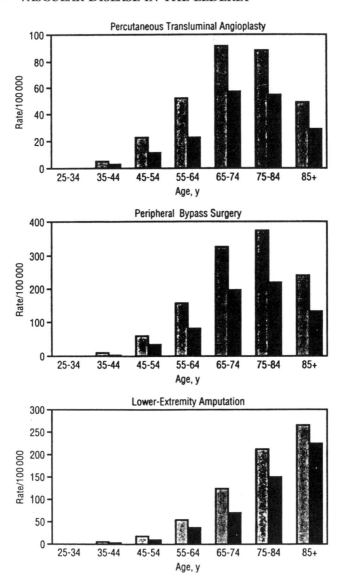

Figure 28. *Influence of age and gender on utilization of angioplasty, bypass, and amputation.* The histogram depicts the rate of procedure utilization (procedures per 100,000 per year) for individual age groups. **Solid black bars** represent men; **stippled bars** represent women. Note that the highest rate of angioplasty is in those aged 65 to 74, the highest rate of bypass is in those aged 75 to 84, and amputation rates are highest in those 85 and older. The data is drawn from all nonfederal hospitals in Maryland over a 2-year period. (Reproduced with permission from Reference 165.)

tion rates were stable actually implies efficacy, as more amputations would have been expected as the population age structure shifted to a higher mean age over one decade. Proper assessment of the efficacy of revascularization based on population measurements requires age-adjusted rates of procedure utilization (e.g., procedures per 100,000 persons aged 50 to 60 per year).

Revascularization or Amputation?

With critical ischemia, the alternative to revascularization is amputation. Given the potential results of revascularization, the proposition that vascular surgery for PAOD is better than amputation may seem self-evident. Nonetheless, the fact that a procedure can be performed is not a convincing argument that it should be. Some argue, based on comparative costs, morbidity, and mortality, particularly in the aged, that amputation is superior. Proponents of primary amputation (i.e., amputation without prior limb salvage revascularization) point to the relative costs of the procedures, claiming that amputation is cheaper, due to the frequent and costly secondary procedures required to maintain graft patency. Proponents of amputation claim that amputation has a lower morbidity and mortality for elderly or high-risk patients. Successful amputation is definitive, sparing patients further operations and allowing them to get along with their lives without the specter of continuing intensive care for an ailing limb. Finally, some data suggests that the final level of amputation required after failed arterial reconstruction is often higher than would have been necessary if limb salvage had not been attempted.

Supporters of revascularization point to overall high rates of limb salvage after revascularization for critical ischemia, and note the devastating impact of major amputation on quality of life and the poor chances for rehabilitation after major amputation, particularly in the aged. Supporters of revascularization argue that it is, in fact, safer and less costly than amputation, both in elderly and young patients.

To some degree, the debate between the two camps is more apparent than real, as many amputations resulting from PAOD, at least in the United States, are performed by vascular surgeons capable of limb salvage surgery. The vascular surgeon always hopes to choose the optimal course for each individual patient, balancing the risks, benefits, and costs. For any given patient, the decision between arterial reconstruction and amputation is based on physiological status and risk for anesthesia, functional status, and the condition of the limb. Revascularization is not pursued in bedridden patients who do not already ambulate, and similarly is avoided in severely demented or incapacitated patients. The issue is clouded for patients with limited mobility, perhaps from a previous contralateral amputation. Are greater efforts to salvage the newly threatened limb justified or, based on the previous result with the amputated limb, is limb salvage relatively unlikely? How does one objectively define a patient in whom revascularization is too risky? Is it the first attempt at revascularization that carries the most risk, or is it the tendency to persistently pursue limb salvage, once started down that path, that puts the patient in harm's way? To some degree, these questions are unanswerable, as the best method of distinguishing between alternative clinical strategies and random prospective trials has not and probably never will be fully applied to the questions posed by the dichotomy between amputation and limb salvage, given the success of lower extremity revascularization procedures and the ethical issues raised.

In general, with any patient who has limb-threatening ischemia, four questions are raised; the answers determine the choice of amputation or vascular reconstruction: 1) Is the patient technically amenable to revascularization? 2) Has the degree of tissue loss or sepsis in the limb progressed beyond the point of a reasonable hope of limb salvage? 3) Does the patient have sufficient functional capacity that he or she would ambulate or be capable of independently transferring if limb salvage were successful? and 4) Is the patient an unacceptably high risk for vascular surgery compared to amputation?

Whether a patient is technically amenable to revascularization is essentially a question of whether a distal vessel exists that is sufficiently free of disease and large enough to provide adequate runoff for a bypass to deliver blood flow into the ischemic portion of circulation. With femoropopliteal disease, a patent popliteal artery with at least one tibial runoff vessel would suffice for an attempt at femoropopliteal bypass. With tibial obstruction, a distal tibial artery that feeds the pedal circulation should be visualized either by angiography (preoperative or intraoperative) or duplex ultrasound to make the attempt at tibial bypass reasonable. Distal bypass to the inframalleolar or pedal vessels is increasingly advocated by aggressive proponents of limb salvage, but even such distal bypasses require an intact target vessel. When distal bypass is required, the absence of saphenous vein, the optimum conduit, is per se not an argument against limb salvage, as upper extremity veins or PTFE vein composite grafts often provide satisfactory results.

In the past, the presence of systemic sepsis or extensive tissue loss would have pushed clinical judgment toward amputation for life salvage, rather than revascularization for limb salvage. The experience of vascular surgeons in the last 15 years, however, has increasingly demonstrated that cases once deemed hopeless can be successfully managed by limited drainage procedures of the foot, often guided by advanced imaging techniques in combination with broad spectrum antibiotics and timely revascularization. Similarly, severe tissue loss such as large hind foot ulcers are now successfully managed with muscle and myocutaneous pedicle or free flaps, taking advantage of the revascularized distal circulation.[157] Again, cases once deemed hopeless can be now salvaged, although multiple debridements and plastic reconstructions may be necessary.

The patient's functional status remains the major consideration in choosing between amputation and arterial reconstruction. Severely compromised patients, such as those with terminal illness and very limited life expectancy are best managed without revascularization. Patients already bedridden or wheelchair bound from the sequelae of a stroke or a previous amputation often are the simplest cases to resolve—revascularization is avoided as it will usually provide little functional benefit. Even so, there are exceptions. The above knee amputee in a wheelchair, although not ambulatory, may have great difficulty balancing seated after bilateral high AKA, and revascularization to achieve a BKA level on one side may be indicated to preserve the ability to sit. Similarly, unilateral amputees who do not ambulate, may still independently transfer from bed to wheelchair with one intact limb. Such a patient often loses independence and becomes dependent on others for total care after a second amputation. Revascularization may prevent an individual from becoming bedridden or becoming a nursing home inmate.

The question of whether a patient is too high a risk for amputation or revascularization presupposes that vascular surgery is more hazardous than amputation. The conventional wisdom widely ascribed to by those familiar (although not necessarily expert) with these matters is that the longer time required to perform vascular procedures and the greater need for transfusion make lower extremity revascularization more dangerous than amputation. It is conceded that there are patients who are too high a risk even for a haircut, much less several hours of anesthesia and surgery, and amputation is the best strategy in these often moribund individuals.

The worst controversy surrounds the typical patient for whom the question of amputation versus limb salvage is usually raised. This would generally be an elderly individual greater than 70 who has limited activity and significant medical problems such as pulmonary or cardiac disease. The assessment of risk for patients like this is imprecise, and should not be solely based on objective scales at the expense of the judgment and experience of the physicians taking care of the patient. Further, the risks of amputation appear great because the patients undergoing the procedure tend to have more advanced vascular disease and more comorbid diagnoses than revascularization candidates. In many cases, amputation is performed on patients who have already suffered graft failure, carrying many implications regarding the risks for the procedure. Arterial anatomy that precludes bypass and decreased functional status are both surrogate markers for increased anaesthetic risk from CAD and other medical problems. As a consequence, comparison of the risk of arterial reconstruction versus amputation is seriously confounded by the significantly greater medical problems of the amputation group. An additional confounding factor is that when amputation is deemed necessary, the patient is more likely to present with life-threatening sepsis, making the overall risks higher.

Accordingly, and not surprisingly, retrospective studies examining perioperative mortality show that revascularization has lower mortality, being 2% to 4%, compared to about 15% with amputation. When the risks are stratified on the basis of age (Tables 2, 3, and 4), two trends are evident. The overall risk of 30-day mortality in the elderly is greater than younger patients with either amputation and revascularization. Second, when the risk of amputation is compared to limb salvage, at any age the latter remains the apparently safer option.

Ouriel et al[177] offered the best available analysis of the situation (Table 8), retrospectively classifying patients undergoing either procedure as low, intermediate, or high risk, depending on cardiac risk factors (Goldman scale) and the American Society of Anaesthesiologists classification of operative risk (ASA scale). With low- and intermediate-risk patients, amputation and revascularization had comparable low mortalities (0% to 3%). In contrast, high-risk patients had significantly greater (p<0.05) 30-day mortality with amputation than bypass (16% versus 6%). With all risk categories, revascularization yielded significantly improved prospects for rehabilitation and decreased length of stay.

Despite the caveat that amputation patients and revascularization patients are not identical in risk, the available evidence does not support the proposition that amputation is actually safer, even in high-risk or elderly patients.

An interesting question is which of the two options has better long-term survival (Tables 4 and 8). In Ouriel et al's study,[177] 29% of high-risk amputees were alive at 3 years compared to 76% of high-risk bypass patients. This comparison is confounded, however, by the fact that the bypass patients were, on the average, 1.5 years younger than the amputees. The lack of long-term survival data indexed by preoperative risk and adjusted for age make it impossible to quantify differences in long-term mortality related to amputation versus revascularization. Some authors have speculated that amputation has a negative impact on survival independent of risk factors due to patients becoming bedridden, which causes increased thromboembolism and perhaps a hypercoaguable state accelerating coronary and cerebrovascular thrombosis. The emotional and psychological impacts of amputation could also conceivably play a role. Perhaps psychic depression and melancholy induced by amputation have a direct mortal impact on health. Another possibility is that health providers for amputees, perceiving a diminished quality of life, are less aggressive in providing optimal care.

In general, about half of PAOD amputations can be satisfactorily achieved below the knee.[139,141,144,145,150,158] Some data indicate that in patients who immediately or ultimately fail bypass and then require amputation, the incidence of AKA is 10% to 20% higher than that seen with patients managed with primary amputation.[159] The possibility that failed bypasses cause more AKAs (with an adverse impact on rehabilitation) is cited by some proponents of primary amputation. This is an ongoing controversy which cannot be settled on the basis of the available data. The reported series have generally sketchy data characterizing the degree of ischemia present. It should be appreciated that even with primary amputation, about 10% to 20% of patients selected for BKA will still ultimately require revision to higher levels. Second, patients selected for revascularization may have more severe ischemia, as concern

Table 8
Results of Amputation Versus Revascularization Stratified for Risk Factors

Risk Group	Number	Mean Age	Procedure	30-Day Mortality (%)	Mean Length of Stay (days)	Rehabilitation (%)
Low	22	57	Amputation	0	19	77
	47	56	Revascular	0	10	98
Intermediate	74	72	Amputation	3	22	76
	110	70	Revascular	3	12	88
High	62	72	Amputation	16	31	44
	47	73	Revascular	6	14	72

(Reproduced with permission from Reference 177.)

that a BKA will not heal may lead to a decision to attempt bypass; consequently, the requirement for AKA after failed bypass may signify the initial severity of ischemia. Similarly, the patient who experiences several years of limb salvage, but ultimately requires amputation after graft thrombosis, may have experienced progression of disease in the interval, and be more ischemic when the graft fails than at the time of the original revascularization.

Increasingly, centers are adopting policies in which virtually every patient with limb threat is revascularized and secondary revascularization interventions are aggressively employed.[76,155,158] Reports from these centers indicate that most attempts at limb salvage lead to amputation-free survival. About 75% of these aggressively treated patients either die within 5 years with the threatened limb intact, or are alive at 5 years with a salvaged limb. With these results, the negative impact of a greater risk for AKA after graft thrombosis is outweighed by the preservation of mobility and independence achieved in successfully salvaged patients. Approximately 80% of the successful limb salvage patients will have preservation of mobility and independence compared to 30% amputees.[158,169] In this context, it seems foolish to forgo limb salvage for the majority of patients if only a minority will ever suffer from a higher level of amputation than might otherwise have been achieved.

Table 9 summarizes data from studies that looked at the relative cost and length of primary amputation versus revascularization. Several features are noteworthy. First, in general, the cost of uncomplicated arterial bypass or primary amputation is almost the same, being within a few percent different. Length of stay is also about the same when complications do not intervene, although this is somewhat more difficult to compare, as whether rehabilitation is conducted on an inpatient or outpatient basis varies among centers. Significantly, when either revascularization or amputation leads to complications, such as amputation after a failed bypass, or revision of a primary BKA to AKA, the total cost of treatment approximately doubles, and length of stay increases. The data refutes the contention that primary amputation is significantly cheaper than revascularization or requires less time in hospital during the initial treatment.

A study by Mackay et al[160,161] looked at long-term costs of treatment for critical ischemia and is summarized in Table 10. One hundred six PAOD patients were treated at an academic medical center with either primary amputation or revascularization over a 5-year period with a mean follow-up of 25 months. There were 78 initial vascular reconstructions and 28 primary amputations. Total hospital charges, number of admissions, and total days in hospital were determined for each patient and averages determined. Over the period of follow-up, patients selected for revascularization had comparable mean total hospital charges, mean number of hospital admissions, and mean total hospital days ($40,769; 2.4 admissions; 67 days) compared to primary amputation patients ($40,600; 2.2 admissions; 85 days). Successfully revascularized patients (44/78=56.5%) had significantly lower charges and hospitaliza-

Table 9
Costs of Amputation Versus Revascularization for Limb Salvage

Author (Year)	Type of Procedure	(Number)	Mean Costs/Charges ($)	Mean Hospital Stay (Days)
Mackey[138] (1986)	all bypass grafts	(21)	27,100	28
	all amputations	(18)	26,100	49
Raviola[161] (1988)	all bypass grafts	(94)	23,500	18
	uncomplicated bypass	(66)	20,300	15
	bypass requiring revision	(12)	25,600	18
	bypass requiring amputation	(8)	42,200	31
	all primary amputation	(53)	24,700	21
	uncomplicated amputation	(41)	20,400	18
	complicated amputation	(12)	40,600	31
Gupta[180] (1990)	limb salvage revascularization	(424)	20,600	23
	major amputation	—	—	19
Cheshire[159] (1992)	distal bypass	(70)	16,700	60
	amputation after bypass	(60)	21,700	

Table 10
Long-Term Costs of Amputation Versus Revascularization

Category (Number)	Cumulative Mean Number of Hospital Admissions	Mean Number of Days in Hospital	Total Costs/Charges ($)
Successful bypass (44)	1.8	43	28,300
Unsuccessful bypass (34)	3.1	97	56,800
Primary amputation (28)	2.2	85	40,600

The data is drawn with permission from Reference 138 and reflects cumulative costs and hospital days for patients having successful initial bypass, those ultimately requiring amputation after failed bypass procedure, and those undergoing initial primary amputation. Mean period of follow-up was 25 months.

tions ($28,300; 1.8 admissions; 43 days) than those patients (34/78= 43.5%) requiring amputation after graft failure ($56,809; 3.1 admissions; 97 days). The mean period of limb salvage in those who ultimately failed revascularization and went on to amputation was 256 ± 55 days compared to 778 ± 78 days in those with continued success.

A more recent British study by Cheshire et al[159] looked at the costs of successful versus unsuccessful distal bypass (tibial and pedal bypass) and included the costs of secondary revascularizations and amputations due to graft failure. Only 3% of the 130 total subjects (mean follow-up was 34 months) had primary amputation. Data on the costs of amputation were accrued from approximately 45% of patients undergoing attempt at limb salvage who ultimately failed and required amputation. The average patient age was 69 in the bypass group compared to 67 in the group of amputees (most of whom had an initial bypass). The average total cost for all distal bypass procedures was $16,700 versus $21,700 for amputations (the latter sum includes bypass and amputation costs). Mean length of hospital stay was 60 days in the bypass group and 67 days in the amputation group. Both groups had equal long-term survival (80% at 3 years). Functionally, the results were much better in the bypass group compared to amputees. Only 13% of all patients in whom bypass was attempted were wheelchair or bed bound, versus 38% of all amputees. Fifty-two percent of all patients in whom bypass was attempted and 79% of successfully bypassed patients were mobile outside the home compared to 31% of the amputees. The additional costs attributed to amputation included rehabilitation and prosthesis costs, but no attempt was made to account for nursing home placement or other assistance. Autologous vein grafts led to fewer secondary patency procedures than PTFE which consequently was about 25% more expensive. The authors of this study concluded that preservation of mobility was achieved in 80% of the bypass patients compared to 31% of the amputees at a lower ultimate cost for limb salvage efforts compared to amputation. One particularly important finding of this study is that overall long-term costs entailed by bypass followed by amputation are not much higher than those entailed with successful bypass.

The net import of all these studies is that successful revascularization is cheaper than primary amputation. The exact savings is dependent on the rate of successful limb salvage, with more savings achieved with better limb salvage results. It is important to realize that even though reports from aggressive centers indicate that successful salvage is achieved in 75% of patients, in these studies, the patient who dies with limbs intact is considered a success. In fact, in many series, about 40% of long-term survivors after bypass have experienced limb loss, so much of the potential savings achieved with limb salvage are due to the patients who die before incurring additional expenses related to amputation.

One factor that is very difficult to incorporate into cost estimates is the cost of long-term care for amputees requiring placement in nursing homes. Couch et al[141] suggests that about one third of amputees require nursing home placement. In 1996, 1 month of nursing home care represents approximately $3,000 of expenditure. Assuming that one third of amputees are placed in nursing homes after hospital discharge, even ultimately failed revascularizations lead to significant savings. Based on Mackey's data, each ultimately failed revascularization patient enjoyed an average of 8 months of limb salvage. If one third of these patients were spared nursing home placement for that 8 months, almost $7,800 per patient was saved by the attempt at revascularization. Similarly, a savings of $36,000 is achieved for every year of limb salvage that keeps a patient out of a nursing home.

Detailed calculations of the relative costs of amputation and revascularization are difficult, as it is not clear what fraction of patients treated by each modality will ultimately require nursing home placement, independent of whether revascularization or rehabilitation are successful. Similarly, available analyses do not completely account for all costs and charges, such as surgeons fees and home health costs. From the perspective of the overall system, survival free of amputation is certain to be regarded as representing a savings, but survival itself is a cost, as survivors incur further health care expenses. As a consequence, increased mortality associated with amputation might be regarded also as a savings.

The most important economic measure which should be applied to the evaluation of these issues is amputation-free survival, for which no reliable cost estimates are available. Calculation of the cost of 1 year of amputation-free survival requires knowledge of the costs incurred for therapy, subsequent care, and the chances of progressing to amputation and/or death. Despite uncertainty regarding these figures, the author believes that the available data clearly shows the cost of 1 year of amputation-free survival to be the same or less than 1 year of survival after amputation. This conclusion indicates that revascularization is cost-effective as it leads to better functional results in patients at a lower cost than is associated with amputation.

Quality of Life

Quality of life is difficult to assess as it relies on patients filling out questionnaires and subjectively assessing their health and emotional status, and these methods are not standardized. Three studies looking at quality of life outcomes after limb salvage surgery have been reported in the English literature. They used different sets of questionnaires to assess quality of life after revascularization; two compared successful limb salvage patients to amputees.

Gibbons et al looked at functional status, well-being, and symptom relief in PAOD patients after infrainguinal bypass.[162] One hundred fifty-six patients completed questionnaires before and 6 months after bypass. The overall limb salvage rate at 6 months was 97%, with total graft patency of 95%; mean age was 66. Ulcers and sores were found to be significantly (p<0.05) improved compared to the baseline preoperative assessment. Similarly, ischemic pain with walking was significantly decreased. Vitality, mental well-being, and the ability to carry out the routine activities of daily living were all noted to be significantly improved based on the questionnaire responses. Preoperative factors such as diabetes, smoking, age, and level of bypass did not influence the changes in measured quality of life. The only independent factor predictive of the change in questionnaire responses was the overall preoperative health status. Patients who functioned better before surgery had significantly more improvement in the quality of life measurement at 6 months than those with poor health status prior to surgery.

Duggan et al assessed quality of life at an average follow-up interval of 18 months in 38 patients (average age 72).[163] Surprisingly, they found that overall health was subjectively rated as worse in both amputees and successfully salvaged patients at the follow-up interval compared to baseline questionnaire results. Limb salvage patients had slightly better overall quality of life scores than amputees, but the differences were not significant. One conclusion of this study was that a better instrument for assessing outcomes was needed.

Albers et al using yet a third questionnaire, studied 61 consecutive patients (mean age 63) presenting with limb threat who were managed either with amputation, revascularization, or conservatively without any intervention.[164] Patients initially managed conservatively and who never required any surgery showed significant improvement in quality of life scores at 1 year compared to baseline. Similarly, patients who required vascular reconstruction and achieved limb salvage had significantly higher scores at 1 year than baseline. Patients undergoing primary amputation or secondary amputation after failed bypass had significantly lower scores than patients whose legs were preserved, but their 1-year scores were not significantly different than baseline.

Two of these studies showed significant improvement in quality of life after limb salvage, but one did not. The patients in the first two studies were younger, suggesting that it is more difficult to demonstrate improved quality of life in older patients because of their increased risk of severe comorbid diagnoses. If the initial health status is poor, less subjective improvement may be expected, even with successful limb salvage, as the problems related to other diagnoses will overshadow the benefit of limb preservation. This is consistent with the conclusion of Gibbons et al's study, where the overall initial health status was the main factor predictive of improvement in health status accomplished by limb salvage.

Influence of Age in Management of Peripheral Arterial Occlusive Disease

We have seen that with increasing age, the chance of developing claudication or limb threat increases, putting elderly patients at the greatest risk for needing amputation or revascularization. Figure 28 show how utilization of angioplasty, bypass, and amputation were influenced by gender and age.[165] Men were more likely than women at all ages to receive treatment for PAOD by a factor of approximately 1.7. Those between the ages of 65 and 74 had the highest rate (70 per 100,000) for angioplasty. Those between ages 75 and 84 had the highest rate (250 per 100,000) for bypass surgery, and those over 85 had the highest rate (225 per 100,000) for amputation. Poorly insured or uninsured patients, as well as African-Americans, had higher rates of amputation and lower utilization of revascularization methods. Women were found to have lower age-adjusted rates for any intervention, but if requiring revascularization, were just as likely as men to have angioplasty or have an amputation. The study illustrates an age-related progression of disease severity and a higher prevalence in men at all ages.

When the influence of age on hospital charges and length of stay incurred for management of PAOD were analyzed by Munoz et al,[166] age emerged as an independent factor predictive of increased resource consumption. Patients aged 80 to 84 admitted with a primary diagnosis of PAOD had mean hospital charges of $19,091 compared to $11,597 for those aged 55 to 64. The mean length of stay for those aged 80 to 84 was 23.7 days compared to 14.2 days for those aged 55 to 64. The older patients had more procedures performed on the average (8.7 versus 6.5). They were not significantly more likely to be admitted through the emergency department or require intensive care unit therapy. The difference between the younger and older patients was not simply related to the number of comorbid diagnoses, as the 55- to 64-age group had a nearly identical mean diagnosis related group (DRG) case mix index (based on the total DRGs and their weighted index per patient) of 1.91 compared to 1.94 for the

80 to 84 group. Similarly, the average number of ICD-9 CM diagnoses for the younger group was 2.22 compared to 2.05 for the older patients. Overall hospital mortality was 20.3% for those aged 80 to 84 compared to 7.4% for those aged 55 to 64. These data indicate that older patients with PAOD have higher risks than young patients, and consume more resources.

Although not surprising, these findings disagree with earlier data regarding the influence of age. In an analysis of hospital charges for Medicare patients admitted for diseases other than PAOD, elderly patients (>80) did not have increased charges compared to younger patients.[166] One implication of these findings is that some inequities in reimbursement policies would be corrected by taking into account the increased severity of disease manifestation in older patients with PAOD, recognizing that DRG indices or ICD-9 coding methods do not adequately factor in the influence of age on resource consumption when PAOD is the primary diagnosis. More importantly, the difference in resource consumption related to vascular versus nonvascular diseases in the aged highlights the critical role that atherosclerosis plays as a cause of morbidity and mortality.

Table 11 is a synopsis of the available studies of limb salvage arterial surgery in patients over age 80. These studies represent the best available data regarding the results of limb salvage in the very elderly. Over 90% of these patients underwent arterial surgery for limb salvage rather than claudication, with about half having tissue loss or gangrene. Several trends in the results are evident. First, there is good agreement in the operative mortality data, with the finding that, except for femoral embolectomy, 30-day mortality was 5% to 6%. The 19% mortality found with embolectomy[167] is consistent with this procedure being disproportionately required for emergencies and associated with increased cardiac risks (which were in fact evident). Second, the overall limb salvage rates reported are in good agreement, ranging from 80% to 92% at 1 year, and 71% to 83% at 3 years. Ignoring the embolectomy data, one finds remarkable congruence in the reported 1- and 3-year survival rates, being 78% to 92%, and 54% to 59%, respectively.

Limb salvage and graft patency data derived from O'Mara et al's study of octogenarians undergoing distal bypass are shown in Figure 29. These results were not significantly different from those found with younger patients, nor was the survival of patients over age 80 requiring bypass significantly different than those under 80 (data not shown). Consistent with the expected impact of PAOD, however, the survival of octogenarians requiring infrainguinal bypass has been shown by Cogbill et al[168] to be reduced compared to age matched controls (Figure 30). Initially, the difference in survival curves was not significant, but by 5 years, the difference is markedly and significantly different. In this study, the average life expectancy of the octogenarian who required bypass for limb threat was about 4 years, compared

Table 11
Results of Limb Salvage in Octagenarians

Author (Year)	Number of Patients	Mean Age	Number of Procedures	Procedure Types	Operative Mortality	Limb Salvage	Survival
Scher[170] (1986)	168	84	182	13% inflow 13% angioplasty 85% infraing bypass	5%	80% 1 year 71% 3 year	78% 1 year 54% 3 year
O'Mara[181] (1987)	34	85	40	tibial bypass	5%	91% 1 year 81% 3 year	91% 1 year 54% 3 year
Cogbill[168] (1987)	46	84	54	infraing bypass	0%	95% 1 year 87% 5 year	85% 1 year 30% 5 year
Edwards[171] (1982)	21	84	25	embolectomy	19%	89% *	67% 1 year 25% 3 year
	55	84	85	7% inflow 5% embolectomy 107% infraing bypass	5%	89%	—
Friedman[169] (1989)	50	84	69	16% inflow 84% infraing bypass	3%	92% 1 year 83% 3 year	92% 1 year 59% 3 year

* unspecified interval

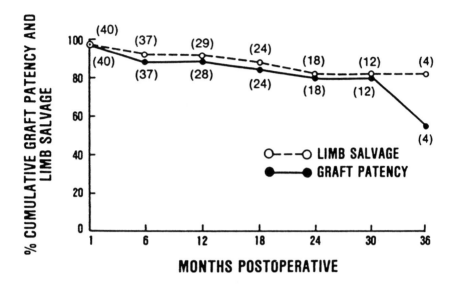

Figure 29. *Limb salvage and graft patency rates in octagenarians.* The patency and limb salvage rates were not significantly different from those found with patients younger than 80. (Reproduced with permission from Reference 181.)

to an average life expectancy at 80 of 7.9 years and a life expectancy at 85 of 5.9 years.[171]

The incidence of secondary revascularization procedures required for these very elderly patients was not particularly high. In Friedman et al's series, 20% of the patients ultimately had revisions or thrombectomies.[169] Scher et al reported that secondary revascularization procedures were undertaken in 8% of the patients.[170] In Edward et al's series, 18% of the patients subsequently underwent secondary operations to restore graft patency.[171]

The tabularized data do not show functional results, as these were not reported in a standardized fashion. Scher et al found that over 50% of patients in whom limb salvage was attempted survived 2 or more years with the threatened limb intact, and 76% of the patients who died after attempted limb salvage had the threatened limb intact at death.[170] O'Mara reported a similar result; 67% of the patients experienced amputation-free survival after distal bypass with a mean follow-up of 21 months.[181] Of eight patients dying more than 30 days after surgery, 75% had a functional and intact limb at death.[171] In Cogbill et al's series,[168] of 18 survivors at the conclusion of the study period, 83% had experienced limb salvage, with graft patency confirmed in 78%. Only one surviving patient was bedridden and 13 were fully ambulatory at 5 years. Two thirds of the survivors lived at home and only one third were nursing home residents.[167]

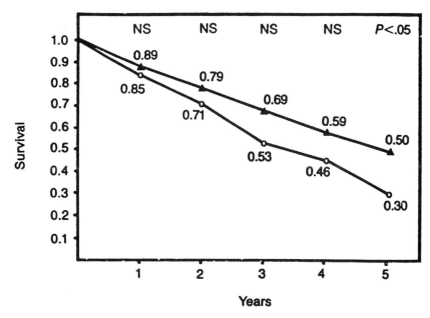

Figure 30. *Cumulative survival after infrainguinal bypass in octagenarians.* Survival after infrainguinal bypass for limb salvage in octagenarians **(circles)** is plotted in comparison to survival of age matched controls **(triangles). NS** indicates not significant. The difference in survival at 5 years was significant. (Reproduced with permission from Reference 168.)

Conclusions

Infrainguinal arterial occlusive disease has increasing prevalence with increasing age. Claudicators have a moderate (20% to 40%) chance of progressing to limb threat, influenced by risk factors such as smoking and diabetes, and the severity of signs and symptoms at initial presentation. Their long-term survival is less than age matched controls because of increased CAD and cerebrovascular disease. In the absence of limb threat, medical management could be as good as endoluminal or surgical interventions for maintaining quality of life, despite few studies demonstrating the natural history of claudicators treated by different modalities. Advances in endoluminal techniques have led to increased utilization of angiographic diagnosis and therapy for both functional and critical ischemia. With limb threat, bypass is the mainstay of surgical intervention, and yields the best long-term results of any therapy, although endoluminal methods have an important primary and adjunctive role in limb salvage efforts.

The data presented in this chapter strongly support devoting resources to limb salvage efforts, not only for younger patients, but also for the very elderly. The results of revascularization surgery are similar in terms of graft patency and limb salvage in older patients (>80) compared to younger ones, although perioperative mortality is modestly higher. The chances of maintaining or improving the functional status of patients with limb threat is good at all ages, and does not seem to be decreased by advanced age independent of other factors.

Although diminished compared to the population without PAOD, the lower life expectancy found with advanced age and PAOD is not so low as to preclude limb salvage efforts. As noted above, life expectancy is approximately 4 years in octogenarians requiring bypass. The available evidence indicates that life expectancies after bypass and rates of limb salvage are only modestly reduced in the very elderly compared to the average patient with PAOD. Amputation in the elderly remains, based on the available data, more dangerous than limb salvage, and age alone cannot be used as a persuasive argument to forgo limb salvage in favor of amputation. This is particularly important to stress, as the chances of successful rehabilitation after amputation decline with age due to decreased cardiovascular reserve. In the majority of the elderly patients subjected to bypass surgery, limb salvage is achieved with attendant improvement in ambulation and mobility.

The data presented regarding the overall costs of limb salvage, including the costs of secondary revascularizations and delayed amputations, when combined with the good results reported for bypass indicate that the cost benefit of bypass compared to amputation applies to patients independent of their age. Elderly patients do, however, require greater consumption of resources to achieve limb salvage because they have more severe comorbid diagnoses, particularly CAD and cerebrovascular disease. Quality of life analysis of the benefits of limb salvage may be confounded by the other problems associated with aging, such that the benefits of preserving independent mobility are masked by the increasing severity of other problems that are present.

Many questions still remain to be studied. The natural history of PAOD after endoluminal therapy needs further delineation. Whether endoluminal therapy is justified for moderate degrees of PAOD is an open question, as the risks, particularly those of provoking intimal hyperplasia with catheter trauma, may well outweigh the benefits. Future clinical research should examine in more detail the costs of different management options with comprehensive accounting for costs, such as surgeons fees and nursing home care. As new methods of improving blood flow in ischemic limbs becomes available, prognostic factors will need to be identified which predict failure or success. Better data on age-adjusted rates of amputation and revascularization, which take into account level of amputation and revascularization, are required to properly assess policies regarding use of vascular interventions. There also is a need for improved standardization in reporting rehabilitation results.

Further advances in therapy, such as effective drugs for treating intimal hyperplasia, coated stents, and improved thrombolytic techniques are imminent. Undoubtedly, the future will continue to see the same revolutionary changes that have marked the last decades.

References

1. Gaius Suetonius Tranquillus: *The Twelve Caesers.* Translated by Robert Graves. Harmondsworth, England: Penguin Books, Ltd.; 205, 1979.
2. European Working Group on Central Leg Ischemia: Second European consensus document on chronic critical leg ischemia. *Circulation* 84(5):IV-1-IV-26, 1991.
3. Rivers SP, Vieth FJ, Ascer E, et al: Successful conservative therapy of severe limb threatening ischemia: the value of nonsympathectomy. *Surgery* 99:759-762, 1986.
4. Widmer LK, Greensher A, Kannel WB: Occlusion of peripheral arteries: a study of 6400 working subjects. *Circulation* 30:836-842, 1964.
5. Rose GA, Ahmeteli M, Ceccacci L, et al: Ischemic heart disease in middle-aged men: prevalence comparisons in Europe. *Bull Org Mond Sante'* 38:885-895, 1968.
6. Hale WE, Marks RG, May FE, et al: Epidemiology of intermittent claudication: evaluation of risk factors. *Age Aging* 17:57-60, 1988.
7. Balkau B, Vray M, Eschewege E: Epidemiology of peripheral arterial disease. *J Cardiovasc Pharmacol* 23(suppl 3):S8-S16, 1994.
8. Kannel WB, Skinner JJ, Schwartz MJ, Slaurtleff D: Intermittent claudication: incidence in the Framingham Study. *Circulation* 91:875-883, 1970.
9. Kannel WB, McGee DL: Update on some epidemiology features of intermittent claudication: the Framingham Study. *J Am Geriatric Soc* 33:13-18, 1985.
10. Schroll M, Munck O: Estimation of peripheral arteriosclerotic disease by ankle blood pressure measurements in a population study of 60-year-old men and women. *J Chron Dis* 34:261-269, 1981.
11. Newman AB, Sutton-Tyrell R, Rutan GH, et al: Lower extremity arterial disease in elderly subjects with systolic hypertension. *J Clin Epidemiol* 44:15-20, 1991.
12. Postiglione A, Cilerano J, Gallotta G: Prevalence of peripheral arterial disease and related risk factors in elderly institutionalized subjects. *Gerontology* 388:330-337, 1992.
13. Boyd AM: The natural course of arteriosclerosis of the lower extremities. *Angiology* 11:10-14, 1960.
14. Naschitz JE, Ambrosio DA, Chang JB: Intermittent claudication: predictors and outcome. *Angiology* 39(Pt 1):16-22, 1988.
15. Rosenbloom MS, Flanigan DP, Schuler JJ: The risk factors affecting the natural history of intermittent claudication. *Arch Surg* 123:867-870, 1988.
16. McDaniel MD, Cronenwett JL: Basic data related to the natural history of intermittent claudication. *Ann Vasc Surg* 3:273-276, 1989.
17. Kacy SS, Wolma FJ, Flye MW: Factors affecting the results of below knee amputation in patients with or without diabetes. *Surg Gynecol Obstet* 155:513-518, 1982.
18. Gupta SK, Vieth FJ: Is arterial reconstruction cost-effective compared with amputation? In: Greenhalgh RM, Jameson CW, Nicolaides AN (eds). *Limb Salvage and Amputation for Vascular Disease.* Philadelphia: WB Saunders, Co.; 447-452, 1988.
19. Hughson WG, Monn JI, Garrod A: Intermittent claudication: prevalence and risk factors. *Br Med J* 275:1379-1381, 1978.
20. Juergens IL, Barker NW, Hines EA: Arteriosclerosis of veterans: a review of 520 cases with special reference to pathogenic and prognostic factors. *Circulation* 21:188-199, 1960.
21. Myers KA, King RB, Scott DF, et al: The effect of smoking on the late patency of arterial reconstructions in the legs. *Br J Surg* 65:267-271, 1978.

22. Clyne CA, Arch PJ, Carpenter D, et al: Smoking, ignorance, and peripheral vascular disease. *Arch Surg* 117:1062-1065, 1987.
23. Gutman M, Kaplan O, Skornick Y, et al: Gangrene of the lower limbs in diabetic patients: a malignant complication. *Am J Surg* 154:305-308, 1987.
24. Krolewski AS, Warram JH, Rand LI, Khan CR: Epidemiologic approach to the etiology of type 1 diabetes mellitus and its complications. *N Engl J Med* 317:1390-1398, 1987.
25. Jonason T, Ringqvist I: Diabetes mellitus and intermittent claudication: relation between peripheral vascular complications and location of the occlusive atherosclerosis in the legs. *Acta Med Scand* 218:217-221, 1985.
26. Blankenhorn D, Hadis H: Arterial imaging and atherosclerosis reversal. *Arterioscler Throm* 14:177-199, 1994.
27. The Diabetes Control and Complications Trial Research Group: The effect of intensive treatment of diabetes on the development and progression of long-term complications in insulin-dependent diabetes mellitus. *N Engl J Med* 329:977-986, 1993.
28. Hallett JW JR, Greenwood LH, Robison JG: Lower extremity arterial disease in young adults: a systematic approach to early diagnosis. *Ann Surg* 202:647-652, 1985.
29. Jonason T, Ringquist I: Factors of prognostic importance for subsequent rest pain in patients with intermittent claudication. *Acta Med Scand* 218:27-33, 1985.
30. Paroito IM, Kim G-E, Davidson T, Crowley JG: Intermittent claudication: its natural course. *Surgery* 78:795-799, 1975.
31. Cronenwett JL, Warner KG, Zelenock GB, et al: Intermittent claudication: current results of nonoperative management. *Arch Surg* 119:430-436, 1984.
32. Zierler RE, Strandness DE: Nonimaging physiologic tests for assessment of extremity arterial disease. In: Zwiebel WJ (ed). Introduction to Vascular Ultrasound. Philadelphia: WB Saunders, Co.; 201-222, 1992.
33. Kohler TR, Nance DR, Cramer MM, et al: Duplex scanning for diagnosis of aortoiliac and femoropopliteal disease: a prospective study. *Circulation* 76:1074-1080, 1987.
34. Seldinger S: Catheter replacement of the needle in percutaneous arteriography. *Acta Radiol* 39:368-371, 1953.
35. Lavtin EM, Freeman NJ, Schoenfeld AH, et al: Radiocontrast-associated renal dysfunction: a comparison of lower-osmolality and conventional high-osmolality contrast media. *AJR* 157:59-65, 1991.
36. Sreeram S, Lumsden AB, Miller JS, et al: Retroperitoneal hematoma following femoral arterial catheterization. *Am Surg* 59:94-98, 1993.
37. Oweida SW, Roubin GS, Smith RB, Salam AA: Postcatheterization vascular complications associated with percutaneous transluminal coronary angioplasty. *J Vasc Surg* 12:310-315, 1990.
38. Tabbara MR, White RA, Cavaye DM, Kopchok GE: In vivo human comparison of intra-vascular ultrasound and angiography. *J Vasc Surg* 14:496-499, 1991.
39. Taylor LM, Porter JM: Natural history and nonoperative treatment of chronic lower extremity ischemia. In: Rutherford RB (ed). *Vascular Surgery*. Philadelphia: WB Saunders, Co.; 762, 1995.
40. Junger M, Frey-Schnewlin G, Bollinger A: Microvascular flow distribution and transcapillary diffusion at the forefoot in patients with peripheral ischemia. *Int J Microcirc Clin Exp* 8:3-24, 1989.
41. Gokal R, Dornan TL, Ledingham JG: Peripheral skin necrosis complicating beta-blockage. *Br Med J* 197:721-722, 1979.

42. D'Angelo Y, Villa S, Mysllvvlec M, et al: Defective fibrinolytic and prostacyclin-like activity in human atherosclerotic plaques. *Thromb Haemostas* 39:535-536, 1978.
43. Conrad MC: Abnormalities of the distal vasculature as related to ulceration and gangrene. *Circulation* 38:568-581, 1968.
44. Bertuglia S, Colantvoni A, Coppini G, Intagletta M: Hypoxia or hyperoxia induced changes in arteriolar vasomotion in skeletal muscle microcirculation. *Am J Physiol* 24:H362-H371, 1991.
45. Nash GB, Thomas PRS, Dormandy JA: Abnormal flow properties of white cells in patients with severe ischemia of the leg. *Br Med J* 296:1699-1701, 1988.
46. Fingerle J, Johnson R, Clowes AW, et al: Role of platelets in smooth muscle cell proliferation and migration after vascular injury in rat carotid artery. *PNAS USA* 86:8412-8416, 1989.
47. Fanelli C, Aronoff R: Restenosis following coronary angioplasty. *Am Heart J* 119:357-368, 1990.
48. McIntyre KE: The diabetic foot and management of infectious gangrene. In: Moore WS, Malone JM (eds). Lower Extremity Amputation. Philadelphia: WB Saunders, Co.; 18-78, 1989.
49. Criqui M, Langer R, Fronek A, et al: Mortality over a period of 10 years in patients with peripheral arterial disease. *N Engl J Med* 326:381-386, 1992.
50. Taylor LM, Porter JM: Current status of the reversed saphenous vein graft. In: Bergan JJ, Yao T (eds). *Arterial Surgery: New Diagnostic and Operative Techniques.* New York: Grune & Stratton, Inc.; 494, 1987.
51. Turnipseed WD, Berkoff HA, Belzer FO: Postoperative stroke in cardiac and peripheral vascular disease. *Ann Surg* 192:365-368, 1980.
52. Ahn SS, Baker JD, Walden K, Moore WS: Which asymptomatic patients should undergo routine screening carotid duplex scan? *Am J Surg* 162:180-184, 1991.
53. Hertzer NR, Beven EG, Yang JR: Coronary artery disease in peripheral vascular patients: a classification of 1000 coronary angiograms and results of surgical management. *Ann Surg* 199:223-233, 1984.
54. Tischler MD, Lee TH, Hirsch AT, et al: Prediction of major cardiac events after peripheral vascular surgery using dipyridamole echocardiography. *Am J Cardiol* 68:593-597, 1991.
55. Boucher CA, Brewster DC, Darling DC, et al: Determination of cardiac risk by dipyridamole thallium before peripheral vascular surgery. *N Engl J Med* 312:389-394, 1985.
56. Booth DC: Current and future role of prophylactic coronary bypass and coronary angioplasty before major vascular surgery. In: Kazmers A (ed). *Cardiac Risk Assessment Before Vascular Surgery.* Armonk, NY: Futura Publishing Co., Inc.; 239-250, 1994.
57. Ernst E, Flalka VA: Review of the clinical effectiveness of exercise therapy for intermittent claudication. *Ann Intern Med* 113:153-159, 1993.
58. Hiatt WR, Regensteiner JG, Hargararten ME, Wolfel EE, Brass EP: Benefit of exercise conditioning for patients with peripheral arterial disease. *Circulation* 81:602-609, 1990.
59. Hiatt WR, Regensteiner JG: Nonsurgical management of peripheral arterial disease. *Hosp Prac* 28:59-82, 1993.
60. Antiplatelet Triallists Collaboration: Final report of second cycle. *Br Med J* 296(6618):320-331, 1988.
61. Goldhaver S, Manson J, Hennekens C, et al: Low dose aspirin and subsequent peripheral arterial surgery in the Physician's Health Study. *Lancet* 340:143-145, 1992.

62. Janson L, Bergquist D, Boberg D, et al: Prevention of myocardial infarction and strokes in patients with intermittent claudication: effects of ticlodipine: results from STIMS, the Swedish Ticlodipine Multicentre Study. *N Engl J Med* 301:962-966, 1979.
63. Connolly JE, Kwaan JHM: In situ saphenous vein bypass. *Arch Surg* 17:1551-1557, 1982.
64. Cameron HA, Walker PC, Ramsay LE: Drug treatment of intermittent claudication: a critical analysis of the methods and findings of published clinical trials, 1965-1985. *Br J Clin Pharmacol* 26:569-576, 1988.
65. Porter JM, Cutler BS, Lee BY, et al: Pentoxyfylline efficacy in the treatment of intermittent claudication: multicenter controlled double-blind trial with objective assessment of chronic occlusive arterial disease patients. *Am Heart J* 104:66-71, 1982.
66. Belch JJF, McKay A, McArdle B, et al: Epoprostenol (prostacyclin) and severe arterial disease: a double-blind trial. *Lancet* i:315-317, 1983.
67. Norgren L, Alwamark A, Anggrist KA, et al: A stable prostacyclin analog (iloprost) in the treatment of ischemic ulcers of the lower limb: a Scandanavian-Polish placebo-controlled, randomized multicenter study. *Eur J Vasc Surg* 4:463-467, 1990.
68. Kunlin J: Le traitement de l'arteite obliterante par la greffe veineuse. *Arch Mal Coeur* 42:371-372, 1949.
69. Campbell CD, Brooks DH, Webster MW, et al: The use of expanded microporous polytetrafluoroethylene for limb salvage: a preliminary report. *Surgery* 79:485-491, 1976.
70. Sauvage LR, Berger K, Wood SJ, et al: An external velour surface for porous arterial prostheses. *Surgery* 70:940-953, 1971.
71. Andrus G, Harris RW, Salles-Cunha SX, et al: Arm veins for arterial revascularization of the legs: arteriographic and clinical observations. *J Vasc Surg* 4:416-427, 1986.
72. Dardik H, Ibraham IM, Dardik I: Successful arterial substitution with modified human umbilical vein. *Ann Surg* 183:252-258, 1976.
73. Rosenberg N, Thompson JE, Keshishian JM, VanderWerf BA: The modified bovine arterial graft. *Arch Surg* 111:222-226, 1976.
74. Taylor RS, Loh A, McFarland RJ, et al: Improved technique for polytetrafluoroethylene bypass grafting: long-term results using anastomotic vein patches. *Br J Surg* 79:348-354, 1992.
75. Jarrett F, Berkoff HA, Crummy AB, et al: Femoro-tibial bypass grafts with sequential technique. *Arch Surg* 116:709-714, 1981.
76. Taylor LM, Edwards JM, Porter JM: Present status of reversed vein bypass grafting: 5-year results of a modern series. *J Vasc Surg* 11:193-205, 1990.
77. Bergamini TM, Towne JB, Bandyk DF, et al: Experience with in situ saphenous vein bypasses during 1981 to 1989: determinant factors of long-term patency. *J Vasc Surg* 13:137, 1991.
78. Donaldson MC, Mannick JA, Whittemore AD: Femoral-distal bypass with in situ greater saphenous vein: long-term results using the Mills valvultatome. *Ann Surg* 213:457-465, 1991.
79. Whittemore AD: Infrainguinal bypass. In: Rutherford RB (ed). *Vascular Surgery*. Philadelphia: WB Saunders, Co.; 808-811, 1995.
80. Cutler BS, Thompson JE, Lleinsasser LJ, et al: Autologens saphenous vein femoro-popliteal bypass: analysis of 298 cases. *Surgery* 79:325-831, 1976.
81. Tilanus HW, Obertop H, Van Urk H: Saphenous vein or PTFE for femoropopliteal bypass: a prospective randomized trial. *Ann Surg* 202:780-782, 1985.

82. Hall KV: The great saphenous vein used "in situ" as an arterial shunt after extirpation of vein valves. *Surgery* 51:492, 1962.
83. Leather RP, Powers SR, Karmody AM: A reappraisal of the in situ saphenous vein arterial bypass: its use in limb salvage. *Surgery* 86:453-461, 1979.
84. Harris PL, How TV, Jones DR: Prospectively randomized clinical trial to compare in situ and reversed saphenous vein grafts for femoropoplital bypass. *Br J Surg* 74:252-255, 1987.
85. Wengerter KR, Veith FJ, Gupta SK, et al: Prospective randomized multicenter comparison of in situ and reversed vein infrapopliteal bypasses. *J Vasc Surg* 13:189, 1991.
86. Veith FJ, Gupta SK, Ascer E, et al: Six-year prospective multicenter randomized comparison of autologous saphenous vein and expanded polytetrafluoroethylene graft in infrainguinal arterial reconstruction. *J Vasc Surg* 3:104-114, 1986.
87. Quinones-Baldrich WJ, Prego AA, Vcelay-Gomez R, et al: Long-term results of infrainguinal revascularization with polytetrafluoroethylene: a 10-year experience. *J Vasc Surg* 16:209-217, 1992.
88. Rosenthal D, Evans D, McKinsey J, et al: Prosthetic above- knee femoropopliteal bypass for intermittent claudication. *J Cardiovasc Surg* 31:462-468, 1990.
89. McCollum C, Kenchington G, Alexander C, et al: PTFE or HUV for femoropopliteal bypass: a multi-center trial. *Eur J Vasc Surg* 5:435-443, 1991.
90. Dardik H, Miller N, Dardik A, et al: A decade of experience with the glutaraldehyde-tanned human unblical cord vein graft for revascularization of the lower limb. *J Vasc Surg* 7:336-346, 1988.
91. Welch M, Durrans D, Car HMH, et al: Endothelial cell seeding: a review. *Ann Vasc Surg* 6:473-484, 1992.
92. Rafferty TD, Avellone JC, Farrell CJ, et al: A metropolitan experience with intrainguinal revascularization: operative risk and later results in northeastern Ohio. *J Vasc Surg* 6:365-371, 1987.
93. Rutherford RB, Jones DN, Bergent S, et al: The efficacy of dextran 40 in preventing early postoperative thrombosis following difficult lower extremity bypass. *J Vasc Surg* 1:765-773, 1984.
94. Donaldson MC, Mannick JA, Whittemore AD: Causes of primary graft failure after in situ saphenous vein bypass grafting. *J Vasc Surg* 15:113, 1992.
95. Gordon IL, Pousti TJ, Stemmer EA, et al: Inguinal wound fluid collections after vascular surgery: management by early reoperation. *South Med J* 88:433-436, 1995.
96. Gelkin M, Valeri R, Hobson RW: Intra-arterial urokinase increases skeletal muscle viability after acute ischemia. *J Vasc Surg* 4:161-168, 1989.
97. Comerota AJ, White JV, Grosh JD: Intraoperative, intra-arterial thrombolytic therapy for salvage of limbs in patients with distal arterial thrombosis. *Surg Gynecol Obstet* 169:283-289, 1989.
98. Brewster DC, Chin AK, Herman GD, Fogarty TJ: Arterial thromboembolism. In: Rutherford RB (ed). *Vascular Surgery*. Philadelphia: WB Saunders, Co.; 662, 1995.
99. Abbott WM, Maloney RD, McCabe CC, et al: Arterial embolism: a 44-year perspective. *Am J Surg* 143:460-464, 1982.
100. Jarrett F, Detmer E: Arterial thromboemboli: factors affecting mortality and morbidity. *J Cardiovasc Surg* 22:454-461, 1981.
101. Dos Santos JC: Sur la de obstruction des thromboses arterielle anciennes. *Mem Acad Chir* 73:409-411, 1960.
102. Cannon JA, Barker WF: Successful management of obstructive femoral arteriosclerosis by endarterectomy. *Surgery* 38:48-54, 1955.

103. Sobel S, Kaplitt MJ, Reingold M, et al: Gas endarterectomy. *Surgery* 59:517-521, 1966.
104. Inahara T, Mukherjee D: Femoral and popliteal thromboendarterectomy. In: Rutherford RB (ed). *Vascular Surgery.* Philadelphia: WB Saunders, Co.; 835-847, 1995.
105. Bernhard VM, Ray LI, Militello JM: The role of angioplasty of the profunda femoris artery in revascularization of the ischemic limb. *Surg Gynecol Obstet* 142:840-844, 1976.
106. Towne JB, Bernhard VM, Rollins DL, et al: Profundaplasty in perspective: limitations in long-term management of limb ischemia. *Surgery* 90:1037-1046, 1981.
107. Campbell WB: Sympathectomy for chronic arterial ischemia. *Eur J Vasc Surg* 2:357-364, 1988.
108. Rutherford RB, Shannon FL: Lumbar sympathectomy. In: Rutherford RB (ed). *Vascular Surgery.* Philadelphia: WB Saunders, Co.; 874-883, 1995.
109. Cronenwett JL, Lindenauer SM: Hemodynamic effects of sympathectomy in ischemic canine hind limbs. *Surgery* 87:417-424, 1980.
110. Beran RD, Tsuro H: Functional and structural changes in the rabbit ear artery after sympathetic denervation. *Circ Res* 49:478-485, 1981.
111. Rutherford RB, Valenta J: Extremity bloodflow and sympathectomy and exercise. *Surgery* 69:332-344, 1971.
112. Welch GH, Leiberman DP: Cutaneous blood flow in the foot following lumbar sympathectomy. *Scand J Clin Lab Invest* 46:621-626, 1985.
113. Perrson AV, Anderson LA, Padberg FT Jr: Selection of patients for lumbar sympathectomy. *Surg Clin North Am* 65:393-403, 1985.
114. Walker PM, Johnston KW: Predicting the success of a sympathectomy: a retrospective study using discriminant function and multiple regression analysis. *Surgery* 87:216-221, 1980.
115. Dotter CT, Judkins MP: Transluminal treatment of arteriosclerotic obstruction: description of a new technic and a preliminary report of its application. *Circulation* 30:654-656, 1964.
116. Grontzig A: Die perkutane rekavalisation chrovisher artelieller verschlusse (Dotter-Privzip) mit einem nemen doppelumingen dilations katheter. *Rofo* 124:80-86, 1976.
117. Wilson SE, Wolfe GL, Cross AP, et al: Percutaneous transluminal angioplasty versus operation for peripheral arteriosclerosis. *J Vasc Surg* 9:1-8, 1989.
118. Martin EC: Introduction. *Circulation* 83(2)(suppl I):1, 1991.
119. Rutherford RB, Durham J: Percutaneous balloon angioplasty for arteriosclerosis obliterations: long-term results. In: Yao JST, Pearce WH (eds). *Technologies in Vascular Surgery.* Philadelphia: WB Saunders, Co.; 329-325, 1992.
120. Johnston KW, Rae M, Hogg-Johnston SA, et al: Five-year results of a perspective study of percutaneous transluminal angioplasty. *Ann Surg* 206:403-413, 1987.
121. Stokes KR, Strunk HM, Campbell DR, et al: Five-year results of iliac and femoropopliteal angioplasty in diabetic patients. *Radiology* 174:977-982, 1990.
122. Krepel VM, van Andel GJ, van Erp WFM, et al: Percutaneous transluminal angioplasty of the femoropopliteal artery: initial and long-term results. *Radiology* 156:325-328, 1985.
123. Gordon IL, Conroy RC, Tobis JM, et al: Determinants of patency after percutaneous angioplasty and atherectomy of occluded superficial femoral arteries. *Am J Surg* 168:115-119, 1994.

124. Adar R, Critchfield GC, Eddy DM: A confidence profile analysis of the results of femoropopliteal percutaneous transluminal angioplasty in the treatment of lower-extremity ischemia. *J Vasc Surg* 10:57-67, 1989.

125. Tamora S, Sniderman KW, Beinart C, et al: Percutaneous transluminal angioplasty of the popliteal and its branches. *Radiology* 143:645-648, 1982.

126. Greenfield AJ: Femoropopliteal, popliteal, and tibial arteries: percutaneous transluminal angioplasty. *AJR* 135:927-935, 1980.

127. Palmaz JC, Garcia OJ, Schatz RA, et al: Placement of balloon-expandable intraluminal stents in iliac arteries: first 171 procedures. *Radiology* 174:969, 1990.

128. Richter G: Balloon-expandable Palmaz stent placement versus PTA in iliac artery stenosis and occlusions: long-term results of a randomized trial. Presented at the *Society Of Cardiovascular and Interventional Radiologists*, Washington, DC, 1992.

129. Gordon IL, Conroy RC, Tobis JM, Nimon M: Stenting occluded femoral arteries. Presented at the *5th International Endovascular Symposium*, Sydney, Australia, 1995.

130. Tobis JM, Conroy R, Deutsch LS, et al: Laser assisted versus mechanical recanalization of peripheral occlusions: a randomized trial. *Am J Cardiol* 68:1079-1086, 1991.

131. Ahn SS, Auth D, et al: Removal of focal atheromatous lesions by angioscopically guided high-speed rotary atherectomy. *J Vasc Surg* 7:292-300, 1988.

132. Simpson JB, Selman MR, Robertson GC: Transluminal atherectomy for occlusive peripheral vascular disease. *Am J Cardiol* 61:96G-101G, 1988.

133. Wholey MH, Jarmolowski RR: New reperfusion devices: the Kensey catheter, the atherolytic reperfusion wire device, and the transluminal extraction catheter. *Radiology* 172:947-952, 1989.

134. Nakamura S, Conroy RM, Gordon IL, et al: A randomized trial of transcutaneous extraction catheter atherectomy in femoral arteries: intravascular ultrasound observations. *J Clin Ultrasound* 23:461-471, 1995.

135. Ouriel K, Comerota AJ: Thrombolytic therapy in the management of peripheral arterial occlusion. In: Ouriel K (ed). Lower Extremity Vascular disease. Philadelphia: WB Saunders, Co.; 295-320, 1995.

136. Ouriel K, Shortell CK, DeWeese JA, et al: A comparison of thrombolytic therapy with acute operative revascularization in the treatment of acute peripheral arterial ischemia. *J Vasc Surg* 19:1021-1030, 1994.

137. ISIS-2 (Second International Study of Infarct Survival) Collaborative Group: Randomized trial of intravenous streptokinase, oral aspirin, both, or neither among 17,187 cases of suspected acute myocardial infarction. *Lancet* II:349-360, 1988.

138. Mackey WC, McCullough JL, Conlon TP, et al: The costs of surgery for limb threatening ischemia. *Surgery* 99:26-34, 1986.

139. Gregg RO: Bypass or amputation: concomitant review of bypass arterial grafting and major amputations. *Am J Surg* 149:397-402, 1985.

140. Bunt IJ, Malone JM: Amputation or revascularization in the >70-year-old. *Am Surg* 60:349-352, 1994.

141. Couch NP, David JK, Tilney NL, Crane CC: Natual history of the leg amputee. *Am J Surg* 133:469-471, 1977.

142. McIntyre KE: The diabetic foot and management of infectious gangrene. In: Moore WS, Malone JM (eds). *Lower Extremity Amputation.* Philadelphia: WB Saunders, Co.; 19, 1989.

143. Powell TW, Burnham SJ, Johnson G: Second leg ischemia: lower extremity bypass versus amputation in patients with contralateral extremity amputation. *Am Surg* 50:577-580, 1984.
144. Whitehouse FW, Jurgensen C, Block MGP: The later life of the diabetic amputee. *Diabetes* 17:520-521, 1980.
145. Keagy BA, Schwartz JA, Koth M, et al: Lower extremity amputations: the control series. *J Vasc Surg* 4:321-326, 1986.
146. Burgess EM, Marsden FW: Major lower extremity amputations following arterial reconstruction. *Arch Surg* 108:655-660, 1974.
147. Nicholas CG, Myers JL, Demuth WE: The role of vascular laboratory criteria in the selection of patients for lower extremity amputation. *Am Surg* 195:469-473, 1982.
148. White RA, Nolan L, Harley D, et al: Noninvasive evaluation of peripheral vascular disease using transcutaneous oxygen tension. *Am J Surg* 144:68-75, 1982.
149. Waters RL, Perry J, Chambers R: Energy expenditure of amputee gait. In: Moore WS, Malone JM (eds). *Lower Extremity Amputation.* Philadelphia: WB Saunders, Co.; 250-260, 1989.
150. Harris KA, van Schiel, Carroll SE, et al: Rehabilitation potential of elderly patients with major amputations. *J Cardiovasc Surg* 32:463-467, 1991.
151. Houghton AD, Taylor PR, Thurlow S, et al: Success rates for rehabilitation of vascular amputees: implications for preoperative assessment and amputation level. *Br J Surg* 79:753-755, 1992.
152. Creasy TS, McMillan PJ, Fletcher EWL, et al: Is percutaneous transluminal angioplasty better than exercise for claudication: preliminary results from a prospective trial. *Eur J Vasc Surg* 4:135-140, 1990.
153. Jeans WD, Danton RM, Baird RN, Horrocks M: The effects of introducing balloon dilatation into vascular surgical practice. *Br J Surg* 59:457-459, 1986.
154. Gallino A, Mahler F, Probst P, et al: Percutaneous transluminal angioplasty of the arteries of the lower limbs: a 5-year follow-up. *Circulation* 70:619-623, 1984.
155. Schmidtke I, Roth VJ: Relapse treatment of percutaneous transluminal dilatation. In: Dotter CT, Gruntzig AR, Schoop W, et al (eds). *Percutaneous Transluminal Angioplasty Technique: Early and Late Results.* Beilin: Springer-Verlag; 131-139, 1983.
156. Vieth FJ, Gupta SK, Wengerter KR, et al: Changing arteriosclerotic disease patterns and management strategies in lower limb-threatening ischemia. *Ann Surg* 211:402-411, 1990.
157. Tunis SR, Bass EB, Steinberg EP: The use of angioplasty, bypass surgery, and amputation in the management of peripheral vascular disease. *N Engl J Med* 3125:556-562, 1991.
158. Cronenwett JL, McDaniel MD, Zwalak RM: Limb salvage despite extensive tissue loss: free tissue transfer combined with distal revascularization. *Arch Surg* 124:609-615, 1989.
159. Cheshire NJW, Wolfe JHN, Noone AM, Davies LD: The economics of femoro-crural reconstruction for critical leg ischemia with and without autologous vein. *J Vasc Surg* 15:167-179, 1992.
160. Kazmers M, Bhagwan S, Evans WE: Amputation level following unsuccessful distal limb salvage operations. *Surgery* 87:683-687, 1980.
161. Raviola CA, Nichter LS, Baker JD, et al: Cost of treating advanced leg ischemia. *Arch Surg* 123:495-496, 1988.

162. Gibbons GW, Burgess AM, Guadagnoli E, et al: Return to well-being and function after infrainguinal revascularization. *J Vasc Surg* 21:35-45, 1995.
163. Duggan NM, Woodson J, Slott TE: Functional outcomes in limb salvage vascular surgery. *Am J Surg* 166:188-191, 1994.
164. Albers M, Fratezi AE, DeLuccia N: Assessment of quality of life patients with severe ischemia as a result of infrainguinal arterial occlusive disease. *J Vasc Surg* 16:54-59, 1992.
165. Tunis SR, Bass EB, Klag MJ, Steinberg EP: Variation in utilizations of procedures for treatment of peripheral arterial disease. *Arch Intern Med* 153:991-998, 1993.
166. Munoz E, Cohen J, Chang J, et al: Socioeconomic concerns in vascular surgery: a survey of the role of age, resource consumption, and outcome in treatment cost. *J Vasc Surg* 9:479-486, 1989.
167. Jencks SF, Kay T: Do frail, disabled, poor, and very old medicare beneficiaries have higher hospital charges? *JAMA* 257:198-202, 1987.
168. Cogbill TH, Landercasper J, Strott PJ, et al: Late results of peripheral vascular surgery in patients 80 years of age or older. *Arch Surg* 122:581-586, 1987.
169. Friedman SG, Kerner BA, Friedman MS, Moccio CG: Limb salvage in elderly patients: is aggressive therapy warranted? *J Cardiovasc Surg* 30:848-851, 1989.
170. Scher LA, Vieth FJ, Ascer E, et al: Limb salvage in octogenarians and nonagenarians. *Surgery* 99:160-164, 1986.
171. Edwards WH, Mulherin JL, Rogers DM: Vascular reconstruction in the octogenarian. *South Med J* 75:648-652, 1982.
172. Rosenblatt MS, Quist WC, Sidawy AN, et al: Results of vein graft reconstruction of the lower extremity in diabetic and nondiabetic patients. *Surg Gynecol Obstet* 171:331-335, 1990.
173. Moody AP, Edwards PR, Harris PL, et al: In situ versus reversed vein femoropopliteal vein grafts: long-term follow-up of a prospective, randomized trial. *Br J Surg* 79:750-755, 1992.
174. Plecha FR, Bertin EJ, Avellone JC, et al: The early results of vascular surgery in patients 75 years of age and older: an analysis of 3259 cases. *J Vasc Surg* 2:769-774, 1985.
175. Huston CC, Bivins BA, Ernst CB, Griffin WO: Morbid implications of above knee amputations. *Arch Surg* 115:167-169, 1980.
176. Rush DB, Huston CC, Bivins BA, Hyde GL: Operative and late mortality rates for above-knee and below-knee amputations. *Am Surg* 41:36-38, 1981.
177. Ouriel K, Fiore WM, Geary JE. Limb-threatening ischemia in the medically compromised patient: amputation or revascularization. *Surgery* 104:667-672, 1988.
178. Hobson RW, Lynh TG, Zafor J, et al: Results of revascularization and amputation in severe lower extremity ischemia. *J Vasc Surg* 2:174-185, 1985.
179. Vieth FJ, Gupta SK, Sampson RH, et al: Superficial femoral and popliteal arteries as inflow sites for distal bypasses. *Surgery* 90:980-990, 1981.
180. Gupta SK, Vieth F, Ascer E, et al: Cost factors in limb threatening ischemia due to infrainguinal arteriosclerosis. *Eur J Vasc Surg* 3:151-154, 1988.
181. O'Mara CS, Kilgore TL, McMullan MH, et al: Distal bypass for limb salvage in very elderly patients. *Am Surg* 53:66-70, 1987.
182. Jonason T, Ringqvist I: Mortality and morbidity in patients with intermittent claudication in relation to the location of the occlusive atherosclerosis in the leg. *Angiology* 186:310-314, 1985.
183. Waters RL, Lusford BR: Energy expenditure of normal and pathologic gait: application to orthotic prescription. In: *American Academy of Orthopaedic Surgeons: Atlas of Orthotics.* 2nd Ed. St. Louis: CV Mosby; 151-159, 1985.

Chapter 22

Management of Thoracic and Thoracoabdominal Aortic Aneurysms in the Elderly

Jean M. Panneton, MD
Larry H. Hollier, MD

Repair of descending thoracic aneurysm (DTA) or thoracoabdominal aortic aneurysm (TAAA) has remained, over the years, a tremendous physiological challenge for patients. Such complex aortic reconstructions involve transient ischemia to many organ systems, and the potential for complications is high. Obviously, the elderly patient may be more at risk for perioperative morbidity and mortality depending on the presence or absence of significant comorbid factors. Furthermore, it is likely that due to population aging and the increased incidence of DTAs and TAAAs, surgeons will have to deal more frequently with the management of these aneurysms in elderly patients. From these considerations arise the importance of careful preoperative evaluation in order to select appropriate candidates for DTA or TAAA repair among the elderly. This patient selection must balance the risk of death from rupture of DTA or TAAA versus the risk of operative mortality and morbidity, such as respiratory failure, need for dialysis, or paraplegia. In this chapter, we review the management of DTA and TAAA pertinent to the elderly population. We also briefly describe our surgical approach to minimize operative risks and improve surgical results of DTA or TAAA repair in the elderly.

Incidence

In a stable American community, the relative incidence of DTAs and TAAAs has been shown to increase with advancing age.[1] In this study, the incidence of DTA was found to be 5.3 per 100,000 person-years.[1] This increased incidence in DTAs combined with the demo-

From: Aronow WS, Stemmer EA, Wilson SE (eds). *Vascular Disease in the Elderly*. Armonk, NY: Futura Publishing Company, Inc., © 1997.

graphic phenomenon of population aging, will undoubtedly make DTA and TAAA a more prevalent problem in the elderly. Thus, vascular surgeons will be frequently faced with an elderly patient with DTA or TAAA, and will have to deal with the decision whether to proceed with surgical repair. In a recent exhaustive review of the literature, we have established that patients with nondissecting TAAA had a median age varying from 64.5 to 68.5 and mean age varying from 58 to 70.5 years.[2] On the same type of review, but for patients with dissecting DTA or TAAA, the mean age was 60.4 years.[3] In our experience, the age of patients operated for TAAA ranged from 31 to 88 years old.[4] In the largest series on TAAA repair, 12% of patients were more than 70 years old.[5] In a more recent series, up to 26% of patients operated for TAAA were between 70 and 85.[6] Schepens and collaborators reported that 30% of their patients undergoing TAAA repair were more than 70 years old.[7] Furthermore, a recent series of 72 consecutive patients operated for TAAA reported that 21% were older than 75.[8] DTA repair series have also shown that the relative proportion of patients older than 70 is quite high, such as 23% in Livesay et al's series.[9] Thus, repair of DTA and TAAA is already being done in a significant proportion of elderly patients and will likely be done more frequently.

Etiology

The etiology of TAAA is mainly divided into two diseases: atherosclerosis and dissection. Atherosclerotic medial degenerative disease accounts for about 82% of TAAA, whereas dissection accounts for another 17%.[2] Other diseases, such as Marfan syndrome, Ehlers-Danlos syndrome, Takayasu's disease, and mycotic or traumatic aneurysms, account altogether for less than 5%.[2] DTA have three main etiologies: atherosclerotic in 55% to 66% of cases, dissection in 23% to 29%, and chronic post-traumatic in 5% to 9%.[9-11] There have been no specific reports on the influence of age on the etiology of DTA or TAAA, but we can deduct from the analysis of the literature that dissecting DTA or TAAA occur and are repaired in a younger age group than atherosclerotic degenerative DTA or TAAA.[2,3]

Prognosis

Knowledge of the natural history of thoracic aneurysms is essential to enable the surgeon to balance the risk of surgery versus the risk of death from rupture. The average expansion rate of thoracic aneurysms has been established at 0.4 cm per year.[12] This expansion rate is quite similar to the one for infrarenal abdominal aortic aneurysms. In the classic series from Crawford and DeNatale, patients with unoperated TAAA had a 2-year survival rate of only 24%, with 50% of death caused from rupture.[13] This dismal statistic was also found for patients with DTAs and TAAAs as shown by Bickerstaff and collaborators, with a 2-

year survival of 29% and a 5-year survival of only 13% with 77% of death from rupture.[1] Also, Pressler and McNamara have shown a 2-year survival rate of only 50% in patients with unoperated nondissecting DTA or TAAA.[14] From these different studies, we can conclude that the natural history of DTA or TAAA is poor and the 2-year survival rate may vary from 24% to 50%. Patients with nondissecting aneurysm may have an average 2-year survival rate around 40% to 50%. In a recent series on the outcome of patients with nondissecting TAAA managed nonoperatively, rupture did not occur in aneurysm less than 5 cm.[15] The 2-year survival rate was 78%, probably because the dissecting aneurysms were excluded and the aneurysms were smaller than the ones in other reported series. Another important aspect in the natural course of patients with TAAA is that nearly 10% present with rupture and about half the patients will become symptomatic; emergent repair will be required in 26% of patients.[2]

Finally, the prognosis of patients with DTA or TAAA is most certainly related to the impact of associated comorbid factors. These associated risk factors are very common: hypertension in 70%; coronary artery disease in 35%; chronic obstructive pulmonary disease (COPD) in 35%; visceral occlusive disease in 25%; chronic renal failure in 20%; and cerebral vascular disease or peripheral vascular disease in 15% each.[2] The prevalence of these comorbid factors can be expected to increase in the subset of elderly patients with DTA or TAAA. Such a high prevalence of comorbid factors dictates the need for careful preoperative evaluation of these organ systems to fully assess the physiological status of the patient. This will give a better idea of the patient's physiological tolerance than will chronological age alone.

Indications and Contraindications for Surgical Repair

The decision whether to operate on an elderly patient with DTA or TAAA is based on the knowledge of the natural history of the aneurysm and the medical condition of the patient. The risk of rupture is related to the maximum diameter of the thoracic aneurysm. It has been determined that we can probably safely observe patients with TAAA less than 5 cm.[15,16] Elective repair is definitely recommended for aneurysm of or greater than 6 cm in maximal diameter. Elective repair of aneurysm greater than 5 cm, but smaller than 6 cm should be considered carefully in elderly patients. In Crawford et al's study on ruptured aneurysm of the DTA and TAAA, 13% of these aneurysms experienced rupture within an estimated aortic diameter between 5 and 6 cm.[16] Thus, even if only a small proportion of ruptured DTA or TAAA occur in these intermediate size aneurysms, it would be reasonable in elderly patients to recommend elective repair of between 5 and 6 cm DTA or TAAA, only if risk factors are absent or moderate. Elderly patients presenting with a ruptured DTA or TAAA should not be denied an attempt at surgical repair based solely on their advanced age. In Crawford et al's study on ruptured DTA and TAAA, age, by univariate or multivariate analysis, was not a significant predictor of early death after emergent repair.[16]

Patients with aneurysms less than 5 cm in maximal diameter should be observed with serial chest and abdominal computed tomography (CT) scan at 6-month intervals. Elderly patients should be considered for elective repair of large DTA or TAAA. Patients with very advanced age, such as octogenarians, should not be denied elective repair if a large aneurysm is present. The contraindications for elective repair should be based on physiological assessment of the patient and not simply on advanced chronological age. Significant ischemic heart disease, such as unstable angina and unreconstructable coronary disease, is a definite contraindication for surgical repair. A recent myocardial infarction should cause one to defer surgery for at least 3 to 6 months until a new cardiac assessment with functional coronary testing is redone. Severe left ventricular dysfunction, such as left ventricular ejection fraction less than 20%, is usually a contraindication to surgical repair. Severe valvular insufficiency, such as aortic or mitral regurgitation, is another contraindication and should be corrected before elective repair is considered. Severe COPD, as confirmed by forced expiratory volume in 1 second of less than 1 liter, also usually contraindicates elective repair. Chronic renal failure or severe hypertension should mandate the assessment of renal arteries to determine if renal revascularization is required either as a preoperative percutaneous transluminal angioplasty, or as a concomitant procedure during TAAA repair. Preoperative renal dysfunction will undoubtedly increase both surgical mortality and the potential need for postoperative dialysis. Finally, the presence of severe dementia or malignancies with a shortened life expectancy should be considered contraindications for both elective and emergent repairs.

Risk of Surgery

In our experience with TAAA repair, advanced age has been correlated with increased perioperative mortality (p = 0.003) and with increased risk of perioperative myocardial infarction (p = 0.01).[17] The impact of advanced age on postoperative mortality, renal failure, paraplegia, and respiratory failure has been studied by many authors (Table) for TAAA repair[5-7,17-23] and for DTA repair.[9,24,25] As shown in the Table, the majority of series have established a correlation between advanced age and early postoperative death. In Crawford et al 's series, patients ages 71 to 86 had a 12% operative mortality, whereas the operative mortality was 9% for those 60 to 66 years and 67 to 70 years.[5] In this study, they found that for each yearly increase in age, the odds ratio for 30-day death was 1.05. However, no significant difference was found

Table
Correlation of Age with Postoperative Mortality and Morbidity after TAAA and DTA repair

Authors	Mortality	Renal Failure	Paraplegia	Respiratory Failure
Svensson et al[5]	yes	yes	yes	—
Coselli[6]	no	yes	no	—
Schepens et al[7]	no	yes	no	—
Hollier et al[17]	yes	no	no	—
Crawford et al[18]	yes	no	no	—
Fox et al[19]	yes	—	—	—
Svensson et al[20]	—	—	—	no
Money et al[21]	—	—	—	yes
Svensson et al[22]	—	no	—	—
Acher et al[23]	—	—	no	—
Livesay et al[9]	yes	yes	no	—
DeBakey et al[24]	yes	—	—	—
Kazui et al[25]	no	no	no	no

TAAA = thoracoabdominal aortic aneurysm
DTA = descending thoracic aneurysm

in a recent study from Coselli; 30-day operative mortality rate was 7.1% for ages 72 to 85 compared to 5.5% for ages 62 to 71.[6]

The data concerning the influence of advanced age on postoperative renal failure is more conflicting (Table). In our own experience, we have found that advanced age does not correlate with an increased risk of renal failure.[17] In Crawford et al's initial experience with TAAA repair, the need for dialysis was 10% among patients 71 to 86, which was not significantly different from the younger age groups.[18] However, increasing age was later found to correlate significantly with an increased incidence of renal dysfunction in the postoperative period.[5] Likewise, in Coselli's series, the age group 72 to 85 years had a 13.3% incidence of renal failure, compared to 5.8% for the younger age groups.[6] Schepens et al established that the risk for postoperative dialysis was related to advanced age and that each yearly increase in age increased the risk by 1.2.[7] In the largest series of patients who underwent DTA or TAAA repair, Svensson and collaborators studied the factors associated with the occurrence of postoperative acute renal failure.[22] In this study, patients between ages 75 and 87 had a 34% incidence of renal dysfunction (creatinine >2 mg/dL) and a 9.6% incidence of need for postoperative dialysis. This renal dysfunction and need for dialysis was shown by univariate analysis to be significantly increased in this older age group.[22] However, by multivariate analysis, age was not found to be an independent predictor of acute renal failure requiring dialysis, nor of renal dysfunction. Instead, the level of preoperative renal dysfunction (defined as increased creatinine above 1.5 mg/dL) and other factors such as postoperative complications were found to be the best independent predictors of renal failure.[22]

All series but one confirmed that advanced age does not correlate with an increased risk of postoperative paraplegia after DTA or TAAA repair.[6,7,9,17,18,23,25] The one exception is the study by Svensson and collaborators, wherein, by multivariate analysis, for each yearly increase in patient age, the odds ratio for postoperative paraplegia is 1.02.[5]

In the Ochsner Clinic experience with TAAA repair, the risk of postoperative respiratory failure was found to be higher in older patients. Patients with respiratory failure had an average age of 72 years compared to patients without respiratory failure with an average age of 65.5 years.[21] However, in the study by Svensson and associates,[20] advanced age was not found to correlate with an increased risk of postoperative respiratory failure. Instead, they found by multivariate analysis that the presence of preoperative COPD and a history of smoking, as well as cardiac and renal postoperative complications, were independent risk factors for respiratory failure.[20]

The conclusion from analysis of the Table is that advanced age seems to be correlated with an increased risk of perioperative mortality and also postoperative complications such as renal or respiratory failure. However, stepwise logistic regression analysis often shows that advanced age itself is not an independent predictor, but that other preoperative factors such as ischemic heart disease, chronic renal failure, and COPD, are more accurate predictors of postoperative mortality or morbidity.

Preoperative Assessment and Surgical Technique

Adequate preoperative evaluation is the most important step in the management of elderly patients with DTA or TAAA. Computerized tomography of the chest and abdomen is used routinely to define aneurysm extent (Figure 1). Furthermore, we believe that CT scanning is the best available method to determine the diameter of the aneurysm, which will dictate the need for operation or for conservative observation. Magnetic resonance imaging (MRI) also provides excellent definition of the aneurysm, and provides coronal and sagittal planes. Because advanced age per se is not a contraindication for DTA or TAAA repair, a thorough physiological assessment of these elderly patients is mandatory. Besides the standard blood tests, routine evaluation includes: carotid duplex ultrasound; baseline electrocardiogram and functional cardiac testing by dipyridamole thallium scan or dobutamine echocardiogram; measurements of left ventricular ejection fraction; and arterial blood gas and pulmonary function test. Renal artery imaging by magnetic resonance angiogram or spiral CT with three-dimensional reconstruction is performed if visceral vessel occlusive disease is suspected (Figure 2). Carotid endarterectomy is performed for severe carotid stenosis greater than 70% to 80% diameter reduction even in asymptomatic patients.

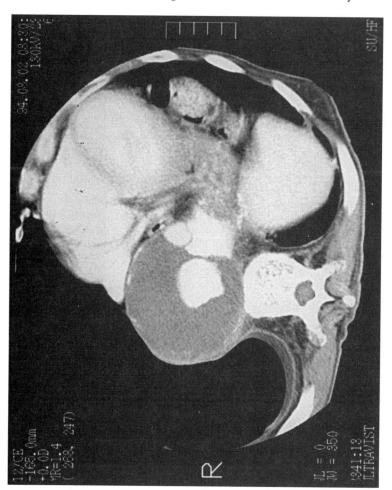

Figure 1. Chest CT scan at the level of the hiatus showing a large dissecting thoracoabdominal aortic aneurysm with a maximum diameter of 8.5 cm.

We believe that routine screening with duplex ultrasound (Figure 3) and prophylactic carotid endarterectomy for high-grade stenosis have decreased the incidence of postoperative stroke in our patients.[26] A coronary angiogram is performed if a patient has significant angina or if the functional study suggests significant coronary artery disease. If possible, severe coronary artery stenoses are treated preoperatively by percutaneous transluminal angioplasty or by coronary artery bypass grafting. If visceral vessel occlusive disease is confirmed by imaging, appropriate lesions are treated by percutaneous transluminal angioplasty, or if not, these occlusive lesions are dealt with usually by transaortic endarterectomy during TAAA repair. Finally, perioperative pulmonary management is based on the severity of the COPD and its response to bronchodilators, antibiotics, or steroids. We follow the rec-

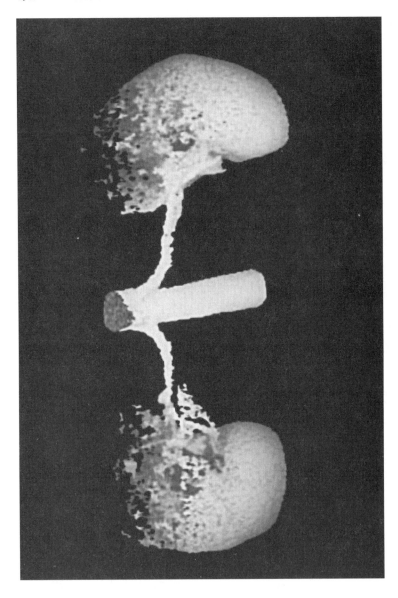

Figure 2. Spiral CT scan of the abdominal aorta with three-dimensional reconstruction showing patent renal arteries.

ommendations for severe COPD management as stated by the Mayo Clinic group.[27]

Our surgical technique for DTA or TAAA repair has evolved over the years and is based on invasive monitoring including: the use of transesophageal echocardiogram for elderly patients with marginal left ventricular function; avoidance of double thoracotomy technique to decrease the risk of respiratory failure; the use of mannitol, renal dose dopamine infusion, and cold perfusion of the kidneys to protect against

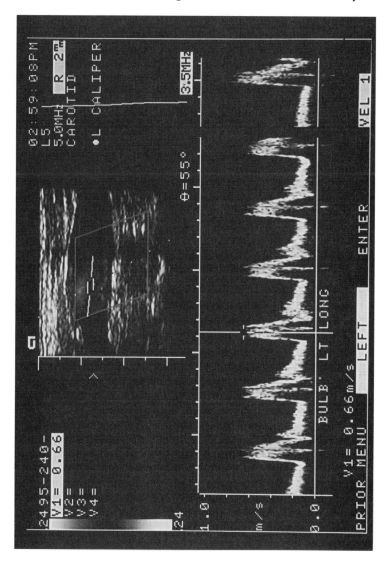

Figure 3. Carotid duplex ultrasound showing in the **top portion** a longitudinal gray scale image of the left carotid bulb, with only minimal plaque and normal origin of the internal carotid artery. The **bottom portion** shows moderate spectral broadening and normal velocity.

postoperative renal failure, especially in elderly patients with increased creatinine value preoperatively; and finally a multimodality approach for spinal cord protection.[28] This multimodality approach for spinal cord protection is based on: expeditious surgery; high proximal aortic pressure; routine intercostal artery reimplantation; distal aortic perfusion for extensive aneurysms; cerebral spinal fluid pressure monitoring and drainage for up to 3 days; moderate systemic hypothermia; and systemic steroids, mannitol, and thiopental. This multimodality approach provides therapeutic interventions at the different steps in the ischemic and reperfusion injury cascade of spinal cord ischemia, as we have previously reported.[4]

Long-Term Survival

Long-term survival is obviously influenced by the age of the patient when DTA or TAAA repair is done. Schepens and collaborators found a 2-year survival of 67% and 5-year survival of 39% for patients over 65.[7] Finally, in Coselli and Crawford's experience, 1-year survival was 68% and 5-year survival was 44% for those 70 to 86 years compared, to a 1-year survival of 80% and 5-year survival of 59% for those from 55 to 69.[29] The extent of long-term survival after DTA or TAAA repair even among elderly patients is definitely superior to the natural history of those aneurysms. Preoperative renal dysfunction or coronary artery disease and postoperative renal failure or paraplegia have a much more important impact on long-term survival then advanced age alone.

Summary

Elderly patients with DTA or TAAA should not be denied repair based on the criteria of advanced age alone. Instead, they should be carefully assessed preoperatively for their physiological status. Associated risk factors are identified and if possible modified by careful preoperative preparation. The decision to operate an elderly patient with DTA and TAAA is based on the size of the aneurysm and the patient's physiological condition. Patients are excluded if the aneurysm is smaller than 5 cm, or if their operative risk is found to be prohibitive due to associated comorbid factors. Operative results and late survival justify surgical repair of DTA and TAAA even in elderly patients if operative candidates are carefully selected.

References

1. Bickerstaff LK, Pairolero PC, Hollier LH, et al: Thoracic aortic aneurysms: a population-based study. *Surgery* 92:1103-1108, 1982.
2. Panneton JM, Hollier LH: Nondissecting thoracoabdominal aortic aneurysms: part I. *Ann Vasc Surg* 9:503-514, 1995.
3. Panneton JM, Hollier LH: Dissecting descending thoracic and thoracoabdominal aortic aneurysms: part II. *Ann Vasc Surg* 9:596-605, 1995.
4. Hollier LH, Money SR, Naslund TC, et al: Risk of spinal cord dysfunction in patients undergoing thoracoabdominal aortic replacement. *Am J Surg* 164:210-214, 1992.
5. Svensson LG, Crawford ES, Hess KR, et al: Experience with 1509 patients undergoing thoracoabdominal aortic operations. *J Vasc Surg* 17:357-370, 1993.
6. Coselli JS: Thoracoabdominal aortic aneurysms: experience with 372 patients. *J Card Surg* 9:638-647, 1994.

7. Schepens MAAM, Defauw JJAM, Hamerlijnck RPHM, et al: Surgical treatment of thoracoabdominal aortic aneurysms by simple crossclamping. *J Thorac Cardiovasc Surg* 107:134-142, 1994.
8. Rice K, Hollier LH, Money SR, et al: Financial impact of thoracoabdominal aneurysm repair. *Am J Surg* 166:186-190, 1993.
9. Livesay JJ, Cooley DA, Ventemiglia RA, et al: Surgical experience in descending thoracic aneurysmectomy with and without adjuncts to avoid ischemia. *Ann Thorac Surg* 39:37-46, 1985.
10. DeBakey ME, McCollum CH, Graham JM: Surgical treatment of aneurysms of the descending thoracic aorta. *J Cardiovasc Surg* 19:571-576, 1978.
11. Crawford ES, Walker HSJ III, Saleh SA, et al: Graft replacement of aneurysm in descending thoracic aorta: results without bypass or shunting. *Surgery* 89:73-85, 1981.
12. Dapunt OE, Galla JD, Sadeghi AM, et al: The natural history of thoracic aortic aneurysms. *J Thorac Cardiovasc Surg* 107:1323-1333, 1994.
13. Crawford ES, DeNatale RW: Thoracoabdominal aortic aneurysm: observations regarding the natural course of the disease. *J Vasc Surg* 3:578-582, 1986.
14. Pressler V, McNamara JJ: Thoracic aortic aneurysm: natural history and treatment. *J Thorac Cardiovasc Surg* 79:489-498, 1980.
15. Cambria RA, Gloviczki P, Stanson AW, et al: Outcome and expansion rate of 57 thoracoabdominal aortic aneurysms managed nonoperatively. *Am J Surg* 170:213-217, 1995.
16. Crawford ES, Hess KR, Cohen ES, et al: Ruptured aneurysm of the descending thoracic and thoracoabdominal aorta. *Ann Surg* 213:417-426, 1991.
17. Hollier LH, Symmonds JB, Pairolero PC, et al: Thoracoabdominal aortic aneurysm repair. *Arch Surg* 123:871-875, 1988.
18. Crawford ES, Crawford JL, Safi HJ, et al: Thoracoabdominal aortic aneurysms: preoperative and intraoperative factors determining immediate and long-term results of operations in 605 patients. *J Vasc Surg* 3:389-404, 1986.
19. Fox AD, Berkowitz HD: Thoracoabdominal aneurysm resection after previous infrarenal abdominal aortic aneurysmectomy. *Am J Surg* 162:142-144, 1991.
20. Svensson LG, Hess KR, Coselli JS, et al: A prospective study of respiratory failure after high-risk surgery on the thoracoabdominal aorta. *J Vasc Surg* 14:271-282, 1991.
21. Money SR, Rice K, Crockett D, et al: Risk of respiratory failure after repair of thoracoabdominal aortic aneurysms. *Am J Surg* 168:152-155, 1994.
22. Svensson LG, Coselli JS, Safi HJ, et al: Appraisal of adjuncts to prevent acute renal failure after surgery on the thoracic or thoracoabdominal aorta. *J Vasc Surg* 10:230-239, 1989.
23. Acher CW, Wynn MN, Hoch JR, et al: Combined use of cerebral spinal fluid drainage and naloxone reduces the risk of paraplegia in thoracoabdominal aneurysm repair. *J Vasc Surg* 19:236-248, 1994.
24. DeBakey ME, McCollum CH, Crawford ES, et al: Dissection and dissecting aneurysms of the aorta: 20-year follow-up of 527 patients treated surgically. *Surgery* 92:1118 1134, 1982.
25. Kazui T, Komatsu S, Yokoyama H: Surgical treatment of aneurysms of the thoracic aorta with the aid of partial cardiopulmonary bypass: an analysis of 95 patients. *Ann Thorac Surg* 43:622-627, 1987.
26. Panneton JM, Hollier LH: Treatment of carotid disease in patients undergoing thoracic or abdominal aortic surgery. In: Caplan L, Moore W, Nicolaides A, Shifrin E (eds). *Cerebrovascular Ischaemia, Investigation and Management.* London: Med-Orion Publishing, Co; 197–206, 1996.

27. Hallett JW Jr, Bower TC, Cherry KJ, et al: Selection and preparation of high-risk patients for repair of abdominal aortic aneurysms. *Mayo Clin Proc* 69:763-768, 1994.
28. Panneton JM, Hollier LH: Clinical approach for thoracoabdominal aortic aneurysm repair. *Intl J Angio* 6:60–66, 1996.
29. Coselli JS, Crawford ES: Thoracoabdominal aortic aneurysms. In: Yao J, Pearce W (eds). *Long-Term Results in Vascular Surgery.* East Norwalk, CT: Appleton & Lange; 135-147, 1993.

Chapter 23

Abdominal Aortic Aneurysms in the Elderly:

Special Considerations

John Menezes, MD
Samuel Eric Wilson, MD

Introduction

The rationale for repair of abdominal aortic aneurysms (AAA) in elderly patients rests on the premise that mortality from rupture will be reduced by an elective procedure, performed with minimal operative mortality, while the quality of life will be maintained postoperatively. As the North American population continues to age, the potential number of patients greater than age 65 who have AAAs has increased. These epidemiological trends create the dilemma of what recommendations should be made for repair of aneurysms, specifically the maximum aortic diameter which is safe in the elderly, who often have significant comorbidity. The risk/benefit ratio for aneurysm repair is different than for younger patients in that aneurysm size and rate of growth must be measured against the patient's remaining life expectancy.

In this chapter, we present an analysis of the prevalence of aortic disease in the older population, and the characteristics of aneurysms peculiar to the elderly which may predispose them to rupture. We also consider which preoperative studies are most useful to the surgeon in deciding who is best suited for repair.

Epidemiology

The North American population has an increasing number of men and women over 65 years of age. An estimated 25 million people in the United States are between the ages of 65 and 85, and by the year

From: Aronow WS, Stemmer EA, Wilson SE (eds). *Vascular Disease in the Elderly.* Armonk, NY: Futura Publishing Company, Inc., © 1997.

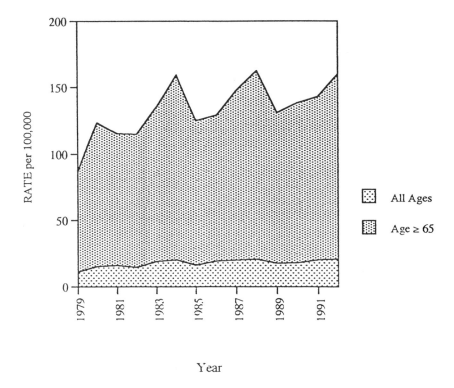

Figure 1. Rate of aortic aneurysm listed for all ages compared with incidence in patients over 65 years of age. (Reproduced with permission from Reference 2.)

2025, this number will rise to approximately 58 million individuals.[1] Today, the life expectancy of a nonagenarian is still almost 5 years.

Recent epidemiological data suggest that aneurysmal disease is becoming a major problem for the aged. Between 1979 and 1990, there was little change in death rates from AAAs. However, in 1991 alone, there were 16,696 deaths attributed to aneurysm, with persons greater than 65 years of age accounting for 14,037 deaths.[1] Additionally, it has been suggested that a single screening of men age 65 to 74 years of age might yield an incidence of 2% to 3% for aneurysms of 4.0 cm or greater.[2] The proportion of the United States population greater than age 65 with AAAs as compared with all age groups is shown in Figure 1. This index has increased from 80 per 100,000 in 1979 to 150 per 100,000 in 1991.[1]

The correlation between advancing age and prevalence of AAAs was demonstrated for both men and women in an epidemiological study of 5,419 subjects age 55 years and older in Rotterdam, The Netherlands, between 1989 and 1993. For example, Table 1 shows in men the increasing rates of aortic aneurysm with age, when an aneurysm is defined as a distal aortic diameter greater than 35 mm, or a dilatation of 50% or more.[3]

Table 1
The Prevalence of Aortic Aneurysm Increases Greatly with Age in the Dutch
Population

Age Group	Prevalence
55 to 59	0.8%
60 to 64	3.1%
65 to 69	3.8%
70 to 74	4.4%
75 to 79	8.3%
≥80	10.3%

(Reproduced with permission from Reference 31.)

The Ad Hoc Committee on Reporting Standards of the Society of Vascular Surgery and the North American Chapter of the International Society for Cardiovascular Surgery define an aneurysm as a permanent localized dilatation of an artery having at least 50% increase in diameter compared to the expected normal diameter of the artery in question.[4] As greatest cross-sectional diameter is the principle measure by which the decision to operate is based on, one would expect information on "normal" aortic measurements to be known according to age. Few studies, however, have related aortic diameter to age. Pearce et al studied the computed tomography (CT) scans of 398 patients between the ages of 17 and 87 with nonvascular disease (e.g., malignancy or infection) to determine the relationships between aortic diameter and age, gender, and body surface area at five levels of the thoracic and abdominal aorta.[4] An additional 16 patients with known aneurysms, matched for age, were compared to discover if these relationships persisted in those with aneurysms. The relationships between age, body surface area, and aortic diameter according to data from Pearce is shown in Figure 2.

Other studies have also found a significant correlation between age and aortic expansion for both the normal aorta and that with aneurysmal disease.[3,5,6] Dixon et al studied 257 normal aortas between the ages of 30 and 80 years and found that progressive expansion of the distal aorta occurs with advancing age, more rapidly in men than in women.[5] Interestingly, it was also confirmed that calcification of the aorta usually does not begin before the fourth decade and that severe calcification becomes significantly more prevalent in women in their seventh and eighth decades as compared to men (20% versus 5%; $p < 0.05$).[5]

In general, these studies confirm that the normal aorta, with aging, undergoes a natural expansion of the infrarenal diameter. In Pearce's study, the data suggest that body surface area should also be taken into account in assessing diameter, although no "normal" aorta, even at the upper limit of body surface area, exceeded 2.5 cm in diameter.[3,4]

The explanation for age-related expansion of the aorta is multifactorial. In one study of 100 normal aortas, Schlatman and Becker found

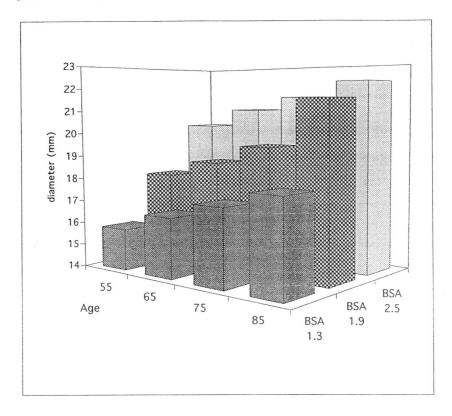

Figure 2. Infrarenal aortic diameter according to age and body surface area (BSA). (Reproduced with permission from Reference 4.)

histological changes which included wall fibrosis, elastin fragmentation, and cystic medial necrosis. Ninety-five of the 100 specimens showed evidence of elastin fragmentation, the exceptions being children.[7] The most significant etiological factor may be depletion of the elastin content of the aortic wall with aging. The process is twofold in that elastin is not regenerated, while enzymes that degrade elastin persist in the aortic wall.[8]

The quantity of elastin also diminishes in gradient fashion from the elastic thoracic aorta to the infrarenal aorta, perhaps accounting for the predominance of aneurysms in this location.[8]

Risk factors that accelerate the atherosclerotic process also appear to have an influence on infrarenal aortic dilatation. Zarins et al examined the relationship between atherosclerotic plaque formation in 30 male cadaver aortas. Enlarged abdominal aortas had a twofold greater plaque area and reduced media thickness, while also exhibiting a regression of internal elastic lamina.[6] In the Rotterdam epidemiological study, among 12 preoperative risk factors correlated with the presence of AAA,

only current tobacco use and mean serum cholesterol were significant—
both major risk factors for atherosclerosis.[3]

Preoperative Tests

Determination of aortic diameter is accomplished through several
modalities. Physical examination by an experienced clinician is perhaps 97% specific and 30% sensitive for AAA, but tends to overestimate
the size and is only a gross estimate at best.[9] Noninvasive imaging is
more accurate for following changes in diameter from year to year.
Ultrasound is the most effective tool for AAA screening since it is safe,
inexpensive, and is close to 100% sensitive and specific.[9] CT scanning
is more accurate in terms of inter- and intraobserver agreement, but
significant variations in diameter reading can occur without a standard
approach. Lederle et al showed in a study of male veterans who had
abdominal ultrasound and CT evaluation of aortic aneurysm, that the
variation between these modalities could be as much as 0.5 cm in 33%
of readings; ultrasound measurement averaged 0.27 cm less than the
diameter determined by CT. Agreement between CT readings was more
accurate, and was significantly improved when standardizing measures
such as calipers and magnifying glasses were instituted (Figure 3).[10]

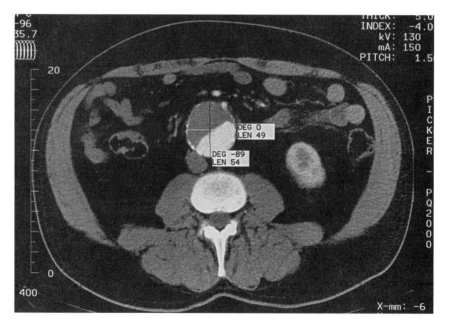

Figure 3. Computed tomography (CT) provides an accurate measurement of aortic
diameter; it shows thrombus within the aneurysm, relationship to renal arteries, and
distal extent of aneurysm. CT is useful to confirm exact growth discovered on screening ultrasound.

Angiography is the most accurate for the delineation of concomitant renovascular disease and definition of the anatomy and extent of collaterals in mesenteric vessels, as well as lower extremity runoff. It cannot, however, measure extraluminal diameter and has the drawbacks of invasiveness and expense.

A new modality rivaling angiography and superior to magnetic resonance angiography is spiral (helical) CT, or computed tomographic angiography (CTA). It is a noninvasive technique compared with conventional angiography, employed with approximately 120 cc of contrast, given by a single peripheral venous injection, and can render an infinite number of three-dimensional reconstructions.[11] The detail is sufficient to accurately assess pathology of renal and mesenteric vessels and their anatomical relationships, in addition to revealing the true and false lumens of a dissecting aneurysm. Drawbacks to CTA include the overestimation of stenosis, important with respect to renovascular disease, and a lower resolution than conventional angiography; plus, so far, it has not been used to evaluate distal runoff (Figures 4A-C, and Figure 5).[11]

Natural History of Abdominal Aortic Aneurysms

The natural history of untreated AAAs is one of progressive enlargement to rupture for a significant number of patients. The rate of aneurysmal expansion varies from 0.1 cm per year to as much as 0.48 cm per year,[12-14] and the rate of expansion is accelerated as the size of the aneurysm increases.[12,14] In a prospective study over 6 years of 600 patients, Guirguis et al[12] found that the median expansion rate was 0.2 cm per year among those with aneurysms less than 4 cm, while those patients with aneurysms greater than 4 cm experienced expansion at rates between 0.3 and 0.8 cm per year. These observations are particularly applicable to elderly patients whose aneurysms tend to be larger.

As aneurysms enlarge, the incidences of rupture increase. In Darling's classic autopsy study, the rate of rupture for aneurysms less than 4 cm was 9.5%; for 4 to 5 cm, 23%; and for those 5 to 6 cm in diameter, 25%.[15] Similarly, in a recent report from the Mayo Clinic, Hallett et al reported that at 5 years after initial assessment, the risk of rupture was nearly 5% for aneurysms less than 5 cm, approximately 25% for aneurysms 5 to 7 cm, and 50% or more for aneurysms greater than 7 cm.[13]

Szilagyi, in 1972, showed that in patients refused operation, rupture can occur unpredictably within 8 years of diagnosis. Among those considered unfit for surgery whose aneurysms subsequently ruptured, the cumulative incidence of rupture was 39% within 1 year of diagnosis and 69% within 2 years.[16]

Rates of Comorbid Disease

A thorough preoperative assessment of comorbidity in the elderly helps the surgeon to determine who is best suited for repair; it also

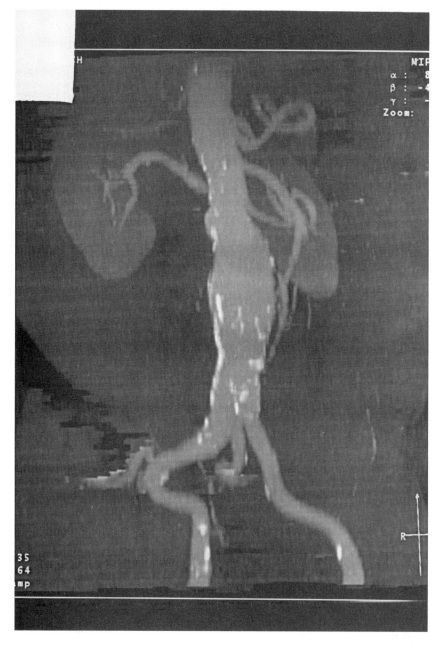

Figures 4A-C. Spiral CT demonstrates a small aortic aneurysm on anterior to posterior view (**A**), lateral view (**B**), and the appearance postoperatively of an aortoiliac.

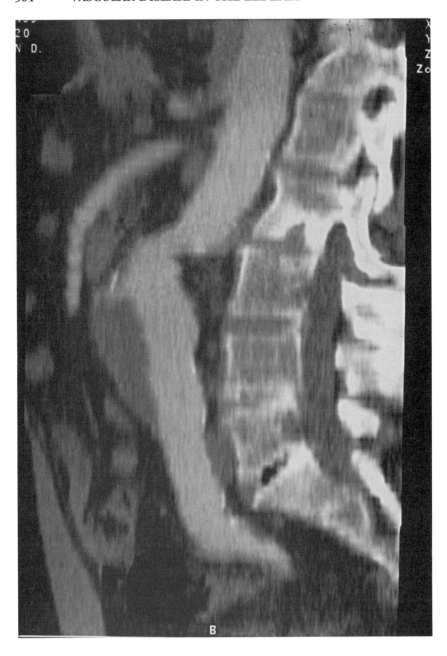

Figure 4B.

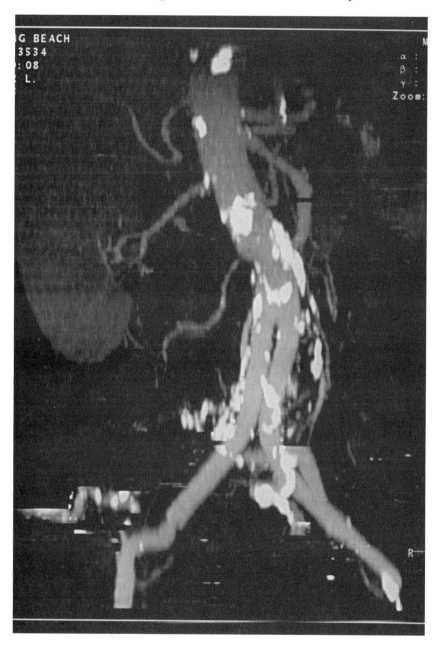

Figure 4C.

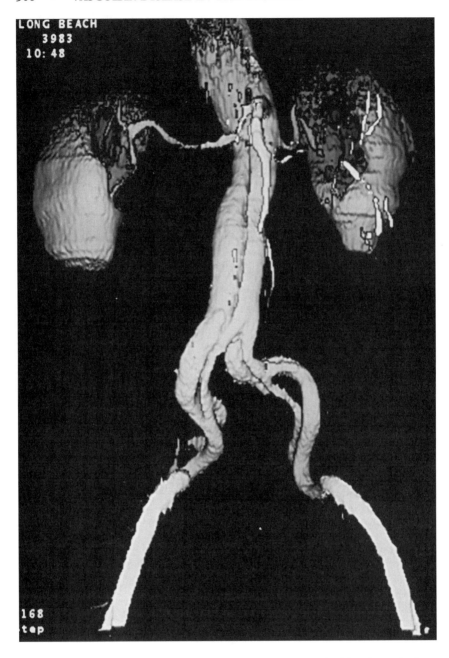

Figure 5. Spiral CT of abdominal aorta demonstrates the double channel of an intramural dissection extending to the iliac arteries.

helps to defer others for observation until a critical size is reached, when repair becomes imperative even with risk factors. The prevalence of systemic disease in the older population presenting for aneurysmectomy is shown in Table 2.

Severe coronary artery disease (CAD) is relatively common in patients with an AAA, and it remains the most significant determinant influencing both early and late mortality.[13,17-23] Therefore, the risk of repair of an AAA is directly related to the magnitude of perioperative cardiac stress and cardiac condition.

Major hemodynamic changes occur with aortic cross-clamping and unclamping during aneurysm repair. Acute infrarenal aortic occlusion produces an immediate rise in pulmonary artery wedge pressure, left ventricular wall stress, peripheral vascular resistance, and a decrease in stroke volume and cardiac output. Patients who have ischemic heart disease or decreased reserve secondary to prior myocardial infarction (MI) may develop signs of acute ventricular decompensation.[24]

Alternatively, unclamping the aorta produces the stress of "declamping shock," with an abrupt decrease in central volume and peripheral resistance that can create a profound arterial hypotension which has occasionally progressed to intractable shock.[24]

Volume shifts also cause additional stress, particularly in aortic surgery during which patients experience the combined effects of blood loss, evaporative losses, and large shifts of volume from the intravascular space into retroperitoneum and intestinal sequestration of fluid. Anesthetic management of these problems can involve large and rapid infusions of volume, vasodilator therapy, and vasoconstrictive therapy.[24]

Identification of significant CAD allows stratification of patients into those who need no preoperative measures, those in whom coronary artery bypass or angioplasty is necessary, and those who have such advanced disease that no revascularization is feasible. Risk assessment can be achieved by objective tests such as exercise stress testing, echocardiography for wall motion, nuclear medicine studies of differential cardiac perfusion and ventricular function, and coronary angiography.

Clinical methods such as the Goldman index are useful in categorizing those at higher risk, but may fail to identify occult disease or those at lesser risk who may still require preoperative measures. In a prospective study of 95 patients undergoing elective aortic aneurysm repair, McEnroe et al assessed cardiac risk with dipyridamole-thallium scintigraphy (DTS), B-mode echocardiographic assessment of ejection fraction (EF), and classification according to the Goldman criteria.[25] Dipyridamole dilates coronary vessels, producing a homogeneous uptake of thallium in normally perfused myocardium, while ischemic muscle shows delayed uptake or areas of redistribution. Infarcted areas show no uptake. In McEnroe's study, DTS was used to identify patients with perfusion defects; a consulting cardiologist then determined those in particular need of coronary artery bypass grafting prior to AAA repair. No correlation could be determined between diminished EF and postopera-

Table 2
Comorbidity in Elderly Patients Who Have Abdominal Aortic Aneurysm

Author	Interval	Mean Age	N†	CAD†	% With Preoperative History Of:				
					CVD	COPD	DM	HTN	Cr > 1.5
Berstein & Chan[5]	1970–1981	69	728	30	13.3	18.1			12
Berstein et al[4]	1978–1985	71.3	123	19.7	4.9	20.5	8.1	45.1	12.2
Dean et al[12]	1985–1992	>80	34	18	21	21		35	18
Guirguis et al[19]	1984–1990	70.4	208					23	
Bayazit et al ¥[3]	1986–1994	65	125	53.0	4	35	2	50	12
McEnroe et al ¥[26]	1987–1990	69	95	36.0			15		
Poulias et al[32]	1967–1993	68.3	672	27.6	4.8		5.8	38.4	3.8
Golden et al ¥[18]	1973–1989	69	500	48.0	7.4	27.4	8	47.6	8.4

CAD = coronary artery disease; CVD = cerebrovascular disease; COPD = chronic obstructive pulmonary disease; DM = diabetes mellitus; HTN = hypertension; Cr = creatinine

¥ Studies primarily examining CAD

* Study of high-risk patients

† n = number

tive MI or ischemia; in fact, all events occurred in those with ventricular EF greater than 50%. All cardiac events and the preponderance of those with reversible defects (i.e., significant ischemic disease) belonged to Goldman class I and II, which would otherwise have predicted a 1% and 5% risk of a postoperative cardiac death, thus, underestimating the true extent of cardiac risk in these patients. Neither the Goldman index nor the DTS was a good predictor of early cardiac morbidity and mortality.[25] White et al, however, in a study of 96 patients undergoing elective repair, did show a significant correlation between Goldman class and long-term survival. Goldman classes III and IV, the presence of cerebrovascular disease or creatinine concentration greater than 3 mg/100 mL all had a significant negative effect on 5-year survival.[23]

DTS is highly specific in determining those with low cardiac risk, since 96% of normal scans had no cardiac morbidity; however, it is less beneficial as a general screen for who may benefit from either percutaneous transluminal coronary angioplasty (PTCA) or coronary artery bypass prior to aortic surgery. It is also useful in identifying a small subset of patients in whom occult disease is not otherwise suspected based on Goldman's index. No cardiac morbidity or mortality occurred among patients undergoing intervention for reconstructible disease, suggesting that in patients who have significant reversible disease, preoperative correction of reconstructible CAD should be pursued.[25] Patients with fixed defects, who were not suitable for revascularization, exhibited a high rate (46%) of postoperative ischemia, MI, or death.[25]

A recent prospective study in the *New England Journal of Medicine* of 457 patients undergoing elective aortic repair, asserts that DTS may not be useful as a general screening tool to determine those at greatest risk for cardiac morbidity and mortality. (Of note in this study is the exclusion of patients with severe correctable disease). While the odds ratio of 1.5 for fixed thallium defect did not reach significance in predicting adverse cardiac outcome, age greater than 65 years and the presence of several clinical predictors did. In patients with either definite CAD or age greater than 65 years, the cardiac complication rate was 24%; with both present, the rate rose to 39%.[17] This suggests that DTS may not be useful as a general screen, but for those particularly at risk, and especially the elderly, it is a useful tool in the selective management of patients prior to AAA repair.

The protection of preoperative angioplasty or bypass for CAD was also demonstrated in Bayazit's study of 145 patients, all of whom underwent coronary angiography prior to surgical treatment of AAA. Coronary artery bypass grafting was performed in 24 patients and PTCA in 4. Overall, early mortality after aneurysm repair was 4%, with three of five deaths occurring in the inoperable cardiac disease category.[18]

Other studies have suggested the benefit of preoperative revascularization in selected patients.[20,26] Golden et al studied 500 patients stratified into three groups based on clinical (e.g., angina) and objective (e.g., EKG, DTS) evidence of CAD. The third group, with greatest cardiac

Table 3
Postoperative Mortality of Ruptured Aneurysm in Elderly Patients

Author	Interval	N†	Age	30-Day Mortality (%)
Crawford[9]	33-yr span	11	>80	27
Dean et al[12]	1985–1992	11	>80	91
McCready et al[24]	1980–1989	38	>80	63
Glovicski et al[17]	1980–1989	57	>80	56
Chalmers et al[6]	1985–1990	25	>80	56
Paty et al[27]	1978–1991	25	>80	24
Coghill et al[8]	1987	9	>80	78

† N = number

risk, underwent coronary artery bypass and experienced no MI or death within 30 days of vascular surgery.[20]

Elmore et al retrospectively evaluated the benefit of PTCA among 100 patients (from a 2,452 patient cohort) receiving preoperative revascularization. While those candidates for PTCA had significantly less CAD than those requiring surgical bypass, the postoperative rate of MI was 0%.[26]

Pulmonary disease is a major source of postoperative morbidity, which requires preoperative assessment in elderly patients. Pulmonary function tests, room air blood gases, treatment with bronchodilators, and for the most severe a short course of corticosteroid, encompass preoperative measures; postoperative plans include early activity out of bed, incentive spirometry, and epidural pain control. A retroperitoneal approach can also minimize pulmonary complications. Long-term survival, however, was not significantly affected by pulmonary disease per White et al, nor by the independent presence of diabetes, peripheral vascular disease, or aneurysm size. A combination of any of any three risk factors did significantly affect survival.[23]

Morbidity and Mortality

Rupture of an AAA in elderly patients is associated with high morbidity and mortality (Table 3). Dean et al in a risk/benefit analysis of the elderly undergoing operation for rupture, discovered a subset of elderly patients in whom mortality was 100%. Rupture was lethal in patients 80 or older who had pronounced hypotension and hemodynamic instability, despite aggressive resuscitation and postoperative intensive care management. For this subset in whom rapid intervention to recover hemodynamic stability was unsuccessful, the approach of observation was suggested.[27]

Table 4
Mortality of Elective Repair and Late Survival

Author	Internal	N†	Age	Early Mortality	5-Yr Survival
Bernstein et al[4]	1978–1985	63	>70	0.8%	67%
Crawford[9]	1981, 25 yrs	43	>70		43
Dean et al[12]	1985–1992	34	>80	5.6%	67%
Hollier et al[21]	1986	106	high risk	5.7%	
Chalmers et al[6]	1985–1990	35	>80	0.0%	§
Paty et al[28]	1978–1991	77	>80	3.0%	63%
McCabe et al[24]	1981	122	>70	5.7%	
Coghill et al[8]	1987	23	>80	4.3%	
Poulias et al[32]	1967–1993	NS	80		65%
*			70		82%
White & Wilson[38]	1972–1984	96	>60	3.1%	67%
			>70		50%
Aune et al ¥[1]	1974–1993	227	72	35.0%	61%
Bernstein & Chan[5]	1970–1981	99	high risk		64%

§ median survival 3 yrs 10 months
* Second age group with Poulias
¥ Study of symptomatic/imminent rupture of AAA
† N = number
NS = not stated

Mortality and Late Survival After Elective Repair of Abdominal Aortic Aneurysm

The goal is to prevent rupture by elective repair of an AAA before the risk of progressing comorbidity becomes prohibitive, and at the same time provide additional years of quality life. Current practice affords a low operative mortality combined with a significant 5-year survival (Table 4).

Surgical selection continues to improve in parallel with operative and postoperative management so that the mortality rate has continued to decline over the last 20 years.[22,28]

Bernstein et al's prospective study of 78 patients greater than age 70 undergoing elective repair of AAA, showed that for those between 70 and 79 years of age, the probability of surviving 5 years was 67%. Patients greater than age 80 had a 66% 5-year survival. This was comparable to the age-matched survival of the general population (69%),[28] and has been confirmed in other studies of aneurysm repair in the elderly.[19,28,30]

Quality of life is also maintained. In all of the above studies examining long-term survival, a general patient satisfaction with outcome was described. Currie et al examined this aspect with a standardized questionnaire evaluating the quality of life in octogenarians who had undergone repair, as compared to normal subjects of a similar age. Responses showed no significant difference in life satisfaction, with a majority being able to walk for distances outside their homes and reporting few restrictions in their enjoyment of life for someone their age.[30] Dissatisfaction was more related to the availability of family support.

Recommendations

The life span in North America continues to lengthen. Today, on average, a 65-year-old can expect to live an additional 15 years, a 75-year-old will live 10 more, and an 80-year-old, 7; it is currently projected that 40% of our population will survive to age 80.[1] The authors recommend that elderly patients with minimal comorbidity or with correctable disease be referred for repair of AAAs greater than 5 cm, with an expectation of operative mortality near 5% and a 5-year longevity greater than 50%. In older patients with aneurysms greater than 6 cm and/or nonremediable cardiac risk or multi-system disease, careful counseling of the patient is advised, after weighing individual risk factors, with a leaning toward repair.

As preoperative evaluation and postoperative care improve, mortality should continue the decline began over the last 20 years. New modalities such as CTA allow effective, less invasive, and safe techniques for preoperative evaluation. Assessment of CAD, the most significant factor in both early and late outcome, can help stratify patients into groups who would benefit from preoperative PTCA or coronary artery bypass surgery. We anticipate that innovative methods for aneurysm repair such as percutaneous endoluminal graft placement, by reducing operative mortality and postoperative morbidity, will extend treatment to an even greater segment of the older population.

References

1. Peter BA: Vascular disease in the elderly patient. *Surg Clin North Am* 74:199–216, 1994.
2. Gillum R: Epidemiology of aortic aneurysm in the United States. *J Clin Epidemiol* 48:1289–1298, 1995.
3. Pleumeekers HJ, Hoes AW, van der Does E: Aneurysm of the abdominal aorta in older adults. The Rotterdam Study. *Am J Epidemiol* 142:1291–1299, 1995.
4. Pearce WH, Slaughter MS, LeMaire S: Aortic diameter as a function of age, gender, and body surface area. *Surgery* 144:691–697, 1993.
5. Dixon AK, Lawrence P, Mitchell RA: Age-related changes in the abdominal aorta shown by computed tomography. *Clin Radiol* 35:33–37, 1984.
6. Zarins CK, Weisenberg E, Koleltis G: Differential enlargement of artery segments in response to enlarging atheroslerotic plaques. *J Vasc Surg* 7:386–394, 1988.
7. Schlatmann TJM, Becker AE: Histologic changes in the normal ageing aorta: implications for dissecting aortic aneurysm. *Am J Cardiol* 39:13–20, 1977.
8. Robert L, Jacob MP, Frances C: Interaction between elastin and elastases, and its role on the aging of the arterial wall, skin, and other connective tissues: a review. *Mech Ageing Dev* 28:155–166, 1984.

9. Frame PS, Fryback DG, Patterson C: Screening for abdominal aortic aneurysm in men ages 60 to 80 years. *Ann Intern Med* 119:411–416, 1993.
10. Lederle FA, Wilson SE, Johnson GR: Variability in measurement of abdominal aortic aneurysms. *J Vasc Surg* 21:945–951, 1995.
11. Rubin GD, Walker PJ, Napel S: Three-dimensional spiral computed tomographic angiography: an alternative imaging modality for the abdominal aorta and its branches. *J Vasc Surg* 18:656–664, 1993.
12. Guirguis EM, Graeme G: The natural history of abdominal aortic aneurysms. *Amer J Surg* 162:481–483, 1991.
13. Hallet JW, Bower TC, Cherry KJ: Selection and preparation of high-risk patients for repair of abdominal aortic aneurysms. *Mayo Clin Proc* 69:763–768, 1994.
14. Sterpetti AV, Schultz RD, Feldhaus RJ: Abdominal aortic aneurysms in elderly patients: selective management based on clinical status and aneurysm expansion rate. *Am J Surg* 98:472–483, 1985.
15. Darling RC, Messina CR, Brewster DC: Autopsy study of unoperated abdominal aortic aneurysms: the case for early resection. *Circulation* 56(3.2):161–164, 1977.
16. Szilagyi DE, Elliot JP, Smith RF: Clinical fate of the patient with asymptomatic abdominal aortic aneurysms and unfit for surgical treatment. *Arch Surg* 104:600, 1972.
17. Baron JF, Oliver M, Michele B: Dipyridamole-thallium scintigraphy and gated radionuclide angiography to assess cardiac risk before abdominal aorrtic surgery. *Engl J Med* 330:663–668, 1994.
18. Bayazit M, Gol MK, Battaloglu B: Routine coronary arteriography before abdominal aortic aneurysm repair. *Amer J Surg* 170:246–250, 1995.
19. Bernstein EF, Chan EL: Abdominal aortic aneurysm in high-risk patients: outcome of selective management based on size and expansion rate. *Ann Surg* 200:255–262, 1994.
20. Golden MA, Whittemore AD, Donaldson MC: Selective evaluation and management of coronary artery disease in patients undergoing repair of abdominal aortic aneurysms: a 16-year experience. *Ann Surg* 212:415–420, 1990.
21. Henderson A, Effeney D: Morbidity and mortality after abdominal aortic surgery in a population of patients with high cardiovascular risk. *Aust N Z J Surg* 65:417–420, 1995.
22. Poulias GE, Doundoulakis D, Skoutas B: Abdominal aneurysmectomy and determinants of improved results and late survival. *J Cardiovasc Surg* 35:115–121, 1994.
23. White GH, Suresh MA, Wilson SE: Cardiac risk index as a predictor of long-term survival after repair of abdominal aortic aneurysm. *Am J Surg* 156:103–107, 1988.
24. Clark NJ, Stanley TH: Anesthesia for vascular surgery. In: Miller RD (ed): *Anesthesia* New York: Churchill Livingstone, Inc., 1876–1881, 1994.
25. McEnroe CS, O'Donnell TF, Yeager A: Comparison of ejection fraction and Goldman risk facto analysis to dipyridamole-thallium 201 studies in the evaluation of cardiac morbidity after aortic aneurysm surgery. *J Vasc Surg* 11:497–504, 1990.
26. Elmore JR, Hallett JW, Gibbons RJ: Myocardial revascularization before abdominal aortic aneurysmorrhaphy: effect of coronary angioplasty. *Mayo Clin Proc* 68:637–641, 1993.
27. Dean RH, Woody JD, Cam EE: Operative treatment of abdominal aortic aneurysms in octogenarians: when is too much too late? *Ann Surg* 6:721–728, 1993.
28. Crawford ES, Stowe C: True aneurysms of the aorta and iliac arteries. In: Moore ES (ed). *Vascular Surgery: A Comprehensive Review*. New York: Grune & Stratton, Inc., 269, 1983.

29. Bernstein EF, Dilley RB, Randolph H: The improving long-term outlook for patients over 70 years of age with abdominal aortic aneurysms. *Ann Surg* 207:318–322, 1988.
30. Currie IC, Scott DJ, Robson AK: Quality of life of octogenarians after aneurysm surgery. *Ann R Coll Surg Eng* 74:269–273, 1992.
31. Aune S, Amundsen SR: The influence of age on operative mortality and long-term relative survival following emergency abdominal aortic aneurysm operations. *Eur J Endovasc Surg* 10:338–341, 1995.
32. Chalmers RT, Stonebridge PA, John TG: Abdominal aortic aneurysm in the elderly. *B J Surg* 80:1122–1123, 1993.
33. Cogbill TH, Landercasper J, Strutt PT: Late results of peripheral vascular surgery in patients 80 years of age and older. *Arch Surg* 122:581, 1987.
34. Gloviciczki P, Pairolero PC, Mucha P Jr: Ruptured abdominal aortic aneurysms: repair should not be denied. *J Vasc Surg* 15:242–243, 1992.
35. Hollier LH, Reigel MM, Kazmier FJ: Conventional repair of abdominal aortic aneurysm in the high-risk patient: a plea for abandonment of nonresective treatment. *J Vasc Surg* 3:712–717, 1986.
36. McCabe CJ, Coleman WS, Berewster DC: The advantage of early operation for abdominal aortic aneurysm. *Arch Surg* 116:1025–1029, 1981.
37. McCready RA, Siderys H, Pittman JN: Ruptured abdominal aortic aneurysms in a private teaching hospital: a decade's experience. *J Vasc Surg* 15:242–243, 1992.
38. Morris GE, Hubbard CS, Quick CR: An abdominal aortic aneurysm screening program for all males over the age of 50 years. *Eur J Vasc Surg* 8:156–160, 1994.
39. Paty PS, Lloyd WE, Benjamin BC: Aortic replacement for abdominal aortic aneurysms in elderly patients. *Am J Surg* 166:191–193, 1993.

Chapter 24

Predictors of Mortality Following Vascular Surgery in the Elderly

Waleed Hassanein, MD
Kwan Hur, MS
Jennifer Daley, MD
William Henderson, PhD
Shukri F. Khuri, MD

Vascular disease increases with advancing age, and is a major cause of morbidity and mortality in the elderly; it exerts its toll on both physical functioning and health-related quality of life.[1,2] The impact of advancing age on postoperative mortality after vascular surgery has not been adequately appreciated, partially because of the lack of large prospective studies that have attempted to elucidate the predictors of postoperative mortality in vascular surgery. The National VA Surgical Risk Study was launched in April of 1991 with the goals of identifying the predictors of morbidity and mortality following major surgery, and developing risk-adjusted models of morbidity and mortality which would allow the comparative evaluation of the quality of surgical care among various provider facilities.[3] An analysis of phase I data from this study has been recently completed.[4] These data included preoperative, intraoperative, and outcome information on 87,087 major surgical operations that were performed in 44 VA medical centers between October 1, 1991 and December 31, 1993. The database included eight major noncardiac surgical specialties, with vascular surgery accounting for 12.5% of the database (10,929 operations). This chapter describes the vascular surgery database in the National VA Surgical Risk Study, focusing primarily on the predictors of 30-day mortality after vascular surgery in the elderly. In line with the definition used in this book, "elderly" denotes patients over 60 years of age.

From: Aronow WS, Stemmer EA, Wilson SE (eds). *Vascular Disease in the Elderly.* Armonk, NY: Futura Publishing Company, Inc., © 1997.

Methods

A detailed description of the methods used in the National VA Surgical Risk Study has been previously published.[3] The study was conducted in 44 VA medical centers which were closely affiliated with university medical centers. Preoperative, intraoperative, and postoperative data were prospectively collected by dedicated clinical nurse managers on major operations performed under general, spinal, or epidural anesthesia. Two traveling coordinators visited each center to review study procedures and to collect data to estimate interexaminer reliability. Preoperative data were collected directly from the medical chart or obtained from a surgical risk assessment profile completed by the surgical resident caring for the patient and verified by the nurse. Preoperative laboratory values within 2 weeks of the index operation and closest to the time of operation were acquired automatically from the laboratory software in each center's computer system. Postoperatively, either the lowest, the highest, or both values of selected laboratory data were obtained automatically. Intraoperative variables were taken from the automated surgery software operative log and from the anesthesia record. The index operation was defined as the first eligible operation performed on the patient. Other operations performed under the same anesthetic by the same or a different surgical team were also recorded. Each case was classified into one of eight major subspecialities based on the subspeciality of the attending surgeon. Vascular surgery operations were classified based on a combination of the subspeciality of the attending surgeon and the current procedure terminology (CPT-4) codes.

To account for differences in the complexity of operations performed between medical centers within a subspecialty, groups of subspecialists were asked to rank the complexity of each index operation CPT-4 code, independent of the patient risk factors, on a scale from 1 to 5. The average score for each index operation was used as a measure of the complexity of that operation (complexity score).

Patients were followed for 30 days after operation. Thirty-day operative mortality was defined as death from any cause inside or outside of the hospital occurring within 30 days of the index operation. Postoperative complications included 21 selected postsurgical events recorded in the 30 days after operation. The nurse obtained outcome information by chart review, interviews with care providers, reports from morbidity and mortality conferences, and communicating with each patient on the thirtieth postoperative day by letter or by telephone.

The nurse input all data into a special Surgical Risk Assessment module in the hospital's computer system. No later than 45 days postoperatively, these data were automatically transmitted to the statistical coordinating center for editing and analysis. A list of the specific variables collected for the study and their frequency in the initial database may be found in a previous publication.[3]

In the statistical analyses, the means of continuous risk variables were compared between patients who died or survived at 30 days post-

operative using Student's t-test. Categorical risk variables were compared using the Chi-square test. Factors with two-tailed p-values less
than 0.05 on univariate tests were considered candidate variables for
multivariate analysis. Forward stepwise logistic regression analysis
with entry and removal criteria set at the 0.05 level was used with
30-day mortality (yes/no) as the dependent variable, and the patient
preoperative risk factors, demographics, preoperative laboratory values,
and the operation's complexity score as the independent variables.
Odds ratios (OR) were calculated based on the estimated model parameter coefficients and standard errors, respectively. The logistic regression
models were used to estimate the probability of 30-day postoperative
mortality for each patient.

Characteristics of Elderly Patients Undergoing Vascular Surgery

Of 87,078 operations which comprised phase I of the database,
there were 10,929 operations that were classified as peripheral vascular.
For the purpose of this chapter, the vascular operations were divided
into two groups according to the age of the patients. Group I comprised
the operations performed in patients over 60 years (n = 8,478), while
group II comprised the operations performed on patients under 60 years
(n = 2,451). As shown in Table 1, older patients tended to have a higher
incidence of hypertension requiring medications, and diabetes mellitus
requiring insulin or oral hypoglycemic medications. A patient was considered to be a smoker if he or she had smoked within 2 weeks prior
to the operation. Accordingly, 45% of the older patient group were

Table 1
Selected Clinical Characteristics and Type of Operation

Parameters	Group I ≥60 Years Old n (%)	Group II <60 Years Old n (%)	P
Age distribution (n)	8,478	2,451	<0.0001
Associated comorbidity:			
— Hypertension requiring medications	4,998 (58.9)	1,205 (49.2)	<0.0001
— Diabetes mellitus[1]	2,303 (27.2)	620 (25.3)	0.0695
— Smoking history 2 weeks prior to surgery	3,792 (44.7)	1,612 (65.8)	<0.0001
Elective vs. emergency operations:			
— Elective cases	7,485 (88.3)	2,109 (86.1)	
— Emergent cases	993 (11.7)	342 (13.9)	0.0031

Number in brackets indicates group percentages. [1] Requiring insulin or oral hypoglycemic medications.

Table 2
Most Prevalent Peripheral Vascular Surgery Performed

Operations	Group I ≥60 Years Old n (%)	Group II <60 Years Old n (%)	P
Carotid endarterectomy	1,387 (16.4)	269 (10.9)	<0.0001
Femoropopliteal bypass	721 (8.5)	262 (10.7)	0.002
Above the knee amputation	712 (8.4)	125 (6.1)	<0.0001
Aortofemoral bypass	522 (6.2)	244 (9.9)	<0.0001
Below the knee amputation	495 (5.8)	131 (5.3)	0.408
Femoro-anterior tibial bypass	274 (3.2)	78 (3.2)	0.957
Abdominal aortic aneurysm repair	273 (3.2)	40 (1.6)	<0.0001
Common femoral artery aneurysm repair	212 (2.5)	53 (2.16)	0.388
Carotid aneurysm repair	144 (1.7)	33 (1.3)	0.268
Carotid thrombectomy	92 (1.1)	19 (0.8)	0.222

Number in brackets indicates group percentages.

smokers, in contrast to 66% of the younger patient group. (This definition of smoking was abandoned in the subsequent phase of data collection because it excluded the more complex patients who might have been too sick to smoke prior to their operations.) The older patient group had a lower percentage of operations performed on emergency basis (Table 1).

Table 2 lists the 10 most common vascular surgical procedures performed in both groups. Carotid endarterectomy and femoral-popliteal bypass were the most frequent operations in both patient groups. The older patient group had a higher incidence of above knee amputation (AKA) and abdominal aortic aneurysm (AAA) repair, a reflection of the natural progression of vascular disease with age. In contrast, the younger patient group had a higher incidence of aorta-bifemoral and femoral-popliteal bypass procedures, reflecting the improved potential for limb salvage in the younger patient population.

Outcome of Elderly Patients Undergoing Peripheral Vascular Surgery

There were significant differences in the outcome of vascular surgery between the two patient groups. The older patient group had longer postoperative lengths of stay, a higher incidence of postoperative complications, and a higher 30-day mortality rate (Table 3). In the younger patient group, the median length of stay was 7 days, in contrast to 10 days in the older patient group. The distribution of the postoperative length of stay in both groups is shown in Table 3. Thirty-one percent of the older patient group developed one or more complications postop-

Table 3
Outcomes Following Peripheral Vascular Surgery

Variables	Group I ≥ 60 years n (%)	Group II < 60 years n (%)	P
Length of postoperative stay (days)			
0–5	2,061 (24.3)	722 (29.5)	<0.0001
6–10	2,444 (28.8)	831 (33.9)	<0.0001
11–20	1,921 (22.7)	461 (18.8)	<0.0001
21–30	739 (8.7)	182 (7.4)	0.047
Patients with 1 or more complications	2,665 (31.4)	565 (23.1)	<0.0001
Most common post-op Complications:			
— Wound infection	2,202 (25.9)	546 (22.3)	0.0002
— Failure to wean off the ventilator >48 hours	533 (6.3)	84 (3.4)	<0.0001
— Graft failure	278 (3.3)	90 (3.7)	0.3755
30-day mortality rate	445 (5.3)	58 (2.4)	<0.0001

Numbers in brackets indicate within group percentages.

eratively, in contrast to 23% of the younger patient group (p<0.0001). The three most common complications following peripheral vascular surgery in both groups were wound infection, failure to wean off the ventilator 48 hours after the operation, and graft failure. As shown in Table 3, there was a higher incidence of wound infection and failure to wean in the older patient population. The incidence of graft failure was similar in both groups. The 30-day postoperative mortality rate was also significantly different between the two groups: 5.3% in the older patient group, and 2.4% in the younger patient group (p<0.0001).

Predictors of Thirty-Day Postoperative Mortality Following Vascular Surgery in the Elderly

Multivariate analysis revealed 17 preoperative variables to be independent predictors of 30-day mortality in elderly patients undergoing vascular surgery. Table 4 lists these variables in the order of their decreasing importance in the model. Preoperative dependency on a ventilator, emergent versus elective nature of the operation, and the American Society of Anesthesiologists (ASA) classification assigned by the anesthesiologist, were the most important predictors of mortality. Four laboratory values which reflected the preoperative renal, hepatic, and nutritional status of the patients were also important predictors of mortality. They were blood urea nitrogen, serum creatinine, serum albumin, and SGOT. The serum albumin was analyzed as a continuous variable,

Table 4
Order of Entry of Predictors of Variables Predictive of 30-Day Postoperative
Mortality for Peripheral Vascular Surgery Patients ≥60 years old

Variable	β Coefficient	Odds Ratio
Ventilator dependent	1.145	3.145
Emergency status	0.996	2.707
ASA class	0.618	1.857
DNR status	1.083	2.954
BUN >40 mg/dL	0.391	1.479
Albumin g/dL	−0.512	0.599
Esophageal varices	2.366	10.657
Complexity score	0.329	1.391
History congestive heart failure	0.455	1.577
Creatinine >1.2 mg/dL	0.340	1.405
SGOT >40 IU/L	0.374	1.454
Age	0.027	1.028
History of COPD	0.299	1.349
On dialysis	0.617	1.855
Hypertension requiring medication	0.278	1.321
Preoperative pneumonia	0.606	1.834
Impaired sensorium	0.335	1.398
Intercept	−7.255	

DNR = Do not resuscitate status
COPD = Chronic obstructive pulmonary disease

while the other three laboratory values were dichotomous (Table 4). The variables predictive of 30-day mortality in the patients over 60 years were similar to the variables identified in the model that included all patients undergoing peripheral vascular surgery. The c-index in the latter model was 0.91, indicating that the models were highly predictive of 30-day postoperative mortality.[4]

Using the information contained in Table 4, one can use the Logit equation to calculate the expected operative mortality of a given elderly VA patient undergoing peripheral vascular surgery, based on the patient's preoperative characteristics. The Logit equation:

$$TE\ (X) = \frac{\exp(\beta_1 X_1 + \beta_2 X_2 + ... + \beta_n X_n + C)}{1 + [\exp(\beta_1 X_1 + \beta_2 X_2 + ... + \beta X_n + C)]}$$

where β is the regression coefficient for each variable (Column 2 in Table 4) and X is the value of the variable. (For dichotomous variables, the X is either 1, indicating the presence of the variable, or zero, indicating the absence of the variable.) C is the intercept for the model which is shown in Table 4. Examples of using the Logit equation to calculate the expected mortality rates of specific patients have been presented by Hammermister et al.[5]

Conclusion

The VA has developed, for the first time, a prospective national database of patients undergoing major surgery, including peripheral vascular surgery. Analysis of phase I of this database reveals that patients over 60 years have a significantly longer postoperative hospital stay, and have a significantly higher incidence of 30-day postoperative morbidity and mortality.

The VA has also developed models highly predictive of 30-day mortality following vascular surgery. A total of 17 preoperative variables have been identified as independent predictors of mortality following vascular surgery in patients over 60 years of age. The most important of these predictors are ventilator dependency, emergency status, and ASA class. Using the Logit equation, one can now estimate the expected mortality of any given elderly patient undergoing peripheral vascular surgery in the VA.

References

1. Stemmer EA, Aronow WS, Wilson SE: Peipheral vascular disease in the elderly: Part I. *Clin Geriatr* 3:17-29, 1995.
2. Stemmer EA, Aronow WS, Wilson SE: Peripheral vascular disease in the elderly: Part II. *Clin Geriatr* 3:16-33, 1995.
3. Khuri FS, Daley J, Henderson W, et al: The national veterans administration surgical risk study: risk adjustment for the comparative assessment of the quality of surgical care. *J Am Coll Surg* 519-531, 1995.
4. Khuri SF, Daley J, Henderson W, et al: Risk adjustment of the postoperative mortality rate for the comparative assessment of the quality of surgical care: results of the national VA risk study. *N Engl J Med* (submitted 1996).
5. Hammermister KE, Johnson R, Marshall G, Grover FL: Continuous assessment and improvemnt in quality of care: a model from the Department of Veterans Affairs Cardiac Surgery. *Ann Surg* 3:281-90, 1994.

Chapter 25

Venous Disease in the Elderly

Fernando E. Kafie, MD
Russell A. Williams, MD

Pulmonary embolism (PE) and deep vein thrombosis (DVT) are common clinical problems associated with significant morbidity and mortality. The National Institutes of Health Consensus Conference estimated that as many as 50,000 people die annually of PE, and that between 300,000 and 600,000 hospitalizations each year in the United States are associated with PE and/or DVT.[1] Despite their clinical importance, much of the fundamental epidemiology has not been described. Studies have shown increased risk in the elderly and men. PE and DVT have lower incidences on the coasts of the United States than in the interior of the country.[1] Recurrent PE tends to be uncommon. As expected, a diagnosis of PE is associated with high mortality over the short-term, but after 12 months the excess risk of death disappears. Previous studies by Lillienfield, Anderson, and Gillum showed an increasing risk of PE with increasing age. All three also confirmed an increased risk of DVT for males.

Venous thromboembolism is the third most common cardiovascular disease after ischemic heart disease and stroke.[2] The reported incidences of DVT and PE have not changed in the last 30 years.[3] In addition, the mortality rate from PE has not diminished during the last generation. The failure of physicians to use adequate DVT prophylaxis in medical and surgical patients has resulted in these bleak statistics. Failure to use DVT prophylaxis occurs, despite literature that has demonstrated that prophylaxis reduces the incidences of DVT and PE.

The risk of the development of DVT and its primary complication, PE, is a major concern following multisystemic injury, particularly in those patients with extremity and pelvic fractures. A variety of methods have been suggested for the prophylaxis of this phenomenon, but no single one has shown clear effectiveness following injury.

Graduated compression stockings (GCS) have been used to increase blood flow from the distal part of the limb to the proximal femoral vein.

From: Aronow WS, Stemmer EA, Wilson SE (eds). *Vascular Disease in the Elderly.* Armonk, NY: Futura Publishing Company, Inc., © 1997.

Theoretically, this reduces the potential for stasis and localized venous thrombosis. Two types of GCS are available: above the knee and below the knee. There is no appreciable difference noted in their use in the prevention of postoperative DVT. The true effectiveness of the use of these GCS was only a very modest reduction, by approximately 11%, in postoperative DVT in elective surgical series. Their effectiveness with patients following trauma has not been documented. Also, the use of GCS is limited in patients with extremity fractures because of external appliances and casts.

Autopsy findings indicate that 73% of cases of PE are not detected clinically.[4] DVT is the source of PE in more that 90% of cases.[5] Because more than 50% of patients with leg symptoms prove to have a diagnosis other than DVT, the need for improved diagnosis and therapeutic techniques is clear. Reliance of history and physical exam on the diagnosis of DVT is extremely unreliable. There are a number of reasons for the lack of clinical diagnostic accuracy. First, the history is often poor, the complaints are vague, and the symptoms are nonspecific. Physical signs may be quite subtle and frequently are mimicked by other pathological conditions. Second, venous obstruction is not as readily detected as arterial obstruction, which usually can be recognized by simple examination of the peripheral pulses.

The two most frequent symptoms in patients with acute PE are dyspnea and pleuritic chest pain. One or both of these symptoms are present in the vast majority of patients as shown in Table 1. The obvious problem facing the clinician is that neither of these two symptoms is specific for PE. Dyspnea and pleuritic chest pain are present in a wide variety of cardiac and pulmonary diseases.

Table 1
Incidence of Pleuritic Pain and Dyspnea in Patients with Angiographically
Documented Pulmonary Embolism

Study	Number of Patients	% with Pleuritic Pain	% with Dyspnea
Bell et al	327	74	84
Dalen	124	57	77
PIOPED Study	117	66	73

Calf Deep Vein Thrombosis

Low risk of PE is also erroneously assumed in isolated calf DVT. Most investigators believe that isolated calf DVT need not be treated. A review of the English language literature by Philbrick and Becker[6] regarding the natural history of isolated calf DVT revealed propagation in up to 20% of cases. If proximal propagation occurs, there is a 50% chance of the thrombus embolizing to the pulmonary vasculature, yielding a 10% risk of PE associated with calf DVT. There is extensive evidence that treatment with standard anticoagulation (heparin and warfarin) prevents extension, embolization, and recurrence of DVT. Therefore, all patients with isolated calf DVT should be treated. If the patient has an increased risk of bleeding with anticoagulants, serial duplex ultrasonography is a reasonable alternative to identify the 20% of calf DVT that may propagate to the proximal veins.

Causes of Deep Vein Thromboses

The underlying causes of DVT may be categorized as clinical conditions, hereditary blood defects, and acquired blood defects. It has long been appreciated that certain clinical circumstances, such as trauma, stasis, cancer, surgery, pregnancy, nephrotic syndrome, sepsis, cardiac disease, burns, use of estrogen-containing compounds, and other medical conditions, are associated with pathological thrombus formation. In 1845, Virchow recognized that three major factors play a role in thrombus formation: 1) change in blood flow; 2) changes in the circulating blood; and 3) changes in the vessel wall. Virchow's early observations provide a model for the study of thrombus formation, and the many mechanisms by which changes in these three factors lead to thrombosis have been elucidated. A number of acquired and hereditary blood protein defects of coagulation have been well characterized. Approaching not only the thrombotic process, but also the underlying causes, enhances the possibility of successful primary treatment and secondary prevention of recurrent events.

Clinical Presentation

The clinical presentation of patients with DVT varies greatly. Individuals recognized to be at high risk have a history of previous thrombotic events of any cause; recent surgery (especially orthopedic); prolonged bed rest or immobilization predisposing to venous stasis, as may occur after trauma or a serious medical illness; serious burns; acute or chronic heart disease, resulting in congestive heart failure with associated poor peripheral perfusion and venous stasis; internal malignancy of any type; certain hematologic malignancies; bacterial, fungal, or viral septicemia (especially with shock); and inherited or acquired blood defects predisposing to thrombosis. Recognizing these special groups of patients as being at high risk is essential to diagnosis because the presenting signs and symptoms may be minimal, misleading, or absent until an undiagnosed DVT results in life-threatening PE. In all cases in which the diagnosis is suspected, an objective diagnostic technique should be employed. At least 50% of PEs occur in patients not suspected of having DVT.[7]

Although the majority of DVTs occur in infrapopliteal veins, the major source of PE is proximal DVT.[8] The chief and classic complaint in a patient with DVT is the recent onset of a painful, swollen leg. The location of swelling depends on the location of the thrombus. The entire leg distal to the site of the thrombosis is usually swollen in complete iliofemoral thrombosis; in calf vein or partial venoocclusion, swelling may be more localized.

Localized pain due to focal inflammation at the site of thrombosis may indicate the specific area of DVT; however, significant pain and tenderness may occur with superficial venous thrombosis and other clinical conditions as well, making the complaint of leg pain unreliable.

Upper extremity swelling and pain have fewer specific causes, and this complaint may be somewhat more reliable as an indicator of thrombosis of the axillary-subclavian system. Because DVT is frequently misdiagnosed before serious complications occur, the presenting complaint is all too often referable to the occurrence of a PE. The first presentation of DVT may be cardiovascular collapse, cardiorespiratory arrest, or sudden death.[8] More classic symptoms of PE include the sudden onset of chest pain (typically pleuritic), shortness of breath, diaphoresis, and anxiety.

The physical examination of patients with DVT, although recognized to reveal certain classic features, has also been well proved to be misleading and frankly in error at least 50% of the time.[9] The clinical diagnosis of acute DVT is hardly more accurate than tossing a coin.[11] The classic signs of edema, erythema, increased warmth, a palpable cord, positive Homan's sign, and tenderness actually occur relatively infrequently. Hull et al[10] noted that in symptomatic patients, only 59% of those with leg pain, tenderness, and swelling; 22% with pain and tenderness; and 11% with isolated leg swelling were ultimately demonstrated to have DVT.

Because there is at least a 50% error in diagnosis of DVT based on clinical findings alone, multiple diagnostic modalities have been developed to allow greater accuracy, lower cost, less discomfort to the patient, and the greatest possible sensitivity and specificity. All diagnostic modalities are compared with the gold standard of ascending contrast venography. Many semi-invasive and noninvasive techniques have been devised to supplement or replace ascending contrast venography in the objective diagnosis of DVT (Table 2).

Impedance Plethysmography

Venous impedance plethysmography (IPG) has been used for the diagnosis of DVT for more that 20 years. The popularity is owed to its noninvasive method and low cost. IPG analyzes the flow variability between patent and obstructed veins. Thrombi occluding the major veins of the leg decrease venous compliance and increase venous outflow resistance. IPG methods for diagnosing DVT depend on recognition of these physiological effects. All IPGs measure volume change (specifically of the calf).

Table 2
Comparison of Objective Tests for Diagnosing Venous Disease

Test	Proximal		Calf		SVT	VI*
	SN	*SP*	*SN*	*SP*		
Invasive						
X-ray phlebography	+	+	+	+	+	±
Semi-invasive						
Radionuclide phlebography	+	+	−	−	−	−
Iodine^{125}-fibrinogen uptake	±	±	+	±	−	−
Noninvasive						
Doppler ultrasonography	+	+	±	±	+	+
Impedance plethysmography	+	+	−	−	−	−
Duplex, color flow scanning	+	+	+	+		

* SN = sensitivity; SP = specificity; SVT = superficial vein thrombosis; VI = valvular incompetence

Before the advent of duplex scanning, IPG was the most widely used and most investigated noninvasive test for DVT. The sensitivity and specificity of IPG for proximal DVT are 96% and 83%, respectively.[12] The major limitation of IPG appears to be poor sensitivity in the detection of calf thrombi because thrombi that are nonobstructing may not be detected by IPG.

IPG is inadequate in the evaluation of asymptomatic patients, such as those undergoing surveillance for DVT after hip surgery. Thrombi may be present in proximal veins, which are detectable by venography or ultrasound, but do not substantially interfere with venous hemodynamics. Calf thrombi may be present, which have little impact on the collective rate of venous outflow. IPG is an acceptable tool for evaluating the symptomatic patient with proximal DVT.

Patients with abnormal studies may be anticoagulated and followed with repeat evaluation. Borderline or normal studies may be followed clinically without treatment, but with repeat IPG to look for propagation of initially undetected calf thrombi into the proximal veins. False-positive results may be expected in the presence of any condition that impairs venous outflow, such as pregnancy and pelvic tumors, which cause extrinsic compression; prior DVT with inadequate recanalization or collateral blood flow; and congestive heart failure. False-negative results may occur in patients with nonocclusive thrombi and calf DVT with extensive collateralization.

Iodine-125 Fibrinogen

The use of fibrinogen as a radioisotope is derived from the hypothesis that deposition of fibrin in an organizing clot could be detected by labeling the fibrinogen precursor of fibrin. Radio-labeled fibrinogen is injected into the peripheral vein, and the extremities are scanned at 24 and 72 hours for evidence of local accumulation. Hot areas are those with active formation of fibrin clots. This technique is useful in the calf, but is unreliable for the thigh[13] and requires such a length of time to perform as to be of questionable utility in clinical decision making. The use of fibrinogen for the procedure exposes the patient to radiation and the risk of acquiring a blood-borne infection. False-positive results occur in areas of hematomas or wounds. The cost of the test is significant. The overall sensitivity and specificity of this test are 73% and 71%, respectively.[14]

Ascending Contrast Venography

Venogram remains the gold standard for the diagnosis of DVT. Hull et al[10] in 1981 noted that in 160 consecutive patients studied with contrast venography for suspected DVT, only 1.3% of those with negative studies were subsequently proved to have thrombi. It is also likely that the cases reported by Hull were in fact thrombosis induced by the venogram rather than primary diagnostic errors.

The technique involves the injection of iodinated contrast media into a small peripheral vein of the affected extremity. Venograms are reliable in any portion of the venous system, including the calf, thigh, and ileofemoral system. Positive findings for acute DVT include the visualization of intraluminal filling defects, nonfilling or absence of venous segments, and abrupt termination of contrast flow. Chronic venous occlusion is identified by irregular, tortuous, narrow, recanalized-appearing vessels with corkscrew collaterals and incompetent perforators. Intravenous injection of the contrast is associated with at least a 2% to 4% risk of developing DVT from the procedure.[10] This risk is minimal, however, when compared to the risk of failure to diagnose DVT. Contrast venography involves considerable expense and requires the services of a specially equipped radiology suite, special equipment, and skilled radiologist and technical staff.

Doppler Ultrasound

Doppler ultrasonography has been used for the last 20 years in the evaluation of venous patency. When compared to contrast venography, Doppler studies have a 94% accuracy. Errors in diagnosis all occur with below the knee thrombi.

The technique involves the use of a detector placed over the posterior tibial, popliteal, superficial femoral, and common femoral veins. The diagnosis is made by the audible interpretation of the venous velocity signals.

Although Doppler ultrasound has proved to be of value in the diagnosis and management of symptomatic patients with proximal

DVT, accuracy is low in asymptomatic and calf DVT.[15] Ultrasound is most accurate for evaluation of the veins of the proximal upper and lower extremities, and less reliable in the distal veins, including the calf. In the clinical application of ultrasound imaging, it has been suggested that when calf DVT is strongly suspected but not detected, proper management should include antiplatelet therapy and local measures, or none at all, with repeat ultrasound analysis at daily to several day intervals until the clinical indications of DVT have passed, or until proximal propagation is actually detected.[16]

Real-Time Ultrasound with Color Doppler

Patent veins are characterized by normal phasic flow signals and obliteration of the venous lumen by direct compression with the Doppler probe, which is normally seen adjacent to the associated artery. With occlusive thrombi, Doppler signals are absent, and the lumen cannot be compressed with direct pressure. Nonocclusive clots result in partial obliteration of the lumen with pressure and continuous rather than phasic venous signals. The calf veins are evaluated by foot compression and monitoring of signals from the posterior tibial vein. Evidence of thrombosis includes the ultrasound findings of lack of movement of the venous valves and walls with direct pressure and with maneuvers such as respiration and Valsalva. Fresh blood clots may appear the same as flowing blood when viewed with the ultrasound; however, the Doppler which detects flow, allows this critical distinction. Fresh clots are also more compressible and less echogenic than older clots.

Laboratory Evaluation

Of the many laboratory studies available to assess the status of the coagulation system, only the antithrombin III (AT III) level is of clinical value. AT III level is predictably diminished to a degree generally corresponding to the severity of thrombosis. Values in single calf thrombosis may drop to 109% of normal AT III values. In iliofemoral thrombosis, levels as low as 80% range would be expected. In patients with combined DVT and pulmonary embolus, the AT III level may drop to 66% of normal.

In clinical practice, the AT III level should be obtained in patients suspected of having DVT as a diagnostic adjunct and to assess the suitability for heparin therapy. Because the effectiveness of heparin therapy depends on adequate levels of AT III, it is clearly important to be aware of the AT III level before instituting therapy. If the AT III level is below 60% of normal, a hereditary deficiency must be suspected. In the absence of adequate levels of AT III, heparin does not produce a sufficient anticoagulant effect. Levels of AT III above 60% are associated with an appropriate therapeutic response to heparin, whereas patients with levels below 40% or less do not respond to heparin.

Treatment

Elevation of the affected extremity enhances venous outflow, and local heat improves microcirculation. Range of motion exercises also improve venous flow through patent veins not involved in the thrombotic process. Venous flow may be further aided by the application of elastic stockings. These must cover the length of the affected extremity, and care must be used to avoid creating a tourniquet effect caused by bunching up of stocking.

The development of the thrombolytic agents streptokinase (SK), urokinase (UK), and recombinant tissue plasminogen activator (tPA) has revolutionized the treatment of arterial and venous thrombosis. The use of thrombolytic agents in life-threatening PE has a well-founded clinical basis. Thrombolytics have been shown to be the therapy of choice in patients with acute massive PE complicated by hemodynamic instability.[17] Pulmonary capillary injury and diffusion capacity resolve more quickly with UK or SK than with standard heparin therapy. However, there is no clear reduction in morbidity or mortality.[18]

Thrombolytic therapy has also been applied, with impressive results, to DVT. Numerous trials have established the efficacy of thrombolytics for the lysis of acute DVT. Thrombolytics in comparison to standard heparin therapy offer the advantage of better preservation of the venous valves and, thus, fewer sequela of chronic venous insufficiency (CVI) and the postphlebitic syndrome.[19] Accumulated data suggests that significantly more patients will regain patency of the venous system when treated with thrombolytic therapy than with anticoagulation; however, 50% will not respond well to lytic therapy and will be considered failures. The goal of thrombolysis for DVT is preservation of venous function, which includes restoring patency of the deep venous system and maintaining valvular function. The damaging effects of thrombosis on the venous valves have been well known since they were first described by Edwards and Edwards in 1937. Thrombosis leads to pathological destruction of the valves which results in incompetence and venous hypertension. The final outcome of venous hypertension is pain, edema, hyperpigmentation, and ulceration. Thrombi present for 2 weeks are good candidates for thrombolysis; after 4 weeks, therapy is not justified, as the likelihood of successful lysis diminishes with time.

The only thrombolytic regimen approved by the Food and Drug Administration to treat DVT is SK administered as a 250,000 U followed by a 100,000 U/hour infusion for 24 to 72 hours. At least partial clot lysis occurs in approximately two thirds of patients treated with SK.[20] Thrombolysis is achieved 3.7 times more often among SK-treated patients when compared to heparin.[21]

Oral anticoagulation with warfarin inhibits the hepatic production of the vitamin K-dependent factors. The level of anticoagulation is monitored by the use of the prothrombin time (PT), which provides an in vitro measure of the rapidity of clotting in the presence of a thromboplastin substrate. Anticoagulation with warfarin generally requires about 36 hours of therapy because the initial doses are bound to plasma proteins and only gradually accumulate in the liver. Therapy with warfarin may begin simultaneously with heparin and the heparin therapy is stopped at the time the PT becomes therapeutic, facilitating early discharge from the hospital with no sacrifice of efficacy or increased risk of recurrent thrombosis. To compensate for the differences in the PT and rate of bleeding complications between patients in different geographic locations, the International Normalization Ratio (INR) has been developed, which allows comparison of the prothrombin substrate in use to an international standard so the test result is, in actuality, reported as though the test was performed using the World Health Organization (WHO) primary standard thromboplastin.[22] The currently recommended PT INR for therapeutic oral anticoagulation for DVT is 2.0 to 3.0.[22]

Because the onset of effective anticoagulation may take several days, warfarin alone it is not useful as an initial therapy for DVT. In patients with protein S and protein C deficiencies, the primary problem may even be made worse, thus further limiting the protein C and S action to inhibit thrombosis. Cutaneous necrosis has been observed in patients receiving warfarin with protein C or S deficiency.[23] It is recommended that heparin be started concomitantly, and the warfarin which is begun at a low dose be increased in small increments until the levels of vitamin K-dependent factors are substantially reduced before heparin is discontinued.[24]

The use of heparin in the treatment of DVT has been generally accepted practice for more than 50 years. Heparin inhibits the ongoing process of thrombosis by accelerating the activity of AT III against serine proteases with resulting inhibition of factors II, X, and IX. Additional important effects of heparin include antiplatelet and anti-inflammatory activity.[25]

Antiplatelet therapy has not been a mainstay of treatment for acute DVT. The primary use of the antiplatelet agents, aspirin, dipyridamole, and lulfinpyrazone, has been in the treatment of arterial disease, especially for the prevention of coronary and cerebrovascular thrombosis. These potent inhibitors of the cyclooxygenase system have been used in venous disease in patients with superficial thrombophlebitis, as well as uncomplicated DVT below the popliteal fossa.[25] When used for superficial thrombophlebitis or DVT below the popliteal fossa, the risk for cephalad propagation of thrombosis must be kept in mind.[22] The potential for gastrointestinal side effects with the use of aspirin is significant.

In patients with uncomplicated DVT due to a known cause that has resolved, a decision regarding the duration of therapy is based as much on the response to treatment of the underlying risk factor as the clinical coarse of the DVT. In patients with acute DVT, therapy with heparin should begin immediately and continue for the time necessary for a stable therapeutic PT INR to be achieved. The total duration of therapy in the uncomplicated patient should be 1 month, assuming that the patient has no increased risk of DVT during this time period. In the patient with DVT and PE, similar guidelines should be followed, but a total of 3 months of anticoagulation is recommended. Patients with continued risk factors and a history of DVT and/or PE should remain on indefinite anticoagulation.

The treatment of DVT or PE is complicated primarily by recurrent or progressive thrombosis or hemorrhage resulting from therapy. Despite appropriate treatment, failures still occur in 10% of patients.

Hemorrhage is the primary adverse outcome resulting directly from treatment. Hemorrhagic complications with the use of warfarin are recorded to be as high as 50%, but with the proper use of the PT INR may be as low as 6%.[26] Hemorrhage in patients using heparin drugs occurs at a much lower rate than in patients on warfarin.[27]

Heparin-induced thrombocytopenia is an infrequently seen, but serious, complication of heparin therapy.[28] Even the low doses used in heparin flushes are enough to cause antibody formation. Treatment includes the discontinuation of heparin. The antibodies clear in about 48 hours and platelets return to normal. The greatest problem with thrombocytopenia is the risk of paradoxic thromboembolism, which occurs in 50% of heparin-induced thrombocytopenic patients. Among these patients, 50% develop new DVT, extension of a preexisting clot, or pulmonary thromboembolism. The patient who requires continued anticoagulation in the face of heparin-induced thrombocytopenia should be treated with warfarin or antiplatelet agents.

Long-term treatment with heparin at doses of 10,000 U/day or more may result in osteoporosis; however, this complication is rare. Heparin does not cross the placental barrier, therefore, it is safe to use in pregnancy.[29] Warfarin is absolutely contraindicated in pregnancy and may cause fatal hemorrhage in the fetus.[29] Heparin and warfarin doses must be adjusted in the presence of hepatic or renal disease.

PE and DVT are common problems in the elderly. Both increase with age, but the effects of race and sex are small. Current treatment patterns appear to be effective in preventing both PE and DVT, and recurrence of PE. Both are associated with substantial 1-year mortality, suggesting the need to understand the role of associated conditions, as well as the indications for prophylaxis and the methods of treatment.

Prevention

Venous thromboembolism is a frequent complication of the primary illness in hospital patients. Apart from the immediate risk to life, the late sequelae of extensive DVT must be considered: swelling of the legs, varicose veins, ulceration, and other trophic changes. Not only should venous thromboembolism be prevented, but prophylactic measures now available make prevention a practical proposition. Two thirds of deaths from PE occur within 30 minutes after the embolic event—too brief a period for any benefit to be derived from thromboembolic therapy, which has been shown to be highly effective in producing rapid lysis of emboli.[30] Furthermore, approximately 80% of PE occur without premonitory signs of peripheral venous thrombosis, and, consequently, treatment with heparin and oral anticoagulants to prevent embolism is often not given. Thus, to adopt a policy of treating massive PE or its precursor, peripheral venous thrombosis, is to expose patients to an unacceptable risk of fatal complications.

Dextran

Dextran is a partially hydrolyzed glucose polymer produced from the bacteria leuconostoc mesenteriodes. There are two dextran preparations suitable for clinical use: dextran 70 and dextran 40. A number of studies have demonstrated that dextran infusion started during surgery and continued in the postoperative period is effective in reducing the incidence of DVT and PE.

Complications from dextran therapy include pulmonary edema in patients with limited cardiac reserve, occasional renal failure, mild allergic reactions, and rare anaphylactic responses. Dextran is expensive and must be given intravenously, and its use is restricted to hospitalized patients during the acute phase of their illness.

Oral Anticoagulants

Oral anticoagulants, properly employed and started well before operation are the most effective and proved method of preventing venous thrombosis. Embolism is quite frequent in patients with heart disease, particularly in those with congestive cardiac failure. Among such patients, oral anticoagulation therapy was effective in reducing the incidence of DVT by approximately 80%, as compared with untreated controls. A major drawback of oral anticoagulation therapy is the risk of massive hemorrhage during and after operation, despite laboratory control of the dosage given. The risk of hemorrhage and the need for strict laboratory control have undoubtedly contributed to the relatively low level of acceptance of this form of prophylaxis among surgeons generally, at least in the United States and the United Kingdom.[31]

Low-Dose Heparin

Low-dose heparin, given subcutaneously, has been claimed to prevent thrombosis without increasing the risk of hemorrhage. The results of 77 clinical trials of low-dose heparin prophylaxis in a variety of patient populations have now been reported.[32] Trials showed evidence of a significant reduction in the incidence of DVT in patients receiving heparin. However, there was clear and consistent evidence for an increased risk of bleeding after administration of subcutaneous heparin in nearly 13,500 patients for whom bleeding data were available.[32]

Low-Molecular Weight Heparin

Low-molecular weight heparin represents the most significant development in antithrombotic therapy. Several authors have concluded on the benefits of low-molecular weight heparin in the prevention of DVT. However, there is no convincing evidence that in general surgery patients, low-molecular weight heparin compared with standard heparin generates a clinically important improvement in the benefit to risk ratio. Low-molecular weight heparins may be preferable for orthopedic surgery patients, in view of the large risk of reduction for venous thrombosis.

Graduated Compression Stockings

GCS produce a higher femoral vein flow than uniform compression.[33] Among low-risk, general surgery patients, GCSs can reduce the frequency of venous thrombosis by more than half compared with no prophylaxis.[34] GCS should be considered as first-line prophylaxis against PE among all hospitalized patients, except for those with peripheral vascular disease whose condition may be worsened by vascular compression.

Intermittent Pneumatic Compression Boots

Intermittent pneumatic compression (IPC) boots are devices that provide intermittent inflation of air-filled cuffs that prevent venous stasis in the legs and appear to stimulate the endogenous fibrinolytic system. The reduction in thrombosis rates of the legs are seen even when the GCSs are placed on the arms, suggesting a fibrinolytic mechanism of action.

Inferior Vena Cava Interruption

Inferior vena cava interruption is accomplished by the use of a filter device that mechanically blocks the embolization of leg thrombi into the lungs, thereby preventing a PE. Inferior vena cava filters are used as a prophylactic measure only in patients that are at extremely high risk for PE. The indications for insertion of a vena caval filter are shown in Table 3.

Table 3
Indications for Vena Caval Filter

1. Recurrent thromboembolism in spite of adequate anticoagulation.
2. Documented thromboembolism in a patient who has a contraindication to antico-agulation.
3. Complication of anticoagulation that forces therapy to be discontinued.
4. Chronic pulmonary embolism with associated pulmonary hypertension and cor pulmonale.
5. Immediately following pulmonary embolectomy.
6. Relative-patient with more than 50% of the pulmonary vascular bed occluded who cannot tolerate any additional embolism, or a patient with a large free-floating ileofemoral thrombus on venogram.

Despite major advances in the prevention, detection, and management of DVT and PE, morbidity and mortality still remain high. Physicians should be better informed in matters of prevention and treatment. A high index of suspicion is a must; early and aggressive therapy will prevent the fatal complication of PE and possibly the long-term sequela of CVI.

Venous Insufficiency

In spite of adequate anticoagulation and bed rest for patients with acute DVT, approximately 50% will develop CVI. With resolution of the DVT, there is a persistent deformity and incompetence of the veins. The result is an unrestrainned column of fluid that transmits pressures of greater than 100 mm Hg to the venules, promoting the extravasation of fluid and proteins. These fibrinous deposits are poorly cleared by the body's reticuloendothelial system, resulting in low oxygen tension and poor nutrient supply. The thickened subcutaneous tissue, along with the extravasation of red cells and deposits of hemosiderin, lead to the formation of a "brownish edema." Legs with CVI are at high risk for infection and cellulitis. The poor local transfer of nutrients and oxygen make this environment a setup for chronic, nonhealing ulcers.

Before the development of current techniques for noninvasive testing for venous disease, evaluation depended on physical examination. A clinical test of values in the deep and superficial venous system is the Trendelenburg compression test (Figure). In the Trendelenburg test, the limb is elevated to evacuate the veins; then pressure by hand or tourniquet is applied to the saphenofemoral junction. With the patient standing, the lower leg is observed for the rate of filling of the varicosities. Gradual filling occurs in normal patients when the perforating veins are competent. Rapid filling occurs if the perforators are incompetent. The second phase of the test consists of release of the pressure to

Figure. There are four possible results of the Trendelenburg compression test. The patient has been lying down with leg elevated; he then stands up with compression over the saphenofemoral junction.

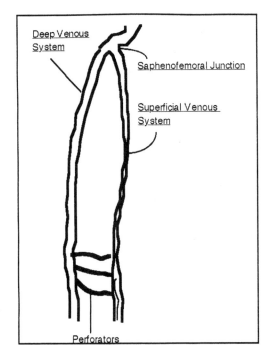

1. *Competent perforators and saphenofemoral junction.* There is a gradual filling of the veins from below over a 30-second period, and there is continued slow filling after release of the hand.

2. *Incompetent saphenofemoral junction.* There is gradual filling of the veins from below over a 30-second period, and on release there is a rapid retrograde filling of the saphenous vein.

3. *Incompetent perforators.* There is rapid (<30 s) filling of the veins from below, and a continued slow filling after release of the hand.

4. *Incompetent perforators and saphenofemoral junction.* There is rapid (<30 s) filling of the veins from below and on release there is a rapid retrograde filling of the saphenous vein.

see if the upper thigh varices fill rapidly, indicating incompetence of the saphenofemoral valve.[35]

Direct measurement of venous pressure by needle and strain gauge provides the most accurate assessment of venous hemodynamics. There are also various noninvasive tests that can be used to asses the venous system. Doppler, IPG, and duplex scanning can all be used with good accuracy to determine venous incompetence.

The most important aspect of management of patients with CVI is the education of the patient and the family in preventing venous stasis ulcers. The emphasis on the importance of GCS cannot be understated. Frequent leg elevation above the heart and the avoidance of prolonged sitting or standing should also be stressed. Once venous ulcers have formed, there is often a long and frustrating recovery phase. This is definitely a field where prevention is vital.

References

1. National Institutes of Health Consensus Conference: Prevention of venous thrombosis and pulmonary embolism. *JAMA* 256:744-749, 1986.

2. Goldhaber SZ: Pulmonary embolism and thrombolysis: a clarion call for international collaboration. *J Am Coll Cardiol* 19:246-247, 1992.

3. Lindblad B, Sternby H, Bergqvist D: Incidence of venous thromboembolism verified by necropsy over 30 years. *Br Med J* 302:709-711, 1991.

4. Landefeld CS, Chren M-M, Myers A, et al: Diagnostic yield of the autopsy in a university hospital and a community hospital. *N Engl J Med* 318:1249, 1988.

5. Oster G, Tuden RL, Colditz GA: A cost effectiveness analysis of prophylaxis against deep vein thrombosis in major orthopedic surgery. *JAMA* 257:203, 1987.

6. Philbrick JT, Becker DM: Calf deep venous thrombosis: a wolf in sheep's clothing? *Arch Intern Med* 148:2131-2138, 1988.

7. Clagett GP, Salzman EW: Prevention of venous thromboembolism in surgical patients. *N Engl J Med* 290:93, 1974.

8. Kistwer RL, Ball JJ, Nordyke RA, et al: Incidence of pulmonary embolism in the coarse of thrombophlebitis of the lower extremities. *Am J Surg* 124:169, 1972.

9. Johnson WC: Evaluation of newer techniques for the diagnosis of venous thrombosis. *J Surg Res* 16:473, 1974.

10. Hull R, Hirsh J, Sackett DL, et al: Clinical validity of a negative venogram in patients with clinically suspected venous thrombosis. *Circulation* 64:622, 1981.

11. Cranley JJ, Canos AJ, Sull WJ: The diagnosis of deep venous thrombosis. *Arch Surg* 111:34, 1976.

12. Heijboer H, Cogo A, Buller HR, et al: Detection of deep vein thrombosis with impedance plethysmography and real-time compression ultrasonography in hospitalized patients. *Arch Intern Med* 152:1901, 1992.

13. Harris WH, Salzman EW, Athanasoulis C, et al: Comparison of 125 I fibrinogen count scanning with phlebography for detection of venous thrombi after elective hip surgery. *N Engl J Med* 292:665, 1975.

14. Comerota AJ, Katz ML, Grossi RJ, et al: The comparative value of noninvasive testing for diagnosis and surveillance of deep vein thrombosis. *J Vasc Surg* 7:40, 1988.

15. Davidson BL, Elliot CG, Lensing AWA: Low accuracy of color Doppler ultrasound in the detection of proximal leg vein thrombosis in asymptomatic high-risk patients. *Ann Intern Med* 117:735, 1992.

16. Chance JF, Abbitt PL, Tegtmeyer CJ, et al: Real-time ultrasound for the detection of deep venous thrombosis. *Ann Emerg Med* 20:494, 1991.

17. Bell WR: Thrombolytic therapy: a comparison between urokinase and streptokinase. *Semin Thromb Hemostas* 2:1, 1975.

18. Sharma GVRK, Burleson VA, Sasahara AA: Effect of thrombolytic therapy on pulmonary-capillary blood volume in patients with pulmonary embolism. *N Engl J Med* 303:842, 1980.

19. Bick RL: *Disorders of Hemostasis and Thrombosis: Principles of Clinical Practice.* New York: Thieme; 45-89, 1985.

20. Rogers LQ, Lutcher CL: Streptokinase therapy for deep vein thrombosis: a comprehensive review of the English literature. *Am J Med* 88:389-395, 1990.

21. Goldhaber SZ, Buring JE, Lipnick RJ, Hennekens CH: Pooled analysis of randomized trials of streptokinase and heparin in phlebographically documented acute deep venous thrombosis. *Am J Med* 76:393-397, 1984.

22. Hirsh J, Dalen J, Deykin D, et al: Oral anticoagulants: mechanisms of action, clinical effectiveness, and optimal theraputic range. *Chest* 102:312S, 1992.

23. Altman P, Rouvier J, Gurfinkel E, et al: Comparison of two levels of anticoagulation therapy in patients with substitute heart valves. *J Thorac Cardiovasc Surg* 101:427, 1991.

24. Broekmans AW, Bertina RM, Loeliger EA, et al: Protein C and the development of skin necrosis during anticoagulation therapy. *Thromb Haemost* 49:244, 1983.
25. Bick RL: Antithrombotic therapy. In: *Disorders of Thrombosis and Hemostasis: Clinical and Laboratory Practice.* Chicago: ASCP Press; 291, 1992.
26. Pederson OM, Aslaksen A, Vik-Mo H, et al: Compression ultrasonograph in hospitalized patients with suspected deep thrombosis. *Arch Intern Med* 151:2217, 1991.
27. Ansell J, Slepchuk N, Kumar R: Heparin-induced thrombocytopenia: a prospective study. *Thromb Haemost* 43:61, 1980.
28. Flessa HC, Kopstrom AB, Glueck HL, et al: Placental transport of heparin. *Am J Obstet Gynecol* 93:570, 1965.
29. Hall RG, Pauli RM, Wilson KM: Maternal and fetal sequelae of anticoagulation during pregnancy. *Am J Med* 68:122, 1980.
30. Donaldson GA, Williams C, Schnnez JG, et al: A reappraisal of the application of the Trendelenburg operation to massive fatal pulmonary embolism. *N Engl J Med* 268:171-174, 1963.
31. Gruber UF, Saldeen T, Brolcop T, et al: Incidence of fatal postoperative pulmonary embolism after prophylaxis with dextran 70 and low dose heparin: an International Multicentre Study. *B Med J* 280:69-72, 1980.
32. Collins R, Scrimgeour A, Yusef S, et al: Reduction in fatal pulmonary embolism and venous thrombosis by perioperative administration of subcutaneous heparin: overview of results of randomized trials of general, or orthopedic and urological surgery. *N Engl J Med* 318:1162-1173, 1988.
33. Sigel B, Edelstein AL, Savitch L, et al: Type of compression for reducing venous stasis: a study of lower extremities during inactive recumbency. *Arch Surg* 110:171-175, 1975.
34. Jeffery PC, Nicolaides AN: Graduated compression stockings in the prevention of postoperative deep vein thrombosis. *Br J Surg* 77:380-383, 1990.
35. Schwartz S, Shires T, Spencer F: *Principles of Surgery.* 6th Ed. London: McGraw-Hill, Inc.; 989-1003, 1994.

Chapter 26

Quality of Life in Older Patients With Cardiovascular Disease:

Effects of Therapeutic Interventions

Donald D. Tresch, MD
Wilbert S. Aronow, MD
Edward A. Stemmer, MD
Samuel Eric Wilson, MD

The assessment of therapeutic outcomes has always been a concern of the individual physician. However, in the recent medical climate of incresed attention to cost-containment and cost-effective therapy, outcome assessment has become a topic of major interest to both the medical profession and the general public. The issue is especially pertinent in older patients, in general, and is specifically important in patients with cardiovascular disease, of which the majority are older. Older patients consume a major portion of the national health care expenditures, and commonly have chronic diseases in which therapeutic goals are markedly different than those in younger patients with acute illnesses. Cardiovascular disease is one of the most prevalent disorders in the older population and is one of the most common disorders that disables older persons.[1] Furthermore, advances in knowledge of cardiovascular disease and increased technology have resulted in an impressive range of diagnostic procedures and therapies, including drugs and surgical techniques that can be used to manage older patients with these disorders. Thirty years ago, objective assessment of vascular disease was not possible and surgery on patients over age 80 was infrequent or inconceivable. Today, various noninterventional methods of assessing vascular disease are possible, and vascular surgery or angioplasty is commonly performed in patients over 80 years of age. With this available array of highly technical and expensive diagnostic and therapeutic options, it is imperative that physicians objectively demon-

From: Aronow WS, Stemmer EA, Wilson SE (eds). *Vascular Disease in the Elderly.* Armonk, NY: Futura Publishing Company, Inc., © 1997.

strate that older patients benefit from such interventions, and that such interventions are cost-effective.

Assessment of Therapeutic Interventions

Over the years, the usual traditional measurements of therapeutic outcomes mainly included objective endpoints of morbidity and mortality, parameters that focused on the underlying disease and the prolongation of life. Such measurements do provide valuable information for physicians; however, in older patients measures of physiological end points and mortality, as measurements of therapeutic outsomes, are extremely limited. Physiological measurements in older patients do not equate with functional status. For example, in older patients with chronic heart or pulmonary disorders, capacity as measured in an exercise laboratory is only weakly similar to that level of exercise capacity realized in daily living.[2] Another problem with the measurement of only physiological parameters as assessment of therapeutic outcomes is the marked heterogeneity of the older population, with the wide variety of functional capacity and subjective satisfaction among older patients. Older patients with the same level of motor abilities by objective testing and similar rating of pain will have extremely different emotional well-being, and will function at different levels and roles in their daily activities. Some may return to their employment, demonstrating a high level of satisfaction with their lifestyle, while others may retire and suffer major depression. Assessment of survival and prolongation, alone, as a measurement of therapeutic outcome in older patients is inappropriate. Only marginal life-exending benefits can be anticipated from any intervention in very old patients, and the main focus of therapeutic interventions in these patients should be the maintenance or improvement of quality of life. This concept of quality of life versus prolongation of life is particularly important in older patients with chronic illnesses and limited functional abilities. The concept is not only important when assessing therapeutic outcome, but has implications when considering initiation, as well as termination of therapy.

Health-Related Quality of Life

Quality of life is subjective and a concept that is difficult to define; frequently, ambiguity occurs. Quality of life is dependent on the functional state of the patient, although functional status is only one of the dimensions that contributes to a patient's preception of overall health and quality of life. Quality of life also includes more complex constructs of aptitudes, motivation, skills, financial security, and pleasures that are acquired as a result of social relationships, environmental conditions, and even cultural opportunities. Due to the complexity which involves assessment of quality of life, the term *health-related quality of life* (HRQL) has been introduced in an attempt to narrow the focus upon that aspect of a person's quality of life which is influenced by the person's health status.[3,4] Dimensions commonly associated with a patient's HRQL include, at minimum, physical and social functioning, mental and psychological well-being, and overall life satisfaction. More specific, some investigators define HRQL as those attributes valued by patients, including: resultant comfort or sense of well-being; the extent to which they are able to maintain reasonable physical, emotional, and intellectual function; and the degree to which they retain their ability to participate in valued activities within the family, workplace, and community.[5]

A common instrument used in the United States to assess HRQL is the Medical Outcomes Study, a 36-item short-form health survey (SF-36).[3,6] This instrument was designed to be used as a general survey or a disease-specific survey, which may be self-administered, or administered by telephone, or during a personal interview. The SF-36 includes one multi-item scale that assess eight health concepts (Table)[6,7]: 1) limitations in physical activities because of health problems; 2) limitations in social activities because of physical or emotional problems; 3) limitations in usual role activities because of physical health problems; 4) bodily pain; 5) general mental health (psychological distress and well-being; 6) limitations in usual role activities because of emotional problems; 7) vitality (energy and fatigue); and 8) general health perceptions.

Table
SF-36 8 Health Concepts

Measure	Definition
1. Physical functioning	Extent to which health interferes with a variety of activities (e.g., sports, carrying groceries, climbing stairs, and walking).
2. Social functioning	Extent to which health interferes with normal social activities, such as visiting friends, during the past month.
3. Role limitations due to physical problems	Extent to which health interferes with usual daily activity such as work, housework, or school.
4. Bodily pain	Extent of bodily pain in the past 4 weeks.
5. General mental health	General mood or effect, including depression, anxiety, and psychological well-being during the past month.
6. Role limitations due to emotional problems	Extent to which emotional health interferes with daily functioning.
7. Vitality	Extent to which health interferes with level of energy; degree of fatigue.
8. General health perceptions	Overall ratings of current health in general.

(Adapted with permission from Reference 7.)

Other instruments that have been developed to measure HRQL include the Sickness Impact Profile,[8] the Nottingham Health Profile,[9] the Quality of Well-Being Scale,[10] and the McMaster Health Index Questionaire.[11] Although these instruments have proved to be dependable and reliable, the SF-36 is usually preferred due to its less time-consuming questionnaire, which is more practical to administer.

Health Related to Quality of Life in Older Patients

It is important when considering HRQL in older patients to realize that health states may have different values for persons at different stages of life.[12] Due to these different values, overall health perception may be determined by different factors in older patients than in younger patients. This will be partially related to the difference in role responsibilities at different ages.[13] A disability may be easier to accept for the older patient whose family is not dependent upon his or her employment wages, compared to the middle-aged patient who is the sole wage earner in the family. Disability also may be easier to accept in older age due to the person's life plan and desires. In certain older persons, it has been demonstrated that increasing dependency may not mean decreasing satisfaction with the quality of one's life. Mangiene and associates[14] in a study of older patients found that despite poorer role function, poorer energy and fatigue scores, and poorer physical function, older patients had similar global health perceptions when compared to younger patients. The investigators concluded that overall health perception in older patients may be determined by different factors than in younger patients, and the usual global measures of HRQL may not capture critically important dimensions of health in older persons.

Another aspect that needs to be emphasized when considering therapeutic interventions in older patients is that patient perception of HRQL may be markedly different than that perceived by the patient's physician or other members of the health team who provide the patient's care. In a recent study by Berlowitz and associates,[15] older nursing home patients' physicians and nurses were asked to complete a questionnaire detailing their perception of the patient's HRQL, which was then compared to an identical questionnaire completed by the patient. In general, the physician's and nurse's assessment correlated weakly with the patient's self-assessment. The patient's physical functioning, general health perception, energy and irritability, role limitations, and mental health were all scored significantly lower by the physician and nurse. Other studies[16] have demonstrated similar results when comparing older patient's self-assessment of HRQL, compared to a family member's perception of the patient's HRQL. These studies suggest that older patients' caregivers, including physicians and family members, tend to judge patients' HRQL much lower than is usually assessed by the patients. Furthermore, studies[16,17] have also demonstrated a failure of agreement between older patients' spouses or physicians and patients in reference to treatment preferences. Older patients usually prefer more therapies, than patients' spouses or physicians would have predicted.

On the basis of the results of these studies, it appears that older patients are able to cope with disabilities in such a manner that their quality of life is not severely diminished. Or it may be that disabilities considered by the patient's physician or family to be detrimental to quality of life are not perceived in a similar manner by the older patient. In an early study, Sugarbaker and associates[18] demonstrated that patients with sarcoma considered limb amputation to have a lesser negative impact on their quality of life, than limb-sparing surgery and irradiation, which was a different response than that expected by the patients' physicians.

Assessment of Therapy in Older Patients With Cardiovascular Disorders

In general, studies specifically designed to assess effects of therapeutic intervention on HRQL in older patients with cardiovascular disorders are sparse. Coronary artery bypass grafting (CABG), however, has received significant attention in both the United States and Europe in reference to its effect on HRQL in older patients. This interest most likely relates to the increasing use of this therapeutic intervention in the very old population, and its effect on the increasing cost of medical care. Having established by repeated studies[19] that patients 65 years and older undergoing CABG could expect good outcome in terms of operative mortality and long-term survival, the next step was to establish if the HRQL was maintained or improved in these older patients. In a recent study in Great Britain,[20] HRQL was assessed pre- and postvalvular or CABG surgery in patients 65 years or older. Using the Nottingham Health Profile,[9] improvement in health status in all six dimensions of the profile, which included physical mobility, pain, energy, sleep, social isolation, and emotional behavior, occurred at 3 months after surgery, and the improvements were either maintained or further enhanced at 1 year (Figure 1). Scores on the Hospital Anxiety and Depression Scale[21] indicated that prior to surgery, 42% of the patients had above normal anxiety levels, which were reduced to 13% at 3 months and 17% at 1 year after surgery. Patients with above normal depression presurgery were also significantly improved after surgery. In reference to activities of daily living and social activities, marked improvement was noted after surgery in patient performance of daily household activities, and in such activities as shopping and gardening (Figure 2).

Similar results have been reported by American studies. In one study of patients, over 65 years of age, who had CABG performed at six academic medical centers in California and Massachusetts, HRQL measurements were assessed pre- and postoperatively, and were com-

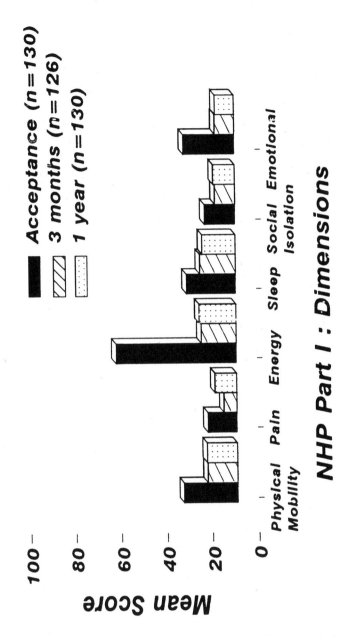

Figure 1. Nottingham Health Profile. Part I. Mean scores before and after cardiac surgery. (Reproduced with permission from Reference 20.)

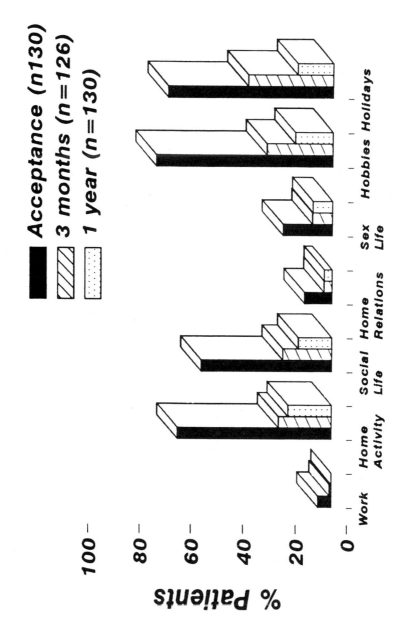

Figure 2. Nottingham Health Profile. Part II. Percent of patients with problems related to health before and after cardiac surgery. (Reproduced with permission from Reference 20.)

pared to HRQL of younger CABG patients.[22] At follow-up of 3 and 12 months, both age groups demonstrated significant improvement in performance of activities of daily living and none of the HRQL scores, except mental health, were significantly different between the age groups. Older patients reported better mental health. The one activity that did not demonstrate improvement in either age group was employment. Another study which demonstrated improved measurements of HRQL in older CABG patients was the Brigham and Women's Hospital (BWH) Study.[22] In this study, improvements in HRQL measurements 6 months after CABG were as great or greater in patients 70 years or older, compared to younger CABG patients (Figure 3).

In order to determine if HRQL benefits of CABG in very old patients are maintained over a long period of time, Belgium investigators performed a study in which patients, 74 years or older, were followed for approximately 5 years after undergoing CABG.[23] At the time of follow-up, the patients were all older than 80 years, with a mean age of 82. The HRQL of these very old patients was determined and compared to a group of younger CABG patients. Quality of life was assessed by physiological and functional status, performance of social roles, and general satisfaction. As in the studies of 3-month and 1-year follow-up periods, self-perception of HRQL was no different between the two age groups at 5 years follow-up, with approximately 75% of each group perceiving their health to be excellent or good. At the time of 5-year follow-up, the entire population of both age groups were living at home, and older patients had similar social interaction scores as younger patients. More older patients, however, perceived a lower dependability of social support and felt more lonely, and depression was more common in older patients. In contrast, older patients were significantly more satisfied with their CABG experience and were more satisfied with their living conditions. No difference in performance of activities of daily living was noted between the age groups. The older CABG patients in this study were also compared to two general populations of older persons in whom CABG was not performed. In comparison to an American "geriatric" population, greater than 60 years of age, the CABG group had better self-health perception, reported better improvement in health during the 5 years following CABG, and had better social resources scores on the Older American Resource Schedule (OARS).[25] When compared to a Dutch group of non-CABG older patients, over 80 years of age, the CABG group, as was found when compared to the American "geriatric" population, demonstrated better scores on performance of household activities and daily activities of living.

In addition to the studies assessing HRQL in older CABG patients, a few studies have attempted to assess the effects of peripheral vascular surgery upon HRQL in older patients. In a study of a small number of older patients, with an average of 67 years, investigators at Yale University examined the effects of complex peripheral vascular surgery (bilateral renal artery revascularization) on patients' HRQL.[7] On the SF-36 questionnaire, at mean follow-up of 36 months, over 80% of the patients

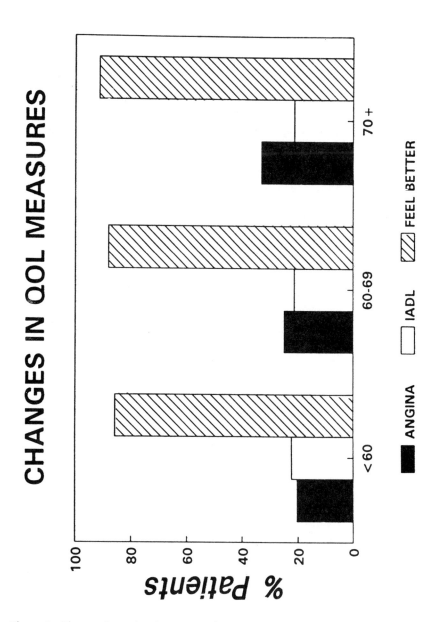

Figure 3. Changes in angina, instrumental activities of daily living (IADL), and reports about feeling better in different age groups of patients in Brigham and Women's Hospital Study. (Reproduced with permission from Reference 22.)

rated their health as good to excellent, with 80% rating it the same as or better than before surgery; 78% of patients had no physical disabilities, and 90% remained as socially involved as they had been preceding surgery. These favorable results were obtained even though preoperatively the majority of patients had a high incidence of morbidity, including coronary artery disease, renal insufficiency, and refractory hypertension. In another study of peripheral vascular surgery, Seabrook and associates[26] found somewhat different results than those reported by the Yale University investigators. In Seabrook's study, 70 patients with a mean age of 69, underwent lower extremity arterial reconstructive surgery for limb-threatening ischemia. As in the Yale University study, the patients had a high incidence of morbidity prior to the arterial reconstructive surgery. At 46 months mean follow-up, functional capacity and HRQL were assessed by SF-36 questionnaire in the surgical patients and compared to a gender and age-matched control group of older patients. Compared to the control group, the surgical group had significantly decreased functional capacity, in that they were unable to walk as far, more frequently required assistance in using the bathtub or shower, and were less likely to do strenuous activities, such as shoveling snow, mowing the lawn, or vacuum cleaning. Despite this difference in functional abilities, the surgical patients reported a sense of well-being similar to the control group, who were without vascular disease. There was no significant difference between the revascularized older patients and the control group in their reponses when asked to identify if they were in "good health" or "poor health," worried about their state of health, were "generally happy," or whether they felt they had an adequate amount of energy.

Summary

Assessment of the benefits of therapeutic intervention is an important aspect of medical care. Such assessment will become even more important as changes in the delivery of medical care evolve. Assessment of therapeutic outcomes is especially pertinent in the care of older patients and particularly applies to patients with cardiovascular disorders, of whom the majority are over 65 years of age. Assessment of therapy in these patients requires evaluation of more than morbidity and mortality, with measurement or quality of life being a major component of the evaluation. Quality of life measurements are possible and have been shown to be beneficial in assessing older patients, even though health states will have different values for persons at different stages of life. Studies have demonstrated that certain therapeutic interventions are beneficial in improving HRQL in older patients with cardiovascular disease. Further studies, however, are necessary to assess other therapeutic interventions. One of the major challenges of the medical profession in the twenty-first century will be to demonstrate that our interventions objectively improve older patients' HRQL. Only by demonstration of a favorable effect on older patients' HRQL will we be able to justify the continuous use of these therapies.

References

1. Williams TF: Rehabilitation in old age. In: Abelles RB, Gift HC, Ory MG (eds). *Age and Quality of Life.* New York: Springer Publishing Co., Inc.; 121-132, 1994.
2. Guyatt GH, Thompson PJ, Berman LB, Sullivan MJ, Townsend M, Jones NL, et al: How should we measure function in patients with chronic heart and lung disease? *J Chron Dis* 38:514-517, 1985.
3. McHorney CA, Ware JE Jr, Raczek AE: The MOS 36-item short-form health survey (SF-36). II. Psychometric and clinical tests of validity in measuring physical and mental health constructs. *Med Care* 31:247-263, 1993.
4. Guyatt GH, Fenny DH, Patrick DL: Measuring health-related quality of life. *Ann Intern Med* 118:622-629, 1993.
5. Wenger N, Furberg CD: Cardiovascular disorders. In: Spilker B (ed). *Quality of Life Assessments in Clinical Trials.* New York: Raven Press; 335-345, 1990.
6. Ware JE Jr, Sherbourne CD: The MOS 36-item short-form health survey (SF-36). I. Conceptual framework and item selection. *Med Care* 30:473-483, 1992.
7. Lacey KO, Meier GH, Krumholz HM, Gusberg RJ: Outcomes after major vascular surgery: the patient's perspective. *J Vasc Nurs* 13:8-13, 1995.
8. Croog S: Current issues in conceptualizing and measuring quality of life. In: *Quality of Life Assessment: Proceedings of a Workshop Sponsored by the Office of the Director.* National Institutes of Health: October 15-17, 1990.
9. Hunt SJ, McEwen J, McKenna, et al: Subjective health of patients with peripheral vascular disease. *Practitioner* 226:133-136, 1982.
10. Kaplan RM, Bush JW, Berry CC: Health status: types of validity and the index of well-being. *Health Serv Res* 11:478-507, 1976.
11. Chambers LW, MacDonald LA, Tugwell P, et al: The McMaster Index Question-naire as a measure of quality of life for patients with rheumatoid disease. *J Rheumatol* 9:780-784, 1982.
12. Kappel K, Sandow P: QUALYS, age, and fairness. *Bioethics* 6:297, 1992.
13. Faden R, German PS: Quality of life: considerations in geriatrics. In: Sachs GA, Cassel CK (eds). *Clinics in Geriatric Medicine.* Philadelphia: WB Saunders, Co.; 541-551, 1994.
14. Mangione CM, Marcantonio ER, Goldman L, Cook EF, et al: Influence of age in measurement of health status in patients undergoing elective surgery. *J Am Geriatr Soc* 41:377-383, 1993.
15. Berlowitz DR, Du W, Kazis L, Lewis S: Health-related quality of life of nursing home residents: differences in patient and provider perceptions. *J Am Geriatr Soc* 43:799-802, 1995.
16. Pearlman RA, Uhlmann RF, Jecker NS: Spousal understanding of patients quality of life: implications for surrogate decision making. *J Clin Ethics* 3:114, 1992.
17. Uhlmann RF, Pearlman RA: Perceived quality of life and preferences for life-sustaining treatment in older adults. *Arch Intern Med* 151:495, 1991.
18. Sugarbaker PH, Barofsky I, Rosenberg SA, Gianola FJ: Quality of life assessment of patients in extremity sarcoma clinical trials. *Surgery* 91:17023, 1982.
19. Shimshak TM, McCallister BD: Coronary artery bypass surgery and percutaneous transluminal coronary angioplasty in the elderly patient with ischemic heart disease. In: Tresch DD, Aronow WS (eds). *Cardiovascular Disease in the Elderly Patient.* New York: Marcel Dekker, In.; 323-344, 1993.

20. Caine N, Tait S, Wallwork J: Survival and health-related quality of life of elderly patients undergoing cardiac surgery. In: Walter PJ (ed). *Coronary Bypass Surgery in the Elderly.* The Netherlands: Kluwer Academic Publishers; 155-166, 1995.
21. Zigmond AS, Snaith RP: The hospital anxiety and depression scale. *Acta Psychiatr Scan* 67:361-370, 1983.
22. Cleary PD, Guadagnoli E, Ayanian JZ: Health-related quality of life after coronary revascularization in older patients. In: Walter PJ (ed). *Coronary Bypass Surgery in the Elderly.* The Netherlands: Kluwer Academic Publishers; 167-177, 1995.
23. Walter PJ, Mohan R, Cornelissen C: Health-related quality of life five years after coronary bypass surgery at age 75 or above. In: Walter PJ (ed). *Coronary Bypass Surgery in the Elderly.* The Netherlands: Kluwer Academic Publishers; 195-210, 1995.
24. Blazer DG: Social support and mortality in an elderly community population. *Am J Epidemiol* 115:684-694, 1982.
25. Seabrook GR, Freischlag JA, Towne JB: Measuring long-term functional outcome and quality of life as a determinant of success for vascular surgery. Presented at the 18th Annual Meeting of the Midwestern Vascular Surgical Society, Cincinnati, OH, 1994.

Index